# Leprosy in
# Medieval England

# Leprosy in Medieval England

CAROLE RAWCLIFFE

THE BOYDELL PRESS

First published 2006
The Boydell Press, Woodbridge

Reprinted in paperback 2009
ISBN 978 1 84383 454 0

The Boydell Press is an imprint of Boydell & Brewer Ltd
PO Box 9, Woodbridge, Suffolk IP12 3DF, UK
and of Boydell & Brewer Inc.
668 Mt Hope Avenue, Rochester, NY 14620, USA
website: www.boydellandbrewer.com

A CIP catalogue record of this publication is available
from the British Library

Typeset by Pru Harrison, Hacheston, Suffolk

# Contents

# List of Illustrations

## Maps

The author and publishers are grateful to all the institutions listed for permission to reproduce the materials in which they hold copyright. Every effort has been made to trace the copyright holders; apologies are offered for any omission, and the publishers will be pleased to add any necessary acknowledgements in subsequent editions.

*To my mother and father*

# Acknowledgements

It is now the best part of fourteen years since I was asked to write a short article on the leper hospitals of medieval Norwich, never dreaming that a few days' research in the local archives would develop into such a major project, or, indeed, such a large book. That I have been able to devote so much time to the complex and challenging subject of historical responses to leprosy is largely due to the support of the Wellcome Trust, which provided generous funding in the form of a University Award, and thus enabled me to begin work in earnest a decade ago. Since then, both the AHRC and the University of East Anglia have allowed me the research leave necessary to complete the enterprise. Throughout this period the staff of many libraries and record offices have proffered expert help and advice. I am particularly grateful for the patience and courtesy extended by librarians and archivists at the British Library, the Wellcome Institute, the Warburg Institute and the Institute of Historical Research, London; the Bodleian Library, Oxford; the Norfolk Record Office and at my own University Library. I would, in particular, like to thank Mr David Harris at UEA for his unfailing good humour and efficiency in dealing with a stream of requests for interlibrary loans that ranged from the recondite to the macabre.

So many people have provided me with references, advice and suggestions that it is impossible to thank them all. My colleagues, Dr Steven Cherry and Dr Larry Butler, Miss Irene Allen of LEPRA and Mr Tony Gould made the initially daunting task of writing an introductory chapter on the nineteenth century far easier. Dr John Arnold, Professor Martha Carlin, Dr Andrew Cunningham, Professor Christopher Dyer, Mr T.A. Heslop, Dr Jonathan Hughes, Dr Piers Mitchell, Dr Peter Murray Jones, Dr Nigel Ramsey and Professor Robert Swanson have been liberal with information and ideas. Dr Hannes Kleineke has risen nobly to the challenge of hunting out hitherto unknown presentments for leprosy. I have greatly profited from Dr John Henderson's expertise on medieval hospitals and Professor Nicholas Vincent's encyclopaedic knowledge of twelfth- and thirteenth-century sources. With his customary skill, Phillip Judge turned my rough sketches and lists of hospitals into maps. Professor F.O. Touati, whose work on leprosy in medieval France constitutes a benchmark against which any national study must now be set, kindly provided me with copies of his many publications. An invitation to speak at a conference on medieval hospitals and *leprosaria* at the University of New Mexico, Albuquerque, in 2003 afforded me the opportunity to meet Professor Luke Demaitre, and discuss his research in the most convivial surroundings.

I am indebted to archaeologists as well as historians. The York Archaeological Trust and the Norfolk Museums and Archaeology Service have permitted me to consult their unpublished excavation reports. Dr John Magilton likewise made available his forthcoming study of the hospital of St Mary Magdalen and St James, Chichester. Professor Roberta Gilchrist first alerted me to the importance of material culture in the study of the medieval hospital, and has since been characteristically generous with assistance.

My research postgraduates at UEA will recognise in these pages many of the topics that have arisen during supervision sessions, seminars and long conversations about health and disease in medieval England. Their enthusiasm and interest have proved invaluable, and I do not think I could have produced this book without them. Its view of reactions to the medieval leper does not entirely accord with that of my own tutor at Sheffield University in the 1960s, Professor R.I. Moore, which is, I hope, the best compliment one can pay to an inspiring teacher.

As this book neared completion and deadlines loomed, I experienced an increasing sympathy for the beleaguered William Caxton, who ended his long *Recuyell of the Historyes of Troye*, in 1475, on a deeply personal note. He felt it was time to call a halt, 'for as moche as in the wrytyng of the same my penne is worn, myn hande wery and not stedfast, myn eyen dimmed with ouermoche lokyng on the whit paper, and my corage not so prone and redy to laboure as hit hath ben'. Having, like Caxton, 'promysed to dyuerce gentilmen and to my frendes' that I would one day complete what must have seemed an interminable undertaking, I can only thank the same 'frendes' for their unflagging – if sometimes bemused – encouragement. It has been a pleasure to collaborate with Ms Caroline Palmer and Mr Peter Clifford of Boydell & Brewer on the publication of this book. In his capacity as publisher's reader, Mr Peregrine Horden made several perceptive and helpful suggestions, which have greatly improved the text. To Ms Elizabeth Danbury, Dr Linda Clark, Ms Heather Creaton-Brooke and Mr Alasdair Hawkyard, I am, as always, grateful for companionship and kindness. The ever gallant Professors Christopher Harper-Bill and John Charmley have proved the most supportive and understanding of colleagues. Only Peter Martin really knows how much I owe him, not least for reading and re-reading multiple drafts of every single chapter. In common with the medieval leper, he has endured his purgatory here on earth, and must surely have secured a martyr's crown. It is customary to dedicate one's first book to one's parents, which I did almost thirty years ago. Neither my mother nor my father can, alas, now manage to read every word, as they were then able to do, for, like Caxton, their sight has faded. But they are more stoical than he, and this book is another affectionate tribute to them both.

Carole Rawcliffe
Norwich
January 2006

# Abbreviations

| | |
|---|---|
| BAR | British Archaeological Reports |
| *BHM* | *Bulletin of the History of Medicine* |
| *BIHR* | *Bulletin of the Institute of Historical Research* |
| BL | British Library |
| *CCR* | *Calendar of Close Rolls* |
| *CIM* | *Calendar of Inquisitions Miscellaneous* |
| *CLR* | *Calendar of Liberate Rolls* |
| CLRO | Corporation of London Record Office |
| *CPR* | *Calendar of Patent Rolls* |
| *CRR* | *Curia Regis Rolls* |
| CS | Camden Society |
| *DNB* | *Dictionary of National Biography* |
| *EEA* | *English Episcopal Acta* |
| EETS | Early English Text Society |
| *EHR* | *English Historical Review* |
| *HMC* | *Historical Manuscripts Commission* |
| *HR* | *Historical Research* |
| *JHM* | *Journal of the History of Medicine* |
| LAO | Lincoln Archives Office |
| *MED* | *Middle English Dictionary* (Ann Arbor, 1956–) |
| *MPIME* | C.H. Talbot and E.A. Hammond, *The Medical Practitioners in Medieval England* (London, 1965) |
| NRO | Norfolk Record Office |
| *PL* | *Patrologia Latina* |
| *PPL* | C.A. Roberts, M.E. Lewis and K. Manchester, eds, *The Past and Present of Leprosy* (BAR, International Series, mliv, 2002) |
| PRO | Public Record Office (National Archives) |
| RO | Record Office |
| RS | Rolls Series |
| *SHM* | *Social History of Medicine* |
| *VCH* | *Victoria County History* |

# Introduction

> *The problem of leprosy is not for the idle-minded. It is full of intricacy and difficulty. The facts are apparently conflicting, and they can be reconciled, if at all, only by great patience and attention to detail. For those, however, who can bring to the task a fair share of patience, a moderate knowledge of history and geography, and a good memory, the labour will not be without interest, nor, I think, without its reward. However repulsive the disease itself in some of its phases may be, there is nothing whatever of that nature about its study. It is a sort of aristocrat among diseases . . . and the history of its prevalence, increase, and decline in different regions of our globe, is interwoven with civilisation itself.*
>
> Jonathan Hutchinson, On Leprosy and Fish-Eating, 1906[1]

Regarded today as an affliction of almost mythical status, remote from the European experience, leprosy manifests scant respect for geographical boundaries. Despite the steady progress of global campaigns for its elimination, it still remains a serious health problem in over twenty countries, notably India, where an estimated 100,000 new cases occur every year alone. Significantly, some of the earliest evidence of the disease, dating from about 600 years before the birth of Christ, survives from the subcontinent, although China and the Nile Valley may lay claim to an even longer history of infection. Moving gradually westwards, leprosy appears to have reached Italy with Pompey's victorious legions in 62 BC, and then to have travelled north as the Roman Empire expanded across the Alps.[2] The first skeletal evidence of its presence in England apparently comes from a fourth-century Romano-British cemetery in Dorchester, although it was not until the Norman Conquest that institutional provision was made for those who had contracted the disease.[3] Having become endemic throughout Europe by the high Middle Ages, it then began slowly to retreat, so that by the late nineteenth century only a few small pockets, in Scandinavia, Greece, the Iberian Peninsula and the Balkans, remained of what had once ranked as the scourge of medieval society.

Now known as Hansen's disease in order to alleviate the sense of stigma

---

1   J. Hutchinson, *On Leprosy and Fish-Eating; A Statement of Facts and Explanations* (London, 1906), p. 1.
2   M.F. Lechat, 'The Palaeoepidemiology of Leprosy: An Overview', *PPL*, pp. 157–62; M.D. Grmek, *Diseases in the Ancient Greek World* (Baltimore, 1989), chapter six; C. Roberts and K. Manchester, *The Archaeology of Disease* (second edn, Stroud, 1995), pp. 145–8; K. Manchester, 'Leprosy: The Origins and Development of the Disease in Antiquity', in D. Gourevitch, ed., *Maladie et maladies: Histoire et conceptualisation* (Paris, 1992), pp. 31–49.
3   C. Roberts and M. Cox, *Health and Disease in Britain* (Stroud, 2003), p. 120.

experienced by its victims, leprosy remains something of a medical enigma. We still do not know precisely why so many people who are regularly exposed to it enjoy immunity, while a small minority do not. For, contrary to popular myth, the risks of succumbing to infection are generally slight.[4] Nor do most sufferers today experience the dramatic loss of physical extremities and horrific disfigurement so often described in sensationalist literature. On the contrary, the symptoms appear diverse, may take the best part of a decade or even longer to develop and are notable for their ability to replicate those of other diseases. From the mid twentieth century onwards, clinicians have distinguished five different forms of leprosy according to the degree of resistance offered by the body's defensive cells to the *Mycobacterium leprae* that spreads it.[5] Skin and nerve cells are commonly first affected, giving rise to discoloured lesions or patches of various sizes, shades, textures and elevation, which are often marked by a loss of sensation. During the initial indeterminate stage, the disease can enter long periods of remission, but as it develops it becomes possible to establish a position on a broad spectrum between the tuberculoid (high resistance) and lepromatous (low resistance) types. Although tuberculoid leprosy is far less virulent than the lepromatous strain, it can none the less prove acutely debilitating if left untreated with drugs such as the sulfone-based antibiotics that first became available in the 1940s.[6] Earlier forms of treatment, including chaulmoogra oil, were at best palliative.

Because the infection tends to be restricted to single or few specific sites, the discoloured, dry and hairless lesions characteristic of tuberculoid leprosy are not always visible to the casual observer. They can, moreover, vanish over time. But by then, as a result of the battle between white blood cells and bacteria, permanent injury may well have been sustained by any adjacent nerves. In severe cases, neural damage, with attendant swelling, pain and ulceration, is more widespread, ultimately anaesthetising those parts of the face or extremities that have been invaded by the bacilli. Unable to sweat, the skin grows dry and fissured. Since they cannot be felt, these cuts, sores and abrasions easily become infected, leading to the eventual loss of fingers and toes through a combination of trauma, sepsis and the absorption of bone. Fingers may also assume a claw or talon shape as the nerves thicken and contract and the blood supply diminishes during periods of extreme reaction. Yet tuberculoid leprosy often remains relatively benign and specifically localised; it may heal spontaneously at an early stage, or

---

4  K. Manchester, 'Tuberculosis and Leprosy: Evidence for Interaction of Disease', in D.J. Ortner and A.C. Aufderheide, eds, *Human Palaeopathology: Current Syntheses and Future Options* (Washington DC, 1991), pp. 23–35, at p. 26.

5  That is tuberculoid, borderline tuberculoid, dimorphous or indeterminate, borderline lepromatous and lepromatous, the most malign and progressive stage. R.H. Thangaraj and S.J. Yawalkar, *Leprosy for Medical Practitioners and Paramedical Workers* (Basle, 1986), pp. 38–9, provide a chart of the most common symptoms to be found in each type.

6  The following account is based on D.S. Ridling and W.H. Jopling, 'A Classification of Leprosy According to Immunity: A Five Group System', *International Journal of Leprosy*, xxxiv (1966), pp. 255–61, and W.H. Jopling, *Handbook of Leprosy* (first edn, London, 1971), pp. 7–31. A lucid account of Hansen's disease in the medieval context may be found in P. Mitchell, 'An Evaluation of the Leprosy of King Baldwin IV of Jerusalem', in B. Hamilton, *The Leper King and his Heirs* (Cambridge, 2000), pp. 245–58. See also, the section on 'Clinical Leprosy' in *PPL*, pp. 17–66.

eventually 'burn out' leaving its victim free of *Mycobacterium leprae*, but still vulnerable to secondary infections, including gangrene or septicaemia.

Whereas tuberculoid leprosy tends to prompt an early reaction as the body's immune system fights off the invader, the lepromatous strain moves far more slowly. Encountering little or no resistance, the bacteria spread throughout the body, only gradually revealing themselves through systemic nerve and tissue damage. Because of the very high concentration of bacilli, lesions begin to spread across the skin, which grows waxen and nodular. Leathery, ulcerated areas may also develop. The face may assume a classic, heavy leonine appearance: the *facies leprosa*, so accurately described in medieval medical texts. If the palate and larynx are infected the voice will grow hoarse and rasping; the nasal cartilage may erode, causing the bridge of the nose to collapse; and the eyes may deteriorate so badly through corneal ulceration (caused by an inability to blink) as to induce blindness. In men, infection of the testicles can lead to sterility. Once the disease has penetrated the bone marrow, the skeletal frame weakens, becoming liable to fracture. Because of widespread ulceration, sufferers from lepromatous leprosy are even more likely to experience the complications resulting from injury and cross-infection described above. It was, for example, observed in nineteenth-century Madras that death was usually caused by dysentery, renal failure, oedema, bronchitis or diarrhoea, although admission to a *leprosarium*, where sores could be cleansed and dressed and dietary needs met, might prolong life for years. Elsewhere tuberculosis took an even heavier toll. Colonial administrators also noted that patients were frequently subject to other 'offensive skin diseases', such as psoriasis or eczema.[7] Conversely, however, individuals with lepromatous leprosy seldom present all its symptoms, and may well be 'borderline' or indeterminate cases with very few. In areas where Hansen's disease has long been established and the population has developed a degree of immunity it rarely assumes such an extreme form.[8]

Leprosy thus adopts a truly protean shape, from the benign to the malignant, which may vary dramatically from one individual, generation or locality to the next. Nor can a diagnosis necessarily remain fixed; borderline and indeterminate cases are prone to move in either direction, becoming more or less tuberculoid or lepromatous as levels of resistance rise or fall. Despite these many challenges, medieval medical practitioners identified a list of symptoms that still figure prominently in today's textbooks, and devised a battery of sophisticated tests to detect them.[9] Palaeopathological evidence confirms that advanced cases, at least, were clearly identified during the later Middle Ages. Excavations at a handful of *leprosaria*, such as those at Naestved in Denmark and Chichester in Sussex, have unearthed the skeletal remains of both lepromatous and tuberculoid cases in

---

7   J. Buckingham, *Leprosy in Colonial South India: Medicine and Confinement* (Basingstoke, 2002), pp. 13–14.

8   E. Silla, *People Are Not the Same: Leprosy and Identity in Twentieth-Century Mali* (Portsmouth and Oxford, 1998), pp. 19–21.

9   L. Demaitre, 'The Description and Diagnosis of Leprosy by Fourteenth-Century Physicians', *BHM*, lix (1985), pp. 327–44. This valuable article provides a corrective to S.N. Brody's dismissal of medieval physicians and their diagnostic abilities: *The Disease of the Soul: Leprosy in Medieval Literature* (Cornell, 1974), pp. 35–51.

significant numbers.[10] Since death must often have occurred *before* the bones were affected, we may reasonably assume that some of their apparently 'healthy' neighbours bore recognisable signs of infection too.[11]

Yet concepts of the disease then had little in common with the biomedical model described above.[12] Based upon Greek humoral theory, the complex nosology employed by medieval physicians distinguished four specific types of *lepra*, which were attributed to the corruption of phlegm, black bile, choler and blood within the human body. Divine will, hostile planetary forces, poor diet, corrupt air, dirt, sexual misconduct, prolonged contact with the leprous and heredity were among the many factors deemed likely to trigger or aggravate such conditions. Opinions about the risks – and, indeed, the means – of transmission from one person to another changed dramatically between the eleventh and fourteenth centuries, although it was generally agreed that particular individuals would be predisposed to the disease and could thus take positive steps to avoid it.[13] Contrary to the trenchant views of nineteenth-century polemicists, fears of contagion (as understood today) were slow to develop, and never universal.[14]

Outside the medical literature, definitions of what constituted *lepra* were not only tantalisingly imprecise, but also subject to a range of shifting social, cultural, moral and even linguistic imperatives. So too were attitudes to segregation, which were heavily influenced by the Church's interpretation of scripture, as well as by the development of the English common law and of urban and manorial custom. The adoption of an increasingly specialist vocabulary from the late eleventh century onwards heralded a more rigorous and systematic approach to the identification of suspects, as did the popular dissemination of scientific theories about public health and the environment during the later Middle Ages. Yet 'misdiagnosis' (as viewed from a purely *modern* perspective) of such a polymorphous disease must often have continued in towns and villages where fear of pestilence and mistrust of the rootless poor escalated during periods of crisis.

Nor do hospital foundations offer much hope to the eager statistician. The early spate of endowments was driven by a theological rather than a medical

---

10  V. Møller-Christensen, *Bone Changes in Leprosy* (Copenhagen, 1961); J. Magilton, 'The Leper Hospital of St James and St Mary Magdalen, Chichester', in C.A. Roberts, F. Lee and J. Bintoff, eds, *Burial Archaeology: Current Research, Methods and Developments* (BAR, British Series, ccxi, 1989), pp. 249–65. For an analysis of the British evidence and a discussion of the interpretative problems facing the palaeopathologist, see Roberts and Cox, *Health and Disease*, pp. 267–72; and the section on 'History and Palaeopathology of Leprosy Worldwide' in *PPL*, pp. 123–259.

11  Recent research suggests that between 29 and 54 per cent of advanced cases will result in skeletal damage: K. Manchester, 'Tuberculosis and Leprosy in Antiquity: An Interpretation', *Medical History*, xxviii (1984), pp. 162–73, at p. 171.

12  The impact of the 'bacteriologic' view of disease, not least upon the writing of medical history, is perceptively discussed in A. Cunningham, 'Transforming Plague: The Laboratory and the Identity of Infectious Disease', in idem and P. Williams, ed., *The Laboratory Revolution in Medicine* (Cambridge, 1992), pp. 209–44. See also, J. Arrizabalaga, 'Problematizing Retrospective Diagnosis in the History of Disease', *Asclepio*, liv, fasc. 1 (2002), pp. 51–70; and S. Cohn, *The Black Death Transformed: Disease and Culture in Early Renaissance Europe* (London, 2001), p. 62.

13  See chapter two, below.

14  F.O. Touati, 'Contagion and Leprosy: Myth, Ideas and Evolution in Medieval Minds and Societies', in L.I. Conrad and D. Wujastyk, eds, *Contagion: Perspectives from Pre-Modern Societies* (Aldershot, 2000), pp. 179–201.

agenda, and tells us more about the spiritual aspirations of patrons and benefactors than it does about the actual incidence of leprosy. In sharp contrast to the profusion of manuscript sources available for many French leper houses, the great majority of English *leprosaria* are poorly documented, with the result that such fundamental questions as the date of foundation and the size of the establishment often remain unanswered.[15] Since we can only make an educated guess at the number of English hospitals functioning at any given time, and have no means of telling how many 'real lepers' lived in them, rather than electing to lead an alternative existence elsewhere, the prospect of calculating infection rates from this source seems remote. We should also bear in mind that levels of immunity to the *Mycobacterium* appear to have risen as the community built up its resistance, although the impact of this process is hard to judge. For all these reasons, attempts to establish the incidence of Hansen's disease in medieval Britain by counting heads and estimating percentages are not only dangerously speculative, but also of limited value to the social historian of medicine.[16] The latter's interest – and the theme of this book – focuses upon the ways in which medieval men and women responded to *what they believed* to be leprosy.[17]

Even today, however, these ideas and reactions are still being viewed through a distorting lens that was first trained upon 'the leprosy problem' by nineteenth-century physicians, polemicists and missionaries. We begin, therefore, with some of the fantasies and misapprehensions about 'the medieval leper' propagated during a period when microbiologists, colonial administrators and evangelicals turned to the past for evidence to support their own campaigns for mandatory segregation. The powerful image of ostracism, forcible detention and rampant fear of contagion fostered by an increasingly influential and vociferous medical lobby soon seized the imagination of poets and novelists on both sides of the Channel. The results still permeate the pages of scholarly as well as popular studies of Hansen's disease, which inevitably present the leper as a marginal figure, shunned throughout the ages by his or her fellow man.

---

15 F.O. Touati, *Archives de la lèpre* (Paris, 1996), pp. 89–150, provides an impressive inventory of manuscript sources for the Senonaise. The problems facing the historian of English hospitals are considered in C. Rawcliffe, 'Passports to Paradise: How English Medieval Hospitals and Almshouses Kept their Archives', *Archives*, xxvii (2002), pp. 2–22.

16 Calvin Wells' estimate in *Bones, Bodies and Disease* (London, 1964), p. 94, of one case in every two hundred Europeans during the twelfth and thirteenth centuries apparently derives from figures produced for India in the 1950s, when the disease was at its peak and the statistics were at their most reliable: J. Mehta, 'Social Reactions in the Past and Present of Leprosy', *PPL*, pp. 21–3. They represent an optimum figure for F.O. Touati, whose work on the archdiocese of Sens suggests a somewhat lower rate: *Archives de la lèpre*, p. 80; *Maladie et société au moyen âge* (Paris, 1998), pp. 294–300. Charles Creighton, *A History of Epidemics in Britain, I, from AD 664 to the Great Plague* (London, 1894, reprinted 1965), chapter two, on the other hand, felt that the medieval 'leper' must, in most cases, have been 'misdiagnosed'.

17 The importance of transcending a narrow biomedical understanding of disease in a historical context was stressed in the 1970s by R.W. Lieban, 'The Field of Medical Anthropology', in D. Landy, ed., *Culture, Disease and Healing: Studies in Medical Anthropology* (New York, 1977), pp. 13–31. It has subsequently been reiterated by, *inter alios*, M. MacDonald, 'Anthropological Perspectives on the History of Science and Medicine', in P. Corsi and P. Weindling, eds, *Information Sources in the History of Science and Medicine* (London, 1983), pp. 61–80; P. Horden, 'Ritual and Public Health in the Early Medieval City', in S. Sheard and H. Power, eds, *Body and City: Histories of Urban Public Health* (Aldershot, 2000), pp. 17–40; and D. Harley, 'Rhetoric and the Social Construction of Sickness and Healing', *SHM*, xii (1999), pp. 407–35.

With a few notable exceptions, most of the Victorian campaigners who used evidence drawn from the medieval past were generally dismissive of the attempts then made by theologians, physicians and surgeons to explain and treat leprosy. The symbiotic relationship between religion and medicine, and the overwhelming influence of the Catholic Church in matters to do with sickness and health, smacked of popish superstition to Anglicans living in an age of untrammelled scientific progress. Yet it constitutes the bedrock upon which any serious study of pre-modern medicine must be founded, and is crucial to an understanding of medieval attitudes to extreme human suffering. In chapter two we move back in time from the world of the laboratory and the microscope to one in which disease was seen, first and foremost, as an act of God, intended to punish, reform or even reward the sufferer, who might remit the pains of purgatory through the patient acceptance of earthly torments. The eager reception in the West of a growing corpus of Classical medical theory, transmitted through the medium of Arab and Hebrew commentators, was greatly facilitated by the ease with which its principles of balance and moderation accorded with profoundly held Christian beliefs. Even so, although sexual promiscuity and other forms of indulgence were believed to precipitate the onset of leprosy in vulnerable individuals, factors such as heredity, extreme anxiety, bad air and celestial forces lay beyond personal control and thus escaped moral censure.

From the presumed causes of *lepra*, we progress in chapter three to the diverse, often ambivalent, responses that such a potentially debilitating disease was liable to provoke. The close connection made between spiritual and physical health explains why these ranged from generosity, compassion and even envy to horror at the overt manifestation of sin. As Caroline Walker Bynum has remarked, 'there is something profoundly alien to modern sensibilities about the role of [the] body in medieval piety'.[18] Twenty-first-century readers may well find the more extravagant reactions to leprous men and women described in these pages disconcerting, if not distasteful. Yet the desire to kiss their disfigured faces and wash their ulcerated feet appears entirely understandable in a society suffused with images of the repentant Magdalen and an increasingly blood-stained, tormented Christ. Once again, theological developments, of which the most notable hinged upon the doctrine of purgatory and the concept of a treasury of merit upon which all sinners might draw, explain how the leper came to be regarded as an especially persuasive agent for the salvation of patrons and carers. The close identification between Christ and the leper made by prominent figures such as Queen Matilda (d. 1118) and Hugh of Lincoln (d. 1200) prompted a fashion for conspicuous acts of abasement before the most physically repugnant individuals. Even so, the sick were eventually transformed from objects of veneration into little more than ciphers whose principal value lay in their usefulness to others. At the same time, a growing awareness of theories about the dangers of corrupt air and the risks of transmission fostered less positive reactions to symptoms that came to personify disorder, dismemberment and economic collapse.

---

18   C. Walker Bynum, *Fragmentation and Redemption: Essays on Gender and the Human Body in Medieval Religion* (New York, 1992), p. 182.

Having considered the religious and social *milieu* in which medieval ideas about disease flourished, we then ask how lepers were actually identified, and what might be attempted, in practical terms, to arrest the process of physical decay. The diagnosis and medical treatment of *lepra*, which have hitherto received comparatively little attention in a specifically English context, are considered in chapters four and five. These deal with the dissemination of medical knowledge throughout society, and examine the increasingly sophisticated methods used not only to detect but also to avert, or at least postpone, the onset of what was invariably regarded as a terminal disease. The prominent role of the monk at the shrine and the priest in the confessional, as well as that of the medical professional and the lay 'expert', comes under scrutiny, as does the growing repertory of drugs and *materia medica* on which the patient might draw. Some of the diagnostic procedures and remedies for *lepra* may strike the modern reader as outlandish. But it is important to recognise that, far from being 'primitive' and 'beyond comprehension',[19] medical responses to the disease fell within the remit of a highly developed system of humoral management that embraced all manner of disorders from acne to cancer (with which *lepra* was often compared). We can readily appreciate why leprosy held such a fascination for medieval practitioners, who were obliged to marshal an armoury of cures in their efforts to combat this 'vniuersal corrupcioun of membres and of humours'.[20] In short, their struggle with the disease provides a valuable, sometimes unique, insight into the evolution of practice and theory over a period of almost four hundred years.

We move in chapter six to the question of segregation, which so preoccupied nineteenth-century physicians and colonial administrators. Often misunderstood, and frequently divorced from their historical background, the various measures established by canon and common law for the containment and support of lepers were less uniform and prescriptive than is generally supposed. Far from acting as detention centres for the forcible removal of suspects from society, *leprosaria* could prove extremely selective in the matter of admissions. Most of the larger, more affluent houses were, for example, run on vocational lines, demanding a voluntary oath of chastity, poverty and obedience, as well, perhaps, as a substantial contribution towards funds. Tonsured and clad in a religious habit, their inmates enjoyed a similar status to professed nuns and monks, while still retaining a degree of contact with the outside world. Yet, as we shall see, familiarity with advice literature on the regimen of health in general, and on environmental risks in particular, made people increasingly nervous about mixing with confirmed lepers. A clear distinction between the 'wild' and the 'tame' had long been made, especially in continental Europe. The upheavals of the fourteenth century, which began with mounting population pressure, famine and growing fears of vagrancy, followed by the lethal impact of successive outbreaks of plague, witnessed a more consistent attempt on the part of

---

[19] C. Roberts, 'Leprosy and Leprosaria in Medieval Britain', *MASCA Journal*, iv (1986), pp. 15–21, at p. 16.

[20] M.C. Seymour, ed., *On the Properties of Things: John Trevisa's Translation of Bartholomaeus Anglicus de Proprietatibus Rerum* (3 vols, Oxford, 1975–88), i, p. 423.

urban authorities to exclude those who appeared either physically or *morally* leprous. As might be expected, the poor, the itinerant and the disreputable bore the brunt of such measures, since the better off could always retreat to private quarters or take refuge in a hospital.

The last chapter begins at the gates of one such *leprosarium*, which bore little relation to the type of penal establishment envisaged by nineteenth-century advocates of mandatory segregation. On the contrary, ejection was a common punishment for serious breaches of discipline, while activities such as begging, pilgrimage, horticulture and visits to friends and family meant that hospitalised lepers were a common sight in the streets and lanes of medieval England. Whereas the more remote, rural houses reflect a desire for the eremitical life, far from the temptations of the world, suburban hospitals were closely integrated into the economic, social and religious fabric of neighbouring towns and cities. Nor is the common assumption that leper hospitals showed scant concern for the welfare of their patients supported by the surviving evidence. Measures for both physical and spiritual care were clearly important to founders and early benefactors. A combination of difficult economic circumstances (that affected many other charitable institutions) and an apparent fall in the number – and perhaps the status – of diagnosed lepers occasioned a sharp decline in levels of institutional provision during the fourteenth and fifteenth centuries. Yet this should not obscure the fact that considerable thought was initially given to the needs of inmates, not least because their welfare was so intimately connected with the spiritual health of patrons and carers.

The fact that so many late medieval leper hospitals either disappeared, began taking other types of patient or changed their function altogether sits oddly with the obvious – and in some cases growing – concern leprosy still provoked. We conclude by addressing this apparent paradox, which can best be understood by examining *lepra* in its proper social and cultural context rather than concentrating too narrowly upon the uncertain history of *Mycobacterium leprae*. Although it was clearly in retreat, the disease continued to epitomise the most profound fears and anxieties of a population whose dread of purgatory was matched by a more immediate desire to regulate the urban environment and eliminate any potential risks to public health.

*   *   *

One of the many attractions – and formidable challenges – of medieval medical history is its interdisciplinarity. The study of leprosy ranges across a number of fields, from topography, archaeology and palaeopathology to religious history, iconography and literature. The French historian, F.O. Touati, has developed this comprehensive methodology with particular success. His seminal study of leprosy in the province of Sens, *Maladie et société au moyen âge* (1998), has done most to challenge entrenched opinions about medieval responses to the disease, and offers what may, appropriately, be termed a *histoire totale* for the region.[21]

---

[21] F.O. Touati, 'Histoire des maladies, histoire totale?', *Sources: Travaux Historiques*, xiii (1988), pp. 3–14, stresses that the history of disease demands 'la globalité de la recherche'.

Luke Demaitre has simultaneously transformed our knowledge of medical approaches to *lepra* in a series of pioneering articles, which redeem the rather battered image of the medieval practitioner through a close study of significant texts.[22] It is none the less important to stress that the English experience of living with leprosy was often very different from that encountered in the parts of Europe with which these two authors are principally concerned. Attitudes to the disease did not evolve uniformly at the same pace, or even in the same way, and such practical matters as diagnosis, legal status and institutional provision varied considerably from one country to another. The notorious connection between the heretic (who was spiritually diseased) and the leper, which made such a striking impact in France, seems, for instance, to have had less resonance in a country spared the 'creeping contagion' of Catharism.

As we shall see, the English were bound by the same strictures of canon law, and shared the same theological beliefs as the rest of Western Christendom. The medical texts of Haly Abbas (al-Maǧūsi), Avicenna (Ibn Sīna) and other 'masters' were copied and studied with as much avidity in England as they were in France and Italy. Indeed, the two celebrated physicians, Gilbertus Anglicus and John of Gaddesden, produced detailed summaries of the existing literature on *lepra* that were widely cited by their peers across the Channel. Translations into English of textbooks by leading continental practitioners, such as Lanfrank of Milan, Bernard Gordon and Guy de Chauliac, ensured that surgeons and other interested laymen who did not read Latin could master the basics of diagnosis and treatment. But the way medicine and surgery were taught and practised, and the limited influence of the faculties of medicine at Oxford and Cambridge set England apart from her continental neighbours. Comparatively few suspect lepers would, for example, have been examined or treated by a graduate physician: a fact that raises interesting questions about the transmission of medical knowledge in a population blessed with remarkably high levels of literacy.

Nor, on balance, did hostility towards, or at least suspicion of, the vagrant or 'uncloistered' leper develop as early in England as was apparently the case in France. As we shall see in chapter one, a tendency to apply sweeping generalisations across time and place can prove extremely misleading. When that evidence has been extrapolated from a work of literature, particular sensitivity is required. One celebrated example, frequently cited by historians as proof that lepers were widely regarded as subhuman, will here suffice.[23] A late twelfth-century version of *The Romance of Tristan* by the French poet, Béroul, recounts how the adulterous queen, Yseut, is condemned to the stake by her husband. A hideous band of lepers ('you never saw anyone so ugly, nor so tumorous, nor so deformed') arrives on the scene and proposes a more terrible, and appropriate, fate. Their leader, Yvain, brazenly accosts King Mark:

22 Listed in the bibliography at the end of this book.
23 See, for example, Brody, *Disease of the Soul*, pp. 179–86; N. Orme and M. Webster, *The English Hospital, 1070–1570* (New Haven and London, 1995), p. 26. The present author herself pleads guilty to this offence: C. Rawcliffe, *Medicine and Society in Later Medieval England* (Stroud, 1995), pp. 15–16.

Give us Yseut, so that we can share her in common. No lady ever endured such an end. Sire, we burn with so much lust! There is no lady in the world who could survive our embraces, not even for a single day. Our ragged clothes stick to our bodies; with you she was accustomed to luxury, to beautiful furs and pleasures . . . If you give her to us lepers, when she sees our squalid hovels and shares our dishes, and has to sleep with us, and when, instead of your fine food, Sire, she has only the scraps and crumbs that are given to us at the gates . . . when she sees *our* court, with all its discomforts, she would rather be dead than alive.[24]

Although it takes place in some mythical part of Cornwall, Béroul's tale is, of course, the product of an individual imagination and a particular courtly *milieu*. In describing the 'burning lust' and wretched appearance of the lepers, the poet provides a dramatic counterpoint to the heroine's own sexual licence and love of luxury. Her soul is as leprous as the bodies of her potential abductors. Béroul also reflects the mounting sense of unease then being voiced by leading clergy in and around Paris about the threat posed by bands of lepers and other misfits, who lived outside the norms of society.[25] There is no evidence whatsoever to suggest that gangs of armed and marauding lepers, over a hundred strong, ever rampaged through the English countryside (or, indeed, that anyone feared they might do so). Educated members of the Anglo-Norman elite, such as Hugh of Lincoln, were certainly aware by this date of medical assumptions that *lepra* might well provoke the sexual appetite because of its destabilising effect upon the body's humoral balance.[26] On the other hand, the tendency to stigmatise *certain* lepers as promiscuous and threatening developed much later, partly in response to growing fears of vagrancy and social unrest from the early fourteenth century onwards. It was, significantly, a largely urban phenomenon.

That a disease so loaded with imagery and symbolism should appeal to the authors of chivalric romance is hardly surprising, and tells us a great deal about its place in the medieval consciousness. Perhaps for this very reason, historians and anthropologists have tended to select the most lurid passages for indiscriminate application across the map of Europe, thereby creating a stereotype that finds less support in the legal, administrative or medical record.[27] In order to avoid such unhelpful generalisations I have concentrated heavily (but not exclusively) upon the stories, poems, homilies and didactic texts that are known to have circulated widely among English readers and listeners, often in vernacular adaptations made for them from French or Latin. These were, in turn, the inspiration for countless sermons and admonitions in the confessional. A more comprehensive, if somewhat negative, guide to representations of leprosy in medieval European literature as a whole may be found in S.N. Brody, *The Disease of the Soul* (1974).

Other specialist monographs have made the task of writing a national study

24  Béroul, *The Romance of Tristan*, ed. N.J. Lacy (New York, 1989), pp. 56–9.
25  J. Avril, 'Le IIIe Concile du Latran et les communautés de lépreux', *Revue Mabillon*, lx (1981), pp. 21–76, pp. 63–4, 70.
26  See below, pp. 123, 144.
27  S. Harper, *Insanity, Individuals and Society in Late-Medieval English Literature* (New York and Lampeter, 2003), pp. 18–20, makes a similar point about writing on mental illness in the medieval period.

far easier. Institutional provision for lepers has, for example, attracted a good deal of attention over the last few years. In particular, readers who wish to learn more about the English Order of Lazarus and the surprisingly limited facilities it offered the sick are referred to David Marcombe's recent study of *Leper Knights*, which investigates this topic in depth.[28] Detailed information about other English medieval *leprosaria* of pre-fourteenth-century foundation that have so far been documented, excavated and mapped may be found in A.E.M. Satchell's Oxford DPhil thesis on 'The Emergence of Leper-Houses in Medieval England' (1998). This excellent survey, which contains a comprehensive gazetteer of some 300 hospitals and their dates, is shortly to be published, and provides the most reliable list of early foundations currently available.

It remains to add a word about the controversial question of vocabulary. As will become depressingly apparent in the course of chapter one, the terms 'leper' and 'leprosy' still carry a unique stigma that campaigners have sought for decades to eradicate by eliminating their use from scientific and popular discourse. The battle has been only partially successful. Over forty years have passed since Harold Wilson described the Tory, Peter Griffiths, as 'a parliamentary leper' after the notorious Smethwick by-election of 1964, and was duly castigated by *The Times* for his offensive language. 'Ruder things may have been said in the House, but they do not spring to mind', remarked one political correspondent, attacking the Prime Minister for 'a degree of bitterness and venom which even he has seldom equalled'.[29] Few gave any thought to the effect that Wilson's words might have had upon sufferers from the disease, whose status as malignant pariahs went largely unquestioned in what was then England's most influential newspaper. Even today, sections of the more reputable British media, as well as the tabloid press, persistently revert to an offensive stereotype of 'the outcast leper' that remains firmly entrenched in the late nineteenth century.[30]

My own use of words that are now deemed unacceptable by people who have contracted, or are involved in the treatment of, Hansen's disease therefore requires an explanation. Although, as we shall see, medieval *leprosi* (lepers) and those who cared for them were acutely conscious of the psychological harm that thoughtless or derogatory speech might cause, they continued to deploy a nomenclature that now seems highly questionable. The Latin terms *leprosus*, *leprosa* and *lepra*, along with their English equivalents of 'lepur' and 'leprosie', figured most prominently. Since the beaten and crucified Christ was frequently said to have been *quasi leprosus* (like a leper), this usage had positive as well as negative implications and had yet to acquire much of the opprobrium later heaped upon it by Victorian segregationists. Moreover, as must already be

---

[28]  D. Marcombe, *Leper Knights: The Order of St Lazarus of Jerusalem in England, c.1150–1544* (Woodbridge, 2003).

[29]  *The Times*, 4 November 1964, p. 12. Wilson's remark was clearly prompted by an inflammatory election address in which Griffiths had asserted that, 'because most blacks have leprosy, they are building two secret leper hospitals in the town': *The Times*, 13 October 1964, p. 18.

[30]  Headlines, culled at random, from a long and recent list: 'Smokers are often treated like lepers' (*Daily Telegraph*, 27 May 2005, p. 27); 'Prisoners are treated like lepers in society' (*Guardian*, 11 May 2005, p. 2); 'Today's graffitists are social lepers' (*The Times*, 16 April 2005, p. 20); 'House builders are used to being the City's lepers' (*The Times*, 13 February 2005, p. 6).

apparent, to describe medieval lepers as 'sufferers from Hansen's disease' would not only be anachronistic but also inherently misleading. It would, in fact, undermine the entire rationale of this book, which is to study *lepra* in all its manifestations and diagnostic complexity through the eyes and speech of medieval men and women. They knew nothing of Hansen and his microscope, and were strangers to our particular sensibilities. When referring to leprosy in a late nineteenth- and twentieth-century context, I have adopted what is currently regarded as a more appropriate vocabulary. It is, of course, only then that a blanket equation with Hansen's disease may safely be made.

# 1

## Creating the Medieval Leper:
## Some Myths and Misunderstandings

*But everyone is free to interpret history their own way, since history is no more than the reflection of the present upon the past, and that is why it is always being rewritten.*

Gustave Flaubert to Madame Roger des Genettes, November 1864 [1]

Readers of the new scientific journal, *Janus*, must have been disconcerted to learn, in the 1897 number, of yet another medical menace creeping stealthily upon the civilised world. Convinced that the West faced a threat to its very survival, the American physician, Albert S. Ashmead, did not mince his words. Members of the scientific community should heed the lessons of the past, however brutal, before time ran out. Unambiguously entitled 'Leprosy Overcome by Isolation in the Middle Ages', his short but trenchant polemic constituted a clarion call to arms. At that distant time, he argued,

> . . . leprosy spread in every civilised country of Europe, and continued to spread until strenuous efforts were made to bring the diseased parts out of contact with the healthy community. In this no charitable regard was had to the victims of the scourge: the weal of the sane majority alone was considered. It is from this point of view that it behooves us to judge the conduct of the church. The Order of Lazarus was founded, and lazarettoes built in great numbers: the work and purpose of the Order were to segregate and govern the afflicted and dangerous part of humanity. The thing was necessary, was an unavoidable consequence of the resolve of healthy mankind, to remain so: it was not so much charity, as one might believe. The community wanted this work to be done, and . . . these middle age people . . . through isolation were fortunate enough finally to overcome the disease. [2]

1 R. Dumesnil, J. Pommier and C. Digeon, eds, *Oeuvres complètes de Gustave Flaubert. Correspondance: supplément 1864–1871* (Paris, 1954), p. 19. Part of this chapter forms the basis of an article on 'Isolating the Medieval Leper: Ideas and Misconceptions about Segregation in the Middle Ages', in P. Horden, ed., *Freedom of Movement in the Middle Ages* (Donington, forthcoming).

2 A.S. Ashmead, 'Leprosy Overcome by Isolation in the Middle Ages', *Janus*, i (1896–97), p. 558. See also, idem, 'What a Leprosy Conference Should Be', *The Lancet*, cl, issue 3859 (14 August 1897), p. 414. Ashmead's isolationist ideas, based upon what he considered to be strict medieval principles, were elaborated in his *Suppression and Prevention of Leprosy* (Norristown, Pennsylvania, 1897). They did not gain universal acceptance: see, for example, A. Davidson's review in *Janus*, ii (1897–98), pp. 191–2, and D.A. Zambaco, *Anthologie: La lèpre à travers les siècles et les contrées* (Paris, 1914), pp. 580–81.

Ashmead also launched a frontal attack on Edward Ehlers, the General Secretary to the first International Congress on Leprosy, then due to meet in Berlin. Yet Ehlers, whose stance on forcible segregation seemed dangerously liberal, was no less aware of the need for firm official action. He had recently condemned the closure in 1846 of Iceland's four medieval *leprosaria*, as a result of which, after centuries of vigilance, leprosy had once again become established on the island. 'It had a far better and more preventative influence', he maintained, when 'the population itself dreaded the infection . . . The leprous disease was, in the Middle Ages all Europe over held to be . . . eminently contagious.'[3]

The image of the segregated leper, secure behind the walls of his or her *leprosarium* or, at the very least, banished, with bell or rattle, to the outer margins of Christian society, exerts a powerful hold even today. It lingers on in illustrations such as that commissioned in 1912 by Sir Henry Wellcome from the watercolourist, Richard Tenant Cooper. [plate 1] This celebrated depiction of medieval villagers 'scrambling to get away from a leper' appears, for instance, without further qualification in a popular study of epidemic diseases produced during the late 1990s. The accompanying text observes grimly that 'the world of the medieval leper was outside the safety of walled cities and towns, a world belonging to bandits and other wild creatures'.[4] Yet the painting dates from a time when the fears expressed by Ashmead and his colleagues had embedded themselves in the European psyche, and a large and vociferous medical lobby was systematically propagating the conviction that 'middle age people' had successfully contained leprosy through isolation. Medieval men or women viewing such a picture would have been appalled by the behaviour of its subjects. Accustomed as they were to representations of Christ and His saints consoling lepers, they would have regarded it, perhaps, as a variant on the parable of Dives and Lazarus, in which divine retribution would swiftly follow the rejection of a beggar 'full of sores'.[5] [plate 2]

Any historian attempting to assess the impact of specific diseases on past societies soon becomes aware of the yawning discrepancies which emerge between the historical baggage he or she carries and the complex, often contradictory picture revealed by the original sources. Recent studies of historical responses to plague, the pox and tuberculosis, for example, show how far our perception of these diseases has been moulded, not simply by generations of medical practitioners with their own assumptions and agendas, but also by artists, poets, moral reformers and even journalists.[6] There is, in David Arnold's words, 'an enduring human disposition to read meaning into collective affliction';[7] and we may take

---

3    E. Ehlers, *On the Conditions under which Leprosy Has Declined in Iceland* (London, 1895), pp. 20, 37–8.

4    K.F. Kiple, ed., *Plague, Pox and Pestilence: Diseases in History* (London, 1997), p. 53. As late as 7 April 1999, a contributor to *The Nursing Times* observed that: 'To the average British Nurse, leprosy is probably no more than a plague of ancient folklore, a medieval scourge so disfiguring and contagious that it required those afflicted to ring warning bells.'

5    See chapter three, below.

6    Cohn, *Black Death Transformed*; J. Arrizabalaga, J. Henderson and R. French, *The Great Pox: The French Disease in Renaissance Europe* (New Haven and London, 1997); D.S. Barnes, *The Making of a Social Disease: Tuberculosis in Nineteenth-Century France* (Berkeley, California, 1995).

7    D. Arnold, 'Introduction: Disease, Medicine and Empire', in idem, ed., *Imperial Medicine in Indigenous Societies* (Manchester, 1988), p. 7.

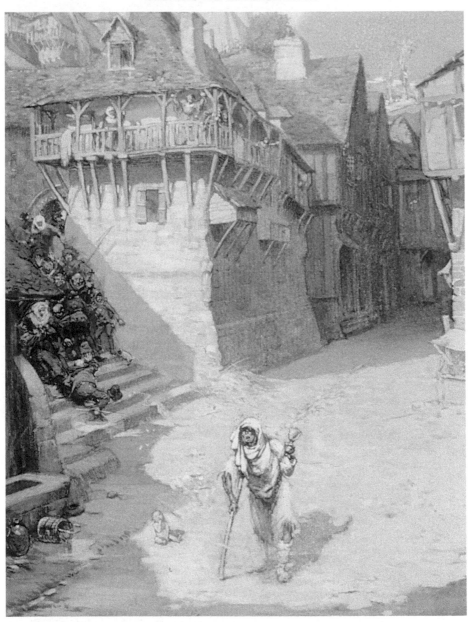

1. Richard Tenant Cooper's watercolour of 'Medieval villagers scrambling to get away from a leper' (1912) reflects the fears of a mass epidemic of leprosy then exercising the European and American medical establishments.

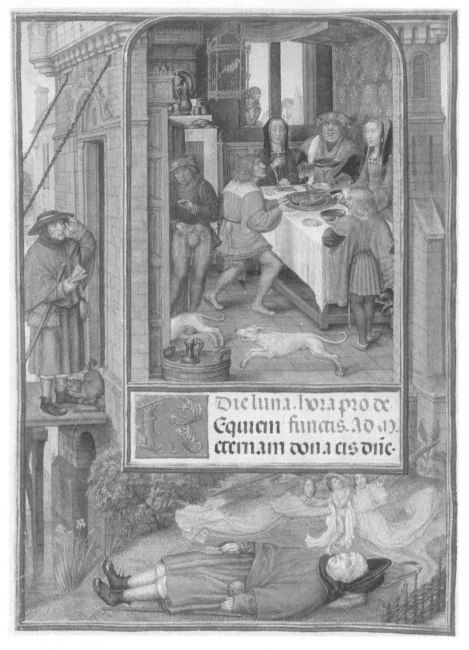

Die luna. hora pro de
Equiem functis. Ad m.
eternam dona eis dnc·

2. This graphic early sixteenth-century illustration of the tale of Dives and
Lazarus depicts the poor beggar as a leper (with rattle), while the gluttony and
wrath of the rich householder are apparent from his groaning table, bloated
features and bright red clothing. Angels transport Lazarus's soul to heaven
(below) after his solitary death.

it as a general rule of thumb that the greater and more dangerous the affliction appears to be, the more earnestly its meaning will be explored and contested. As writers on the topic – and they are legion – frequently remind us, the effects of untreated leprosy on the human body prompt extreme reactions. It is thus hardly surprising that its history, too, has so often been misunderstood, misrepresented, exploited and sensationalised. Just as cancer and AIDS have become the iconic diseases of the late twentieth century, so leprosy has often been projected as representative of 'the Dark Ages', when prejudice and superstition marched hand in hand with ignorance.[8] This process offers some salutary warnings. That a disease called leprosy played a notable part in the medieval imagination, and was accorded significance far beyond the physical threat it actually posed to the population, will become apparent in the course of this book. So too will the fact that responses to it were far more complex, diverse and subject to change over time than the majority of nineteenth- and twentieth-century writers would have us believe. Between them, these leprologists, missionaries and literary lions have, to a notable extent, performed the office of a Dr Frankenstein in cobbling together their monster from miscellaneous body parts. The rest of this chapter traces how such an ill-assorted being was galvanised into life.

## 'This global disaster': the biomedical model

Ashmead and Ehlers were not unusual in their recourse to historical precedents. Indeed, their fascination with medieval leprosy went far beyond the amateur scholarship customarily pursued by medical antiquarians in a more leisurely and lettered age. To understand why they and their colleagues were so drawn to the topic, and to appreciate the powerful and persistent influence their conclusions were to exert, not least upon future generations of archaeologists, historians and anthropologists, we must begin with the bitter controversy about the causes of leprosy, which came to a head in the 1890s.

The publication in 1847 by the Norwegian physician, D.C. Danielssen, and his associate, C.W. Boeck, of a meticulously illustrated atlas of leprosy, *Om Spedalskhed*,[9] drew attention to a problem hitherto largely ignored by the medical profession [**plate 3**]. Clinical experience convinced Danielssen that the disease was not contagious but hereditary: a view shared by many other practitioners who came in regular contact with its victims. The impoverished diet and unhygienic living conditions so often found in vulnerable Scandinavian communities also lent support to what might be termed an environmental or Galenic theory of causation, broadly similar to that adopted by medieval physicians.[10] Besides encouraging further scientific debate, Danielssen's researches

---

8 C.M. Cipolla, *Public Health and the Medical Profession in the Renaissance* (Cambridge, 1976), p. 11, describes 'the Dark Ages' as a period dominated by leprosy. See also, S. Sontag, *Illness as a Metaphor* (London, 1990), p. 59: 'Leprosy in its heyday aroused a similarly disproportionate sense of horror [as cancer in the twentieth century]. In the middle ages, the leper was a social text in which corruption was made visible; an exemplum, an emblem of decay.'

9 Rapidly disseminated in other languages, as, for example, *Traité de la spédalskhed ou éléphantiasis des Grecs* (Paris and London, 1848). This work first identified two basic types of leprosy, nodular and anaesthetic (respectively, lepromatous and tuberculoid).

10 See chapter two, below.

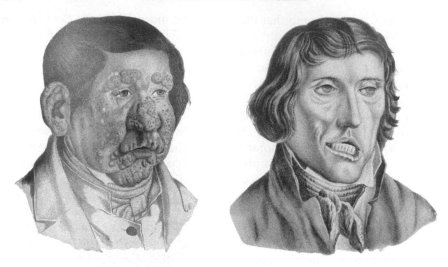

3. Cases of 'nodular' (left, now known as lepromatous) and 'anaesthetic' (now tuberculoid) leprosy depicted with striking realism in D.C. Danielssen and C.W. Boeck, *Om Spedalskhed* (1847)

stimulated a growing enthusiasm for the history of leprosy among his colleagues. This inevitably focused upon the reasons for its virtual disappearance in most of northern Europe during the later Middle Ages and the causes of its subsequent resurgence.[11]

In 1859, for example, the eminent pathologist, Rudolf Virchow, compiled a detailed international questionnaire designed not only to ascertain the scale of the current problem (and the measures already in place to deal with it), but also to survey the historical evidence. Health authorities in countries such as Spain, where pockets of the disease remained, were asked to provide lists of medieval *leprosaria* and to assess their effectiveness. Whereas Virchow and his assistants referred to the 'slow progress' of what looked like a new epidemic, others were less measured. Indeed, within the year, Méndez Alvaro, Secretary to the Spanish Council of Health, published a history of leprosy in Spain from the medieval period onwards, concluding that the 'devastating and repugnant pestilence which populated the Christian world of the Middle Ages with lepers' was again on the march.[12]

Although their interest in the disease was at this stage confined to the further reaches of Empire rather than home turf, members of the British medical

---

[11] Although James Y. Simpson, Professor of Midwifery at the University of Edinburgh, had already published 'Antiquarian Notices of Leprosy and Leper Hospitals in Scotland and England', *The Edinburgh Medical and Surgical Journal*, clvi (1841), part 1, pp. 301–30; clvii (1842), part 2, pp. 121–56, and part 3, pp. 394–429. See P.A. Kalisch, 'An Overview of Research on the History of Leprosy', *International Journal of Leprosy*, xliii (1975), pp. 129–44, for a survey of earlier work.

[12] There were then only about 600 lepers in Spain: J. Bernabeu-Mestre and T. Ballester-Artigues, 'Le Retour d'un péril: La lèpre dans l'Espagne, 1878–1932', *Annales de demographie historique: Epidémies et populations* (Paris, 1997), pp. 115–34, at pp. 116–17, 131. I am grateful to Professor Bernabeu-Mestre for providing me with a copy of this article.

community felt that they, too, had much to contribute. Such a conviction was, for instance, demonstrated by the physician, Robert Liveing, whose Goulstonian lectures for 1873 on *Elephantiasis Graecorum, or True Leprosy*, began with a lengthy examination of historical strategies of containment. This was, in fact, an issue of considerable moment, given the intelligentsia's current preoccupation with the blight of moral and physical degeneracy. A belief that criminals, sick paupers, the insane and others who functioned at the 'lower stages of human evolution' should be institutionalised attracted many converts.[13] A wholehearted advocate of social Darwinism, Liveing informed his audience that draconian measures introduced in medieval Britain through a mistaken fear of contagion had, in fact, proved remarkably successful. This was because they 'destroyed the race of lepers' by preventing them from breeding, and thus passing on their hereditary curse. 'The exclusion of lepers from society', he writes, 'was considered a high moral duty, simply because the disease was believed to be dreadfully infectious.'[14] Having described in lingering detail the funerary ritual of the 'Leper Mass', when the condemned man or woman was reputedly pronounced dead to the world and debarred from human society while standing beside a bier or in an open grave, he went on to urge an immediate return to 'the compulsory segregation of lepers with the view of exterminating the disease . . . as was done in the Middle Ages'.[15] His evocation of the lone medieval leper, debarred from all contact with the healthy and consigned to the living dead, still haunts the pages of scholarly as well as popular literature, along with a persistent but entirely erroneous belief in the ubiquity of the so-called 'Leper Mass'.[16]

Resuscitated (and greatly embellished) in the 1980s as academics and journalists explored the historical context of the AIDS epidemic, this gruesome ritual has, in every sense, enjoyed life beyond the grave.[17] Yet, as several historians have already argued, there is no evidence whatsoever that it was ever enacted in

---

[13] J. Saunders, 'Quarantining the Weak-Minded: Psychiatric Definitions of Degeneracy and the Late-Victorian Asylum', in W.F. Bynum, R. Porter and M. Shepherd, eds, *The Anatomy of Madness, III, The Asylum and its Psychiatry* (London and New York, 1988), pp. 273–96, especially pp. 277–8; E. Shorter, *A History of Psychiatry* (New York, 1997), pp. 93–8.

[14] R. Liveing, *Elephantiasis Graecorum, or True Leprosy* (London, 1873), p. 13. A committee of the Royal College of Physicians had pronounced leprosy a hereditary disease in 1862–63, but, unlike Liveing, had recommended the relaxation of rules for containment: M. Worboys, *Spreading Germs: Disease Theories and Medical Practice in Britain 1865–1900* (Cambridge, 2000), p. 42.

[15] Liveing, *Elephantiasis*, p. 149. This, he urged, should be accompanied by the prohibition of marriage not just of lepers themselves but also of their children, and the *mandatory* sterilisation of all males born to leprous parents.

[16] Liveing must have been influenced by the work of C.N. Macnamara, whose *Leprosy: A Communicable Disease* was first published in Calcutta in 1866. A supporter of the 'hereditary' theory of transmission (ibid., p. 27), Macnamara none the less accepted that the disease might also be communicable. Much of his evidence came from what he believed to be medieval practices: having introduced leprosy to Europe, the 'old Crusaders' eliminated it by 'enforcing absolute and strict segregation', not least through the 'Leper Mass', which is described at length (ibid., pp. 34–7, 40).

[17] See, for example, D.F. Musto, 'Quarantine and the Problem of AIDS', in E. Fee and D.M. Fox, eds, *AIDS: The Burdens of History* (Berkeley, Los Angeles and London, 1988), pp. 68–71; and, for a particularly depressing view of the Middle Ages, K.J. Doka, *Fear and Society: Challenging the Dreaded Disease* (Washington DC, 1984), pp. 26–8. Both authors subscribe to the by then common assumption that Henry II actually *burnt* lepers. See below, p. 39.

medieval England.[18] The most convincing case so far has been advanced by the liturgical scholar, A.J. Collins. His 1960 edition of the *Sarum Missal* reveals that the Mass's first appearance in this seminal text may be dated to printed versions specially designed for the continental market in the 1520s and 1540s, by which time leprosy had all but disappeared from mainland Britain.[19] Apparently copied from a book 'of extremely local circulation', originating in the French diocese of St Flour, the rite seems to have been chosen (along with an equally obscure one preceding the burial of an English king) for its curiosity value. Foreign booksellers liked to entertain their readers, who bought such manuals 'to beguile an idle hour' rather than for practical use. We should be no less cautious in according the Mass a much longer pedigree in continental Europe. Indeed, F.O. Touati, who has done most in recent years radically to challenge received wisdom about medieval leprosy, has dismissed its celebration in France as being so far without any historical foundation.[20] The surviving statutes of *leprosaria* often refer to rituals of admission, but, as we shall see in chapter seven, these were common to *all* medieval hospitals of any size and focused upon the reception of the newcomer into a quasi-monastic community.[21]

Fictitious or not, the morbid spectacle of the 'Leper Mass' appealed to Victorian sensibilities. It was through reading an article on the ceremony in, of all places, *The Isle of Wight County Press* of 4 February 1888, that Alfred, Lord Tennyson, was inspired to write a poem about the repentant wife of a leprous crusader, who follows him into the wilderness after just such a rite of exclusion.[22] Whatever its merits as a work of literature, *Happy: The Leper's Bride* illustrates graphically how tenacious these ideas had already become:

> '*Libera me, Domine!*' you sang the Psalm, and when
> The Priest pronounced you dead, and flung the mould upon your feet,
> A beauty came upon your face, not that of living men,
> But seen upon the silent brow when life has ceased to beat.
>
> The Priest who joined you to the dead, has joined our hands of old;
> If man and wife be but one flesh, let mine be leprous too,

---

18  W. MacArthur, 'Mediaeval "Leprosy" in the British Isles', *Leprosy Review*, xxiv (1953), pp. 8–19, at p. 12; Orme and Webster, *English Hospital*, pp. 29–31.

19  A.J. Collins, ed., *Manuale ad usum percelebris ecclesie Sarisburiensis* (Henry Bradshaw Society, xci, 1958), pp. xx, 182–5.

20  Touati, *Maladie et société*, pp. 39–40, 46–7.

21  F. Bériac, 'Mourir au monde: Les ordines de séparation des lépreux en France au XVe et XVIe siècles', *Journal of Medieval History*, xi (1985), pp. 245–68, lists seven so-called 'rites' for the separation of lepers, mostly parodies of the Dance of Death, circulating among a narrow readership between 1490 and 1550, and stresses that *real* ceremonies of admission to *leprosaria* were essentially welcoming and inclusive. Piera Borradori, whose *Mourir au monde: Les lépreux dans le pays de Vaud* (Cahiers Lausannois d'Histoire Médiévale, vii, 1992) places greater emphasis upon the valedictory nature of such ceremonies, also observes (pp. 39–42) that the Mass of exclusion was never celebrated. So too does Albert Bourgeois, *Lépreux et maladreries du Pas-de-Calais* (Arras, 1972), p. 54. Rituals for admission are also discussed in M. Kupfer, *The Art of Healing* (Pennsylvania, 2003), pp. 142–4.

22  C. Ricks, ed., *The Poems of Tennyson* (3 vols, London, 1987), iii, pp. 189–90, 193–4. The article, by E. Boucher-James, reiterates Dean Milman's view that 'the protection and care afforded by the Church to this blighted race of lepers was among the most beautiful of its offices during the Middle Ages', sentiments which reflect the uneasy combination of late Victorian missionary zeal and eugenics discussed below.

As dead from all the human race as if beneath the mould;
If you be dead, then I am dead, who live only for you.[23]

It would be tedious to rehearse the long – and still growing – list of more recent authors who cite this ritual, usually as evidence of the marginality, stigmatisation and isolation of the medieval leper. Reproduced in full in R.M. Clay's *The Mediaeval Hospitals of England*, which appeared in 1909 and served as the only general history of its kind for the best part of ninety years,[24] it became grist to the mill of writers for the popular market. Books such as Anthony Weymouth's *Through the Leper Squint* and Paolo Zappa's *Unclean! Unclean!* (titles which speak volumes) itemised the list of torments inflicted upon 'the contaminated outcast of the Middle Ages', who was 'relentlessly shut up and forbidden any contact with the outside world'.[25]

Before long, these funerary rites began to attract the attention of anthropologists, archaeologists, historians and sociologists.[26] B.S. Turner's influential study, *The Body and Society: Explanations in Social Theory*, which first appeared in 1984 and was revised twelve years later, offers one example among many.

The outward decay of the leper was a sign of inner profanity. The leper constituted both a moral and physical threat to the community and had to be separated from the population by dramatic rituals and other legal means. The Church's office for the seclusion of a leper did not differ in fundamentals from the office of the dead, since the *separatio leprosorum* defined the leper as a ritually dead person.[27]

---

23 Ricks, *Poems of Tennyson*, iii, pp. 191, 193. Influential missionaries, such as John Jackson, believed that this poem offered an accurate depiction of medieval practices: *Lepers: Thirty-Six Years Among Them, Being the History of the Mission to India and the East 1874–1910* (London, 1910), p. 2.

24 Appendix A, pp. 273–6. The book was reprinted in 1966.

25 A. Weymouth, *Through the Leper Squint: A Study of Leprosy from Pre-Christian Times to the Present Day* (London, 1938), pp. 14–17; P. Zappa, *Unclean! Unclean!* (London, 1933), pp. 70–72. In his introduction to the latter work, Sir Leonard Rogers, founder of the British Empire Leprosy Relief Association, dwells on the cruelty of 'the ancient system of compulsory isolation' (ibid., pp. 9–10). The 'Leper Mass' also featured in serious studies intended for the medical profession. See, for example, G. Thin, *Leprosy* (London, 1891), pp. 237–8; and R. Roose, *Leprosy and its Prevention* (London, 1890), p. 8. C.A. Mercier's Fitzpatrick Lectures to the Royal College of Physicians in 1914 began with a talk on leper hospitals in which he described the Mass at length: *Leper Houses and Medieval Hospitals* (London, 1915), pp. 13–14.

26 See, for a sample of fairly recent titles dealing specifically with Britain, F.F. Cartwright, *A Social History of Medicine* (London, 1977), p. 27; J. Cule, 'The Diagnosis, Care and Treatment of Leprosy in Wales and the Border in the Middle Ages', *Transactions of the British Society for the History of Pharmacy*, i (1970), pp. 29–58, at pp. 35–6; idem, 'The Stigma of Leprosy: Its Historical Origins and Consequences with Particular Reference to the Laws of Wales', *PPL*, p. 151; C. Daniell, *Death and Burial in Medieval England 1066–1550* (London, 1997), pp. 204–5; R. Gilchrist, 'Christian Bodies and Souls: The Archaeology of Life and Death in Later Medieval Hospitals', in S. Bassett, ed., *Death in Towns: Urban Responses to the Dying and the Dead, 100–1600* (Leicester, 1992), pp. 115–16; eadem, 'Medieval Bodies in the Material World: Gender, Stigma and the Body', in S. Kay and M. Rubin, eds, *Framing Medieval Bodies* (Manchester, 1994), p. 48; eadem, *Contemplation and Action: The Other Monasticism* (Leicester, 1995), pp. 39–40; B.L. Grigsby, *Pestilence in Medieval and Early Modern English Literature* (London and New York, 2004), pp. 39–40; M.B. Honeybourne, 'The Leper Hospitals of the London Area', *Transactions of the London and Middlesex Archaeological Society*, xxi (1967), pp. 1–55, at p. 1; P. Richards, *The Medieval Leper and His Northern Heirs* (Cambridge, 1977), reprinted Woodbridge, 2000), pp. 68–9, 137–9; Roberts and Cox, *Health and Disease*, p. 272; S. Rubin, *English Medieval Medicine* (London and Vancouver, 1974), pp. 158–9.

27 B.S. Turner, *The Body and Society: Explorations in Social Theory* (Oxford, 1984), pp. 67–8; (revised edn, London, 1996), p. 89.

In common with most other writers on this subject, Turner also believed that English common law offered a formal mechanism for exclusion. The assumption that a royal writ *de leproso amovendo* had been widely deployed in medieval England for the forcible ejection of lepers from healthy society was based more upon a half-truth than a complete fiction. Twice, in 1346 and 1472, the crown had issued orders for the expulsion of lepers from the streets of London. The first, better-known, missive took the form of a letter close, and was specifically directed against those who frequented the stews, or brothels, of the city, thereby allegedly spreading their disease.[28] The second, described in the London records as a letter, but never enrolled in Chancery, targeted vagrants and followed a serious outbreak of plague. It was presumably sent under the signet of Edward IV, and then copied in the corporation's journal.[29]

In addition, on about half a dozen known occasions, late medieval sheriffs were commanded by royal writ to arrange for the examination of designated suspects, who were to be removed from society in a decent manner should they be pronounced leprous. As we shall see in chapter six, the wording of these documents employs the same standard phrases, but none that were recognised in any medieval formulary or described by contemporary writers on jurisprudence.[30] The first works to identify such a writ by name were the *Registrum omnium breuium*, first published by William Rastall in 1531, and Sir Anthony Fitzherbert's *Novelle natura brevium* of 1534. Both cite a solitary example from London. It concerns one I[ohannes] de N[——], who had persistently gone about in public despite his potentially dangerous condition, and was to be duly examined by experts. The very same example was produced almost a century later by Sir Edward Coke in *The First Part of the Institutes of the Laws of England*.[31] Can we trace this person?

The records of medieval London furnish only one case of direct intervention by the civic authorities to remove a *named* leper. This was in June 1372, in the aftermath of a serious epidemic, and concerned a baker named Iohannes (John) Mayn. Having been repeatedly warned by the mayor and aldermen that he constituted a health hazard, Mayn was finally threatened with the pillory should he continue to mix among healthy people and, presumably, sell his bread. Although no mention is made of any royal writ or other external directive, it is

---

28  H.T. Riley, ed., *Memorials of London and London Life in the Thirteenth, Fourteenth and Fifteenth Centuries* (London, 1868), pp. 230–31; *CCR, 1346–1349*, pp. 61–2. Similar orders were then directed to the bailiffs of King's Lynn. See chapter six for a discussion of the circumstances in which these measures were promulgated.

29  CLRO, Journal 8, fos 19v, 21r; R.R. Sharpe, ed., *Calendar of Letter-Books of the City of London, Letter-Book L* (London, 1912), pp. 102–3.

30  No mention of the writ occurs in E. de Haas and G.D.G. Hall, eds, *Early English Registers of Writs* (Selden Society, lxxxvii, 1970).

31  *The New Natura Brevium of the Most Reverend Judge Mr Anthony Fitzherbert* (London 1677), pp. 520–21; Sir Edward Coke, *The First Part of the Institutes of the Laws of England* (London, 1794), liber II, sect. 201. Rubin, *English Medieval Medicine*, p. 157, dates the writ to 1100, but provides no supporting evidence. Clay, *Mediaeval Hospitals*, p. 52, cites a case of 1220 brought in the *curia regis* as evidence of the writ's usage, but the actual proceedings do not mention it at all. On the contrary, they concern a young man who was pronounced leprous and placed in a hospital as a minor, but left it two years later, and eventually went off on a pilgrimage: *CRR, 1219–1220*, pp. 308–10. Richards, *Medieval Leper*, p. 50, reproduces Clay almost *verbatim*.

possible that one had already been issued and had secured a positive diagnosis.[32] Nineteenth-century writers seem to have ignored this case, which suggests that suspect lepers had to be both intransigent and highly visible before they caused real offence. Instead, they turned to the antiquary, John Stow, who recalls in his *Survey of London* (1598) that he had once heard tell of 'a writte in our Law, *de leproso amouendo*', and then proceeds to describe Edward III's letter close of 1346.[33] Yet, despite its uncertain history, the royal writ, like the 'Leper Mass', soon became a central plank in the segregationists' arguments, figuring prominently as evidence of a draconian and systematic policy of exclusion employed across the nation. Cited by, *inter alios*, Macnamara (1861), Liveing (1873) and Thin (1891) as proof positive of the dynamic strategy they wished to revive, John Stow's passing recollection was transformed into a manifesto for government action.

It is, of course, unlikely that so much emphasis would have been placed either upon an obscure writ or the notorious 'Leper Mass' had the spread of leprosy – or, more accurately, misplaced fears about its contagiousness – not become a burning issue in late nineteenth-century Europe. Advances in the emergent science of microbiology had meanwhile prompted Armauer Hansen, Danielssen's assistant, to begin the search for a living pathogen that could be clinically proved to transmit the disease. In 1873, the year of Liveing's lectures, he successfully isolated *Mycobacterium leprae*, a bacillus found in tissue samples taken from his patients at the hospital of St George in Bergen. Yet all was not plain sailing. The elusive bacillus stubbornly resisted all attempts at cultivation and inoculation, the two other vital tests of infection established in 1884 by the leading exponent of germ theory, Robert Koch. Hansen therefore proceeded with caution. He advocated voluntary segregation of the kind successfully adopted in Norway, where compulsion was regarded as a last, but necessary, resort, should educational measures fail.[34] Others were more dogmatic. H.V. Carter, a surgeon-major in the Bombay Medical Service, who had been visiting Hansen at the time of his discovery, abandoned his support of the 'hereditary' theory to become a militant contagionist. His views encountered considerable opposition among his more conservative colleagues in British India, where the disease was endemic, but were vigorously promoted at home by many influential authors, including the polemicist, H.P. Wright.[35]

As an Anglican clergyman, Archdeacon Wright took a less jaundiced view of the medieval Church's charitable effort than the sceptical Dr Ashmead, but his recourse to dubious historical precedents served exactly the same ends. It was, he stressed, the strict isolation maintained by monastic *leprosaria* that had kept contagious individuals 'well apart from the strong and healthy'.[36] His *Leprosy*

---

32  Riley, *Memorials*, pp. 365–6. A precedent book kept by the clerk of the crown in Chancery during the reign of Henry VIII records two undated writs *de leproso amovendo*, one of which is for the examination of I[——], *leprosus* of London: PRO, C193/1, fo. 24v. I am grateful to Dr Hannes Kleineke for this reference.

33  C.L. Kingsford, ed., *A Survey of London by John Stow* (2 vols, Oxford, 1908), ii, pp. 147–8.

34  He also campaigned for improvements in public hygiene: G.A. Hansen and C. Looft, *Leprosy in its Clinical and Pathological Aspects* (Bristol and London, 1895), p. 124.

35  Buckingham, *Leprosy in Colonial South India*, pp. 8–15, 146–53.

36  H.P. Wright, *Leprosy and Segregation* (London, 1885), p. 92.

*and Segregation* of 1885 fired a broadside for the return to firm medieval principles: 'Whatever were the sanitary shortcomings of our ancestors, the measures
publicly adopted and by authority enforced in Great Britain and in most of
Europe seems [*sic*] to have been co-efficient, to say the least, in eradicating
leprosy'.[37] The book concluded with a lengthy appendix listing the medieval
leper hospitals of the British Isles. Wright's principal concern was the threat to
Europeans, and especially the English, posed by the dark shadow of disease,
promiscuity and racial degeneration moving inexorably westwards from the
expanding colonies. 'May God preserve my country from leprosy!' he prayed
four years later in *Leprosy an Imperial Danger*, a title that fostered patriotism and
paranoia in equal measure.[38] Once again he commended the 'strict isolation'
practised in medieval England, arguing that 'the danger of contact between the
leprous and the healthy' had then never been questioned.[39]

The Archdeacon's renewed plea for enforced segregation can only have intensified the mood of panic spread by the dramatic, and widely publicised, death in
1889 of the Belgian missionary, Father Damien, who had contracted the disease
while working among the lepers of Moloka'i in Hawaii. The impact of what was
widely regarded as the martyrdom of a contemporary saint, who, like his medieval predecessors, had devoted his life to the wretched outcasts of society in their
'living graveyard', is hard to exaggerate.[40] 'In England', one observer reported,
'the news was received with wild outbursts of popular feeling. A wave of enthusiasm swept the land from end to end, and Damien became the hero of the
hour.'[41] At the same time, the chairman of the Epidemiological Society of
London reiterated 'the urgent need for more medical inquiry into the history of
leprosy', in order to support the escalating demand for stricter segregation.[42] If
comparatively few Europeans reflected upon the devastating effects of imperialism upon the health of indigenous populations, their fear of transmission in the
other direction could verge on the hysterical.[43]

Capitalising upon the publicity generated by Damien's death, the
contagionists seized the initiative. A.S. Ashmead, with whose forceful opinions
this chapter begins, was especially concerned about infected Norwegian immi-
grants entering the United States, while the influential French physician,
Professor Edouard Jeanselme, fulminated against the danger posed to 'the
mother race' by leprosy and syphilis in France's African colonies.[44] A distinguished expert on both diseases, Jeanselme represented his country at the Berlin

37  Wright, *Leprosy and Segregation*, pp. 92–3. These ideas are echoed in Thin, *Leprosy*, chapter one.
38  H.P. Wright, *Leprosy an Imperial Danger* (London, 1889), p. ix. Carter had his champions abroad, too.
    Writing anonymously in 1879, 'un missionaire' argued that medieval *leprosaria* were not simply
    authorised to receive lepers, 'but had the right, in the public interest, to force them to enter these
    houses': *La lèpre est contagieuse* (Paris, 1879), p. 26.
39  Wright, *Leprosy an Imperial Danger*, pp. 4, 18. See also his letter on 'The Spread of Leprosy' to *The
    Times*, 8 November 1887, p. 13.
40  P. Moblo, 'Blessed Damien of Moloka'i: The Critical Analysis of a Contemporary Myth', *Ethnohistory*,
    xliv (1997), pp. 691–726.
41  M. Quinlan, *Damien of Molokai* (London, 1909), p. 148.
42  *The Times*, 13 June 1889, p. 10.
43  Arnold, 'Disease, Medicine and Empire', pp. 4–10.
44  Zambaco, *Anthologie*, pp. 646–8.

Congress in 1897, and chaired the third International Congress on Leprosy at Strasbourg in 1923. He was later to produce a substantial, and still often cited, article of 155 pages for the Société Francaise d'Histoire de la Médecine, of which he had been president, entitled 'Comment l'Europe, au moyen age, se protéga contre la lèpre'. Not surprisingly, the 'Leper Mass' and the writ *de leproso amovendo* rank high among the prophylactic measures he describes.[45] His last work, a monumental study of leprosy, begins with an historical overview of the disease, which compares the ritual of isolation with the office of the dead. While admitting that, in medieval Europe, complete segregation had never been achieved, he observes that *leprosaria* were 'above all institutions for sanitary policing, from which therapeutics were totally excluded'.[46]

To an already explosive brew of racialism, social Darwinism, imperialism and religion was thus now added the gelignite of scientific medicine. As we have already seen, dramatic advances in the laboratory, notably in the field of micro-biology, greatly strengthened the hand of the late nineteenth-century medical profession, which had a clear agenda of its own in seeking to colonise the management of leprosy. The impact of an emergent profession fighting hard for recognition at home and abroad is strikingly apparent, for example, in Colombia. Here the number of lepers was deliberately and grossly inflated in order to push through a biomedically driven programme of forcible segregation during the 1890s.[47] Claiming that the disease had reached epidemic proportions, which threatened to undermine the whole fabric of society, the physician, Abraham Aparicio, advocated the forcible removal of all infected persons to a remote island off the Panama coast. He justified this controversial step on the ground that, although the scientific principles behind it had not been fully understood, the medieval policy of mandatory and highly ritualised segregation had rid Europe of the disease. In short, history proved that isolation was the only answer. Readers of, and contributors to, the leading medical journal, *Revista Medica de Colombia*, developed a burning interest in the Middle Ages, shared by the better educated – and as yet voluntary – residents of the existing *leprosarium* at Agua de Dios. One such correspondent accepted that medieval leprosy was indeed highly contagious, having been spread by crusaders on their return from the East, but insisted that the modern strain of the disease was caused by a combination of environmental, dietary and physiological factors, which varied from person to person.[48]

Men who prided themselves on a more judicious use of historical evidence than their opponents championed this conservative aetiology from within the British medical establishment. Both George Newman, MD, and Jonathan Hutchinson, FRCS, for instance, persisted in the belief that poor hygiene, an

45 *Bulletin de la Société Francaise d'Histoire de la Médecine*, xxv (1931), pp. 1–155, at pp. 62–70 (Mass) and 26–7 (writ).
46 E. Jeanselme, *La lèpre* (Paris, 1934), pp. 2–67, quotation at p. 47.
47 An incomplete 1890 census revealed 1,724 cases. By the end of the decade estimates had soared to 30,000, or 0.75 of the population. In order to raise funds, one Italian priest claimed there were almost *twice as many again*: D. Obregón, 'Lepra, Exageración y Authoridad Médica', *Asclepio*, l (1998), pp. 125–48, pp. 138–9.
48 Orbegón, 'Lepra', pp. 133–4, 141–3.

unbalanced diet and humid climate would cause leprosy in individuals with a natural predisposition to the disease. Neither accepted that segregation had been consistently, effectively or even deliberately deployed in the Middle Ages. Maintaining that he had found 'absolutely no evidence at all' of such practices, Newman insisted that medieval leper hospitals were nothing more than 'charitable resorts'. His view of the period was, even so, a gloomy one.[49] The picture of unmitigated squalor, sexual promiscuity and deprivation to emerge from his pages reinforced the disparaging remarks about degenerate native populations so often made by nineteenth- and early twentieth-century colonial administrators and physicians.[50]

Hutchinson took a similar line, blaming the spread of leprosy on poor diet, particularly an excessive consumption of salt fish. He even attacked the redoubtable Robert Koch at Berlin in 1897 and again in 1906 for supporting 'the confuted fallacy' of medieval isolation. This, he claimed, was 'conceivable only in a partisan willing to avail himself of anything which may seem to give support to his theory, or . . . who has never studied the facts and bases his assertions on mere hearsay'.[51] Assembling a mass of evidence from medieval sources in support of his argument, he bewailed the fact that 'the popular imagination is occupied by stories, in prose and poetry, of the outcast leper and of the fearful ceremonies by which he was compelled to renounce the world'.[52] Hutchinson's early research on the connection between diet and leprosy was used by Charles Creighton, another sceptic, who believed that claims regarding the incidence of the disease in medieval England had been consistently and grossly exaggerated. 'The village leper may have been about as common as the village fool', he observed in the first volume of his *History of Epidemics in Britain* (1894), a work notable for its antagonism towards the 'bacteriological bugbear'.[53] He was, however, fighting a losing battle. By the 1920s the orthodoxy was so entrenched that members of the North Nyasa Native Association listened 'with heartfelt awe' as an African hospital assistant explained how effective strict segregation had proved in medieval Britain.[54]

For the residents of United States Marine Hospital Number Sixty-Six, at Carville, Louisiana, 'an enforced isolation which harks back to the Middle Ages' was more than a matter of antiquarian or medical interest.[55] Converted into

49  G. Newman, *On the History of the Decline and Final Extinction of Leprosy as an Endemic Disease in the British Isles* (London, 1895), pp. 66, 70–79, 84–5. The contagionist, W. Munro, *Leprosy* (Manchester, 1879), p. 25, conceded that diet was a crucial factor in lowering or boosting resistance, but was far more bullish about conditions in medieval England. His conviction that its nascent democrats had led the way in exterminating the disease through a combination of strict segregation and innate superiority offers a paradigm of Whiggishness.

50  See, for example, Z. Gussow and G.S. Tracy, 'Stigma and the Leprosy Phenomenon', *BHM*, xliv (1970), pp. 425–49; and Z. Gussow, *Leprosy, Racism and Public Health: Social Policy and Chronic Disease Control* (Boulder, Colorado, 1989).

51  Hutchinson, *Leprosy and Fish-Eating*, p. 280. Although on the conservative wing of the profession, Hutchinson maintained a lively and well-informed interest in the scientific developments of the period: Worboys, *Spreading Germs*, pp. 100–02.

52  Hutchinson, *On Leprosy*, p. 282.

53  Creighton, *History of Epidemics in Britain*, i, pp. 8–14, and chapter two, passim.

54  M. Vaughan, *Curing their Ills: Colonial Power and African Illness* (Oxford, 1991), p. 88.

55  *The Star*, iii, no. 10 (15 October 1933). I am most grateful to Mr Tony Gould for providing me with copies of this journal.

America's national *leprosarium* in 1916–17, when concerns about racial purity and degeneration were at their height, Carville was initially run more as a penal colony than a hospital.[56] Its crusading journal, *The Star*, campaigned tirelessly to lift the stigma associated with leprosy, running, in 1934, a trenchant exchange on the nature and purpose of medieval rites of exclusion. 'Such shocking scenes were common occurances [*sic*] during the Dark Ages', wrote one correspondent, 'but this is the twentieth century [and] still we have not materially changed our attitude toward the leper'. The debate culminated in a bitter and highly controversial attack by the editor, Stanley Stein, upon those missionaries who were still influenced by practices current in 'the darkest period of human history'. 'We are', he maintained, 'still outcasts in their minds, and they still continue to hold the Leper Mass over us, though in a somewhat modified form.'[57] Stein's battle against 'Dark Age ignorance' became justifiably famous, thereby perpetuating an even bleaker view of medieval responses to the disease among those authors who have studied its more recent history.[58]

It was, then, the victorious contagionists who not only created a model of leprosy as a dangerously communicable disease, but also to a notable extent constructed its history. George Orwell's often quoted observation that 'who controls the past controls the future: who controls the present controls the past' applies as much to medicine as to politics.[59] For it is this history, with its emphasis on terror, isolation and repression, which has in so many quarters been accepted at face value, without further qualification or sense of context. However much they may have resisted demands for forcible segregation, few liberals followed Newman, Hutchinson and Creighton in questioning the medieval precedents advanced by their opponents. Writing in 1887 to the Turkish leprologist, D.A. Zambaco, one British physician expressed concern that 'the exaggeration of the theory of contagion is destined to do more harm than good, and can only lead to a return to the ideas of olden days, which condemned lepers to tortures as horrible as the disease itself'.[60] Over a century later, Suzanne Saunders voiced identical sentiments in a robust attack on British responses to leprosy among the aboriginal population of Australia. These, she claimed, were 'largely based on a tradition which had evolved in the medieval world of Western Europe and . . . came to be associated with ostracism, degeneration and criminality'.[61] According to Zachary Gussow, the creation of colonial *leprosaria* sent the disease 'stumbling backwards to the Middle Ages', when 'ancient ideas

---

56  Gussow, *Leprosy, Racism and Public Health*, pp. 15, 131–60.
57  *The Star*, iv, nos 2 (July 1934), 3 (August 1934), 4 (September – October 1934).
58  This reaches its apogee in Sheldon Watts' contention that medieval leprosy was the 'construct' of an insecure ecclesiastical and political elite, which used it as a 'felicitous way' of removing deviants, such as Jews and witches, from society: *Epidemics and History: Disease, Power and Imperialism* (Yale, 1997), pp. 40–83.
59  G. Orwell, *1984: A Novel* (London, 1949), p. 199.
60  Zambaco, *Anthologie*, p. 623. Shortly before this date, the German physician, Eduard Arning, attacked forcible segregation as 'a remnant of medieval barbarism which every professional man ought to oppose': T. Gould, *Don't Fence Me In: From Curse to Cure, Leprosy in Modern Times* (London, 2005), p. 80.
61  S. Saunders, *'A Suitable Island Site': Leprosy in the Northern Territory and the Channel Island Leprosarium 1880–1955* (Darwin, 1989), pp. 1, 58.

of extrusion and asylum' had emerged from a world 'of myths and superstitions' in which 'lepraphobia was institutionalised and incorporated into a host of social and political practices, most of which became ritualistic'.[62] Since just such a picture had, meanwhile, been perpetuated by scholars as influential as Michel Foucault,[63] Mary Douglas[64] and R.I. Moore,[65] its tenacity is hardly surprising. Should we be as sceptical of claims about widespread segregation and ostracism as we ought to be about the 'Leper Mass'?

We may certainly disregard suggestions that medieval *leprosaria* were designed to act as secure units or detention centres, such as those demanded by nineteenth-century contagionists.[66] On the contrary, like most other medieval hospitals and *maisons Dieu*, the larger, earlier houses in particular followed a monastic model, which required voluntary profession, sometimes after a proba-tionary period, on the part of lay brothers and sisters. Those who failed to conform faced eviction.[67] As we have already seen, if they are able to keep reasonably clean and are well nourished, sufferers from Hansen's disease can often survive for years, if not decades, without more sophisticated medical treat-ment. So too can the victims of other disfiguring, but not necessarily terminal, skin conditions. Since they were residents rather than short-stay patients, the men and women who entered such institutions occupied a similar position to the *conversi* who staffed general hospitals for the sick poor or to the elderly and disabled bedesmen of some later medieval almshouses. Most of these people swore oaths of poverty, chastity and obedience, wore a distinctive habit and were bound to a life regulated by prayer and strict religious observance.[68] To a greater or lesser extent they, too, were 'dead to the world', in so far that, like monks or nuns, they had pledged themselves to God.[69] That cloistered lepers were widely held to constitute a type of religious order is, for example, apparent from the

---

62   Gussow, *Leprosy, Racism and Public Health*, pp. 11, 155.
63   M. Foucault, *Madness and Civilisation: A History of Insanity in the Age of Reason* (London, 1971), pp. 1–7.
64   M. Douglas, 'Witchcraft and Leprosy: Two Strategies of Exclusion', *Man*, new series, xxvi (1991), pp. 723–6. Douglas derived her views on medieval leprosy from M.G. Pegg, 'Le corps et l'autorité: La lèpre de Baudouin IV', *Annales*, xlv (1990), pp. 265–87, who argues that the late twelfth century was marked by a draconian policy of ritualised segregation designed to protect the integrity of the social body. The article is notable for its reliance upon authors such as Brody, Clay and Richards.
65   R.I. Moore, *The Formation of a Persecuting Society* (Oxford, 1987), regards lepers as a group subject, like Jews, heretics and other undesirables, to collective isolation and repression from the eleventh century onwards.
66   For example, J.N. Hays, *The Burdens of Disease: Epidemics and Human Response in Western History* (New Brunswick, NJ, and London, 1998), pp. 23–5, describes the 'awful ritual' of the Leper Mass, observing that medieval *leprosaria* were 'prisons for people declared legally dead'.
67   See chapter seven, below.
68   Touati, *Maladie et société*, pp. 409–13; F. Bériac, 'Les fraternités des lépreux et lépreuses', in K. Elm and M. Parisse, eds, *Doppelklöster und andere Formen der Symbiose männlicher und weiblicher Religiosen in Mittelalter* (Berlin, 1992), pp. 203–11. For English examples of hospital regulations as strict, or stricter, than those of any *leprosarium*, see J.A.A. Goodall, *God's House at Ewelme* (Aldershot, 2001), Appendix 1; C. Rawcliffe, *Medicine for the Soul: The Life, Death and Resurrection of an English Medieval Hospital* (Stroud, 1999), pp. 29–33, 241–8; and W.H. Stevenson, ed., *Records of the Borough of Nottingham I* (Nottingham, 1882), pp. 29–33.
69   As the great English jurist, Bracton, ruled, men and women who gave themselves to religion were the 'civil dead' and had renounced the world for ever: S.E. Thorne, ed., *Bracton on the Laws and Customs of England* (4 vols, Cambridge, Mass., 1968–77), iv, p. 310.

Welsh laws of Hywel Dda (preserved from 1200) and the early thirteenth-century *Liber poenitentialis* of Robert of Flamborough, which grouped them alongside Hospitallers and Templars.[70]

It is also worth stressing at this point that rituals involving funerary practices, even the burial place itself, were by no means uncommon in medieval religious life. The twelfth-century female recluse was advised 'to scrape up earth every day out of the grave in which [she] shall rot. God knows, the sight of her grave near her does many an anchoress much good . . . She keeps her death as it were before her eyes, her open grave reminding her of it.'[71] A general reluctance on the part of medical and social historians to set the medieval leper in this broader religious *milieu* has clearly fostered exaggerated beliefs about segregation and exclusion, while also obscuring some important changes in responses to the disease.[72] The men and women who found refuge in institutions supervised by late medieval urban authorities were rarely bound by oaths of profession, and therefore enjoyed the same legal rights as any other member of the community.[73] This aspect of the disease's history was, however, of little interest to the evangelical missionaries of Victorian England, who preferred to envisage a world of abandoned outcasts and heroic saints.

## 'Outside the camp': the missionary model

For Stanley Stein and the other residents at Carville, the 'Leper Mass' was symbolic of a far wider problem. They were angered by the Church's failure to detach itself from a heavy freight of biblical and medieval symbolism, which marked them out as victims of a disease apart. Doubts had already been voiced regarding the identification of Old Testament 'leprosy' with Hansen's disease, although Christian missionaries persistently invoked the image of the 'unclean' leper, expelled from human society by Mosaic law and subsequently condemned to a life beyond the pale.[74] 'While it is true that there are many Good Samaritans among the religious faiths', Stein conceded,

> There is no effort made to put us on equality with those suffering from other diseases much more contagious than our own . . . if the Church would be as

---

70 Cule, 'Diagnosis, Care and Treatment', p. 38 (see also p. 41, where lepers, monks and the blind are classed together); Robert of Flamborough, *Liber poenitentialis: A Critical Edition with Introduction and Notes*, ed., J.J.F. Firth (Toronto, Pontifical Institute of Mediaeval Studies, xviii, 1971), pp. 150–51: 'Personas religiosas voco non solum monachos et canonicos, sed etiam templarios, hospitalarios, *leprosos qui sunt de congregationibus* (de vagis enim non loquor) et illos qui se domibus Dei dederunt et similes.' Significantly, vagrant lepers are exempted from this group.

71 M.B. Salu, ed. and trans, *The Ancrene Riwle* (London, 1955, reprinted Exeter, 1990), pp. 51–2.

72 See A. Uyttebrouck, 'Sequestration ou retraite volontaire? Quelques réflexions à propos de l'hérbergement des lépreux à la léproserie de Terbank-lez-Louvain', in *Mélanges offerts à G. Jacquemyns* (Brussels, 1968), pp. 615–32, notably p. 630, for further confirmation of this point.

73 See pp. 272–3, below.

74 As late as 1970, the medical missionary, S.G. Browne, felt that 'in the providence of God, serious mistranslations of words in the original Scriptures can be overruled, and even the misidentification of biblical "leprosy" has not been an unrelieved misfortune; in point of fact, it has inspired a tremendous volume of disinterested philanthropy': *Leprosy in the Bible* (Christian Medical Fellowship, London, third edn, 1979), p. 4. For Stanley Stein's remarkable career, see Gould, *Don't Fence Me In*, chapter ten; and for the mistranslation of Leviticus, below, pp. 72–8.

energetic in trying to remove the stigma which modern science has shown to be wholly unjustified as it was active during the Dark Ages in instituting fear and horror, leprosy would be rid of the odium that now surrounds it.[75]

Yet, as many recent authors have pointed out, missionary activity among lepers depended for its success, if not its very *raison d'être*, upon the active promotion of an image of ostracism, suffering and victimisation.[76] And in this respect the disease was, indeed, unique, being defined as much in *moral* as physiological terms.[77] Alone among the recipients of colonial medicine, its victims could be removed, voluntarily or by force, from their customary surroundings and subjected to an intensive programme of evangelisation. The female missionary who felt a call to nurse leprosy patients was advised in 1902 that 'she needs to be as skilled in dealing with sick souls as she is in relieving bodily pain'.[78] To a notable extent the leper asylum, with its emphasis upon healing through salvation, was portrayed as the direct successor of the medieval *leprosarium*, and its staff as 'Christian heroes' following in the steps of men such as St Francis of Assisi (d. 1226) and his acolytes.

The lurid propaganda deemed necessary to raise funds for overseas missions not only intensified fears of contagion at home, but also disseminated a monolithic view of historical as well as indigenous responses to leprosy. It certainly tended to misrepresent, or at best homogenise, the way many Asian and African communities had hitherto dealt with 'the leper problem'.[79] John Jackson, an evangelist and early historian of the Mission to Lepers, provides a typical example of this approach:

> In the long procession of ages there is no more truly tragic figure than that of the leper. Inspired both by traditional association and by natural horror, men have shrunk from him as a creature cut off from all the interests of healthy humanity. His cup is full to the brim of bitterness, and includes in it every ingredient of sorrow. Disease both loathsome and lifelong; expulsion alike from home and city; forfeiture of social and legal rights; all these, together with the consciousness that he is an outcast and that life holds for him no hope, combine to make the lot of the leper the very quintessence of misery and despair. Indeed, the very word has

---

75  *The Star*, iv, no. 3 (August 1934).
76  R.S. Kipp, 'The Evangelical Uses of Leprosy', *Social Science and Medicine*, xxxix (1994), pp. 165–78; Watts, *Epidemics and History*, pp. 72–8.
77  In the words of Gussow and Tracy, leprosy was 'thought of less as a disease than as a moral condition . . . colored by the status of the care-takers, the religious, not the physician': 'Stigma and the Leprosy Phenomenon', p. 446.
78  *The Church Missionary Gleaner*, 2 July 1902, cited by Gould, *Don't Fence Me In*, p. 135.
79  See, for instance, C.J. Dutton, *The Samaritans of Moloka'i* (London, 1934), pp. 10, 20–23. Many societies, such as the Hansa of Northern Nigeria, expressed few concerns about cases of leprosy in their midst until the arrival of Western medicine and missionaries: N.E. Waxler, 'Learning to be a Leper: A Case Study in the Social Construction of Illness', in E.G. Mishler, ed., *Social Contexts of Health, Illness and Patient Care* (Cambridge, 1981), pp. 169–93. British authorities in Madras were as appalled as late medieval magistrates by the freedom with which lepers went about their business, while French colonial officials on the Ivory Coast of West Africa complained that 'the mutilated continue to live in contact with all': Buckingham, *Leprosy in Colonial South India*, pp. 32–3; Silla, *People Are Not the Same*, pp. 96–7. A similar situation obtained in Ethiopia: R. Pankhurst, 'The History of Leprosy in Ethiopia to 1935', *Medical History*, xxviii (1984), pp. 57–72; and the Congo: Gould, *Don't Fence Me In*, p. 328.

become the synonym for all that is foul and repulsive. In all eyes and in all lands it has been the same.[80]

Charles Creighton wrote scathingly of the 'halo of morbid exaggeration' that had surrounded the disease in the twelfth and thirteenth centuries, but his remarks were no less applicable to his own age.[81] If the nineteenth-century bacteriologist had created a dangerously communicable disease, the missionary covered it with a glowing patina of evangelical piety. In the words of one such activist, recorded in 1920, lepers could be cured only by the Divine Physician at the moment of resurrection, 'when their poor bodies of humiliation shall be made like unto His glorious body and their sufferings, sorrows and sin will be remembered no more'.[82] As we shall see, these sentiments might have sprung just as readily from the lips of St Hugh of Lincoln (d. 1200) or Jacques de Vitry (d. 1240), although they, at least, regarded the disease as a mark of election, which gave the leper a distinct edge over the common run of sinners, condemned as *they* all were to the fires of hell or purgatory.[83]

Founded in 1874 by Wellesley C. Bailey and a group of friends in Dublin, the Mission to Lepers undertook the dual task of bringing spiritual and physical relief to men and women who had been conspicuously rejected by society. Following a moment of revelation virtually identical to that experienced by the youthful St Francis, Bailey embraced the 'Christ-like work' of spreading 'the consolation of the Gospel' among the most pitiful of Queen Victoria's subjects.[84] By the time of his retirement, in 1914, the Mission had grown far beyond the British Empire, and he was able to reflect, as the early Franciscans might have done, upon the *spiritual* healing his colleagues had accomplished:

> The marvellous contrast in the appearance and condition of those we saw outside our Homes and those inside, made a deep impression on us. On the one hand, starved, unkempt, unclothed, degraded and demoralised, their physical condition appalling; on the other, well fed, comfortably clothed, all their wants attended to, physical condition greatly improved, while they are daily and hourly hearing of the Blessed Saviour Who has done so much for them, *the despised and outcast of the world.*[85]

The death in 1889 of Father Damien had not only generated widespread fears of contagion, but also prompted a wave of charitable donations to further the work

---

[80] Jackson, *Lepers*, p. 1.

[81] Creighton, *A History of Epidemics in Britain*, i, p. 85. He believed that other diseases, such as pellagra, were being neglected because they offered fewer opportunities for ostentatious 'heroism and self-sacrifice': (ibid., p. 110).

[82] W.C. Irvine, 'Christian Teaching and Spiritual Work in Asylums', *Report of a Conference of Leper Asylum Superintendents and Others on the Leper Problem in India* (Calcutta, 1920), pp. 132–5, at p. 135. Such sentiments were voiced even more forcefully in Catholic countries: J. Bernabeu-Mestre and T. Ballester-Artigues, 'Disease as a Metaphorical Resource: The Fontilles Philanthropic Initiative in the Fight against Leprosy, 1901–1932', *SHM*, xvii (2004), pp. 409–21.

[83] See chapter two, below.

[84] A.D. Miller, *An Inn Called Welcome: The Story of the Mission to Lepers 1874–1917* (London, 1964), p. 11.

[85] Miller, *An Inn Called Welcome*, pp. 214–15. See ibid., pp. 40, 49, 103, 165, for similar reflections, and also P.A. Kalisch, 'Tracadie and Penikese Leprosaria: A Comparative Analysis of Societal Response to Leprosy in New Brunswick, 1844–1880', *BHM*, xlvii (1973), pp. 480–512, at p. 507.

of those men and women who were courageous enough to assume his mantle. From a modest £1,628 a year at the close of the 1890s, the Mission's gross receipts had risen to £11,298 by 1899, helped greatly by the publication of a quarterly magazine appropriately entitled *Without the Camp*.[86] Nor was it the only British organisation to take up the cause. Soon after Damien's death, the National Leprosy Fund was established under the sponsorship of the Prince of Wales, and in turn gave rise to the Indian Leprosy Commission. The latter, it is worth noting, dissented from several leading members of the parent body by opposing compulsory segregation.[87]

Among the flurry of publications to appear at this time, George Thin's influential *Leprosy* provided bemused members of the English medical profession with a concise summary of the current state of knowledge and debate. A convinced and eloquent segregationist, Thin acknowledged that the modern missionary, like his medieval predecessor, belonged to a very special breed. During the European Middle Ages, he maintained,

> [Leprosy] had multiplied to such an extent as to have inspired the whole of Christendom with horror and fear. The disgust and terror which it evoked roused the whole populations of these parts to drive the unfortunate lepers from their midst. The genius of Christianity, fortunately, was true to itself, and tempered this act by providing 'lazar houses' for the reception of the unfortunate outcasts. The leper everywhere was met with the cry of 'unclean' and to touch him was considered an act which only supernatural faith could inspire.[88]

That work among lepers represented a unique calling, which brought both the patient and the carer closer to God, was an assumption fostered by missionaries of all nationalities and religious persuasions. It was also portrayed as a particular challenge, or quest, akin to that of the medieval knight errant. Generally – and perhaps justifiably – forgotten now, the work of the American poet, J.R. Lowell, enjoyed considerable popularity in England after the publication of his collected works in 1879. Although it had been written some thirty years earlier, his tale of the chivalrous Sir Launfal, who encounters a leper at the gate of his castle as he sets out in search of the Holy Grail, expressed these sentiments to perfection. Like St Francis, the young man initially recoils in horror at the spectacle before him:

> And a loathing over Sir Launfal came;
> The sunshine went out of his soul with a thrill,
> The flesh 'neath his armour 'gan shrink and crawl,
> And midway its leap his heart stood still
> Like a frozen waterfall;
> For this man, so foul and bent of stature,

---

86  Miller, *An Inn Called Welcome*, pp. 55, 71.
87  Gussow, *Leprosy, Racism and Public Health*, pp. 106–7. It is interesting (but hardly surprising) to note that this upsurge in charitable activity generated a less creditable fear that England would be swamped by leprous asylum seekers, attracted by the prospect of 'comfortable quarters and Royal patronage': *The Lancet*, cxxxv, issue 3481 (17 May 1890), pp. 1064–5.
88  Thin, *Leprosy*, p. 42.

Rasped hard against his dainty nature,
And seemed the one blot on the summer morn –
So he tossed him a piece of gold in scorn.[89]

Eventually after many bitter experiences, he comes to realise, as Francis had done, that the leper, 'lank as the rain-blanched bone' is in fact Christ's representative on earth, and that the Grail resides within the soul of anyone prepared to embrace him. Committed to memory by thousands of Victorian and Edwardian children (including the present writer's own grandmother, who could still recite them with considerable *brio* at the age of eighty), these verses, and many others like them, further consolidated the image of a disease apart.

The rediscovery, or more accurately the reinvention, of St Francis of Assisi during the nineteenth century saw his transformation into a nature-loving exemplar of chivalric virtue, whose appeal transcended denominational boundaries.[90] Margaret Oliphant's popular biography of 1868, which circulated in the Sunday Library of Household Reading, must have inspired many future missionaries. She describes how 'the determination to overcome himself, which is the first duty of the Christian knight', prompted his supreme act of humility. He elected to work among lepers.[91] Commending Francis's 'sincere and practical attempts to realise the kingdom of God on earth', the French Protestant, Paul Sabatier (1894), spoke even more directly to the Wellesley Baileys of Victorian England. Surrounded by a chorus of adoring lepers 'blinded by love', the muscular Christian who emerges from his pages offered a powerful role model to men and women with a religious calling.[92] At the same time, the Abbé Le Monnier introduced English readers to St Francis as political activist and liberator, 'who powerfully ameliorated the condition of the people' in his quest for social reform.[93] This was heady stuff.

Even before his death, Father Damien commanded widespread respect in England as a latter day St Francis. Indeed, among the many tokens of esteem sent to Moloka'i by English admirers was a watercolour of the Saint in ecstasy, which Edward Burne-Jones had painted especially for him.[94] Given that the stigmata Francis received on this occasion are now regarded as early symptoms of Hansen's disease, the gift seems especially poignant.[95] The celebrated press campaign fought in 1890 by Robert Louis Stevenson to clear Damien's name of various posthumous slurs contributed further to an emergent cult. With such an eloquent propagandist to fight his corner, it is hardly surprising that 'this plain,

---

[89] W.M. Rossetti, ed., *The Poetical Works of James Russell Lowell* (London, 1879), pp. 182–91, quotation at p. 186.

[90] A. Cunningham, 'Science and Religion in the Thirteenth Century Revisited: The Making of St Francis the Proto-Ecologist', *Studies in the History and Philosophy of Science*, xxxi (2000), pp. 613–43; xxxii (2001), pp. 69–98. I am most grateful to Dr Cunningham for drawing my attention to this topic.

[91] Mrs [M.] Oliphant, *St Francis of Assisi* (London, 1868), pp. 16–17.

[92] P. Sabatier, *Life of St Francis of Assisi* (London, 1941), pp. 27, 64, 144. The book was translated in 1894.

[93] L. Le Monnier, *History of St Francis of Assisi* (London, 1894), pp. 53–5.

[94] E. Clifford, *Father Damien: A Journey from Cashmere to His Home in Hawaii* (London, 1889), p. 57.

[95] J. Schatzlein and D.P. Sulmasy, 'The Diagnosis of St Francis: Evidence for Leprosy', *Franciscan Studies*, xlvii (1987), pp. 181–217. Damien described himself as being marked with the cross of leprosy, 'with which our Divine Saviour has permitted me to be stigmatised': Gould, *Don't Fence Me In*, pp. 84–5.

noble human brother and father of ours' became a focus of media attention.[96] Commenting adversely upon the indifference to *spiritual* welfare shown by government relief agencies, Anthony Weymouth reflected that it had taken 'the example of one man – cast in the mould of the medieval saints' to achieve a modern miracle.[97] Sanctity and leprosy now became so closely connected that by the close of the nineteenth century the disease seemed to have retreated even further into a remote medieval landscape populated by holy men and disfigured pariahs. An appropriate template was soon constructed. In his account of the 'self-sacrificing effort' of one Lutheran pastor in Bengal, for instance, John Jackson reported that

> This good man dressed the sores of lepers with his own hands (though his doctor's degree was not that of medicine but philosophy), mended their clothes, and even carried them to their graves. No wonder they regarded him as a saint and scarcely stopped short of worshipping him, and it is particularly certain that, had he only died among them, his grave would have become a shrine, so deep was their gratitude and affection . . .[98]

His evocation of the Seven Comfortable Works performed by a humble layman without formal medical training tapped into a long tradition of homiletic literature, eagerly transmitted in Sunday Schools and missions throughout Britain. Tales of medieval men and women who had surrendered their lives to the poor of Christ had considerably more grounding in historical fact than recitations of the 'Leper Mass'. But they did little to soften the relentlessly negative image of a disease that, to all appearances, had always occupied a place on the furthest margins of Christian society.[99]

### 'Leprosies of sin': the literary model

Tennyson and Lowell were not alone in drawing inspiration from such an apparently unpromising source. Growing levels of concern about the perceived dangers of leprosy, as well as a slew of publications describing its physical symptoms and history, inevitably attracted the interest of poets and novelists. The deployment of the disease (usually in its most extreme form) as a metaphor for decay and degeneration was hardly new, but the proliferation of this image during the nineteenth century moved at a striking pace. *The Rime of the Ancient Mariner* (1797) contains a brief but chilling description of 'the nightmare LIFE-IN-DEATH', whose skin appears 'as white as leprosy' as she sails towards the hero across a 'slimy sea'.[100] Coleridge is here drawing upon the language of

---

[96]   'Letter to Dr Hyde', *The Works of Robert Louis Stevenson: Pentland Edition XV* (London, 1907), pp. 350–66, quotation at p. 360; Mobolo, 'Blessed Damien', pp. 702–5.

[97]   Weymouth, *Through the Leper-Squint*, pp. 109–10, and chapter thirteen, passim. In the revised (London, 1889) edition of his *Leprosy: A Communicable Disease*, which was reprinted after Damien's death, C.N. Macnamara made an made an equally unfavourable comparison between the 'richly endowed leper asylums' of medieval Europe and the meagre provision then available in India (ibid, p. 53).

[98]   Jackson, *Lepers*, p. 119.

[99]   See, for example, J. Farrow, *Damien the Leper* (New York, 1937), pp. 89–93.

[100]  Samuel Taylor Coleridge, *The Rime of the Ancient Mariner*, ed. P.H. Fry (Boston, Mass., 1999), p. 43.

the Old Testament, whereas later generations of authors were remorseless in their use of newly published clinical detail. The American general Lewis Wallace quoted these lines at the start of book six of *Ben-Hur: A Tale of the Time of Our Lord* (1880), which rapidly became an international bestseller. His account of the appalling fate of the hero's mother and sister, left to rot in the squalor of a remote colony, did much to reinforce a biblical stereotype of the outcast leper and, indirectly, to support the heroic work of Christian missionaries.

In the interim, readers with a taste for French literature could contemplate even grimmer images of physical decay in the pages of Gustave Flaubert's *Salammbô* (1862). Hannon, the leprous Suffete, whose disease symbolises the collapse of the Carthaginian Empire (as well as much that Flaubert found deplorable in contemporary France), seems to decompose before our eyes. In a novel replete with the imagery of death and corruption, his putrefying flesh, minutely described, conveys an overwhelming sense of physical and spiritual collapse. Even Flaubert's friends found such passages disturbing, while some critics professed nausea.[101] Yet despite – or perhaps because – of the allegations made against it, the book sold well; and, notwithstanding cavils in certain quarters, was generally regarded as an accurate historical record. The author, who prided himself on his meticulous research, was contemptuous of the article on leprosy he had consulted in the *Dictionnaire des sciences médicinales*, preferring to rely upon his own observation of the disease in North Africa.[102] The lasting impression it made upon him is apparent from his unsparing depiction of another, very different, leper in *La légende de Saint Julien l'Hospitalier* (1877). This tale of the penitent medieval hermit, who accidentally murders his parents, ends in an encounter between Julien and a hideously deformed traveller. Overcoming the nausea engendered by his foul breath and repugnant appearance, Julien not only feeds and warms the leper, but folds his freezing body naked in his arms, 'mouth against mouth, breast against breast'. His remarkable compassion receives its due reward, as, duly absolved and forgiven, he is transported ecstatically to heaven in Christ's passionate embrace. A recurring theme in medieval hagiography, the encounter between saint and *Christus quasi leprosus* here assumes an erotic power absent from its precursors. Illustrated editions, such as that produced by L.O. Merson in 1895, left little to the imagination.[103]

The Victorian moralist, Robert Williams Buchanan, almost certainly had Flaubert in his sights when he began campaigning against the miasmic pollution spread by decadent French literature. Perhaps the 'steaming viper's brew' drunk by Hannon inspired him to warn against

The American poet, Nathaniel Parker Willis, likewise adopts the language of Leviticus in 'The Leper', *Complete Works* (3 vols, New York, 1846), iii, pp. 818–19, which describes Christ's encounter with an unclean outcast covered in 'white scales'.

101 A. Green, *Flaubert and the Historical Novel: Salammbô Reassessed* (Cambridge, 1982), pp. 26, 53–4, 60, 63, 125.

102 *Oeuvres complètes de Gustave Flaubert: Correspondance: cinquième série, 1862–1868* (Paris, 1929), p. 58, Flaubert to Sainte-Beuve, December 1862.

103 Gustave Flaubert, *La légend de Saint Julien l'Hospitalier illustrée de vingt-six compositions par L.O. Merson* (Paris, 1895). For medieval English versions of the tale, see A. Brandeis, ed., *Jacob's Well* (EETS, cxv, 1900), pp. 264–5.

> The snake that grovels
> In a host of scrofulous novels,
> Leper even of the leprous
> Race of serpents vain and viprous.[104]

As might be expected, Buchanan was no admirer of Algernon Swinburne, whom he condemned as 'morbid', 'sensual' and, significantly, 'unclean'.[105] The latter's early poem, *The Leper* (1866), which deals with the illicit, and eventually necrophiliac, passion nursed by a humble clerk for a medieval lady of high estate, reputedly prompted Tennyson to write his own, more sanitised (and by his lights optimistic) verses about the stricken crusader and his bride. Swinburne's depiction of a beautiful but promiscuous woman, cursed by God with leprosy and 'cast forth for a base thing' to starve certainly plays upon the familiar themes of sin, suffering and rejection.[106] Indeed, despite their obvious differences, the two poets each projected an image of medieval leprosy strikingly akin to that being advanced by the contagionist lobby.

Popular fiction warmed to the theme. The dramatic appearance of a blind and hooded leper in *The Black Arrow: A Tale of the Two Roses*, must have sent a *frisson* of horror down many young spines. First serialised in 1883, long before its author, Robert Louis Stevenson, made his famous trip to Moloka'i, the story involves a fearful encounter between the hero, his friend and the menacing stranger:

> He had been a tall man before he was bowed by his disgusting sickness, and even now he walked with a vigorous step. The dismal beating of his bell, the pattering of his stick, the eyeless screen before his countenance, and the knowledge that he was not only doomed to death and suffering, but shut out for ever from the touch of his fellow-men filled the lads' bosoms with dismay; and at every step that brought him nearer, their courage and strength seemed to desert them . . . Even Dick became dead-white and closed his eyes, as if by the mere sight he might become infected.[107]

Such, indeed, is the boys' terror, that one of them – admittedly a girl in disguise – faints at the approach of 'their horrible enemy'. In the event, it transpires that the dastardly Sir Daniel Brackley has dressed as a leper in order to escape his enemies, this being an infallible means of avoiding detection.

Although it is set in late eighteenth-century Italy rather than late medieval England, Xavier de Maistre's essay, *Le lépreux de la cité d'Aoste* (1811), also exercised a profound influence on generations of impressionable adolescents. This harrowing account of the experiences of a man condemned to a life of isolation, and of his painful struggle to accept his fate, figured from the late 1870s onwards

---

104   *The Complete Poetical Works of Robert Williams Buchanan* (London, 1901), p. 393.
105   P. Baker, *The Dedalus Book of Absinthe* (Sawtry, 2001), pp. 33–5.
106   *The Poems of Algernon Charles Swinburne, I, Poems and Ballads* (London, 1904), pp. 118–24. Swinburne must have been familiar with Robert Henryson's *Testament of Cresseid*, a late fifteenth-century poem, which develops the theme of lust and pride punished by leprosy and had been in print since 1593. Significantly, Denton Fox's introduction to the standard edition (London, 1968), pp. 39–40, cites Clay as an authority on rituals of exclusion and 'mock-burial'.
107   R.L. Stevenson, *The Black Arrow: A Tale of the Two Roses* (London, 1901 reprint), pp. 85–6.

as a text in the Cambridge local examinations. It rapidly ran through multiple cheap editions and 'cribs', in both French and English. 'My name is a terrible one', warns the anonymous hero, 'the world forgets my family name and the name religion gave me at my birth. I am *the Leper*'.[108] With its stress upon the virtues of Christian piety and resignation in the face of suffering,[109] the work repeated a message already familiar to readers of missionary literature, such as the journal, *Central Africa*:

> I spoke to [the lepers of Lundu] of the life hereafter, and told them that though their bodies were decaying, and though this life did not give them all they hoped for, yet each had a soul to be saved or lost, and that they must try and look forward to the better life beyond the grave, and not dwell too much on their present misfortunes.[110]

On balance, however, the picture of leprosy to emerge from the pages of nine-teenth- and early twentieth-century fiction was intended to shock rather than inspire or even moralise. That a disease so replete with symbolism would appeal to the *fin de siècle* imagination is hardly surprising. In *The Picture of Dorian Gray* (1890–91), for example, Oscar Wilde describes the 'leprosies of sin', slowly eating away at the telltale portrait concealed in the attic. It was, he observes, 'from within, apparently, that the foulness and horror had come . . . the rotting of a corpse in a watery grave was not so fearful'.[111]

A fervent admirer of both Wilde and Stevenson, the French symbolist, Marcel Schwob, drew upon poetry and myth – as well as his own fertile imagination – to create a medieval panorama of outcasts and pariahs. One of his most successful short stories, *Le roi au masque d'or* (1892), tells of a masked king, who, like his ancestors, is leprous. Knowledge of his affliction comes upon him suddenly, on his first expedition from the royal palace. The terrified response of a girl who sees his real face prompts him to look at his reflection in the water of a nearby river. Here, in the dusk, he sees 'a blanched face, tumerous, covered in scales, the skin distended by hideous swellings', and immediately realises the truth.[112] Determined to punish himself for living a lie and for being so defiled, he puts out his own eyes with the clasps of the mask, and staggers off into the night. On the road to 'the city of the wretched' he encounters a kindly young woman, but dies before they arrive. She conceals from him that she, too, is leprous, while he remains unaware that 'the blood from his heart which gushed from his eyes' has cleansed his diseased flesh of all impurity. As a parable on the themes of self-deception, identity and the elusive search for inner knowledge, the tale treats leprosy as yet another mask to be acquired or shed on life's journey. But its

---

108 Kelly's Keys to the Classics, *La jeune Sibérienne et le lépreux de la cité d'Aoste: A Literal Translation from the French* (London, 1886), p. 95.

109 See C.M. Lombard, *Xavier de Maistre* (Boston, Mass., 1977), pp. 71–80, for a discussion of these themes.

110 A.G. de La P[ryme], 'Lundu, the Leper Isle', *Central Africa*, xxvii (1909), p. 214.

111 Oscar Wilde, *The Picture of Dorian Gray*, ed. D.L. Lawler (London, 1988), p. 262.

112 Marcel Schwob, *Le roi au masque d'or, vies imaginaires, la croisade des enfants* (Paris, 1979), p. 50. Shades of the masked and leprous king may be found in Umberto Eco's *Baudolino* (London, 2002), p. 404.

power, of course, lies in the macabre fascination that the disease held for nineteenth-century readers. No other would have produced such an effect. Having, in the meantime, written an introduction to the illustrated edition of Flaubert's *Saint Julien*, Schwob returned to the medieval leper four years later in *Le croisade des enfants*, in which he portrays a tormented figure, 'enclosed on earth in pale damnation'.[113] Rejected, isolated and abandoned by God, he lurks by the roadside intent on 'sucking innocent blood at the throat' from passing children. Sure enough, a young crusader falls into his hands, but since he shows no fear of the disease or loathing for his captor he is allowed to go free. As we shall see in chapter five, many medieval legends explored the theme of human blood as a cure for leprosy, but none enshrine a vampiric creature to rival Schwob's, or suggest that wandering lepers preyed on human flesh. This is a work of pure fantasy.

It was only a matter of time before leprosy – like that other taboo subject, syphilis – would become the theme of a play in its own right. In 1896, fifteen years after the appearance of *Ghosts* (which *The Daily Telegraph* described as 'an open drain; a loathsome sore unbandaged; a dirty act done publicly; a lazar house with all its doors and windows open'), a Parisian theatre staged *La lépreuse* by Henri Bataille. Reputedly based upon a medieval Breton legend, the story tells of an impressionable young man who falls in love with the child of lepers, and is deliberately infected with the disease by the girl and her evil mother. Bataille was no Ibsen, and in places his melodrama lurches uncomfortably towards *Grand Guignol*. Yet at the time it caused a scandal, and was rarely performed after its first outing. Subsequent attempts to turn the 'tragic legend' into grand opera (eventually renamed *L'ensorcelé*) rendered it no more acceptable to the sensibilities of the French bourgeoisie, even though the score by the appropriately named Wagnerite, Joseph Sylvio Lazzari (d. 1944), is commonly regarded as his finest work.[114] Bataille's portrayal of leprosy as a highly contagious disease, which struck terror into whole medieval communities, was not, however, called into question; and it offers the modern reader a remarkable insight into the extent to which the medical opinions discussed in this chapter had become fused with historical myth. 'With a drop of blood from this little finger I can kill a hundred, I can kill a thousand', proclaims the girl, who has been infected through her mother's milk.[115] The theme of contaminated blood, with which Ernest Jeanselme, A.S. Ashmead, A.P. Wright and so many others were then preoccupied, dominates the play until its predictable climax. The final scene of the opera, with its tolling bells, requiem Mass and solemn procession of priests and villagers as the hero and his penitent nemesis are led away from an open grave to endure their living death in a distant leper colony, does, indeed,

---

113 Schwob, *Le roi au masque d'or, vies imaginaires, la croisade des enfants*, p. 293.
114 K. Grön, 'Leprosy in Literature and Art', *International Journal of Leprosy*, xli (1973), pp. 249–83, at pp. 250–52, misidentifies the composer, whose biography appears in S. Sadie, ed., *The New Grove Dictionary of Music and Musicians* (29 vols, London, 2001), xiv, pp. 415–16. A full orchestral score and a reduction for voice and piano were published by Max Eschig (Paris, 1912).
115 Henry Bataille, *Ton sang précédé de la lépreuse* (Paris, 1898), pp. 57–8. Significantly, *Ton Sang*, the companion play, was also about corruption or weakness of the blood.

suggest distant echoes of *Parsifal*, and bears, as we have seen, no closer relation to fact.

## Consolidating the myth

When reflecting on the nature and relative objectivity of historical research, E.H. Carr observed that 'our picture has been pre-selected and pre-determined for us, not so much by accident as by people who were consciously or unconsciously imbued with a particular view and thought the facts which supported that view worth preserving'.[116] In the case of medieval leprosy, the process has proved less a matter of selection than invention – or at least serious distortion. Neither the 'Leper Mass' nor the writ of exclusion, for example, were absolute fictions, although the process of repetition, elaboration and misquotation which has transformed them into planks of a national policy of segregation seems at times to resemble an academic game of Chinese whispers. It would, moreover, be wrong to regard the medical writers, novelists and missionaries of the nineteenth and early twentieth centuries as the worst culprits. Later generations of scholars have, in many respects, compounded the problem by accepting so much ill-documented supposition at face value.

S.N. Brody, whose study of leprosy in medieval literature, *The Disease of the Soul*, has become a principal source for medical and social historians, anthropologists and archaeologists since its appearance in 1974, presents a consistently bleak and intermittently censorious account of responses to the disease.[117] He subscribes uncritically, for example, to the belief that English lepers were burnt at the stake, citing as his source a particularly purple passage from *Eleven Blue Men and other Narratives of Medical Detection* by the writer of popular medical journalism, Berton Roueché. The lines in question are worth quoting *in extenso*:

> Several highly placed lepraphobes, including Henry II of England, his great-grandson Edward I, and Philip V of France, took the position that the recommended ritual was unnecessarily symbolical. The revisions instituted by Henry and Philip were similar. Both chose to replace the religious service with a simple civil ceremony. It consisted of strapping the leper to a post and setting him afire. Edward adhered a trifle more closely to the letter of the ecumenical decree. Lepers, during his reign, were permitted the comforts of a Christian funeral. They were led down to the cemetery and buried alive.[118]

It is easy to see how a fertile imagination might seize upon the many references to 'open graves' and 'mock-burial' which appear in discussions of the 'Leper

---

116  E.H. Carr, *What is History?* (London, 1961), p. 8.

117  Gussow, *Leprosy, Racism and Public Health*, p. 12, for instance, derives his view of medieval leprosy from Brody. The passage in question comes from Zappa's, *Unclean! Unclean!*, thereby perpetuating a circle of misinformation.

118  B. Roueché, 'A Lonely Road', in *Eleven Blue Men and other Narratives of Medical Detection* (New York, 1953), p. 117, cited in Brody, *Disease of the Soul*, p. 69. The story was reprinted for British readers in Roueché, *Annals of Medical Detection* (London, 1954), pp. 131–49. The quotation is on p. 140, and follows a lengthy description of the 'Leper Mass'. Medical journalism demonstrates a predictably morbid fascination with leprosy and its presumed medieval history. See, for example, R. Wilkins, *The Fireside Book of Deadly Diseases* (London, 1994), pp. 87–91.

Mass' and project them even further into the realms of fantasy. The origins of the myth about immolation pose more of a challenge. Although neither Henry II nor King Edward can, by any stretch of the imagination, be described as compassionate men, each took seriously his public responsibilities as a Christian monarch, not least towards the leprous poor. Three possible explanations of this *reductio ad absurdum* suggest themselves, providing yet more examples of the manipulation and abuse of historical sources.

In his *History of Epidemics in England*, Charles Creighton describes an ordi-nance of Henry II that made the importation of illicit religious texts into England a capital offence. Lepers in breach of the decree were allegedly to be burnt, and otherwise healthy laymen hung. He offers no supporting evidence for this statement, but suggests that the 'lepers' in question were, in fact, vagrants.[119] His source probably derives from a couple of campaigning articles written in 1884 for *The Nineteenth Century* by Agnes Lambert. A convinced segregationist, with a predictable interest in the Middle Ages, her admiration for the medieval Church went hand in hand with a desire to dispel 'the dark clouds of leprosy' then louring over Europe.[120] She was also anxious to record all the curbs histori-cally placed upon the movement of infected persons. Citing Lord Lyttelton's *History of the Life of King Henry the Second* (1769–73), she notes that fear of a papal interdict had driven the king to threaten any leper found carrying docu-ments from Rome with the stake.[121] Lyttelton derived his evidence from an anonymous letter to Thomas Becket, the cause of all the trouble, reporting these and other draconian measures as if they had already been put into effect. Dating from October 1169 (not 1166 as he supposed), the letter actually presents an unreliable – perhaps deliberately exaggerated – account of Henry's additions to the Constitutions of Clarendon. None of the independent contemporary sources that describe these new penalties in greater detail mention lepers at all, merely observing that anyone who brought suspect material into the realm would be punished as a traitor.[122]

The finger of unjustified suspicion points at Henry from another direction, too. A few years earlier he had taken firm action against a group of foreign here-tics, who were branded, flogged and left to die in the cold outside the walls of Oxford. The chronicler, William of Newburgh, our principal source for the inci-dent, describes their beliefs as a pestilential disease. This was a common meta-phor among theologians, who, as we shall see, often compared heretic preachers to a *spiritual* cancer or leprosy, gnawing at the soul of the body politic.[123] Appro-

---

119 Creighton, *History of Epidemics in England*, i, pp. 77–8.
120 A. Lambert, 'Leprosy Past and Present: I Present', *The Nineteenth Century*, xc (August 1884), pp. 210–27, quotation at p. 212.
121 A. Lambert, 'Leprosy Past and Present: II Past', *The Nineteenth Century*, xc (September 1884), pp. 467–89. The letter is discussed and quoted in full in George, Lord Lyttelton, *The History of the Life of King Henry the Second* (6 vols, London, 1769–73), iv, pp. 137–8, 473. For a modern edition, see A.J. Duggan, ed., *The Correspondence of Thomas Becket, Archbishop of Canterbury, 1162–1170* (2 vols, Oxford, 2000), i, pp. 334–5.
122 M.D. Knowles, A.J. Duggan and C.N.L. Brooke, 'Henry II's Supplement to the Constitutions of Clar-endon', *EHR*, lxxxvii (1972), pp. 757–71.
123 P. Biller, 'William of Newburgh and the Cathar Mission to England', in D. Wood, ed., *Life and Death in the Northern Church c. 1100–c.1700* (Studies in Church History, Subsidia, xii, 1999), pp. 11–36;

priate prophylactic measures were introduced in the Assize of Clarendon of 1166, which ruled that the home (*domus*) of anyone who harboured a suspect would be demolished, removed outside the town or village and burnt.[124] The idea that buildings might be infected by the creeping contagion of heresy can be traced to a lengthy passage in Mosaic Law dealing with the destruction of 'leprous' dwellings [Leviticus 14, vv. 34–57].[125] Creighton quite possibly took Newburgh's rhetorical language at face value and assumed that any lepers associated with these unwelcome visitors were to be incinerated as well. He may also have had in mind a third royal directive, this time regarding the distribution of largesse by the king's almoner among the poor at coronations. During the thirteenth century, lepers mingled freely among the thousands of other supplicants for relief and were, inevitably, involved in the brawls that broke out on such occasions. In 1236, as a means of imposing order on an unruly rabble, any leper who struck another with a knife was threatened with the stake.[126] No evidence survives of anyone actually being condemned to death as a result of what would, of course, have been an act of treason if committed in the royal presence. It is, indeed, a long step from here to the belief that immolation was widely deployed as a sanitary measure to contain the disease.

Yet lepers *were* once consigned to the flames in significant numbers, and the brutal elimination of whole communities in parts of France during the early fourteenth century has clearly encouraged a mistaken belief that such practices were a recurrent feature of life in England, too. A fatal combination of royal avarice and regional factionalism led, in 1321, to the massacre of Jews and lepers in southern France, and the confiscation by Philip V of the considerable assets of many *leprosaria*.[127] Some historians have described this pogrom as symptomatic of the 'underlying hatred and resentment' towards lepers endemic throughout the European Middle Ages,[128] although it is important to stress that no such institutional victimisation ever occurred in England. Indeed, the Lanercost

D.C. Douglas and G.W. Greenaway, eds, *English Historical Documents, II, 1042–1189* (London, 1953), pp. 329–30.

124 W. Stubbs, ed., *Chronica Magistri Rogeri de Houedene* (4 vols, RS, 1868–71), ii, p. 252. Richards, *Medieval Leper*, p. 50, compares the so-called writ *de leproso amovendo* with that *de heretico comburendo*, introduced by parliamentary statute in the reign of Henry IV. There is no historical basis whatsoever for this analogy, which erroneously perpetuates the association between leprosy and the stake.

125 For the idea that heresy, far worse than leprosy, could linger in the *domus* for generations, see J. Duvernoy, ed., *Le registre d'inquisition de Jacques Fournier, évêque de Pamiers* (3 vols, Toulouse, 1965), ii, pp. 110–11.

126 H. Hall, ed., *The Red Book of the Exchequer* (3 vols, RS, 1897), ii, p. 759: 'ea die habet omnem jurisdictionem circa rixas et delicta pauperum et leprosorum; adeo quod si leprosus alium cultello percusserit, judicare eum ut comburatur'. See also, H. Johnstone, 'Poor Relief in the Royal Household of Thirteenth-Century England', *Speculum*, iv (1929), pp. 149–67, at p. 156.

127 M. Barber, 'Lepers, Jews and Moslems: The Plot to Overthrow Christendom in 1321', *History*, lxvi (1981), pp. 1–17, to which C. Ginzburg, *Ecstasies: Deciphering the Witches' Sabbath* (London, 1990), pp. 33–5, adds further sources. The most judicious reading of these events may be found in Touati, *Maladie et société*, chapter twelve, where the author traces a gradual hardening of attitudes back to the end of the thirteenth century.

128 Sheldon Watts, for instance, regards the pogrom of 1321 as 'the end product of a conjunction of abstractions' formulated from the eleventh century onwards: *Epidemics and History*, pp. 60–63. See also, M. Goodich, *Other Middle Ages: Witnesses at the Margins of Society* (Philadelphia, 1998), pp. 10–11, 110.

Chronicle describes these events as a distinctly continental phenomenon, which happened far away 'in nearly all parts over the sea (*in omnibus fere partibus transmarinis*) as far as Rome'.[129] Reparation was eventually made to some of the dispossessed, while churchmen, such as the bishop of Lausanne, expressed anxiety that 'innocent' lepers should be spared, and urged their congregations to continue giving alms as freely as before.[130] Sweeping generalisations irrespective of place and context have, however, become a hallmark of writing on the English medieval leper, which all too often consigns him or her to a limbo of 'otherness' or 'liminality' without any further qualification.

This is partly because of the impression made upon historians and archaeologists by anthropological research on rites of passage, such as that undertaken in the 1960s among the Ndembu of Zambia by Victor Turner. Such rites, according to Turner, entail a three-fold process of separation from the community, followed by a period of 'limen' (or transition) and either reintegration or irreparable breach. The experiences of medieval pilgrims and religious women have, for example, been reinterpreted in this light, which also casts its beam upon men and women entering *leprosaria*.[131] The concept of liminality can prove extremely helpful in furthering our understanding of the pre-modern hospital, although it is by no means always applicable to it.[132] Caution is certainly in order with regard to the 'Leper Mass', which seems, on the face of things, to offer a platonic expression of the exclusion ritual, whereby its chief protagonist moves, quite literally, from one world to another through the threshold, or *limen*, of his or her open grave. Not surprisingly, it has proved irresistible to anthropologists and sociologists, who have seen no reason to doubt its validity. The blanket equation of leprosy with marginality has been further reinforced over the last two decades by a growing interest on the part of social and cultural historians in men and women who appear deviant or 'transgressive'. It is thus still common to read of the 'ritual degradation' of the leper, 'driven from his home and buried to the neck in a grave'. Such procedures 'for making all lepers into social outcasts' were, we learn in one source, 'summarised in England under the Statute [*sic*] *De leproso amovendo*'.[133] That 'the leper' must inevitably have occupied a similar position to 'the prostitute', 'the witch', 'the heretic', 'the criminal' and 'the Jew'

129  J. Stevenson, ed., *Chronicon de Lanercost, 1272–1346* (Bannatyne Club, lxv, Edinburgh, 1839), p. 241. See also, Thomas Walsingham, *Ypodigma Neustriae*, ed. H.T. Riley (RS, 1876), p. 252.

130  Borradori, *Mourir au monde*, p. 85.

131  V. Turner, 'Betwixt and Between: The Liminal Period in Rites de Passage', in W.A. Lessa and E.Z. Vogt, eds, *Reader in Comparative Religion: An Anthropological Approach* (fourth edn, New York, 1979), pp. 234–43. See also, idem, *The Ritual Process: Structure and Anti-Structure* (Chicago, 1969), pp. 94–130; idem, *Dramas, Fields and Metaphors: Symbolic Action in Human Society* (Ithaca, 1974), pp. 231–71; idem, *Image and Pilgrimage in Christian Culture: Anthropological Perspectives* (New York, 1978), chapter one; idem, 'Social Dramas and Stories about Them', in W.J.T. Mitchell, ed., *On Narrative* (Chicago, 1981), pp. 137–64. Walker Bynum, *Fragmentation and Redemption*, pp. 27–51, offers a perceptive assessment of the value and limitations for medievalists of Turner's approach.

132  C. Rawcliffe, 'The Earthly and Spiritual Topography of Suburban Hospitals', in K. Giles and C. Dyer, eds, *Town and Country in the Middle Ages: Contrasts, Contacts and Interconnections* (Society for Medieval Archaeology, Monograph xxii, 2005), pp. 251–74.

133  M. Hepworth and B.S. Turner, *Confession: Studies in Deviance and Religion* (London, 1992), p. 25. The entry for 'leprosy' in K.F. Kiple, ed., *The Cambridge World History of Human Disease* (Cambridge, 1993), p. 838, reports – with a depressing disregard for syntax – that, during the high Middle Ages, 'considered "dead to society", last rites and services might be said in the leper's pres-

often seems to pass unquestioned. The arguments – and inventions – of nineteenth-century leprologists have thus found a secure place in mainstream historical writing.[134]

Leprosy was not the only 'medieval' disease to have been put under the microscope during the nineteenth and early twentieth centuries. In his recent study of the Black Death, Samuel Cohn blames 'the heavy hand of the Middle Ages on medicine in the halcyon years of microbiological investigation' for hampering research on 'modern' plague and its transmission.[135] As late as the 1920s, he argues, responses to contemporary epidemics were being framed according to an inappropriate medieval model, notwithstanding the many striking differences between the two. Historians, as well as scientists, made valiant efforts 'to square the circle', through the careful manipulation of irreconcilable evidence, thereby elevating modern plague into 'the dreadful scourge' which had haunted fourteenth-century Europe. Nineteenth-century writers on leprosy were even more cavalier with their source material, and they, too, warned of 'a global disaster',[136] whose menace they exaggerated out of all proportion to the risks it actually posed. Yet if, as Stanley Stein so rightly believed, victims of the disease were heirs to a poisoned legacy of stigmatisation and rejection, it was one richly embellished over the previous century, and the 'heavy hand' was as much that of the contagionist and missionary as of the medieval physician or cleric. Armed with a conviction that the West faced an epidemic of devastating proportions, leprologists needed ammunition to support a campaign for segregation and thus, to a notable extent, constructed a medieval leper to serve their purpose. As we shall see in the following chapters, leprosy did, indeed, inspire fear and loathing in medieval England. But it was also regarded as a mark of election, akin to a religious calling, and did not automatically lead either to segregation or vilification. There were, in fact, many leprosies: of bodies and souls, of saints and sinners, of men and metals, of animals and plants. There were tame lepers and wild lepers, rich and poor, cloistered and vagrant, potential and real. Even Christ was believed to have been *quasi leprosus*. Once free from 'the tyranny of modern medicine' and the desire to project our own scientific beliefs back into the past, we can begin to understand how medieval men and women grasped this perplexing diversity.[137] And it is with *their* ideas about causation that we should start.

---

ence, sometimes as the victim stood symbolically in an open grave'. The sources cited include Brody, Clay and Richards.

134 In his pioneering study of *The Margins of Society in Medieval Paris*, trans J. Birrell (Cambridge, 1987), p. 173, for example, Bronislaw Geremek cites Jeanselme and Foucault as his authorities for the segregation of lepers. In a similar vein, see M. Camille, *Image on the Edge: The Margins of Medieval Art* (London, 1992), pp. 132–4; and J. Richards, *Sex, Dissidence and Damnation: Minority Groups in the Middle Ages* (London, 1991), chapter eight.

135 Cohn, *Black Death Transformed*, p. 2, and chapters one and three, passim.

136 Zambaco, *Anthologie*, pp. x–xi.

137 V. Nutton, 'Did the Greeks Have a Word for It? Contagion and Contagion Theory in Classical Antiquity', in Conrad and Wujastyk, *Contagion*, p. 150.

# 2

## The Body and the Soul:
## Ideas about Causation

*'Deo Gratias brought me a note. I don't think Rycker liked me
touching it. I noticed that he didn't shake hands with me when he
said goodbye. What strange ideas people have about leprosy,
doctor.'*
*'They learn it from the Bible. Like sex.'*
*'It's a pity people pick and choose what they learn from the Bible,'*
*the Superior said, trying to knock the end of his cheroot into the
ashtray. But he was always doomed to miss.*

Graham Greene, A Burnt-Out Case, 1974[1]

Henry IV did not enjoy an easy reign. Having usurped the throne of England
from his rival, Richard II, in 1399, he faced a series of plots, betrayals and rebel-
lions, culminating, six years later, in a northern rising led by the archbishop of
York, Richard Scrope. A combination of fear, exasperation and determination to
extirpate the cancer of civil unrest led Henry to take the unprecedented step of
ordering the archbishop's execution outside the walls of York, and thereby
decapitating the Lord's anointed. Retribution followed fast, for within hours of
Scrope's death, on 8 June 1405, Henry fell sick. He soon recovered from what
had, almost certainly, been a psychosomatic disorder, although his health gave
more serious concern in the following year. From then onwards, he suffered
intermittently from debilitating bouts of illness, which aggravated the existing
climate of political instability. The nature of Henry's various maladies has generated considerable debate, in part because of their disruptive effect upon the business of government, but also, more sensationally, because it was widely
rumoured that he had been stricken with leprosy.[2]

By the time of his death, in 1413, chroniclers in both France and England
were describing the effects of this terrible disease upon Henry's face and body.[3]
It was, however, during the Wars of the Roses, some decades later, that more

---

1    Graham Greene, *A Burnt-Out Case* (London, 1974), p. 16.
2    For a judicious assessment of the debate and the evidence, see P. McNiven, 'The Problem of Henry
     IV's Health, 1405–1413', *EHR*, c (1985), pp. 747–72; and D. Biggs, 'The Politics of Health: Henry IV
     and the Long Parliament of 1406', in G. Dodd and D. Biggs, eds, *Henry IV: The Establishment of a
     Regime 1399–1406* (York, 2003), pp. 185–202.
3    M.L. Bellaguet, ed., *Chronique du religieux de Saint-Denys* (6 vols, Paris, 1839–1852), iv, p. 77; F.S.

lurid accounts of his sickness began to circulate, initially in propaganda directed by supporters of the House of York against his grandson, the feeble-minded Henry VI. An unsparing description of 'the great leprous pustules' that had erupted on his face and hands after Scrope's death appears in the *Loci e libro veritatum* of the Yorkshireman, Thomas Gascoigne (d. 1458). Nor was the author any more sympathetic towards Henry's father, the pox-ridden John of Gaunt, who is depicted as the progenitor of a doomed dynasty, putrefaction spreading through his body from his rotting genitals.[4] This crude but effective image was deployed by other opponents of the failing Lancastrian regime. Regarding Henry's disease as condign punishment for usurpation rather than homicide, another northerner, John Hardying (d. *c.* 1465), adopted a note of high drama. On his deathbed, the penitent monarch contemplates

> This wormes mete, this caryon full vnquerte [diseased],
> That some tyme thought in worlde it had no pere,
> This face so foule that leprous doth apere,
> That here afore I haue had suche a pryde
> To purtraye ofte in many place full wyde:
> Of which ryght nowe ye porest of this lande,
> Except only of theyr benignyte,
> Wolde loth to looke vpon I vnderstande.[5]

Whatever Henry's medical problems may have been, leprosy (either as understood by his contemporaries or as defined by modern day specialists) was clearly not among them. Stories about his deformed and contracted body, 'scarse a cubite of length', were demonstrably at variance with the facts, not least as reported by sober eyewitnesses and as later confirmed by his skeletal remains. Yet the myth persisted and was, for a while, conspicuously embellished. Why?

For alchemists and mystics, such as George Ripley (d. *c.* 1490), an Augustinian canon and intimate of several prominent Yorkists, Henry's illness was symbolic of a deep malaise in the body politic. His allegory of a leprous kingdom infected by malignant planets and generations of corrupt blood must have seemed apt enough during the last years of Henry VI. So also did his vision of a healthy young king reborn in the crucible of war, although in the event Edward IV failed to match these lofty expectations.[6] Others adopted a more literal approach. That Henry *ought* to have contracted leprosy seemed axiomatic to his enemies, whose thoughts clearly turned to the Old Testament monarch, Uzziah. According to the Second Book of Chronicles, this warlike ruler had been smitten

---

Haydon, ed., *Eulogium historiarum sive temporis* (3 vols, RS, 1858–63), iii, p. 408; Simpson, 'Leprosy and Leper Hospitals', part 3, pp. 397–9.

4   Struck immediately with a '*horribili et pessimo genere leprae*', Henry appeared eight days later, according to eyewitnesses, with prominent pustules on his hands and face, like nipples ('*quasi capita mamillarum*'): Thomas Gascoigne, *Loci e libro veritatum*, ed. J.H. Thorold Rogers (Oxford, 1881), pp. 137 (Gaunt), 228 (Henry).

5   H. Ellis, ed., *The Chronicle of Iohn Hardyng* (London, 1812), p. 370.

6   J. Hughes, *Arthurian Myths and Alchemy: The Kingship of Edward IV* (Stroud, 2002), pp. 71, 217. The celebrated Yorkist poem known as 'A Political Retrospect' (1462) likewise describes Henry's leprosy as a consequence of 'tyranny and violence': T. Wright, ed., *Political Poems and Songs Relating to English History* (2 vols, RS, 1859–61), ii, p. 267.

with leprosy 'in the forehead' for his presumption in defying the servers in the Temple and burning incense there [26, vv. 16–21].[7] At the height of their quarrel, in 1166, Thomas Becket, the only other English archbishop to be murdered by an angry king, had specifically warned Henry II to heed the fate of Uzziah, who had 'spurned the reverence due to the Lord and wished to usurp for himself... a duty which did not belong to his office, but to that of the priests'.[8]

It is no coincidence that Becket's friend, John of Salisbury, had used the very same biblical *exemplum* to illustrate the devastating consequences of pride, the deadliest of the seven sins, and begetter of all other vices. In his *Policraticus* (1159), a study in the uses and abuses of power, he too refers to Uzziah, whose 'face was filled with his disgrace'. The book begins with another biblical illustration of the 'general leprosy which affects us all', this time in the person of Gehazi, whom John holds out as a terrible warning against the besetting vice of self-love.[9] More generally viewed as the personification of avarice, this venal servant of the prophet Elisha had incurred the wrath of God by fraudulently extracting money from the Syrian commander, Naaman [II Kings 5, vv. 20–27]. Since his master had cured the general of leprosy without any expectation of financial reward, it was, indeed, fitting that Gehazi should be cursed with the same disease. As generations of theologians, preachers and homilists recognised, his affliction was spiritual rather than physical, gnawing into the soul of the contaminated sinner:

> For just as leprosy makes the body ugly and loathsome and repulsive, so the filth of lechery makes the soul spiritually very foul. And the swelling of secret pride is leprosy, which none can hide. And envy and jealousy and felony may be called spiritual leprosy, and the covetousness of simony so apparent in Gehazi. For Gehazi and all his kind, as we may find in the Book of Kings, were sick with simony, which nowadays greatly afflicts the clergy.[10]

Critics of the late medieval Church, among whom the Lollards were most vociferous, regarded the sale of benefices as a malignant disease. 'He that noght lawfulli but bi symonye ordeyneth eni man into holi ordre, he geueth hym not office but lepre', proclaimed one heretical preacher, in a sermon on the theme of 'gostli meselis' (spiritual lepers).[11] But his adversaries gave as good as they got.

---

7    McNiven, 'Henry IV's Health', p. 753, notes that none of the chroniclers who describe Henry's affliction refer directly to Uzziah. By then, however, the comparison must have seemed obvious, since preachers so often used his fate as a warning against pride: W.O. Ross, ed., *Middle English Sermons* (EETS, ccix, 1940, reprinted 1960), p. 211.

8    Duggan, *Correspondence of Thomas Becket*, i, p. 335. Such threats were common. In 1243, Robert Grosseteste, bishop of Lincoln, informed Henry III that his support for a rebellious faction at Bardney abbey was akin to Uzziah's meddling in ecclesiastical affairs: H.R. Luard, ed., *Roberti Grosseteste episcopi quondam Lincolniensis epistolae* (RS, 1861), no. 102. Since Henry was rumoured to suffer from '*morphea, polipo vel quandam specie leprae*', this was a serious allegation: below, n. 27.

9    John of Salisbury, *Policraticus*, ed. C.J. Nederman (Cambridge, 1990), pp. 17, 215. Pride was still equated with spiritual leprosy after the Reformation. William Turner, for example, described 'proud stertuppes' (the *nouveaux riches*) and 'lordely byshoppes' as victims of this 'foule disease': *A New Booke of Spirituall Physik for Dyuerse Diseases of the Nobilite and Gentlemen of Englande* (Emden, 1555), fos 83r–84r.

10   J. Small, ed., *English Metrical Homilies* (Edinburgh, 1862), pp. 129–30. The poem dates from about 1325.

11   G. Cigman, ed., *Lollard Sermons* (EETS, ccxciv, 1989), p. 36. As early as 1167, the German theologian,

At about the same time, a more orthodox cleric addressed his congregation on this very topic, singling out 'the stynkinge lepir of errours & erisies' for attack. 'Lepir is coruptif of clernes, & ter-bi [thereby] it bitokenid wikkid doctrin & falsnis of techyng', he warned, advising his congregation to flee from such a pernicious infection.[12] Both men were drawing on a long tradition that made it easy to diagnose the 'vicius lepir of dedli synne' in almost any activity of which one disapproved. Heresy stood high on the list, especially in continental Europe, where, as we have already seen, an epidemic of Catharism in the twelfth and thirteenth centuries unleashed a stream of violent invective.[13] There were, however, many equally lethal sources of contamination from which poison could spread. Even those who failed to defend the Church from attack, but cravenly kept silent, were 'so thicke of whelkes and bladdres in here soules' that they, too, ranked among the leprous.[14]

This chapter begins by examining the intimate relationship between sin and disease that remained constant throughout the Middle Ages. There was, however, no single, easy answer to the question of human suffering. It might equally be regarded as an enviable opportunity for personal redemption, or even as a mark of divine grace. The moral stature, or spiritual health, of the individual was therefore crucial in determining his or her culpability, for saints as well as sinners might be leprous. To a notable extent, these dual concepts were upheld in the burgeoning medical literature on *lepra* to which we then turn. Many authorities pinpointed a lack of control over the carnal appetites, especially where the lethal troika of sex, food and alcohol was concerned. Yet other presumed causes were understood in terms of evolving theories about heredity, environmental pollution and planetary forces, and thus effectively absolved the individual from personal blame. But in whatever way it was conceived, the aetiology of such a polymorphous disease hinged, in the last resort, upon the unique complexion of the soul as well as the body, and the capacity of both to withstand the onslaught of corruption.

---

Gerhoh von Reichersberg, attacked the avarice that began in Rome and ate through the body of the Church. The pope was a *pontifex leprosus*, or a *leprosus avarus*: H. Bayer, 'Lepra Universalis: Neoplatonism (Catharism) and Judaism as Reflected in Twelfth and Thirteenth Century Literature', *History of European Ideas*, ix (1988), pp. 281–303, at pp. 287, 292.

12 D.M. Grisdale, ed., *Three Middle English Sermons from the Worcester Chapter Manuscript F.10* (Leeds School of English Language Texts and Monographs, v, 1939), pp. 29, 40–41. It is important to stress the preacher's admonition that 'the scabbe e the lepur o dedli synne' was 'more vowler & mor horrible e the sith o God thanne euer was any mesel that euer was maad' (p. 29). Not everyone drew this distinction.

13 R.I. Moore, 'Heresy as a Disease', in W. Lourdaux and V. Verhelst, eds, *The Concept of Heresy in the Middle Ages* (Mediaevalia Louaniensia, first series, iv, 1976), pp. 1–11.

14 'Thei ben contagiouse to alle that ben besides hem; and wolde God that thei dwelde withoute toun as other meselis don, for thei ben worse and more perelous': A.J. McCarthy, ed., *Book to a Mother* (Elizabethan and Renaissance Studies, xcii, Salzburg, 1981), p. 63. For the shifting hierarchy of sins, see L.K. Little, 'Pride Goes before Avarice: Social Change and the Vices in Latin Christendom', *American Historical Review*, lxxvi (1971), pp. 16–49; and for the development of ideas about contagion, below, pp. 90–95.

## The wages of sin

A conviction that the soul was as susceptible to disease as the flesh had long been the stock in trade of political commentators and moralists. The Greek historian, Polybius (d. *c.* 118 BC), had, for example, argued that the malign vapours of evil could destroy the moral faculties in the same way that galloping ulcers consumed the body.[15] Two centuries later Tacitus suggested that the soul of a tyrant such as the Roman Emperor Tiberius would inevitably display bruises and wounds, 'for as the body is scourged by lashes, so is the spirit by cruelty, lust and malice'.[16] Yet, eloquent as they are, these writers were far outdone by their Christian successors, whose religious beliefs hinged upon the certain knowledge that every misdeed would be recorded, judged and punished, either in this world or, even more painfully, the next.

Whether their knowledge was acquired at the most basic level through the parish church, or developed after years of laborious study, medieval men and women were steeped in the Bible. It permeated every aspect of their lives, as an unimpeachable historical record, a source of moral instruction and a guide to spiritual development. Tales of Old Testament kings, prophets and heroes could be read or interpreted at a variety of different levels, from the most literal to the profoundly symbolic, as a profusion of meanings and pointers was teased from the original text. The spots and stains of leprosy thus served as an effective metaphor for various manifestations of sin. But the boundaries separating allegory from the accidents of daily life were often blurred by authors who wished to drive their message home as dramatically as possible.[17] The assumption that spiritual deformity would somehow leave its trace upon the body as well as the soul insidiously found its way into religious and secular literature alike. Such warnings must have been familiar from the pulpit long before accessible vernacular versions of Latin texts began to circulate among the laity. Thus, for example, the story of the Emperor Merelaus (or Jereslaus) and his long-suffering wife first gained currency in a compilation of homilies for preachers known as the *Gesta Romanorum* before being reworked for an educated English readership by various authors, including Thomas Hoccleve (d. 1450). The poet tells how three evil men attempted to seduce this beautiful but intensely devout woman. The first, her brother-in-law, compounded his sin by betraying the emperor and trying to commit incest. He was fittingly transformed into 'as foul a leepre as mighte be'. The second (a faithless steward who also murdered his lord's child) went deaf and blind. The third, a sea captain, lost his mind, while the mendacious servant who betrayed her to him was crippled with gout. All were eventually cured by their intended victim, but not until they had fully confessed 'hire offenses dirke & synnes blake'.[18]

---

[15] J.A.C. Buch, ed., *Ouvrages historiques de Polybe, Hérodien and Zozine* (2 vols, Paris, 1836), i, p. 41.

[16] R. Mellor, *Tacitus* (London, 1994), p. 27.

[17] Grigsby, *Pestilence*, pp. 35, 79–102, itemises the sins associated with leprosy, concluding that the disease must inevitably have been linked with moral corruption.

[18] A. Blamires, ed., *Woman Defamed and Woman Defended* (Oxford, 1992), pp. 270–77; F.J. Furnivall, ed., *Hoccleve's Works: The Minor Poems* (EETS, extra series, lxi, 1892), pp. 140–78. The quotations are from pp. 164, 167. The French version of the tale, which dwells at greater length upon the contrast

Some tales were homelier and thus more appealing to ordinary men and women. Keen to hold the attention of their congregations with lively and appropriate *exempla*, medieval clergy turned to works such as Robert Brunne's advice manual, *Handlyng Synne*. This provided a selection of entertaining moral anecdotes, often with a rustic flavour, which could be used to explain fundamental tenets of the Christian faith to a largely unlettered audience. That of the hermit, St Florens, and an amiable bear who tended his sheep, must have made a deep impression, especially upon the young. Devastated by the death of his 'wylde and stoute' companion at the hand of four jealous monks, the saint calls for retribution:

> As he seyde, so gan hyt falle;
> Gode toke veniaunce on hem alle;
> Meseles [lepers] they waxe than to pyne,
> Here lemes roted before here yne [eyes];
> Aboue the erthe they were stynkyng,
> That to the beres deth were consenting.[19]

Having warned his listeners that 'enuye ys a cursed synne', the priest might then perhaps turn to the biblical tale of Miriam whose criticism of her brother, Moses, led God to strike her briefly with leprosy 'as white as snow' [Numbers 12, vv. 1–16]. Sometimes directly linked with the psalmist's admonition against sinning with one's tongue, this particular instance of divine retribution seemed especially applicable to women [**plate 4**].[20] That leprosy destroyed the human voice may have rendered it an even more appropriate punishment for unbridled speech. But the 'leper of bakbityng' was far from gender specific. As a rider to his solemn warning about heresy, our orthodox preacher moved on to address the dangers of malicious gossip, observing 'how infectif' it was to both sexes.[21] Like generations of churchmen before him, he found the disease a compelling symbol for whatever vices might currently be exercising leading members of the ecclesiastical establishment. As we shall see in the next chapter, their explorations of human frailty often began with Christ's miraculous cure of the sick, and especially of the ten lepers [Luke 17, vv. 12–19], who served as the perfect allegory for contaminated souls in search of spiritual health.[22]

between the Empress's spiritual beauty and her persecutors' physical deformities, is discussed in A. Garnier, *Mutations temporelles et cheminement spirituel* (Paris, 1988).

[19] F.J. Furnivall, ed., *Robert of Brunne's 'Handlyng Synne'* (EETS, cxix, 1901, and cxxiii, 1903, reprinted as one, 1973), pp. 139–40. The preacher may also have drawn a parallel between the ursine shepherd and Christ.

[20] See, for example, Bodleian Library, MS Bodley 618, fo. 12r, 'de continencia locucionis'. The French knight of La Tour-Landry reminded his two young daughters of the fate of Miriam, warning that 'often tymes God ponisshed so the enuyous and the euell spekers': T. Wright, ed., *The Book of the Knight of La Tour-Landry* (EETS, xxxiii, 1868, reprinted 1969), p. 90. See also, B. Dekeyzer, *Layers of Illusion: The Mayer van den Bergh Breviary* (Ghent and Amsterdam, 2004), pp. 76–9.

[21] Grisdale, *Three Middle English Sermons*, p. 40. In *The Faerie Queene*, Edmund Spenser (d. 1599) observes that Envy 'does backbite, and spightfull poison spues/ From leprous mouth on all that euer writt': *Complete Poetical Works*, eds J.C. Smith and E. de Selincourt (Oxford, 1912), book I, canto iv, 32.

[22] H.O. Old, ed., *The Reading and Preaching of the Scriptures, III, The Medieval Church* (Grand Rapids, Michigan, 1999), p. 327; G. Pichon, 'Essai sur la lèpre du haut moyen âge', *Le Moyen Age*, fourth series, xxxix (1984), pp. 331–56, at pp. 337–8; and below, pp. 111–12.

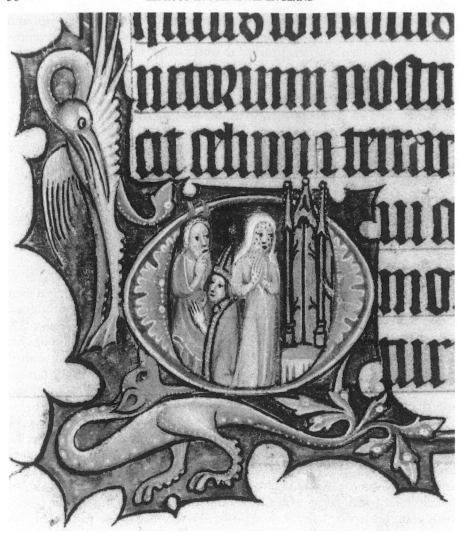

4. In this illumination from a fourteenth-century English psalter, Miriam is struck by leprosy before the tabernacle of the congregation for presuming to criticise her brother, Moses (left, with his traditional horns). Aaron, their priestly sibling, here garbed as a medieval bishop, humbly intercedes on her behalf, for he, too, has murmured against Moses [Numbers 12, vv. 1–16].

Historians have tended to regard this type of writing as a barometer of contemporary responses to the physically sick. Yet a voracious appetite for morality tales did not necessarily preclude a more reflective approach to ideas about the causation of disease. Examples may be gleaned from all periods. One twelfth-century chronicler's account of the presumed leprosy of Bishop Aelfweard of London (d. 1044) reveals a striking degree of objectivity. On the verge of death, the bishop had returned to Evesham abbey, which he had greatly enriched during his time as abbot, only to be repulsed by a faction of horrified monks. Reporting that some clergy regarded the bishop's illness as the result of a sacrilegious attempt to remove the relics of St Osyth from their resting place for display in his cathedral, the writer maintained that it was best not to engage in idle speculation about such things. After all, he reflected, the manifold symptoms of *lepra* that so disfigured his face, rendering it dry, white and scaly, might equally well derive from a multitude of entirely natural causes. A plethora of blood boiling up in the veins, excessive heat, a humoral imbalance or some respiratory impediment to the flow of the vital spirits around the body could undermine human health just as effectively as the wrath of God. Since the author in question was a monk of Ramsey abbey, where Aelfweard (and his not inconsiderable treasure) found a final resting place, it could be argued that he was hardly an unbiased observer.[23] Perhaps he simply wished to demonstrate his familiarity with the most recent medical literature. Significantly, though, others went even further in describing the bishop's enemies as diabolically inspired to traduce his reputation and bring ruin upon a once prosperous house.[24]

Even so, the steady drip of prejudice inevitably had some practical repercussions, as the linguistic distinctions between metaphorical and physical leprosy became increasingly blurred. As Beryl Smalley has observed, symbolic comparisons made between the benighted synagogue and the radiant light of Christianity had less abstract implications for a 'living Jew'.[25] Nor can there be much doubt that the fires of anti-Semitism were further stoked by constant references to Judaism as a type of spiritual, if not bodily, *lepra*.[26] It was certainly far from unusual for chroniclers and propagandists like John Hardyng to infer that their enemies were physically as well as morally tainted. According to Matthew Paris, one of the charges levelled in 1239 against the disgraced former justiciar of England, Hubert de Burgh, concerned treasonous remarks he had reputedly made about his royal master. To describe Henry III as a squint-eyed, cowardly perjurer was offensive enough, but to suggest that he had also contracted 'a type of leprosy' seemed infinitely worse.[27]

Such allegations were, no doubt, the stuff of hearsay and gossip, but they reflect how seriously imputations of leprosy were taken. The waspish Paris was himself an adept at slurs of this kind. Thus, for example, he reported that a nasal polyp from which Bishop d'Aigueblanche of Hereford had been suffering in the late 1250s was either a symptom of morphew or else of *lepra* sent by God as a punishment for the many exactions he had laid upon the English people. Since morphew was commonly regarded as a sign of incipient leprosy, either disease seemed appropriate retribution for the financial abuses and disasters in foreign policy that Paris (and many others) laid at the bishop's door.[28] An ecclesiastical Uzziah, whose presumptuous meddling in international politics had virtually

23  W.D. Macray, ed., *Chronicon Abbatiae Rameseiensis* (RS, 1886), pp. 157–8.
24  W.D. Macray, ed., *Chronicon Abbatiae de Evesham* (RS, 1863), pp. 83–5.
25  B. Smalley, *The Study of the Bible in the Middle Ages* (Oxford, 1952), pp. 2–3, 25–6. Brody, *Disease of the Soul*, pp. 110–23, offers many examples of the allegorical uses of leprosy.
26  Pichon, 'Essai sur la lèpre', pp. 336–8; C. Fabre-Vassas, *The Singular Beast: Jews, Christians and the Pig* (Columbia, New York, 1997), pp. 104, 147.
27  Mathew Paris, *Chronica Majora*, ed. H.R. Luard (7 vols, RS, 1872–84), iii, pp. 618–19.
28  Paris, *Chronica Majora*, v, pp. 622, 679; *DNB*, i, pp. 475–8.

bankrupted the nation, the bishop surely merited chastisement. Two centuries later, Reginald Pecok, another controversial bishop, invited similar obloquy, this time because of his unorthodox religious beliefs. Thomas Gascoigne (whose censorious eye was constantly on the lookout for physical manifestations of sin) remarked that Pecok was physically *disposed* towards the disease (*dispositus ad lepram corporis*) and that many of his ancestors had actually suffered from it. Yet his mind rather than his body had grown leprous through the contagion of heresy.[29]

Not surprisingly, since most of these authors (including Gascoigne) had taken holy orders, the imputation of leprosy tended to follow an act of sacrilege or mark of disrespect to the Church. Robert Fitzpernel, earl of Leicester, was, for instance, allegedly afflicted because he unjustly took possession of an estate lately belonging to Hugh of Avalon, the revered bishop of Lincoln. Having been reluctant to confront St Hugh in his lifetime, he confiscated the property after his death, and 'immediately contracted leprosy' as a result. With undisguised satisfaction, the bishop's biographer reports that he went into a decline and expired without issue almost at once in 1204.[30] Since his elder brother, William, who had died some six years earlier, was later said to have founded the *leprosarium* of St Leonard, Leicester, because he himself suffered from the disease, there may have been a germ of truth in this story.[31] The antiquary, John Nichols, was struck by the fact that their father, another earl Robert, was known as '*blanchemayns*' (white hands), and suggested that their condition might well have been hereditary.[32] In ecclesiastical eyes, however, Fitzpernel's pride and avarice were explanation enough.

It would, none the less, be unwise to assume that medieval men and women ranked leprosy above all other diseases as the ultimate penalty for human sin. There was, after all, a depressingly wide choice. Plague and pox were alike regarded as heavy artillery in the ongoing *bellum Dei contra homines*. Congregations recoiling under the fusillade of pestilence were constantly reminded of their moral shortcomings. Gambling, lechery, shady business dealings and indecent fashions among the young had alike incurred the spectacular displays of divine wrath that swept across Europe from 1348 onwards.[33] So too, ironically, had hostility towards the leprous poor of Christ. Responsibility for an outbreak of pestilence in early fifteenth-century Nuremberg was laid squarely at the door of the mayor, who had refused to allow them into the city for the customary

29  Gascoigne, *Loci e libro veritatum*, p. 29.
30  D.L. Douie and D.H. Farmer, eds, *Magna vita Sancti Hugonis: The Life of St Hugh of Lincoln* (2 vols, London, 1961–62), ii, p. 84. Marcombe, *Leper Knights*, pp. 139–40, speculates that the 'leper head' in Lincoln cathedral may be Fitzpernel's.
31  J.R. Lumby, ed., *Chronicon Henrici Knighton monachi Leycestrensis* (2 vols, RS, 1889–95), i, p. 64. Knighton was a monk of Leicester abbey, and thus presumably well informed about the nearby hospital, which was in fact founded by William's father, Robert, and endowed by both his sons: *HMC, Report on the Hastings Manuscripts I* (London, 1928), pp. 336, 341. William cannot have lived there for long, if at all, as he was still active in 1198: V. Gibbs et al., *The Complete Peerage* (14 vols, London and Stroud, 1910–98), vii, p. 533.
32  J. Nichols, *The History and Antiquities of the County of Leicester* (4 vols, London, 1795–1815), i, part 2, p. 321.
33  R. Horrox, ed., *The Black Death* (Manchester, 1994), pp. 95–157.

religious observances of Holy Week. As might be expected, the practice resumed forthwith, having by the 1490s developed into a major festival, during which food, drink, clothing and spiritual succour were lavished upon these special visitors as an insurance policy against future epidemics.[34] One could never tell where, or precisely how, the blow would strike. Seizing advantage of the chaos caused by the Black Death of 1349, the Scots invaded England, only to fall under the sword of God. According to one chronicler, they were duly punished with *lepra*, just as the English had been afflicted with swellings and buboes.[35] Some preachers considered plague to be a greater curse than leprosy, while most people agreed that the pox outdid them both.[36] But whereas theologians invariably regarded plague as a collective retribution, *lepra* almost always ranked as an individual punishment, incurred, like madness, because of personal misdeeds. It was, significantly, said by English (but not Scottish) chroniclers to have been the cause of Robert the Bruce's lingering death.[37]

For many, the dramatic bouts of insanity that God had visited upon the biblical rulers Nebuchadnezzar and Herod constituted the most dreadful punishment of all. Familiar to medieval audiences from the stage and pulpit, Herod, the personification of both wrath and pride, lay beyond the reach of spiritual as well as earthly medicine. For whereas leprosy attacked the body, madness – especially in the form of demonic possession – destroyed the rational faculties, shattering into pieces that which had been created in the divine image.[38] Still free to make his or her peace with God, to receive the sacraments and to die in the arms of the Church, the leper remained a fully active member of the Christian community. The mentally disturbed, on the other hand, could neither confess nor take communion, and were thus truly segregated from the body of the faithful.[39] Enemies of Charles VI of France, whose violent attacks of madness began in 1392 and continued until his death thirty years later, believed that he had been justly punished for fostering schism within the Church and

---

34  A. Martin, 'The Representation of Leprosy and of Lepers in Minor Art, Particularly in Germany', *The Urologic and Cutaneous Review*, xxv (1921), pp. 445–53, at p. 450.

35  E.M. Thompson, ed., *Chronicon Galfridi le Baker de Swynebroke* (Oxford, 1889), p. 100. An epic life of St Werburge of Chester describes how, among her many posthumous miracles, she defended the city from attack by the marauding Welsh. 'Of the principall doers some raged out of mynde, some smetyn with palsy, some lepre, halt and blynde': Henry Bradshaw, *The Life of Saint Werburge*, ed. C. Horstmann (EETS, lxxxviii, 1887), p. 166.

36  T[homas] S[wadlin], *Sermons, Meditations and Prayers upon the Plague 1636* (London, 1637), pp. 27–8; Arrizabalaga, Henderson and French, *Great Pox*, p. 253; C. Quétel, *History of Syphilis* (Oxford, 1990), pp. 10, 12, 17, 24–5.

37  H. Maxwell, ed., *The Chronicle of Lanercost, 1272–1346* (Glasgow, 1913), pp. 257, 264; Simpson, 'Leprosy and Leper Hospitals', part 3, pp. 400–04. The interminable debate as to whether or not Robert the Bruce suffered from Hansen's disease is set to remain inconclusive, since the evidence is at best ambiguous: M.H. Kaufman and W.J. MacLennan, 'Robert the Bruce and Leprosy', *Proceedings of the Royal College of Physicians*, xxx (2000), pp. 75–80. Of greater interest in the present context is the way contemporary chroniclers reacted to news of his ill health on predictably national lines: R. Nicholson, *Scotland in the Middle Ages* (Edinburgh, 1974), pp. 121–2.

38  P.B.R. Doob, *Nebuchadnezzar's Children: Conventions of Madness in Middle English Literature* (Yale, 1974), pp. 10–17, 103–15. The fourteenth-century *Cursor Mundi* departs from the convention of madness to catalogue a positive lexicon of diseases suffered by Herod, concluding that 'ouer al than was he mesel [leper] plain': R. Morris, ed., *Cursor Mundi, II* (EETS, lix, 1875, reprinted 1966), pp. 678–9.

39  R.C. Pickett, *Mental Affliction and Church Law* (Ottawa, 1952), pp. 54–9.

immorality in his own court. The loyal subjects who documented his fate inevitably sought a different explanation. As in the case of the Ramsey Abbey chronicler, they looked for natural causes, while also suspecting that the king might have been bewitched. But to console themselves, they reflected that illness was a scourge sent by God to chastise those wayward children whom he truly loved.[40] Indeed, far from signalling inner depravity, it might even be seen as a gift, or at the very least a *test*, in which the prize outshone all others. If, as medieval theologians and preachers maintained, extremes of human suffering could represent a mark of election, bringing with them the promise of salvation, the leper and the lunatic alike appeared in an entirely different light.

The high profile of several 'noble' lepers, whose rank and unimpeachable moral character merited a less censorious response, has been seen as a powerful factor in promoting an alternative image of the disease. Although the evidence for such an argument remains impressionistic, it appears that many prominent eleventh- and twelfth-century figures were deemed to be leprous.[41] They clearly helped to break one mould and create another. Baldwin IV, king of Jerusalem (d. 1185), and the early members of the crusading Order of St Lazarus were, for example, more likely to inspire praise than vilification.[42] Baldwin, who died at the age of twenty-three, was so crippled that he had to be carried into battle on a litter. Yet his Frankish followers proved remarkably tolerant of symptoms that rendered him blind, as well as malodorous and disfigured, making no apparent attempt to remove him from power. Quite possibly, as Bernard Hamilton has suggested, their admiration for his chastity and dedication to the crusading ideal overcame whatever initial reservations they might have had.[43] Not all westerners took this view. In an encyclical of 1181 Pope Alexander III maintained that the king was incapable of ruling because he had been 'so severely afflicted by the just judgement of God', although he did not hold him personally culpable for his debility. Rather, the march of leprosy through his young body then seemed to mirror the inroads made by Saladin into a weak and divided crusader kingdom.[44] Yet Baldwin's eventual success against the infidel, achieved against the odds, won him great respect. Referring to God's 'hidden' and mysterious purposes, the English chronicler, William of Newburgh (d. *c.* 1198), drew a sharp distinction between the king's decaying flesh and his virtuous, well-governed soul.[45] Another contemporary, Roger of Howden (d. 1201–02), who actually visited Jerusalem, observed that Baldwin had achieved great success

[40] B. Guenée, *La folie de Charles VI: Roi bien-aimé* (Paris, 2004), pp. 147–8, and passim; Doob, *Nebuchadnezzar's Children*, pp. 46–9.

[41] S.R. Ell, 'Diet and Leprosy in the Medieval West: The Noble Leper', *Janus*, lxxii (1985), pp. 113–29, passim.

[42] S. Shahar, 'Des lépreux pas comme les autres: L'ordre de Saint-Lazare dans le royaume latin de Jerusalem', *Revue Historique*, cclxvii (1982), pp. 19–41. The order was founded for crusaders who became leprous 'by the will of God'. No mention was made of sin or chastisement.

[43] Hamilton, *Leper King*, pp. 241–2. In this instance, Hansen's disease can be diagnosed with reasonable certainty: Mitchell, 'Evaluation of the Leprosy of King Baldwin', pp. 245–58.

[44] Alexander III, *Opera omnia: Epistolae et privilegia*, PL, cc, cols 1294–6. Pegg, 'Le corps et l'autorité, p. 265, translates '*justo Dei judicio flagellatus*' as 'chastised by a just chastisement of God', and argues that, in the West, Baldwin's leprosy must have been equated with sin.

[45] William of Newburgh, *Historia rerum Anglicarum*, ed. R. Howlett (RS, 1885), p. 241.

despite his leprosy, and that many miracles had been worked during his reign.[46] Later generations of Englishmen admired 'the douhty kyng', whose tenacious defence of his beleaguered realm ('neuer in his lyue he lese a fote of lond') put others to shame.[47] But there were additional, even more persuasive reasons, for reassessing the place of the leper in Christian theology.

## The gift of paradise

The Cistercian abbot and theologian, Aelred of Rievaulx (d. 1167), regarded the human body as a necessary but impermanent receptacle for the soul. Delicious food might be served in an ugly, misshapen dish, while the most beautiful golden vessel could just as easily conceal rotting meat. It would be foolish to judge on superficial appearances, when the contents alone mattered.[48] Such weighty considerations prompted Louis IX of France to interrogate his friend, Jean Joinville (d. 1317), about his attitude to spiritual health. On being asked whether he would rather commit a mortal sin or become a leper, the horrified courtier declared that he would sooner commit thirty than endure such a terrible fate. This was the wrong answer. As Louis explained, no earthly disease could be as vile as a soul consumed by even one deadly sin. For, whereas physical leprosy ended with death, diseases of the soul might endure throughout all eternity in the flames of hell.[49] That Louis drew a sharp distinction between the two is apparent from his many visits to *leprosaria*, where he personally fed and tended the inmates. One severely deformed monk, in particular, commanded his admiration. 'The good king comforted this patient', reports his biographer, 'and said that he bore his sickness with admirable patience, and that it was his purgatory on earth; and that it was better that he suffered such a malady here, than that he suffer something else in the world to come.'[50]

However desirable they might appear, health and beauty could easily become a poisoned chalice, brimming over with the sins of pride, lust and avarice. Better by far to be physically repugnant, and thus free from such snares. A life of pain and rejection could, moreover, bring one closer to God. In the words of St Anselm (d. 1109) to the dying bishop of Rochester, 'the progress of the soul grows out of the failure of the flesh'.[51] By focusing the mind upon repentance and atonement, a long stay in the antechamber of Death prepared the soul for a rapid ascent to heaven; it was a spur to salvation. When addressing a community of nuns, Bernard of Clairvaux (d. 1175), no stranger himself to chronic illness, argued that disease should be embraced as a divine gift, pregnant with opportunity.[52] Similar advice was offered a few years later in the *Ancrene Riwle*, a manual for the guidance of female English recluses.

46 W. Stubbs, ed., *Chronica Magistri Rogeri de Houedene* (4 vols, RS, 1868–71), i, p. 275.
47 T. Hearne, ed., *Peter Langtoft's Chronicle* (2 vols, Oxford, 1725, reprinted 1810), i, p. 140.
48 S. Shahar, *Growing Old in the Middle Ages* (London, 2004), p. 54.
49 Jean Joinville, *The Life of St Louis*, ed. and trans. R. Hague (London, 1955), pp. 28–9.
50 Dom. Bouquet, ed., *Vie de Saint Louis par le confesseur de la Reine Marguerite: Rerum Gallicarum et Francicarum scriptores, XX* (Paris, 1840), pp. 96–7. See also, J. Le Goff, *Saint Louis* (Paris, 1996), pp. 869, 880–81.
51 W. Frölich, ed., *The Letters of Saint Anselm of Canterbury I* (Cistercian Studies, xcvi, 1990), no. 53.
52 Bernard of Clairvaux, *Opera ominia: Liber de modo bene vivendi, PL*, clxxxiv, *De infirmitate*, cols

God tests those he loves in the same way as the goldsmith refines gold in the furnace. The base metal vanishes completely, but the pure gold emerges truer and better than ever it was before. Sickness likewise inflicts pain and burning, but just as nothing purifies gold like fire, so nothing cleanses the soul like illness. I mean, of course, the afflictions that God sends, not other types of suffering. For many people make themselves unwell through their own foolishness or ignorance; and they, not God, are thus to blame . . . Sickness is your goldsmith, that in the bliss of heaven gilds your crown. For the greater the sickness the busier is your goldsmith, and the longer it lasts, the brighter your crown will shine.[53]

Sentiments of this kind were not simply directed at women whose sense of vocation might have appeared fleeting or vulnerable to their male guardians. A sense that God had deliberately *chosen* the leper emerges clearly from the many comparisons made between him and the Old Testament icon of righteous suffering, Job. For either might claim that, having been smelted in the divine furnace, they would 'come forth as gold' [Job 23, v. 10].

As recounted in the Latin *Vulgate*, the story of Job dealt with a pious and successful man, whose material goods, children and health were destroyed by Satan – with God's approval – to test the strength of his faith. Having patiently endured a devastating series of blows, including 'sore boils from the sole of his foot unto his crown', and resisted manifold temptations to curse his maker, he was eventually restored to even greater happiness than before. Medieval versions of his life, which glossed over any expressions of rebelliousness, were greatly embellished with a mass of circumstantial detail about the severity of his disease and the humility of his response to unbearable suffering. In keeping with the apocryphal *Testament of Job*, he was, for example, frequently depicted in words and images as a naked, ulcerated beggar seated upon a dung heap outside the city walls, the stench of his sores demanding the use of fumigants by those who visited him.[54] A major contribution to the creation of this image was made by St Gregory the Great (d. 604), whose *Moralia in Job* described him as a model of saintly forbearance, and, at an allegorical level, as the precursor of Christ himself.[55] That he was also believed to represent the suffering Church in its struggle against heresy strikes a very different note from the analogy between heretics and lepers discussed above.[56]

The cult of 'Saint' Job flourished during the later Middle Ages and beyond, since, for obvious reasons, victims of the plague and pox frequently called upon him for help.[57] First and foremost, though, his mortification was that of the leper. In the words of a fifteenth-century verse commentary:

---

1264–5. Bernard lived among, and undoubtedly preached to, the lepers of the Grand-Beaulieu, Chartres, in 1131: N. Bériou and F.O. Touati, eds, *Voluntate Dei leprosus: Les lépreux entre conversion et exclusion aux XIIème et XIIIème siècles* (Testi, Studi, Strumenti, iv, 1991), pp. 21, 58–9.

53   A. Zetterstein, ed., *The English Text of the Ancrene Riwle* (EETS, cclxxiv, 1976), pp. 79–80.

54   L.L. Besserman, *The Legend of Job in the Middle Ages* (Harvard, 1979), pp. 1–89; S. Terrien, *The Iconography of Job through the Centuries: Artists as Biblical Interpreters* (Pennsylvania State University Press, Pennsylvania, 1996), pp. 35–6, 99–102.

55   Gregory the Great, *Morals in the Book of Job*, ed. J. Bliss (4 vols, Oxford, 1844–50), i, pp. 26, 147–8.

56   Terrien, *Iconography of Job*, pp. 74–8.

57   Arrizabalaga, Henderson and French, *Great Pox*, pp. 22–5, 52–4, 87. Job was associated with skin diseases of all kinds: C. Habrich et al., *Aussatz, Lepra, Hasen-Krankheit: Ein Menschheitsproblem im Wandel* (Munich, 1982), nos 2.9–13, 2.18, 4.24.

Thus lykyd god for to proue exprese
His grete meknes with messelry [leprosy],
And for he fand his fayth ay fresch,
He wuns in welth, als is worthy.[58]

The humble leper would, of course, win his wealth in heaven rather than on earth, but might rest assured that he, like Job, was especially beloved of God, and thus confident of a celestial reward if he endured his manifold sufferings with fortitude. Such was the message spread in the early thirteenth century by Jacques de Vitry, two of whose sermons *ad lepros et alios infirmos* survive. A gifted and eloquent preacher, he compared his listeners to bells, which would naturally be struck by any prospective purchaser, just as God was testing them to see if they were true. (Perhaps, at this point, he actually rang one of the bells the residents of *leprosaria* used when they were collecting alms in order to prove his point.) Disease, however terrible, should thus be welcomed as a blessing, not least because it marked the first step on the road to conversion, and thence to spiritual perfection.[59]

Medical practitioners were expected to relay this message. When counselling his colleagues about the diagnostic procedures to be employed in cases of presumed leprosy, the distinguished French surgeon, Guy de Chauliac (d. 1368), stressed how important it was to reassure the patient that his affliction constituted a mark of election rather than a curse. 'Firste, in clepynge [calling upon] Goddes help, he schall comforte ham and saie that this passioun or sekenesse is saluacioun of the soule', ran his advice. A few incautious words about sin might plunge the patient into despair, whereas a message of divine love, emphasising Christ's great compassion for the leprous, would help him to 'stande in pees'.[60] As we shall see in chapter five, recommendations of this kind were soundly based on contemporary medical theory, and may have been followed by practitioners for what we would now call psychosomatic reasons. Even so, they are reiterated, with added force, in the words of Chaucer's parson, in *The Canterbury Tales*, who warned that condemnation or criticism of the sick constituted a 'ful grisly sin'. Jibes directed against the deformed or leprous were, he stressed, tantamount to an attack upon Christ himself. This was because 'peyne is sent by the rightwys sonde [just judgement] of God, and by his sufferance, be it meselrie [leprosy], or mayhem or maladie'.[61]

The beneficial effects of earthly tribulations took an increasingly literal, almost quantifiable, turn as a complex infrastructure of belief slowly took shape in support of the doctrine of purgatory. From the time of St Augustine (d. 430) onwards it was understood that, after death, all but the holy (who went directly

---

58  Besserman, *Legend of Job*, p. 88.
59  Bériou and Touati, *Voluntate Dei leprosus*, pp. 24, 38–42, 101–28. The bell simile is on p. 115.
60  M.S. Ogden, ed., *The Cyrurgie of Guy de Chauliac* (EETS, cclxv, 1971), p. 381. There is, in fact, no evidence to suggest that medieval European practitioners 'added unnecessary fear, loathing and censorship to their accounts of the disease': M.W. Dols, 'Leprosy in Medieval Arab Medicine', *Journal of the History of Medicine and Allied Sciences*, xxxiv (1979), pp. 314–33, at p. 332; and Grigsby, *Pestilence*, pp. 51–3.
61  Geoffrey Chaucer, *The Canterbury Tales*, in L.D. Benson, ed., *The Riverside Chaucer* (Boston, 1987), p. 308.

to heaven) and the eternally damned would undergo a period of purgation from residual sins for which atonement had still to be made. In this way a legion of tarnished, but not irreparably corroded, souls would be made free of imperfection and fit to meet their maker at the Last Judgement. Not surprisingly, religious teaching about this period of cleansing, especially with regard to the various ways by which it might be reduced, greatly strengthened the Church's financial and moral authority.[62] Ideas about the life to come also had a profound impact upon medieval society's attitude towards lepers and the victims of other bodily afflictions. To a notable extent, the responsibility for hastening the passage of an individual soul through its spiritual prison lay with those who remained behind on earth. Masses and prayers of intercession for the departed, which, as we shall see, were such a prominent feature of hospital life, greatly eased this period of transition. But, to employ a well-worn analogy with banking, it was also possible to make deposits in advance, and thus build up one's credit before death. Good works, which naturally included charitable provision for the sick, carried a high premium (unless they engendered pride), to be augmented by other activities, such as pilgrimage and the purchase of indulgences. The patient acceptance of physical debility or extreme hardship likewise appeared to promise a speedy passage through this painful nether world, not only for the sufferer but also those for whom he or she was prepared to intercede. Although, during the later Middle Ages, the purchasing power of these spiritual investments became a matter of precise, almost obsessive calculation, the principles involved were considerably older.

From a comparatively early date, vivid accounts of the process of purgation, such as those to be found in Bede's *Ecclesiastical History* (731) and, even more graphically, *The Revelation of the Monk of Eynsham* (1196), dwell on the 'indescribable stench' and physical torments endured by the wretched souls in question.[63] It is easy to see how leprosy came to be described as purgatory on earth; and, as the map of the nether world gradually assumed a more precise and heavily populated form, actually figured among the many torments inflicted there as well. As it passed through purgatory, a soul still consumed by venial sin would be punished in many ingenious ways, not least being centuries, perhaps even millennia, under the lash of a specific and appropriate disease. The equation varied from one author to another, although, as we shall see, most demonstrated an awareness of current medical literature. Wrath, for instance, might incur madness, heart failure or shaking palsy, while a soul consumed with gluttony or lust would be shackled to *lepra*.[64]

In view of the horrors to come, purgation *before* death began to seem more

---

62   P. Binski, *Medieval Death: Ritual and Representation* (London, 1996), pp. 24–8, 181–99. Purgatory first became a matter of dogma in 1247.

63   J. Le Goff, *The Birth of Purgatory* (Chicago, 1984), pp. 84–91, 91–5, 102–3, 193–201; The Venerable Bede, *Ecclesiastical History of the English People*, eds B. Colgrave and R.A.B. Mynors (Oxford, 1969), pp. 488–99; H. Thurston, ed., 'Visio monnachi de Eynsham', *Analecta Bollandia*, xxii (1903), pp. 225–319.

64   M.W. Bloomfield, *The Seven Deadly Sins* (Michigan, 1952), pp. 176–7, 194–6, 233. In *The Divine Comedy*, Dante's friend, Forese Donati, is punished for his gluttony with 'dry leprosy': D.L. Sayers, ed. and trans., *The Comedy of Dante Alighieri: Purgatory* (Harmondsworth, 1955), p. 248.

like a privilege or mark of divine favour than a curse. 'Thoo thou had all maner of sekenes of bodye all thi liffe tyme', warned the preacher, 'and thoo that thow lyveste an hundreth vyntere [winters], yitt it vere not so grevous as one daye in purgatorie.'[65] Suffering was, as St Hugh of Lincoln recognised, an elevated rung on the ladder of perfection, which bestowed upon the leper a glowing, 'internal splendour'. Whereas 'an eye darkened by arrogance' would never recognise the spiritual beauty of men with 'swollen and livid, diseased and deformed' faces,

> he declared such to be blessed, and called them the flowers of paradise and the lucent pearls in the crown of the eternal king. These, he said, could confidently await the coming of our Saviour, Jesus Christ, who would transform their vile bodies into the glory of His risen body [Philippians III, v. 21]. Those on the other hand must dread the coming of the heavenly judge, who now gloried in the beauty of their bodies . . .[66]

Medieval hagiography reveals many examples of holy men and women who did not simply welcome leprosy as a mark of divine favour, but apparently begged God to inflict it upon them. The eleventh-century English *vita* of the Irish saint, Finian Lobhar (Finianus *leprosus*), describes how he miraculously cured a blind, mute and leprous child by assuming the disease himself and suffering patiently, like Job, under the lash of God.[67] Others evidently sought to atone for past sins. Ralph (d. 1062), the notoriously 'ill-tonsured' monk of Marmoutier, came to repent an early life spent in pursuit of 'knightly sports and frivolities'. After devoting years to the study of medicine, and establishing a formidable reputation for his skills as a physician, he grew concerned about the state of his own spiritual health. 'Spurning earthly glory' for a life of repentance, he 'humbly implored God to afflict his body with incurable leprosy so that his soul might be cleansed of its foul sins'.[68] His prayer was answered. According to Orderic Vitalis, who recounts this tale of conversion in his *Historia Ecclesiastica*, Ralph's nephew, the abbot of St Evroul, gave him an isolated hillside chapel where he might retreat from the world and meditate upon his past misdeeds. Despite his disease – or more probably because it marked him out as a man blessed by God – droves of pilgrims came to consult him about their own personal anxieties.[69] Whereas in his sinful past he had been preoccupied with their perishable bodies, he now acted as a physician of their souls. The moral is unambiguous: leprosy may begin as atonement for worldly pride in physical and intellectual achievements, but can end in a state of grace.

As we shall see, the concept of leprosy as a religious vocation was not, in general, destined to survive beyond the mid thirteenth century. Yet a conviction that illness 'pacientlye and gladly' endured would purify the soul and facilitate its journey through purgatory remained a recurrent theme of English devotional

---

65  Ross, *Middle English Sermons*, pp. 41–2.
66  Douie and Farmer, *Life of St Hugh*, ii, pp. 13–14.
67  *Acta Sanctorum*, viii, March II (16 March), pp. 439–42. Another medieval Irish word for leper was *martar*, one who suffers torment on earth in return for a heavenly palm: G.A. Lee, *Leper Hospitals in Medieval Ireland* (Dublin, 1996), p. 19.
68  M. Chibnall, ed., *The Ecclesiastical History of Orderic Vitalis* (6 vols, Oxford, 1969–80), ii, p. 29.
69  Chibnall, *Ecclesiastical History*, ii, pp. 74–7.

writing until the Reformation.[70] Fears of epidemic disease and the prospect of unshriven, sudden death prompted a spate of late medieval penitential literature extolling the opportunities for spiritual development to be derived from protracted suffering. Perhaps it offered some relief to men and women who had abandoned any hope of earthly medicine. Anxious to make sense of his own failing sight and hearing, the chantry priest, John Audelay (*fl.* 1426), argued, like St Louis, that it was infinitely preferable

> To haue thi payne, thi purgatorye,
> Out of this wor[l]d or that thou dye,
> Fore God ponysshe not twyse truly.[71]

His lines echo earlier verses by the troubadour, Jean Bodel, who fell victim to leprosy soon after taking the cross in 1204. Although due allowance should be made for the literary conventions of the genre, his *Conges d'Arras* provides a moving – and rare – account of the inner turmoil experienced by those who had no choice but to endure their purgatory on earth. Having voluntarily decided to retreat from society, Bodel took the opportunity to solicit accommodation in the nearby *leprosarium* ('a place which has always delighted me') and bid farewell to his many friends (none of whom, including a physician, appear to have expressed the slightest reluctance to mix in his company).[72] Yet, despite the great kindness shown to him as his condition deteriorated, Bodel pulls no punches about the bleak future ahead, or his own initial sense of physical and spiritual isolation. Only after a long struggle does he recognise that leprosy offers a unique path to conversion and redemption. Like the penitential period of Lent, his sufferings will be followed by the festivities of Holy Week. In short,

> Everything will work for the best
> In the course of a hard and bitter life
> To make my soul clean and pure.[73]

Resisting the temptation to curse God, he ends by embracing his disease as an occasion for settling his spiritual debts in full before death.

For many, the leper was not merely elect of God; he *was* God, or at least an earthly reminder that, in putting on 'the kyndely infirmyte of the manhede', Christ had become the most despised and rejected of men.[74] His close similarity to Job, the Old Testament man of sorrows, was reinforced in late medieval iconography by images of His beaten and abused body, which shared many of

---

70  T. Matsuda, *Death and Purgatory in Middle English Didactic Poetry* (Woodbridge, 1997), pp. 167–9, 188.

71  E.K. Whiting, ed., *The Poems of John Audelay* (EETS, clxxxiv, 1931), p. 85.

72  G. Raynaud, 'Les congés de Jean Bodel', *Romania*, ix (1880), pp. 216–47. See also, C. Foulon, *L'oeuvre de Jehan Bodel* (Paris, 1958), part eight.

73  Raynaud, 'Congés', p. 238. M. Zink, 'Le ladre, de l'exile au royaume', *Exclus et systemes d'exclusion dans la littérature et la civilisation mediévales* (Senefiance, v, Aix-en-Provence, 1978), pp. 69–88, compares Bodel's poem with a similar set of verses by his contemporary, Baude Fastoul. The latter's view is more clear cut: for him purgatory on earth will automatically earn its reward in heaven.

74  The quotation is from the Carthusian, Nicholas Love, *The Mirror of the Blessed Life of Jesus Christ*, ed. M.G. Sargent (New York, 1992), pp. 161–2.

the features conventionally deployed in the depiction of lepers [**plate 5**].[75] Meditations upon the passion dwelt at length upon the lacerations inflicted upon 'his fayrest vysage', which 'aperyd more lyke a lepre than a verye man'.[76] Strikingly, whereas to Louis IX a leprous *soul* assumed 'the likeness of the devil', diseased *flesh* came, in theory at least, to share something of the divine.[77] Devotional literature of this kind commanded a wide, often female, readership in fourteenth- and fifteenth-century England. It developed, as we shall discover in chapter four, in tandem with medical texts on the importance of facial symptoms in the diagnosis of *lepra*, and dwells in graphic detail upon the physical brutality involved.

Thus, for example, a tract on the Holy Face, which belonged to the pious East Anglian gentlewoman, Anne Harling (d. 1499), describes how Christ, like Job, was left, friendless, to endure his ordeal:

For he was made so lothely [repulsive], what thorow buffeting and what thorow spitting, that thei on him spittid in his faire face, what for blood that stramed doune from the sharpe pricking croune of thornes that so desfigurid and so gresly made his face that he was mor whaltsum [loathsome] un to se then any mesell [leper]. Herto berith Isaie, the holi profet, witnes wher he saith *reputamus Christum quasi leprosum*, that is we areltiden [regarded] him as a lipor . . . Loke thu then, thu cristen man, in to the face of thi criste, ffor thus was he dight [condemned] all only for the loue of the.[78]

The enduring concept of *Christus quasi leprosus*, to which the author refers, owed its origins to St Jerome's rather free translation of the Book of Isaiah [53, v. 4] from Greek into Latin. In his *Vulgate* text, the verse beginning 'Surely he hath borne our griefs and carried our sorrows' concludes 'and we took him for a leper, and struck by God and humiliated'. Although the original Greek says nothing of leprosy, Jerome was anxious to stress that Christ had, indeed, assumed 'the likeness of sinful flesh' [Romans 8, v. 4] in its most wretched form.[79] This was demonstrably the case after His ordeal at the hands of His tormentors, which left Him covered from head to foot in wounds, bruises and

---

75 G. von der Osten, 'Job and Christ', *Journal of the Warburg and Courtauld Institutes*, xvi (1953), pp. 153–8.

76 A. Barratt, 'Stabant matres dolorosae: Women as Readers and Writers of Passion Prayers, Meditations and Visions', in A.A. MacDonald and others, eds, *The Broken Body: Passion Devotion in Late Medieval Culture* (Groningen, 1998), pp. 61–3. St Bridget of Sweden described Christ after his crucifixion 'as he had semed leprous and bloo, for his een [eyes] were dede and full of blude': R. Ellis, ed., *The Liber Celestis of St Bridget of Sweden* (EETS, ccxci, 1987), p. 22.

77 Joinville, *Life of St Louis*, p. 29.

78 BL, MS Harley 4012, fo. 92r. For Anne Harling, see G. McMurray Gibson, *The Theater of Devotion* (Chicago, 1989), pp. 96–105; and for the devotional context of such literature, R.N. Swanson, 'Passion and Practice: The Social and Ecclesiastical Implications of Passion Devotion in the Late Middle Ages', in MacDonald and others, *Broken Body*, pp. 1–30. One of the legends associated with Elizabeth of Hungary described how she nursed a leper in her bed. When her suspicious husband pulled back the curtains he saw an image of the crucified Christ: C. Gaignebet and J.D. Lajoux, *Art profane et religion populaire au moyen âge* (Paris, 1985), p. 109. See also below, p. 136 n. 136.

79 *Opera omnia: Commentariorum in Isaiam prophetam*, PL, xxiv, cols 506–7; Pichon, 'Essai sur la lèpre', pp. 354–5. According to medieval legend, the Jewish messiah was also 'as a leper', being a poor outcast, stricken with disease: L.B. Philip, 'The Prado *Epiphany* by Jerome Bosch', *Art Bulletin*, xxxv (1953), pp. 267–93; J.J. Brierre-Narbonne, *Le Messie souffrant dans la littérature rabbinique* (Paris, 1940), pp. 14–16, 56.

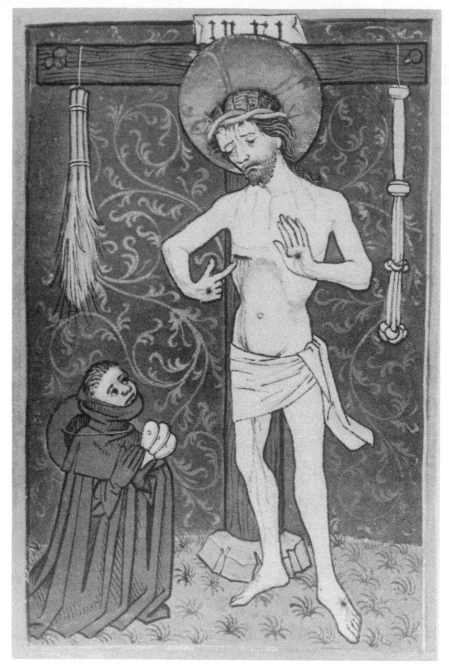

5. Christ assures the leper that, being Himself *quasi leprosus*, He shares his suffering, and can offer the faithful and penitent spiritual health through the blood He shed at the crucifixion. The instruments used to scourge His macerated flesh are depicted on the left and right. The leper is clad in the copious habit of a hospital, his covered hands and mouth reflecting late medieval ideas about contagion through the breath and skin. Like Dives, he carries a rattle for begging.

putrefying sores [plate 16]. As the Books of Isaiah [1, v. 6] and Job [2, v. 7] had prophesied, 'from the sole of his foot to the crown of his head, there is no health in him'. Hagiographers, such as Benedict, abbot of Peterborough (d. *c.* 1194), who recorded many of Thomas Becket's miracles, occasionally use these familiar words to describe extreme cases of *lepra* among pilgrims.[80]

The full implications of Christ's sacrifice were explained in one of Gregory the Great's most famous homilies. This tells the story of a monk named Martyrius, who encountered an exhausted leper on the road and carried him on his shoulders to the monastery gates. On their arrival, the poor creature metamorphosed into Christ and ascended to heaven, assuring the astonished monk that his kindness would be repaid in the next life. Having extolled the virtues of charity and compassion, Gregory observes

> What can be more abject in the flesh of man than the flesh of the leper, harrowed by swollen sores and suffused with nauseous exhalations? But see that He has appeared in the aspect of a leper; and He who is revered above all has not scorned to appear despised beneath all.[81]

Such a powerful story was readily absorbed into the western hagiographic and homiletic tradition. Flaubert's retelling of the legend of St Julian the Hospitaller drew upon one of many versions. Another may be found in the *vita* of the Irish saint, Colman Ela, who received his reward when the detritus left by a 'wretched leper' he carried into church and cleansed with his own tongue was transformed into an ingot of gold bearing an inscription forged by the Holy Trinity.[82] One of the miracles attributed to St Edward the Confessor by the twelfth-century chronicler, Roger of Howden, concerned his cure of a leper, whom he had borne on his shoulders, like Martyrius, in a gesture of humility appropriate to a king.[83] Most famously of all, St Francis's moment of conversion to the mendicant life hinged upon his encounter on the plains near Assisi with a leprous beggar, in whom he is said to have recognised Christ. Henceforward, according to his later biographers, he overcame his previous horror of the disease, and 'rendered humble service to the lepers with human concern and devoted kindness in order that he might completely despise himself, because of Christ crucified, who . . . was despised as a leper'.[84]

---

[80] J.C. Robertson, ed., *Materials for the History of Thomas Becket* (7 vols, RS, 1875–85), ii, pp. 245–6.

[81] *Opera omnia: Homiliarum in Evangelia, PL,* lxxvi, cols 1300–01.

[82] C. Plummer, ed., *Bethada Náem Érenn: Lives of the Irish Saints* (2 vols, Oxford, 1922), ii, pp. 172–3. Colman died in *c.* 610, but the undated *vita* is much later: ibid., i, pp. xxxii–xxxiii. Such tales circulated widely, as, for example, in Brandeis, *Jacob's Well,* pp. 247–8 (where, following Caesarius of Heisterbach, *The Dialogue of Miracles,* ed. H. von E. Scott and C.C. Swinton Bland (2 vols, London, 1929), ii, pp. 31–3, Ela has become a French bishop) and 264–5.

[83] Stubbs, *Chronica Rogeri de Houedene,* i, pp. 110–11. The story does not appear in the earlier, near contemporary, *Vita Ædwardi Regis:* F. Barlow, ed., *The Life of King Edward* (Oxford, 1992). It initially featured a cripple in Aelred of Rievaulx's hagiographical *Life of Edward the Confessor,* ed. J. Bertram (Guildford, 1990), pp. 48–50, but had far greater impact once the subject became leprous.

[84] E. Cousins, ed., *Bonaventure: The Soul's Journey into God; The Tree of Life; The Life of St Francis* (Toronto, 1978), pp. 189–90. The story was first recounted in about 1229 by Thomas of Celano in the *Vita prima* of St Francis, and refashioned in the *Vita secunda* of *c.* 1245 to emphasise the saint's dialogue with Christ rather than a human leper: C. Peyroux, 'The Leper's Kiss', in S. Farmer and B.H. Rosenwein, eds, *Monks and Nuns, Saints and Outcasts: Religion in Medieval Society* (Ithaca and London, 2000), pp. 172–3, 186–8.

The next chapter will explore how healthy men and women sought to exploit the spiritual assets of those whom they believed to command the ear of God, but we may note at this point that suitably penitent lepers were deemed capable of redeeming others as well as themselves. If *Christus quasi leprosus* had unlocked the chains of sin through His passion, might not the men and women he resembled perform a similar miracle? Alice of Schaerbeck (d. 1250), a Cistercian nun, certainly believed that her torments would release sinners from purgatory. Secure in the conviction that she had been chosen as a divine 'vessel of election' and would emerge burnished from the refiner's fire, she dedicated her leprosy to the ransoming of souls already 'subject to long excruciating detention in regions of penalty and for the sinners of this world'.[85] There were, however, limits as to what even the most saintly leper might achieve. The *Gesta Romanorum* tells of a pious young man who 'prayde oure lorde that he wolde sende hym a sekenesse in the stid [instead] of purgatorie'. After fifteen years of epilepsy, leprosy and 'the fyre of helle' (perhaps ergotism) all his sins were duly forgiven. But his efforts to release his late mother from purgation by repeating the ordeal on her behalf were doomed to failure. Her crippling burden of vanity and pride could only be shed through the miracle of the Mass.[86]

The purchase of heavenly bliss was rarely a matter for negotiation or compromise. The sinner had little choice but to accept the consequences of his or her actions, for which atonement would have to be made either in this world or the next. In a pre-Cartesian society, which regarded the human body as a frail but necessary lodging for the soul, it naturally followed that the welfare of one would intimately affect the other. Writers of medical literature were as concerned about gluttony, wrath and sexual indulgence as theologians and homilists, since the consequences of wrongful or reckless behaviour could have a dramatic impact on physical as well as spiritual health. In the second part of this chapter we shall explore the increasingly complex explanations for *lepra* and other degenerative illnesses advanced in a fast expanding corpus of material intended for practical use by physicians and surgeons. It is, however, important to reiterate that the intimate union then existing between medicine and religion would have made such an artificial distinction hard to comprehend.

## A question of balance

When describing attitudes to disease in the Classical world, the medical historian, G.D. Grmek, reminded his readers that beliefs about the causation and nature of illness 'are explanatory models of reality, not its constitutive elements'. In short, they should be regarded as the products of 'a certain medical philosophy or pathological system of reference', which can change radically over time, or from one society to another.[87] Some elements of the 'well articulated

---

85  *Acta Sanctorum*, xx, June II (11 June), p. 476 (her disease is described in the same words as Job's). For Alice, see C. Walker Bynum, *Holy Feast and Holy Fast: The Religious Significance of Food to Medieval Women* (London, 1987), pp. 115–16, 121, 234, 248–9.
86  S.J.H. Herrtage, ed., *The Early English Versions of the Gesta Romanorum* (EETS, extra series, xxxiii, 1879, reprinted 1962), pp. 401–2.
87  Grmek, *Diseases in the Ancient Greek World*, p. 1.

conceptual structure' of the Ancient Greeks, about whom Grmek wrote, lingered on in Western Europe after the collapse of the Roman Empire. Most were, however, recovered piecemeal, from the eleventh century onwards, through Latin translations of Hebrew and Islamic texts, which in many cases represented a significant reworking, development or digest of the originals. This composite 'medical ideology' was transplanted into, and significantly shaped by, the Christian culture where it now flourished. Despite some initial resistance on the part of ascetics, such as Bernard of Clairvaux, the widespread acceptance of Greek and Islamic medical knowledge proceeded apace. This was largely because it fitted – or could be made to fit – so easily into the existing framework of religious belief, most notably with regard to the close association between body and soul, disease and sin.[88]

The Greek view of health hinged upon an essentially simple, but comprehensive, principle of balance. This, in turn, derived from a belief that each individual represented a microcosm of the universe, and thus shared its component parts. Just as the cosmos had been created from earth, water, fire and air, and would become seriously disturbed if one of these *four elements* got out of control, so the human body needed a temperate mixture of coldness, moisture, heat and dryness to function effectively. Hippocrates (*fl*. 400 BC), whom medieval physicians hailed as the father of medicine, was widely believed to have defined and developed this theory of 'interacting qualities' or *humours*, which determined the relative heat and moisture of each individual. The melancholic humour was cold, dry and earthy; the phlegmatic humour cold and wet, like water; the choleric humour hot and dry, like fire; and the sanguine hot, wet and airy [**plate 6**]. To a notable extent, their proper management depended upon diet, 'the first principle of medicine', which assumed overwhelming importance in the preservation of health.[89]

As the product of an ongoing culinary process, the humours were generated from food that had been cooked in the stomach and thence transported to the liver. Under ideal conditions, the bulk of this mixture, done to a turn, would be converted into blood, while the residual uncooked matter became phlegm (potential blood). The foam, or froth, on the top changed into choler, or yellow bile, and the sediment at the bottom into black bile, or melancholia. Reserves of choler and black bile were stored, respectively, in the gall bladder and the spleen, the rest being transported with the blood and phlegm along the *vena cava* into the venous system, and thence to the vital organs and extremities. In a healthy body, surplus matter would be rapidly excreted in sweat, urine or faeces.[90] An excess of any humour could trigger serious illness, although choler and black

---

88  V. Nutton, *Ancient Medicine* (London, 2004), chapters four and sixteen; D.W. Amundsen, *Medicine, Society and Faith in the Ancient and Medieval Worlds* (Baltimore, 1996), chapter seven; and L.I. Conrad et al., *The Western Medical Tradition 800 BC to AD 1800* (Cambridge, 1995), chapters one to five, provide a valuable background to this section.

89  N. Siraisi, *Medieval and Early Renaissance Medicine* (Chicago, 1990), pp. 97–109.

90  These concepts were briskly set out in the *Isagoge*, a ninth-century Arab digest of Galenic medicine, which was available in the West from the late eleventh century, and became a standard text: E. Grant, ed., *A Source Book in Medieval Science* (Cambridge, Mass., 1974), pp. 705–15.

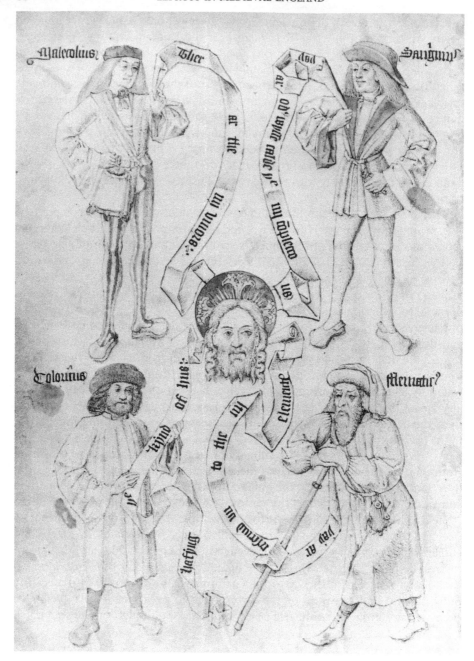

6. Produced for the barber surgeons of York in the late fifteenth century, this depiction of the four humoral types or temperaments (clockwise from the top right hand corner: sanguine, phlegmatic, choleric and melancholic) also reflects the belief that Christ (centre) alone after the Fall possessed a perfect balance and was thus unaffected by any of the physical imperfections resulting from original sin.

bile were deemed the most potentially dangerous. Demonstrating an apt choice of metaphor, one late medieval vernacular text explained:

> that ther be 4 humeros in man and 2 of thaim be frendes and 2 enemys. His 2 frendes be blode and flueme; his 2 enemies ben colre and malencolie. And for [because] they be enemies, kinde [Nature] hath prisoned thaim, wher colre in galle [gall bladder] and malencolie in the milte [spleen]. And if any of thaim breke prisone . . . they engendereth dedely sekenesse. And for blode and fleume ben frendes, kinde hath yeue [given] thaim leue [leave] to goo at large. But thair principal dwelling is in the blode and in the liuer and herte and flueme in the longes.[91]

To a medieval physician, who knew nothing of the circulation of the blood, the veins, arteries and nerves functioned in the same way as a network of rivers, streams and irrigation canals.[92] The venous blood, with its admixture of humours or *natural spirits*, fed and nurtured the entire body, enabling it to grow and reproduce [plate 7]. Some of this blood was transported directly to the heart, the source of natural warmth and thus of life itself. Here it was believed to pass through the septum, from the right ventricle to the left, where the purified or filtered product mixed with air from the lungs. Now transformed into frothy *vital spirits* or *pneuma*, it travelled along the arteries, carrying heat and life to the organs and limbs, any noxious vapours generated in the process being immediately exhaled, thus ridding the body of poison [plate 8]. The vital spirits destined for the brain underwent a further process of refinement on their passage through 'a marvellous network', or *rete mirabile*, at the top of the spine. From the time of its identification by Galen (d. *c.* AD 200), 'the prince of physicians', until Vesalius disproved its existence in the sixteenth century, this remarkable organ was believed to turn arterial blood into 'the finest kind of matter'. Once mixed with air from the nostrils, these *animal spirits* assumed the power not only to activate the motor neurone system (*via* the spinal chord) but also to mediate between 'animal perception' (the evidence of the senses) and the 'divine faculty of reason' [plate 9]. This was because they dwelt in immediate proximity to the soul itself.[93]

Mind and body thus enjoyed a symbiotic relationship, which depended upon the smooth working of this complex, finely tuned physiological system. An imbalance in the humours could have devastating consequences for human behaviour, plunging the body in a downward spiral of mental and physical instability. The *Pantegni* of Haly Abbas (al-Maǧūsī, d. 994), which circulated widely in a late eleventh-century translation by Constantine the African, maintained

---

91  I. Taavitsainen, 'Transferring Classical Discourse Conventions into the Vernacular', in eadem and P. Pahta, eds, *Medical and Scientific Writing in Late Medieval English* (Cambridge, 2004), pp. 52–3.
92  G.K. Paster, 'Nervous Tension: Networks of Blood and Spirit in the Early Modern Body', in D. Hillman and C. Mazzio, eds, *The Body in Parts: Fantasies of Corporeality in Early Modern Europe* (New York and London, 1997), pp. 112–16.
93  R.E. Harvey, *The Inward Wits: Psychological Theory in the Middle Ages and the Renaissance* (Warburg Institute Surveys, vi, 1975), pp. 2–28; N.G. Siraisi, *Taddeo Alderotti and his Pupils* (Princeton, 1981), chapter seven; F.D. Hoeniger, *Medicine and Shakespeare in the English Renaissance* (Delaware, 1992), pp. 72–178.

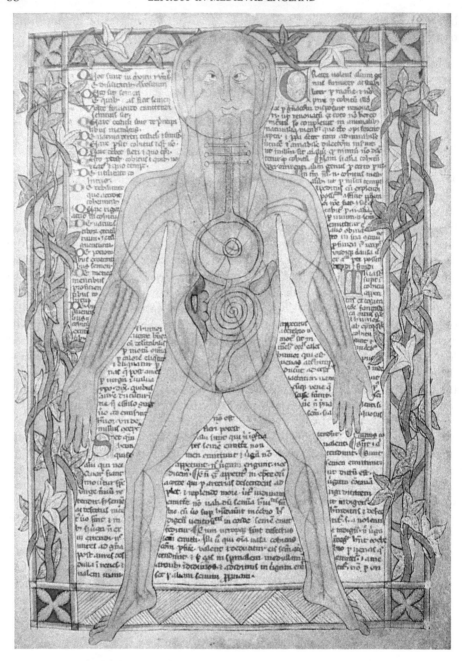

7. From an English-owned medical treatise of *c.* 1292, this diagram of the venous system depicts the stomach, intestines and liver (the leaf-shaped organ on the figure's right side), where the natural spirits (humours) are generated from food. These spirits are duly transported to the principal organs and extremities in the veins, thus providing the nourishment essential for growth and reproduction.

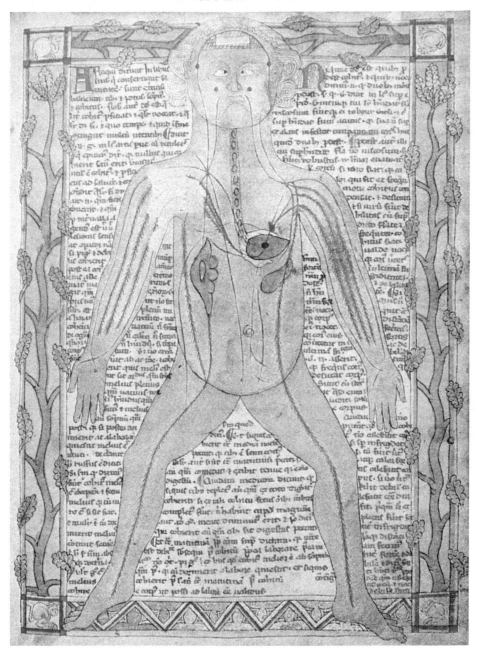

8. On its passage through the heart (the lozenge on the left of the figure's chest), the source of heat and life, some of the venous blood undergoes a process of purification. Then mixed with air from the lungs, it becomes *pneuma* or vital spirit and is carried by the arteries to the rest of the body, which is thus warmed and energised. This drawing of *c*. 1292 depicts the arterial system.

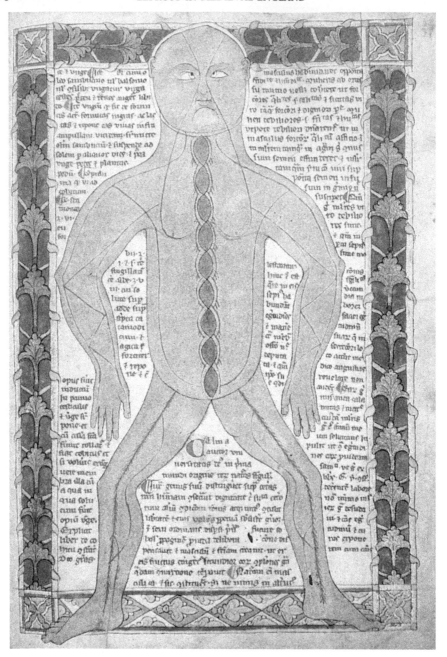

9. A further process of refinement occurs at the base of the skull, as some of the *pneuma* is filtered through a network known as the *rete mirabile*. Once combined with air from the nostrils, it assumes the power to animate the body, *via* the spinal cord and nervous system (illustrated in this textbook of *c.* 1292). The animal spirits not only enable the body to move, but also transmit the evidence of the senses to and from the brain, responding to such information with acute sensitivity.

that truly rational thought was conditional upon physical health.[94] Influenced by such works, theologians came to associate particular complexions with a predisposition towards specific sins as well as diseases: a choleric individual would, for example, be inclined to wrath, while his phlegmatic neighbour would have to fight against the demons of sloth and idleness. Yet this had not been God's initial plan for his creation. Scholars debated at length over the vexed question of Adam's immortality, speculating on the natural span of years he might have enjoyed had he remained in paradise, and the vulnerability of his then perfect constitution (*complexio equalis*) to decay.[95] But all were unanimous in blaming the Fall for the bitter legacy of pain, disease and death to which mankind was now heir.

On their expulsion from the Garden of Eden, Adam and Eve lost the vital humoral balance that had hitherto protected them from sickness. Through his sacrifice on the cross, Christ, who represented a unique state of perfection, had redeemed mankind from the spiritual consequences of original sin, which could henceforward be washed away through baptism.[96] The physical repercussions still remained, however: disease and mortality constituted a grim reminder of the collective punishment visited upon humanity through the disobedience of its first ancestors.[97] Moreover, the body's fragile mechanisms could be further upset in a variety of ways, which all too often involved intemperate, if not overtly transgressive, behaviour.

Whereas Galen had regarded any departure from humoral equilibrium (*discrasia*) as a potentially pathological condition, his Muslim and Christian successors were less prescriptive. In a postlapsarian society, striking variations of individual *temperament* seemed unavoidable. Women's damp, timid and fleshly bodies made them inherently phlegmatic, while men naturally veered towards the sanguine or choleric. Although factors such as diet, environment, heredity and lifestyle could easily upset conventional stereotypes of age and gender, the young of both sexes were held to be warmer and moister than the elderly, who grew progressively colder, drier and more melancholic with the passage of years. Such a process of desiccation was ultimately inimical to survival. According to the Franciscan friar, Bartholomaeus Anglicus (d. 1250):

> He [dryness] gendreth in bodyes ful euel sikenes . . . and is cause of inordynate therst, and maketh the wosons [arteries] rogh, and lettith the voice and maketh it hose [hoarse], and spoyleth the heede of here and maketh it balled, and draweth togidres and maketh croked toon [toes] and fyngres of fete and of hondes, *as it is iseye [seen] in leprous men.*[98]

---

94  *Liber Pantegni* (Lyon, 1515), *theorica*, liber IV, caps 19–20, fo. 17v; Harvey, *Inward Wits*, p. 14. The *Pantegni* fell out of favour more quickly in France than in England: Touati, 'Contagion', p. 193.

95  J. Ziegler, 'Medicine and Immortality in Terrestrial Paradise', in P. Biller and J. Ziegler, eds, *Religion and Medicine in the Middle Ages* (York, 2001), pp. 201–42.

96  Just as Naaman the leper was cleansed in the river Jordan: see below, pp. 125–6.

97  This was still the case in the nineteenth century. Writing in 1882, the Reverend W.M. Thomson compared the 'loathsome and polluting' disease of leprosy, which he believed to be hereditary, with 'man's moral leprosy', transmitted across the generations: G. Lewis, 'A Lesson from Leviticus: Leprosy', *Man*, new series xxii (1987), pp. 593–612, at p. 593.

98  Seymour, *On the Properties of Things*, i, p. 140.

A cold, dry, melancholic temperament therefore seemed the least desirable, although it was not in itself unhealthy. Natural, or 'kindly', black bile played an essential role in the body, thickening the blood, promoting the appetite, removing superfluities and nourishing the spleen and bones.[99] One could not live without it.

There was, however, another, far more malignant and aggressive variety, which (paradoxically, given its chilling effects) resulted from a process of *adustion*, or burning, of excess choler in the digestive tract.[100] This ashen and pernicious humour was feared for its 'deedliche qualities' and capacity to generate 'eueles vncurable, as cancre and lepre'.[101] As any medieval cook knew, the task of keeping an oven at the optimum temperature, so that food was neither charred nor underdone, could prove difficult. Similar considerations held good for the body's own oven, the stomach, which could easily become more like a furnace, thereby causing the liver to overheat in turn. Malfunction of the spleen would then open the floodgates of poison, demanding immediate and effective elimination. Any failure of the body's excretory mechanisms at this stage clearly spelt disaster. An injudicious diet or excessive consumption of alcohol was thus to be avoided by anyone of a vulnerable disposition. So too was exposure to bad air or other toxic substances, such as corrupt semen and menstrual blood. The section of the *Pantegni* devoted to *lepra* begins with a warning against these evils.

Some versions of this short text, which circulated separately as a manual for physicians, became known as *Constantini liber de elephancia*.[102] This was because writers of the Classical and early Christian period had generally used the words '*elephas*', '*elephancia*', or '*elephantiasis*' when they were discussing the disease we have hitherto called *lepra*. Since the vocabulary employed to describe medieval leprosy and its victims was destined to grow even more complex once four humoral sub-types had been identified and a significant body of vernacular literature began to circulate, it is worth pausing for a moment to examine how such a potentially confusing nomenclature developed.

### From *sāra'ath* to *elephancia*

Uzziah, Gehazi and all the other so-called 'lepers' mentioned in the Old Testament were suffering from a skin condition known in Hebrew as *sāra'ath*. Oceans of ink have been spilt in the search for a precise definition of this elusive word, which is widely believed to have embraced an eclectic range of dermatological

---

99   Seymour, *On the Properties of Things*, i, pp. 159–60; R. Klibansky, E. Panofsky and F. Saxl, *Saturn and Melancholy* (London, 1964), pp. 52–4, 98–102.
100  The process of digestion was not confined to the stomach, but continued in the liver and veins, until the natural spirits had been absorbed into the extremities.
101  Seymour, *On the Properties of Things*, i, p. 160.
102  *Liber Pantegni, practica*, liber IV, caps 2–5, fos 93r–94r; A.I. Martín Ferreira, ed., *Tratado médico de Constantino el Africano: Constantini liber de elephancia* (Valladolid, 1996), pp. 28–32, 74–99; E. Montero Cartelle and A.I. Martín Ferreira, 'Le *De elephancia* de Constantin l'Africain et ses rapports avec le *Pantegni*', in C. Burnett and D. Jacquart, eds, *Constantine the African and 'Alī Ibn al 'Abbās al Maǧūsī* (Leiden, 1994), pp. 233–46.

disorders. As we shall see in chapter three, the detailed and ritualistic prohibitions against *sāra'ath* in Mosaic Law itemised a number of imprecise, but far from life threatening, physical symptoms, such as scaly, scabrous and raw skin. Comparisons have, for example, been drawn with favus, psoriasis and eczema, which produce similar effects.[103] It has also been suggested that these biblical injunctions may have served to screen far more serious diseases, such as bejel (endemic syphilis) and perhaps even lepromatous leprosy (as we understand it today), but they were certainly not aimed specifically at them.[104] In short, the exercise confirms, yet again, the difficulties and pitfalls of attempting to diagnose retrospectively over past millennia.

When the Septuagint was translated from Hebrew into Greek in the second century BC, the problem of finding an equivalent word for such a vague term as *sāra'ath* was solved by the use of λέπρά (*lepra*). Associated in the Hippocratic corpus with a range of benign skin conditions characterised by flaky, discoloured patches, λέπρά offered a good match, because it, too, was remarkably comprehensive. Through this route, the word *lepra* entered the Latin *Vulgate*, and eventually became part of the vocabulary of medieval Christians. In describing Christ as a leper, Jerome wished to convey an image of bruised and damaged flesh, marked by the lesions which Hebrew priests had found so alarming.

During the first and second centuries AD, Greek and Roman physicians began writing about an apparently new and far more frightening disease, whose destructive, and almost invariably fatal, effects upon the human body seemed particularly repugnant.[105] Rufus of Ephesus (d. *c*. AD 117), one of the first to provide a coherent account of the symptoms, reports an understandable difficulty over terminology. His immediate predecessors, he observed, had called the early stages '*leontiasis*', because the sick assumed a distinctly leonine appearance. They began to smell very badly, their cheeks collapsed and their lips grew thick. As inevitable degeneration set in, a new name, '*satyriasis*' seemed more appropriate, since its victims developed a distinct resemblance to the satyrs of Greek myth. Not only did their eyebrows swell and their cheeks redden, but they also (he believed) were 'seized with a desire for sex'. Rufus was careful to distinguish this state of heightened arousal from the priapic condition of the same name described by many Greek authors, although, as we shall see, the assumption that some sufferers, at least, would be driven by lust proved remarkably tenacious.[106] Finally, once the entire body was affected, *elephantiasis* set in:

---

103  E.V. Hulse, 'The Nature of Biblical "Leprosy" and the Use of Alternative Medical Terms in Modern Translations of the Bible', *Palestine Exploration Quarterly*, cvii (1975), pp. 87–105, at pp. 96–100.

104  E. Lieber, 'Old Testament "Leprosy", Contagion and Sin', in Conrad and Wujastyk, *Contagion*, pp. 99–136, provides a valuable discussion of recent literature. See also Grmek, *Diseases in the Ancient Greek World*, chapter six.

105  A survey of the principal authors to write about *elephantiasis* may be found in F. Adams, ed., *The Seven Books of Paulus Aegineta* (3 vols, Sydenham Society, London, 1844–47), ii, pp. 6–15; and Simpson, 'Leprosy and Leper Hospitals', part ii, pp. 125–8.

106  This belief puzzles medical historians who wish to draw a precise correspondence between medieval leprosy and Hansen's disease, since the latter is often accompanied by a decline in the sex drive. S.R. Ell, 'Blood and Sexuality in Medieval Leprosy', *Janus*, lxxi (1984), pp. 153–64, at pp. 158–61, suggests that, in periods of remission, sufferers may experience surges of testosterone. But to Rufus, who made a pioneering study of melancholia, this temperament was notable for its inclination to lechery.

Now the symptoms are obvious: they consist of livid and black lumps, looking above all like bruises; some are located on the face, others on the arms, yet more on the legs; many also develop on the back, on the chest and on the stomach. At first these lumps are not ulcerated; later they also ulcerate in the most hideous manner, since this ulceration is accompanied by the swelling of the lips and such terrible putrefaction that, among some, the ends of the fingers fall away, and the ulcers never heal. It seems, therefore, that this is a superficial [i.e. dermatological] disease, because it manifests itself on the skin; but the difficulty of curing it, a difficulty which verges upon the impossible, prompts our opinion that it has a more deep-seated origin, an origin which it is not easy to fathom; it is, moreover, as deep-seated as is that of cancer, according to general opinion.[107]

Aretaeus the Cappadocian (first century AD) compared this devastating disease to an elephant, since 'it is the most powerful of all in taking life; and also for it is filthy and dreadful to behold'.[108] In short it behaved 'like a wild animal', and seemed to trample its victims underfoot with the same brutality. Moreover, the thick, rough, insensitive and fissured skin of its victims looked remarkably elephantine. Aretaeus and others, such as Caelius Aurelianus and Paulus Aegineta (d. 690), who came after him, developed a more detailed picture of *elephantiasis* and its victims, suggesting a range of palliative measures and debating the merits (as well as the feasibility) of segregation.[109]

Well before the end of the seventh century, educated Westerners seem also to have recognised that *lepra* and *elephantiasis* were entirely different.[110] One of the great reference works of the Middle Ages, the *Etymologiarum* of Isidore of Seville (d. 636), defined the former as a scaly skin condition, similar to a mottled herb called *lepida*, in which discoloured red, black or white patches erupted between areas of healthy flesh. *Elephantiasis*, however, gave rise to the elephantine appearance noted above, and to suffering of equal magnitude.[111] M.W. Dols has suggested that such a definition of *lepra* possibly embraced 'the macules and infiltrated lesions of tuberculoid leprosy', while *elephantiasis* may more confidently be equated with the *lepromatous* strain of Hansen's disease as we know it today.[112] Isidore and his contemporaries, on the other hand, thought in terms of degree, regarding *lepra* as, quite literally, superficial, while *elephantiasis* spread inexorably from within the body's deepest recesses.

The Muslim physicians and scientists who inherited and developed much of this late Classical literature observed a similar set of definitions and distinctions. Having considerable experience of both diseases, they greatly expanded the rele-

---

[107] Rufus's account of *elephantiasis* survives only in an encylopaedia by the Byzantine physician, Oribasios (d. 403), and may be found in French translation in J.G. Andersen, ed., *Studies in the Mediaeval Diagnosis of Leprosy in Denmark* (Copenhagen, 1969), pp. 44–5.

[108] F. Adams, ed., *The Extant Works of Aretaeus the Cappadocian* (London, Sydenham Society, 1856), pp. 366–73, 494–8, quotation at p. 368.

[109] Adams, *Seven Books of Paulus Aegineta*, pp. 1–5; Nutton, 'Did the Greeks Have a Word', p. 149.

[110] A degree of confusion in one pseudo-Galenic work of the first century, *Introductio seu medicus*, is almost certainly the result of textual corruption: C.G. Kühn, ed., *Claudii Galeni opera omnia* (20 vols, Leipzig, 1821–33, reprinted Hildesheim, 1964–65), xiv, pp. 757–8; Andersen, *Mediaeval Diagnosis of Leprosy*, pp. 41–2.

[111] W.M. Lindsay, ed., *Isidori Hispalensis episcopi, etymologiarum sive originum libri XX* (2 vols, Oxford, 1911), i, liber IV, cap. 8.

[112] Dols, 'Leprosy', p. 318.

vant pharmacopoeia, while also refining ideas about causation. As might be expected, their approach was based upon the Galenic theory described above, and represented a considerable advance in the proposed aetiology of *elephantiasis* (or *judhām*, as it was generally known in Arabic).[113] It now appeared that an excess of 'unnatural' black bile or adust choler was only the start of the problem. For it could poison each of the 'natural' humours, too, thereby giving rise to four specific sub-types or categories of symptoms, named after an appropriate animal. Al-Maǧūsī outlined this important diagnostic plan in the *Pantegni*:

| humour | type | animal | symptoms |
| --- | --- | --- | --- |
| sanguine blood hot/wet | alopecia | fox bald/mangy | red, hot swellings, corrupt |
| choleric yellow bile hot/dry | leonina | lion fierce/malodorous | yellow *maculae*, pustules, cracked skin |
| melancholic black bile cold/dry | elephancia | elephant strong/thick-skinned | black, cracked skin, tremors, contraction of digits |
| phlegmatic phleym cold/wet | tyria | serpent scaly/sheds skin | white, oil skin, humidity |

If, as often happened, more than one humour had been corrupted, a combination of symptoms would become apparent. The intense dryness and heat generated by putrefied choler and black bile would, for instance, damage the chest and voice, while also causing cracked, dry and ulcerated skin, inflammation and nervous damage.[114] Although it was further developed during the later Middle Ages, this schema provided a basic model that physicians, surgeons and educated laypeople were to follow for centuries.[115] It allowed for infinite permutations of symptoms and proved useful in diagnosing other diseases, too. Mental disturbances fitted especially well into three of the four humoral categories, which accounted for frenzy or acute dementia (choler), deep depression (melancholia) and catatonia or lassitude (phlegm). Here, too, 'unkindly' black bile was seen as the root cause of the initial imbalance.[116]

---

[113] M.W. Dols, 'The Leper in Medieval Islamic Society', *Speculum*, lviii (1983), pp. 891–916.

[114] *Liber Pantegni, practica*, liber IV, cap. 2, fo. 93r; Martín Ferreira, *Constantini liber de elephancia*, pp. 76–81.

[115] Andrew Boorde, *The Breuiary of Healthe* (London, 1552), describes these 'foure kyndes of leprousnes' which 'hath the properties of the beastes' (fo. 69v). One is 'the Olyphant sicknesse' (fo. 43r); another is like a fox, which sheds its hair and is scrofulous (fos 10v–11r); a third is marked by 'corodyng of the fleshe' like a serpent (fo. 112v); and the last, which devours the body with great ferocity, is leonine (fo. 70r). A number of short verses served as mnemonics for the practitioner: Andersen, *Mediaeval Diagnosis of Leprosy*, pp. 51–2; BL, MS Sloane 2272 (part 1), fo. 91v. Even so, some writers, such as the priest, John Mirfield (d. 1407), author of the *Breviarium Bartholomaei*, became confused: BL, MS Harley 3, fo. 21v.

[116] Klibansky, Panofsky and Saxl, *Saturn and Melancholy*, p. 88; Doob, *Nebuchadnezzar's Children*, pp. 23–8; Seymour, *On the Properties of Things*, i, pp. 348–51.

The Latin translators who tackled works such as the *Pantegni* were like explorers venturing into uncharted territory. The term *judhām* posed a particular challenge, since to render it as *elephantiasis* or *elephans* would not only cause obvious linguistic confusion between the disease and its third humoral subtype, *elephancia*, but also with an entirely different medical condition. Caused by a parasitic infestation of the lymph vessels, this chronic and debilitating disorder led to the extreme enlargement of specific body parts (usually the legs or scrotum). It was already known by the Arabs as elephantiasis (*dā' al fīl*), a name it still bears today.[117] Clearly, *judhām* did not trip easily off any Christian tongue and had to be rendered in a more accessible way for readers of Latin. What word would suffice? For Constantine the African and his pupils the obvious answer (or perhaps the result of a genuine misunderstanding) was to call it *lepra*, a familiar name that already encompassed a variety of skin diseases.

Gerard of Cremona (d. 1187) subsequently adopted this solution when he translated the *Canon* of Avicenna (Ibn Sīna, d. 1037) into Latin. Destined to become the most influential medical work in the late medieval West, it offered an 'authoritative compendium of traditional Greco-Roman scientific medicine', which was clearly and coherently organised into such topics as physiology, *materia medica*, pathology, surgery and the production of compound medicines.[118] The fourth book contained a lengthy section on *judhām* (now rendered as *lepra*), which was consistently plundered by the European physicians and surgeons we shall meet in subsequent chapters. It was, for example, Avicenna who devised three progressive categories of causation, the antecedent (production of corrupt matter in the liver), the conjoint (failure to expel it) and additional (factors likely to exacerbate the problem).[119] The impact of the *Canon* on western medical writing was, nevertheless, comparatively slow. In contrast to their continental peers, neither of the small and rather conservative faculties of medicine at Oxford and Cambridge incorporated it in the standard syllabus, although the scholars who trained there would undoubtedly have owned or had access to a copy.[120]

By then, however, the consequences of this mistranslation were already evident. Over time, medieval men and women came to believe that the many 'lepers' of the Old and New Testaments had contracted the disfiguring disease described in the *Pantegni* and other newly available medical texts, rather than something far less aggressive.[121] Such an assumption must have been confirmed by the distressing symptoms often displayed by the residents of local *leprosaria*, whose physical deformity alone sufficed to explain why biblical responses had been so extreme. Even so, a degree of ambiguity – if not outright perplexity –

---

117  Dols, 'Leprosy', p. 326.
118  L.E. Goodman, *Avicenna* (London, 1992), pp. 32–6.
119  Avicenna, *Liber canonis* (Venice, 1507, reprinted Hildesheim, 1964), liber IV, fen. iii, tractatus iii, cap. i, fo. 442v.
120  Rawcliffe, *Medicine and Society*, p. 108. For the greater impact of Avicenna in Italy, see Siraisi, *Taddeo Alderotti*, pp. 24, 62–3, 96–7, 108, 153; and in France, Touati, *Maladie et société*, pp. 148–51. The dissemination of Islamic texts in general is traced in D. Jacquart and F. Micheau, *La médecine arabe et l'occident médiéval* (Paris, 1990).
121  One Salernitan author soon observed that *elephantiasis* was being called *lepra* by the 'vulgar': Grmek, *Diseases in the Ancient Greek World*, p. 172.

about the meaning and derivation of specific terms lingered on, as successive generations of practitioners, encyclopaedists and theologians tried to make sense of such a divergent vocabulary. Monastic chroniclers and hagiographers, who knew their Isidore, spoke of *elephantiasis* when they wished to emphasise the severity of particular symptoms and thereby extol the miraculous powers of a healing saint. Thus, for example, Thomas of Monmouth, the biographer of William, the child martyr of Norwich (d. 1144), reports the apparent cure of a woman whose entire body 'was swollen and ulcerated as though afflicted with elephantiasis (*tanquam elephantino perclusa*)'.[122] With a striking regard for linguistic precision, the Battle Abbey Chronicle describes Abbot Walter de Lucy's 'compassion for lepers and those afflicted with elephantiasis (*leprosorum . . . et elephantiosorum*)', to whom he ministered in the 1160s with true Christian charity.[123]

But the distinction was not long preserved. As medical literature became both more copious and accessible, the terms *elephantiasis* and *elephancia* were deployed either as direct synonyms for *lepra*, or, more specifically, to denote what was generally perceived as its most invasive humoral type. Late medieval English readers accepted the wisdom of 'Constantinus', whose belief that 'eueriche *elefancia* or lepre hath bigynnynge principally of corrupcioun of melancolia' was enough to convince them that the two words described exactly the same chronic condition. The better informed among them also knew that the melancholic strain of the disease 'hath that name of the elephaunt that is a ful grete best and huge, for this euel greueth and noyeth the pacient passinge hugeliche and sore'.[124] At least that was the theory. In practice, however, a good deal of imprecision remained, for one layperson's idea of *lepra* was not necessarily another's. The question of semantics assumes particular importance when we come to examine the foundation of England's earliest leper houses, since we have no means of telling whether the intended inmates were to be leprous in the Levitical or Constantinian sense. Quite possibly the patrons themselves were unclear on this point.

The spread of vernacular texts during the fourteenth century further enlarged the vocabulary of disease, although the meaning of words such as 'mesel' and 'lazar' could vary according to the context in which they were used. The former, for example, generally denoted a leper (as defined by physicians such as Gilbertus Anglicus or Bernard Gordon), but could be employed more loosely in devotional works or poetry to describe any unprepossessing, scrofulous or simply wretched individual.[125] By the same token, a 'lazar', who took his or her name from the diseased beggar 'full of sores' in St Luke's gospel [16, vv. 19–31], might be depicted in various ways, not least as one of the malodorous and unwelcome vagrants who caused so much alarm to the late medieval state.[126]

122  Thomas of Monmouth, *The Life and Miracles of St William of Norwich*, eds A. Jessopp and M. Rhodes James (Cambridge, 1896), p. 148. See also, Robertson, *Miracles*, i, p. 213.
123  E. Searle, ed., *The Chronicle of Battle Abbey* (Oxford, 1980), pp. 260–61.
124  Seymour, *On the Properties of Things*, i, p. 423.
125  *MED, M–N, sub* 'mesel', pp. 360–61; W. Rothwell et al., eds, *Anglo-Norman Dictionary* (London, 1992), p. 421. The word derives from the Latin *miser* or wretched.
126  *MED, I–L, sub* 'laser', pp. 671–2; Rothwell, *Anglo-Norman Dictionary*, p. 380.

Despite these apparent inconsistencies, the identification and naming of diseases was no idle matter, for such words resonated with symbolic overtones and, as we shall see, were far from neutral.

### 'Malencolik mete' and 'fleschelie lust'

In common with other learned members of society, later medieval medical authorities demonstrated a profound veneration for their predecessors. Their work was littered with references to a pantheon of distinguished writers, dominated by Galen, his near contemporaries and the Muslims who had preserved, augmented and glossed this scattered oeuvre. Far from questioning or seeking to escape the parameters of Galenic humoral theory, they developed their arguments through the assiduous citation of past masters, eventually joining this august company themselves. Thus, the English physician, Gilbertus Anglicus, whose *Compendium medicine* (*c.* 1240) contains one of the first systematic accounts of *lepra* to be produced in the West, begins with a conventional description of the malignant effects of black (burnt) choler.[127] He describes how this venomous substance putrefies the entire system from within, dispelling its natural heat and moisture if a natural outlet cannot speedily be found.[128] None the less, he adds, with a deferential nod in the direction of Avicenna, whereas there is now a general consensus about the nature of this terrible disease, the exact process of causation remains a matter of debate. As the *Pantegni* had already warned, the slow and stealthy spread of corruption made it very difficult for a practitioner to identify what might have provoked the initial *discrasia* in each individual patient.[129]

Diet and sex were clearly prime suspects. Hot food, which would have the same effect upon the digestive process as throwing dry kindling on a fire, was clearly to be avoided, especially by those of a choleric disposition. Medieval advice manuals warned against the consumption of onions, lentils, leeks, pepper, red wine and spices by anyone who feared the onset of leprosy.[130] Garlic

---

[127] Gilbertus Anglicus, *Compendium medicine* (Lyon, 1510), fos 336v–345v. The *Compendium* is discussed and dated in F.M. Getz, ed., *Healing and Society in Medieval England: A Middle English Translation of the Pharmaceutical Writings of Gilbertus Anglicus* (Wisconsin, 1991), pp. liii–lvi.

[128] Gilbertus Anglicus, *Compendium medicine*, fos 336v–337r. In *c.* 1267, the Italian surgeon, Theoderic, gave Avicenna (*Liber canonis*, liber IV, fen. iii, tractatus iii, cap. i, fo. 442v) as his source for the view that leprosy was 'an evil condition arising from a bad constitution of the bile throughout the entire body, whereby the skin is corrupted in shape and appearance': E. Campbell and J.C. Colton, eds, *The Surgery of Theoderic* (2 vols, New York, 1955–60), ii, p. 167. Another surgeon, Henri de Mondeville (d. *c.* 1320), described it as 'an evil disease resulting from melancholic matter or from matter rendered into melancholy, corrupted by incorrigible putrefaction': E. Nicaise, ed., *Chirurgie de Maitre Henri de Mondeville* (Paris, 1893), p. 616. Bartholomaeus Anglicanus cited the *Pantegni*, observing that the disease was 'coolde euel and drye, and cometh of blake colera and strong iroted, and is isene in the vttir partie of the body': Seymour, *On the Properties of Things*, i, p. 423. John of Gaddesden (1304) concurred, reiterating Avicenna's belief that *lepra* was 'a common cancer of the whole body': *Rosa Anglica practica medicine a capite ad pedes* (Pavia, 1492), fos 55v–62r, at fo. 55v. All these works circulated widely in later medieval England.

[129] *Liber Pantegni, practica*, liber IV, cap. 2, fo. 93r; Martín Ferreira, *Constantini liber de elephancia*, pp. 74–5.

[130] John of Gaddesden, *Rosa Anglica*, fo. 56r; BL, MS Sloane 963, fo. 53v. For a fuller discussion of diet, see below, pp. 213–26.

seemed particularly dangerous. One devotional text compared it to self-will, which could prove a mixed blessing, for although 'hit is good for to do awey the scabbe, hit breedeth the lepere . . . norschith the frenesye and harmeth the syght'.[131] Gilbertus, and most commentators after him, felt that an unhealthy combination of fish and milk consumed at the same meal would have equally malign effects, through the generation of putrid phlegm.[132] As we saw in the previous chapter, a conviction that leprosy was caused, or at least exacerbated, by just such abuses lingered on until the nineteenth century. Galenic theory was, for example, invoked in a report on 'poor leprous men' on the Faroe Islands, made in 1670. Here it transpired that

> The meat of all, specially of the poorer sort, is half rotten flesh or fish, all their nourishment in Summer being likewise fresh fish and sweet Milk, without any Salt; wherefore he that is not of a strong and good complexion may easily have his blood corrupted, the sickness gnawing then it self throught [sic] the body, before it breketh out.[133]

In the medieval period, too, contaminated foodstuffs, most notably rancid oil and lard, infected pork and rotten fish were believed to breed disease. Since the poor often had little choice but to consume flyblown meat, the responsibility for removing 'pokky' or leprous wares from urban markets lay squarely at the door of local authorities. Late medieval English borough courts moved fast to dispose of 'mesel swynes felische' and other offensive goods, imposing heavy fines upon the stallholders who endangered public health, sometimes even consigning them to prison or the pillory. That such wares may also have seemed 'unclean' and polluted can only have compounded the problem.[134]

The ostensibly callous practice of giving leper houses food which had been condemned as unfit for human consumption seemed entirely logical at the time, since the residents were already riddled with disease and thus able to eat it with impunity.[135] The inmates of St Giles's hospital, Maldon, traditionally claimed the right to all forfeitures of 'bread, ale, flesh and unsound fish' made in the town; and in 1301 the York civic authorities allocated 'any measly meat' confis-

---

131 F.N.M. Diekstra, ed., *Book for a Simple and Devout Woman* (Groningen, 1998), p. 91.
132 Gilbertus Anglicus, *Compendium medicine*, fo. 337r; John of Gaddesden, *Rosa Anglica*, fo. 56r: Bodleian Library, MS Ashmole 1505, fo. 30v; BL, MS Harley 3, fo. 21v; MS Sloane 2272 (part 1), fo. 91v. Each of these authors was echoing Avicenna: O. Cameron Gruner, ed., *Treatise on the Canon of Medicine of Avicenna* (London, 1930), pp. 406–7.
133 L.J. Debes, *A Description of the Islands and Inhabitants of Foeroe . . . Englished by J[ohn] S[tarpin] Doctor of Physick* (London, 1676), pp. 311–12. In 1789, the naturalist, Gilbert White, suggested that improvements in hygiene and diet (except among 'the poorer Welsh who are subject to foul erup- tions') accounted for the virtual disappearance of leprosy from England: *Natural History and Antiq- uities of Selborne* (London, 1906), pp. 187–91. See also Simpson, 'Leprosy and Leper Hospitals', part 3, p. 408.
134 W. Hudson, ed., *Leet Jurisdiction in the City of Norwich during the Thirteenth and Fourteenth Centuries* (Selden Society, v, 1892), pp. 8, 16, 57, 80; Horden, 'Ritual and Public Health', p. 29; and below, p. 283.
135 In 1356, St John's hospital, Oxford, which accommodated the sick poor, was assigned 'all flesh or fish that shall be putrid, unclean, vicious or otherwise unfit' from the market, but the usual recipients of such doles were leprous: G.G. Coulton, *Medieval Panorama* (Cambridge, 1939), pp. 455–6.

cated in the market to local lepers.[136] Across the border, Scottish borough custom likewise decreed that 'corrupt pork and salmon' seized in markets should be assigned immediately to the leprous.[137] Rural communities of lepers, such as those at Thrapston and Cotes in Northamptonshire, fared rather better, as occasional assignments of freshly killed venison that had been abandoned by poachers were made to them, in keeping with forest law.[138] In Scotland, any 'wylde best . . . fundyn dede or wondyt' was likewise dispatched to the nearest house of 'lepir men' or else the poor. Medical authorities considered most game to be potentially risky, as its heavy, melancholic qualities could well destabilise a vulnerable patient. But those who had already lost the fight were at least free from such constraints.[139] The notorious propensity of pork to develop the same 'measly' spots and tubercules as the leper was blamed upon the irregular reproductive cycle of the sow, whose meat appeared particularly unwholesome after she had begun to breed.[140]

Similar considerations applied to women. As we have already seen, they were held to be damper and cooler than men, especially during their childbearing years. Although Classical ideas about the female body and its precise role in the process of generation were far from uniform, the belief that menstruation served to purge corrupt humoral matter which women were too cold or sedentary to eliminate gained widespread currency. It also, according to the Hippocratic corpus, removed excess blood before the system became saturated like a wet sponge and began to malfunction. During pregnancy, this 'plethora' would be transformed into nourishment for the growing embryo, and subsequently into milk for the newly born infant, but retention at other times might prove fatal.[141] The ubiquity of medical remedies to provoke abundant menses testifies to the alarm occasioned by amenorrhoea, which must have been common in times of dearth. Yet, although regular monthly purgation was both natural and essential for women's health, it could prove extremely harmful to others.

Menstruating women were themselves immune to its malignant effects, but men, small children, pregnant women, animals, foodstuffs and even metals appeared to be less fortunate. At least, so Pliny the Elder (d. AD 79), Isidore of Seville and the authors of late medieval advice literature, such as the hugely popular *De secretis mulierum*, maintained. Composed towards the end of the thirteenth century and (wrongly) attributed to Albertus Magnus, this influential text is notable both for its relentless misogyny and the emphasis that it placed

---

136  *CCR, 1402–1405*, pp. 17–18; M. Prestwich, ed., *York Civic Ordinances, 1301* (Borthwick Papers, xlix, York, 1976), p. 13. The importance of fresh food was, however, understood by patrons: below, pp. 327–8.

137  T. Thomson and C. Innes, eds, *The Acts of the Parliament of Scotland* (12 vols, Edinburgh, 1844–75), ii, p. 729.

138  G.J. Turner, ed., *Select Pleas of the Forest* (Selden Society, xiii, 1899), pp. 84, 89; R.M. Serjeantson and W.R.D. Adkins, eds, *VCH Northampton II* (London, 1906), pp. 154, 166.

139  Thomson and Innes, *Acts of the Parliament of Scotland*, ii, p. 692; and below, p. 213.

140  Fabre-Vassas, *Singular Beast*, pp. 55–6, 106. Contaminated pork seemed especially dangerous for those disposed to *lepra*: BL, MS Sloane 282, fo. 129v.

141  H. King, *Hippocrates' Woman: Reading the Female Body in Ancient Greece* (London, 1998), pp. 29–31; M.H. Green, ed., *The Trotula* (Philadelphia, 2001), pp. 19–22.

upon the toxicity of menstrual blood.[142] Suffused with this poison, the 'menstrous eye', for example, contaminates whatever it looks upon, while the woman's noxious exhalations poison the surrounding atmosphere:

> When men go near these women they are made hoarse, so they cannot speak well. This is because the venomous humours from the woman's body infect the air by her breath, and the infected air travels to the man's vocal chords and arteries, causing him to become hoarse.[143]

The author makes no direct connection between the gaze or breath of a menstruating woman and the onset of *lepra*, although it is interesting to observe how strongly the idea of polluted air as a vector of disease had now taken hold. The most serious risk lay, as both the *Canon* and the *Pantegni* had previously pointed out, to any offspring that might be conceived at this inauspicious time.[144] Nurtured from the start on such cold, venomous matter, the embryo was likely to be leprous, epileptic, deformed or at least cursed with red hair. Indeed, although some theologians (and the eminent French surgeon, Henri de Mondeville) argued that Jews were far less likely to contract *lepra* because of the strict Mosaic Law regarding contact with menstruating women and the consumption of pork, late medieval iconography consistently depicted them as redheaded, ulcerated and physically deformed.[145]

Like *sāra'ath*, menstrual blood was regarded as a pollutant by the tribes of Israel, and thus gave rise to a number of stringent taboos. Offenders who broke the absolute prohibition upon coitus at this time were condemned to be 'cut off from among their people' [Leviticus 20, v. 18], although the purpose of such measures was to avoid ritual defilement rather than to protect any potential offspring.[146] The medical connection seems first to have been made by St Jerome in his commentary upon Ezekiel 18, v. 18. The original verse cautions the righteous man not to approach a menstruating woman. He added the further warning that:

> Each month the heavy and torpid bodies of women are revealed through the effusion of unclean blood. If a man has sex with a woman at this time, the foetuses that are conceived are said to absorb the corruption of the semen, so that lepers and sufferers from *elephantia* (*leprosi et elephantiaci*) are born from this conception; and the polluted blood deforms the vile bodies of both sexes through the inadequacy or enormity of the members . . .[147]

---

[142] H.R. Lemay, ed., *Women's Secrets: A Translation of the Pseudo-Albertus Magnus's De secretis mulierum with Commentaries* (Albany, New York, 1992), pp. 15, 18, 36–7, 48, 129; J. Cadden, *Meanings of Sex Difference in the Middle Ages* (Cambridge, 1993), pp. 174–5, 268; D. Jacquart and C. Thomasset, *Sexuality and Medicine in the Middle Ages* (Oxford, 1988), pp. 71–86.

[143] Lemay, *Women's Secrets*, pp. 130.

[144] Avicenna, *Liber canonis*, liber IV, fen. iii, cap. 1, fo. 442v; *Liber Pantegni, practica*, liber IV, cap. 2, fo. 93r; Martín Ferreira, *Constantini liber de elephancia*, pp. 74–5.

[145] P.J. Payer, *The Bridling of Desire: Views of Sex in the Later Middle Ages* (Toronto, 1993), p. 109; Cadden, *Meanings of Sex Difference*, p. 268; Fabre-Vassas, *Singular Beast*, p. 25; Nicaise, *Chirurgie de Henri de Mondeville*, p. 616; R. Mellinkoff, *Outcasts: Signs of Otherness in Northern European Art of the Late Middle Ages* (2 vols, Los Angeles, 1993), i, pp. 147–59, 163–8, 188.

[146] M. Douglas, *Purity and Danger: An Analysis of the Concepts of Pollution and Taboo* (London, 1966, reprinted 1994), chapter three.

[147] Saint Jerome, *Opera omnia: Commentariorum in Ezechielem*, PL, xxv (Paris, 1884), vi, cap. xviii, col.

Jerome's words were reiterated in medieval penitentials, which demanded long and arduous expiation of anyone who confessed to a sin that ranked alongside murder in its enormity.[148] Although, as we shall learn in chapter four, offenders rarely experienced the full force of canon law, the association between menstrual blood, disobedience and physical corruption remained strong, not least because monthly purgation was demonstrably the curse of Eve. There had, after all, been no need for it in paradise.[149] Aimed at a married female readership, one early fifteenth-century book of homilies stressed the physical rather than the moral consequences of engaging in sexual activity at forbidden times:

> That is whan he [her husband] woot that sche hath that yuel that is comune to wommen by certeyn tymes of the monthe. For hit is forboden by God in the olde lawe, for many periles that cometh therof. For as, as seith seint Ierom [Jerome], in suche tyme beth geten mesells [lepers], maimed, vnschapliche, witles, croked, blynde, lame, dowmbe, deef and of many othre mescheues.[150]

Medical anxieties on this score continued long after the Reformation. A popular sixteenth-century *Questyonary of Cyrurgyens*, observed that any child conceived 'in the tyme that the woman hath her floures [period], and that she be nat clene' would be lucky to escape 'lepry', being, at the very least, 'scalled, or touched with suche infecte dyseases'.[151] Indeed, as late as 1720, verses *On the Art of Getting Beautiful Children* warned about the 'foul, leprous spots' likely to disfigure such a 'miscreated thing'.[152]

Could a menstruating woman harm her sexual partner as well as their unborn child? *De secretis mulierum* urged that 'a man should be especially careful not to have sexual intercourse with women who have their periods because by doing so he can contract leprosy and become seriously ill'.[153] Fears of cancer and sterility were also common. Because menstrual blood was deemed to be cold as well as poisonous, men of a phlegmatic or melancholic temperament seemed especially at risk, but all took a gamble by engaging in such illicit activities.[154]

Far more dangerous, though, was coitus with a woman who had previously been impregnated by a leper. Drawing upon the information newly available

---

173. Payer, *Bridling of Desire*, p. 231 n. 126, suggests that Jerome was drawing upon far earlier sources.

[148] Robert of Flamborough, *Liber poenitentialis*, p. 238; St Ivo, *Opera omnia*, PL, clxi, *Decreti pars x*, cols 688–9; Jacquart and Thomasset, *Sexuality and Medicine*, pp. 186–7. Ignoring the medical rationale behind this prohibition, Caesarius of Arles argued that, in addition, sexual activity on a Sunday or a feast day would result in offspring that were leprous, epileptic or possessed by devils: Pichon, 'Essai sur la lèpre', p. 352; Touati, *Maladie et société*, pp. 109–15.

[149] C.T. Wood, 'The Doctor's Dilemma: Sin, Salvation and the Menstrual Cycle in Medieval Thought', *Speculum*, lvi (1981), pp. 710–27; Cadden, *Meanings of Sex Difference*, pp. 72–3.

[150] BL, MS Harley 45, fo. 119v. I am most grateful to Professor Martha Carlin for drawing my attention to this source, which, significantly, has abandoned Jerome's distinction between *leprosi* and *elephantici*.

[151] Robert Copeland, trans., *Questyonary of Cyrurgyens* (London, 1542), sig. Qii verso. This text is based on the 'Lytell Guydo', or *Cyrurgie* of Guy de Chauliac.

[152] P. Crawford, 'Attitudes to Menstruation in Seventeenth-Century England', *Past and Present*, xci (1981), pp. 47–73, at p. 63.

[153] Lemay, *Women's Secrets*, pp. 88, 131.

[154] Cadden, *Meanings of Sex Difference*, p. 286.

from Islamic texts, twelfth-century physicians at the celebrated Italian medical school of Salerno produced a significant corpus of literature on human anatomy.[155] Their findings were encapsulated in a series of questions and answers that initially circulated in Latin among academic readers, such as Adelard of Bath (d. *c.* 1152), who used them in scholastic debates. Eventually, however, they became a matter of common knowledge, providing the interested layman or woman with a useful bedrock of medical information. One set of over three hundred Salernitan questions was compiled by an associate of Hugh de Mapenore (who later became bishop of Hereford) in about 1200, and conveyed current assumptions about the sexual transmission of *lepra* in unambiguous terms. Why was a woman left unharmed after having sexual relations with a leper, when the first healthy man to enjoy her favours thereafter would contract the disease? The reason, set out in three separate answers, hinged upon the inherent density and coldness of the female complexion, which was said to be 'hard and extremely resistant to male corruption'.[156] The toxic semen produced from the contaminated blood of the leper thus remained secure within the thick, protective walls of her uterus. Here it turned into to a clammy and putrid vapour. Since men were believed to be much hotter than women, especially during sex, it followed that the 'attractive force' of the penis would absorb any moisture through the open pores. In this way the poisonous miasma entered her next partner's body, being transmitted from the genitals to the other organs by the natural, vital and animal spirits. 'Thus', notes the author, 'it is said that, in those who become leprous this way, ulcers appear first on the penis and then elsewhere'.[157]

Gilbertus Anglicus warned ominously that, if such a woman were to ejaculate during coitus, the threat to her partner would increase exponentially. Her semen would mix with that left by the leper, rendering it more mobile, and thus increasing the speed of absorption.[158] Galen's belief that both male and female semen was essential for conception ran counter to that of Aristotle, who assigned women a more passive role in reproduction.[159] But the Galenic 'two seed' model was widely accepted by medical practitioners, and in this instance served to make coitus appear even more threatening to men. The immunity apparently enjoyed by females was not, however, complete. Despite its undoubted strength, the uterus was not capable of containing the levels of poison likely to accumulate through frequent sexual activity with lepers over a sustained period.[160]

---

[155] Jacquart and Thomasset, *Sexuality and Medicine*, pp. 16–35; Green, *Trotula*, pp. 3–14.

[156] B. Lawn, ed., *The Prose Salernitan Questions* (Oxford, 1963), pp. 9 (no. 14). See also, pp. 18 (no. 33), 101 (no. 187). Adelard discussed women's immunity in his *Questiones naturales*, which were based on Arab texts: C. Burnett, ed., *Adelard of Bath, Conversations with his Nephew* (Cambridge, 1998), pp. 168–9.

[157] Lawn, *Prose Salernitan Questions*, p. 18 (no. 33).

[158] Gilbertus Anglicus, *Compendium medicine*, fo. 337r–337v.

[159] Cadden, *Meanings of Sex Difference*, pp. 23–4, 34, 93–7; T. Laqueur, *Making Sex: Body and Gender from the Greeks to Freud* (Cambridge, Mass., 1992), chapter two.

[160] Gilbertus Anglicus, *Compendium medicine*, fo. 337v. As the *Lytell Guydo* pointed out, all noxious matter was purged from the uterus on a monthly basis, 'whiche a man can nat do, bycause he hath no receptable whereto hold the sayd immundycytees [poisons]': Copeland, *Questyonary of Cyruryens*, sig. Qii verso.

Many – but certainly not all – of the medieval physicians and surgeons who wrote about *lepra* make some reference to the dangers of sexual congress with women who were known to associate with victims of the disease, or who had contracted it themselves (in which case their semen would also be toxic).[161] In his *Lilium medicine* (1303) the French physician, Bernard Gordon, drew on personal experience when discussing this means of transmission. An English translation of this celebrated work was made for Robert Broke, the master of the royal stillatories, in the second quarter of the fifteenth century and repeats the cautionary tale:

> A countesse that was leprous come to Mounpeleris [Montpellier] and atte last heo was in my cure and a squier that serued here lay by her & brought her with childe. And the man bycome leprous: therefore they sculleth be y-blessyd that beth war of paryles [avoid such risks].[162]

Bernard briefly noted a few prophylactic measures for the elimination of corrupt semen from the uterus, but was less explicit than authorities such as Gilbertus Anglicus, Theoderic, John of Gaddesden and Henri de Mondeville, each of whom devoted some space to this topic. They itemised the symptoms likely to follow an ill-advised sexual encounter, observing that the patient's colour would change dramatically from redness to pallor, or *vice versa*, as his temperature fluctuated from heat to cold and back again. Unpleasant 'crawling' sensations might also be experienced beneath the skin, sometimes accompanied by chills or stiffness. His face would be flushed, and feel as if it were erupting in abscesses.[163] As we shall see in chapter five, it was generally assumed that such conditions might be healed through prompt recourse to medical help, speed being essential.

The renegade Franciscan, Arnaud de Verniolles, one of many flamboyant characters to enliven Emmanuel Le Roy Ladurie's study of life in early fourteenth-century Montaillou, claimed that his face became extremely swollen after visiting a prostitute. Such was his apparent terror at the prospect of contracting leprosy that he vowed never to consort with women again and turned instead to the pleasures of sodomy with young men.[164] Fear that he might fall victim to the pogrom then being waged against the lepers of southern France may perhaps have served further to justify his sexual preferences, although concerns about prostitution as a vector of leprosy were hardly new. One of Thomas Becket's early miracles concerned a man named Odo de Beaumont,

[161] Demaitre, 'Description and Diagnosis', pp. 327–44, assesses the evidence.
[162] Bodleian Library, MS Ashmole 1505, fo. 30v. For more on this MS, see L.E. Voigts, 'The Master of the King's Stillatories', in J. Stratford, ed., *The Lancastrian Court* (Stamford, 2003), pp. 233–52; and for Gordon, L. Demaitre, *Doctor Bernard de Gordon: Professor and Practitioner* (Toronto, 1980).
[163] Campbell and Colton, *Surgery of Theoderic*, ii, pp. 178–9; Gilbertus Anglicus, *Compendium medicine*, fo. 344r; John of Gaddesden, *Rosa Anglica*, fo. 61r–61v; Nicaise, *Chirurgie de Henri de Mondeville*, pp. 624–6. Fifteenth-century regulations for the Southwark brothels forbade women with 'any sikeness of brennynge' (generally believed to be gonorrhoea) and 'the perilous infirmite' from working there, but do not specifically mention *lepra*: J.B. Post, 'A Fifteenth-Century Customary for the Southwark Stews', *Journal of the Society of Archivists*, v (1977), pp. 418–28, at p. 426.
[164] E. Le Roy Ladurie, *Montaillou: Cathars and Catholics in a French Village 1294–1324* (Harmondsworth, 1980), p. 145. Significantly, some of these acts took place in a field near the *leprosarium* at Pamiers, presumably because it was fairly secluded: Goodich, *Other Middle Ages*, pp. 127–8.

who had reputedly become leprous immediately after recourse to a prostitute. Having confessed his sins, embarked on a strict fast and promised to undertake a pilgrimage to Becket's shrine, he was cured. A temporary lapse (evidently of a sexual nature) led to a resurgence of the disease, after which he remained both chaste and chastened.[165]

The Church exploited these fears, sometimes in surprising ways. The *Gesta Romanorum* offered preachers the memorable homily of two knights, Envy and Avarice. The latter wants to acquire Envy's land, and persuades his reluctant wife, who is very beautiful, to offer herself to him as the purchase price. Being himself married to a wretchedly ugly creature, Envy is jealous of his neighbour's good fortune. So much so, that he deliberately contracts leprosy in order to infect Lady Avarice when they sleep together, thereby making her just as undesirable as the hideous Lady Envy. On learning about this cruel deception, Avarice advises his stricken wife to leave for the nearest university town, where she can proposition a passing student. Suspecting nothing (some parables are timeless), he will absorb the poison from her, contract the disease and leave her free from contagion. Since the son of the Emperor is the first to solicit her favours, she deems it prudent to reveal her condition, but he persists and duly cures her *lepra* by assuming it himself. He, in turn, eventually recovers from the disease after a painful course of treatment. It says much for the creativity of the medieval imagination that the student symbolises Christ, the Saviour of mankind, while Lady Avarice is, of course, Eve, who has been infected with the leprosy of original sin.[166] In the present context, though, the story is notable for a choice of a metaphor that reflects widespread ideas about the sexual transmission of an apparently curable type of *lepra*.

Such beliefs were certainly shared by the King's Lynn mystic, Margery Kempe, whose spiritual autobiography records the distress occasioned by her unmarried son's dissolute lifestyle and her wish that God would punish him for failing to remain 'clene'. Sure enough, while he was away on business overseas his 'synne of letchery' incurred its due reward. 'Sone aftyr', she reports with grim satisfaction, 'his face wex ful of whelys and bloberys *as it had ben a lepyr*.' By refusing to see the young man until he 'prayed for grace', Margery ensured that first his soul and then his body would be purged of disease. He duly recovered his spiritual and physical health, never to fall again.[167] She was not the only member of Lynn's merchant elite to express concern on this score, for a few years earlier the expatriate community in Danzig had imposed a series of disciplinary measures on its 'yong men'. 'Kepyng dishaunttyngely to ony onnonest [dishonest] woman' figured prominently on the list of prohibitions.[168]

That many presumed lepers carried no personal blame whatsoever for their

---

[165] Robertson, *Materials*, i, p. 340. Sermons *ad status* preached to the young and to married couples often invoked the threat of leprosy as a means of regulating sexual conduct: J. Bird, 'Medicine for Body and Soul: Jacques de Vitry's Sermons to Hospitallers and their Charges', in Biller and Ziegler, *Religion and Medicine*, pp. 92–3.

[166] H. Oesterley, ed., *Gesta Romanorum* (Berlin, 1872), pp. 507–9.

[167] S.B. Meech, ed., *The Book of Margery Kempe* (EETS, ccxii, 1940), pp. 221–3.

[168] D.M. Owen, ed., *The Making of King's Lynn* (Records of Social and Economic History, new series, ix, 1984), p. 279.

condition was, however, widely acknowledged. They were, as Avicenna observed, often the victims of a hereditary disease. Since both male and female semen constituted a refined form of venous blood, any contaminated humoral matter would naturally be transmitted to such offspring at conception. As it developed, the foetus might be nurtured on infected blood, and the newborn child 'i-fedde with corrupt melke of a leprous norse' or diseased mother.[169] Thomas Gascoigne's snide remark about the Pecok family's history of *lepra* reflects a widespread assumption that the disease, or at least a predisposition towards it, would pass from one generation to the next 'as it were by lawe of heritage'.[170] Nor was the belief that 'a leper begets a leper' simply a matter of popular gossip and innuendo. Physicians and surgeons often began their examination of a suspect by asking 'if he be comen of the kynde [kindred] of lepres', before moving on to investigate his diet and way of life.[171] Observation none the less confirmed that, just as a healthy individual might live among the sick without contracting their disease, so too a leprous person could well produce unblemished issue.[172] How? One explanation for this conundrum focussed upon the other parent. The child of a male leper and a robust woman with a healthy uterus might, for example, escape with nothing more than a mild rash or benign skin condition, which could be managed by a good physician.[173]

Although it clearly alarmed the Church and naturally concerned practitioners, illicit or ill-judged sexual activity constituted only one of many explanations for the onset of *lepra*. Other sins besides lechery posed a risk to health, and other factors, such as diet and environment, were just as likely to determine whether or not the disease developed. It is therefore appropriate to ask why historians have recently paid so much attention to medieval ideas about the venereal transmission of leprosy at the expense of other theories of causation. The transformation of the medieval leper into a 'living symbol of lust and promiscuity . . . infecting society with its rampant sexuality' poses some interesting questions.[174] As we shall see in chapter six, fear of pestilence, unrest and vagrancy encouraged the stigmatisation of 'wild' or transient lepers during the fourteenth and fifteenth centuries. The belief, initially expressed by Rufus of Ephesus and his near contemporaries, that leprosy made its victims unusually

---

169 Avicenna, *Liber canonis*, liber IV, fen. iii, cap. 1, fo. 442v; Gilbertus Anglicus, *Compendium medicine*, fos 337r, 338r; Seymour, *On the Properties of Things*, i, p. 426. By the same token, healthy parents would not beget leprous offspring, since only corruption could generate corruption: Lawn, *Prose Salernitan Questions*, pp.18–19 (no. 34). The previously healthy embryo of a pregnant woman who had sex with a leprous man might, on the other hand, be contaminated by his semen: Bodleian Library, MS Ashmole 1505, fo. 30r; BL, Sloane MS 2272 (part 1), fo. 91v.

170 Seymour, *On the Properties of Things*, i, p. 426.

171 Ogden, *Cyrurgie of Guy de Chauliac*, p. 381; Demaitre, 'Description and Diagnosis of Leprosy', p. 332. It has recently been suggested that between a quarter and half of the children born to parents with lepromatous leprosy will develop some symptoms of the disease (although many heal spontaneously): M.E. Lewis, 'Infant and Childhood Leprosy: Present and Past', *PPL*, p. 163. In some cases, at least, medieval practitioners must have been observing this phenomenon.

172 BL, MS Sloane 2272 (part 1), fo. 91v; Touati, 'Contagion', p. 190.

173 Demaitre, 'Description and Diagnosis', p. 332.

174 Richards, *Sex, Dissidence and Damnation*, pp. 155–6. See also Dols, 'Leper in Medieval Islamic Society', p. 891; Hepworth and Turner, *Confession*, p. 23; and Saunders, *Suitable Island Site*, pp. 1, 58, who assumes that, during the Middle Ages, the 'unwary associate' of any leprous person would also have been tarred with the brush of extreme depravity.

licentious tended to fuel this anxiety. The treatment of fictional characters, such as Robert Henryson's Cresseid, who is already 'maculait', or spotted, with the sin of 'fleschelie lust', as if they were real historical case studies has further consolidated the intimate relationship between sexual licence and leprosy that now features so prominently in mainstream scholarship.[175] Yet it is the protracted debate about the origins of syphilis (the pox), which began in the sixteenth century and still continues today, that has proved especially influential in this regard. It has fostered a persistent belief that most so-called English 'lepers' were not only suffering from venereal disease but were inevitably seen by their contemporaries as the personification of moral depravity.[176]

As initial attempts to explain *elephantiasis* reveal, medical practitioners often found it difficult to accommodate new diseases within the existing framework of humoral theory. This was especially true of epidemics, since their rapid and apparently indiscriminate progress did not immediately accord with the concept of personal balance and *discrasia* described above. The development of ideas about contaminated air and planetary forces, to which we shall presently turn, clearly helped to establish a more plausible aetiology. Both explanations were advanced to account for the outbreaks of pox that swept Europe in the late fifteenth and sixteenth centuries, as, understandably, were others drawn (like many initial attempts at treatment) from the substantial corpus of medical literature on *lepra*. Given the apparent similarity between their respective symptoms, it seemed to many physicians that the two diseases must be closely related. Was the pox actually a new strain of leprosy? Or might it perhaps develop into 'lepre' as part of an ongoing degenerative process? Opinions varied, especially at first.[177] Some writers, including Paracelsus (d. 1541), traced the epidemic back to 'a leprous knight at Valencia', whose encounter with a diseased prostitute had led to the infection of the royal army and thence the rest of Europe. Inevitably, traditionalists blamed the toxic nature of menstrual blood, although scepticism on this score became increasingly apparent.[178] That the pox was spread through the retention of infected semen in the humid bodies of prostitutes won widespread credence, especially as evidence of sexual transmission became increasingly apparent.[179]

The pox soon acquired a distinct literature and aetiology of its own, but the close connection with *lepra* lingered on, not least in the use of iconographic representations traditionally associated with the medieval leper.[180] A shared repertory of patron saints (notably Job) and, most tellingly, a common vocabulary highlighted these perceived similarities. In the interests of hygiene and public order, disused or half-empty *leprosaria* were earmarked as refuges and

175  Henryson, *Testament of Cresseid*, p. 28; and above, pp. 73–4.
176  See, for example, Brody, *Disease of the Soul*, p. 146. Grigsby, *Pestilence*, pp. 42–4, 70–77, 157–77.
177  Ulrich von Hutten, *De morbo Gallico*, trans Thomas Paynell (London, 1533), sig. A 5v, maintained that 'these infirmities be very neighbours one to another' and could thus mutate.
178  W. Schleiner, 'Infection and Cure through Women: Renaissance Constructions of Syphilis', *Journal of Medieval and Renaissance Studies*, xxiv (1994), pp. 499–517. Arrizabalaga, Henderson and French, *Great Pox*, passim, and for specific comparisons with leprosy pp. 14, 25, 79, 85.
179  Amundsen, *Medicine Society and Faith*, p. 331.
180  J. Fabricius, *Syphilis in Shakespeare's England* (London, 1994), pp. 3–5, 259.

dumping grounds for the pox-ridden poor, giving the words 'spital', 'lazar' and 'loathsome leprosie' a whole new meaning.[181] Pistol's reference to the prostitute, Doll Tearsheet, as 'the lazar kite of Cressid's kind' in Shakespeare's *Henry the Fifth* reflects this pejorative shift in usage. So too does the eruption in sixteenth-century Britain of oaths and imprecations combining leprosy and the pox in richly creative, if repetitive, permutations.[182] Evidently unaware of the changing role of former leper hospitals, nineteenth-century contagionists cited the draconian new regulations promulgated for institutions such as Greenside, Edinburgh (1591), and Brigend, Glasgow (1610), as proof positive that the medieval leper was subject to stringent and oppressive controls.[183]

The suggestion that misdiagnosed venereal disease probably accounted for most cases of medieval *lepra* was first raised during the nineteenth century, in part as a reaction against the powerful segregationist lobby. But licentiousness and leprosy were closely linked in the Victorian imagination long before Charles Creighton argued in 1894 that the inmates of English *leprosaria* must generally have been suffering from *lues venerea*.[184] This was largely because of underlying anxieties about the promiscuity and infectiousness of colonial populations. Not even the saintly father Damien escaped innuendoes of this kind, being obliged to undergo an examination for syphilis because of rumours that he had been too familiar with Hawaiian women. As late as the 1940s, British officials and missionaries who succumbed to leprosy strenuously denied any 'irregular or intemperate habits' of the sort customarily associated with native peoples. Their defensive attitude was almost certainly encouraged by the enduring assumption that they had contracted a shameful disease under dubious circumstances.[185]

Meanwhile, a highly selective reading of Bernard Gordon convinced the American physician, J.C. Holcomb, that medieval leprosy must, in fact, have been caused by a strain of congenital syphilis, which mutated in the 1490s into the pox.[186] Holcomb's views had a particular impact on literary scholars such as Denton Fox, editor of *The Testament of Cresseid*, leading him to exaggerate the emphasis placed by medieval practitioners upon the sexual transmission of *lepra*.[187] They subsequently influenced Saul Brody's pessimistic account of the disease, and led Claude Thomasset to maintain that an inherent confusion

---

[181]  The process is well documented in London and Norwich: K.P. Siena, *Venereal Disease, Hospitals and the Urban Poor* (Rochester, New York and Woodbridge, 2004), pp. 64–7; Honeybourne 'Leper Hospitals of the London Area', pp. 4–54; Fabricius, *Syphilis*, pp. 60, 72–3; Rawcliffe, *Medicine for the Soul*, pp. 215–23.

[182]  Henryson, *Testament of Cresseid*, pp. 29–30; G. Hughes, *Swearing: A Social History of Foul Language, Oaths and Profanity in English* (London, 1998), p. 97; Fabricius, *Syphilis*, pp. 41, 63, 65, 109, 257–9. By contrast, the twelfth-century foundation charter of the *leprosarium* at St Albans refers to the '*pauperes Christi, videlicet lazeres*': BL, MS Cotton Nero D I, fo. 193r.

[183]  Simpson, 'Leprosy and Leper Hospitals', part iii, pp. 419–21, 424–5. An early sixteenth-century addition to the cartulary of the leper hospital at Maiden Bradley records a remedy for 'the French Pockes': BL, MS Add. 37503, fo. 62r.

[184]  Creighton, *History of Epidemics in Britain*, i, pp. 72–3; Gussow, *Leprosy, Racism and Public Health*, pp. 111–12.

[185]  Buckingham, *Leprosy in Colonial South India*, pp. 29–30; Gould, *Don't Fence Me In*, pp. 12, 83, 98–90; Gussow, *Leprosy, Racism and Public Health*, p. 95.

[186]  R.C. Holcomb, 'The Antiquity of Congenital Syphilis', *BHM*, x (1941), pp. 148–77, should be read in conjunction with Demaitre, 'Description and Diagnosis', pp. 327–44.

[187]  Robert Henryson, *Testament of Cresseid*, p. 27.

between leprosy and syphilis lay at the root of medieval gynophobia. Thomasset later modified his views, concluding that *lymphogranuloma venereum* offered a more plausible alternative to syphilis, and that many so called 'lepers' must have been suffering from it.[188]

The imposition of a modern biomedical model upon diseases that were experienced and described over half a millennium ago is, as we have already seen, likely to create more myths than it dispels. Particular caution seems advisable where the retrospective diagnosis of *lepra* is concerned. There is now sufficient skeletal evidence to settle once and for all the long-standing controversy about the incidence of syphilis in Europe before Columbus returned from the New World in 1493. Treponemal infections (either endemic or venereal syphilis) were far from unknown, if not evidently widespread, in medieval England. They gave rise in a few well-documented instances to the type of nasal and maxillary damage that figures so prominently in contemporary descriptions of *lepra*. Such cases have, for example, been identified at the Dominican friary at Gloucester and in a Norwich cemetery (closed in 1468), where residents of the local lazar house were also buried.[189] To conclude that sufferers from these infections were routinely 'mistaken' for lepers and wrongly 'confined' in *leprosaria* as a matter of course is, none the less, to make a number of unwarranted and potentially misleading assumptions.

On the one hand, the argument that confirmed lepers were consistently 'misdiagnosed'[190] presupposes an exact correspondence between medieval *lepra* and Hansen's disease that did not – and could not – exist at the time. It ignores the fact that definitions of *lepra*, especially in its early stages, were then sufficiently elastic to embrace at least some venereal infections, the majority of which were apparently deemed curable. Inevitably, too, it establishes an artificial yardstick by which to measure the competence of practitioners whose conceptual framework of disease was radically different from our own. Far from presenting a 'false conclusion', based on 'many wrongly interpreted facts',[191] Bernard Gordon's diagnosis of the leprous countess and her lover accorded perfectly with contemporary medical theory. It is, on the other hand, necessary to reiterate that the distinguished professor and his colleagues advanced many other explanations, which had nothing whatever to do with sexual activity.

188  Brody, *Disease of the Soul*, pp. 181–6; Demaitre, 'Description and Diagnosis', p. 329; Jacquart and Thomasset, *Sexuality and Medicine*, pp. 180–87.

189  A. Stirland, 'Evidence for Pre-Columbian Treponematosis in Medieval Europe', in O. Dutour et al., eds, *L'origine de la syphilis en Europe* (Paris and Toulon, undated, c. 1994), pp. 109–15; and below, pp. 262–3. This evidence undermines G.M.M. Crane-Kramer's assertion that lepers and people with treponemal infections were never buried together: 'Was There a Medieval Diagnostic Confusion between Leprosy and Syphilis', *PPL*, pp. 111–18.

190  C. Roberts, 'Treponematosis in Gloucester, England: A Theoretical and Practical Approach to the Pre-Colombian Theory', in Dutour, *Origine de la syphilis*, p. 106.

191  Jacquart and Thomasset, *Sexuality and Medicine*, pp. 187–8. Attempting to square the circle, Ell, 'Bood and Sexuality', pp. 153–64, argues that medieval assumptions about the transmission of *lepra* would 'represent quite reasonable interpretations of observable phenomena' in cases where a person with Hansen's disease had *also* contracted syphilis. Moreover, since pregnancy may suppress immunity to *Mycobacterium leprae*, its subsequent onset in a woman might well be associated with sexual activity.

## 'A contagiouse sekenesse and infectynge'

The assumption that leprosy was regarded as a highly contagious disease throughout entire Middle Ages was zealously fostered by nineteenth-century physicians on both sides of the 'segregationist' debate. For Robert Liveing and many others, such an apparently unshakeable belief in 'the infectious character of leprosy' was a holy grail to be reclaimed at all costs.[192] Although recent research by historians such as F.O. Touati and Luke Demaitre has effectively undermined the solid edifice created by the likes of Archdeacon Wright and his contemporaries, a conviction that medieval men and women invariably fled the company of lepers because they feared catching the disease still flourishes in academic as well as popular studies of the period.[193] This is partly because of the deceptively similar vocabulary that links us to the past. Words like '*contagio*', 'contagyoun' and 'infectyf' convey a very specific meaning to readers who have been deluged with information about tuberculosis, AIDS and, more recently, SARS and MRSA. Yet medieval writers, whose explanations of health and sickness hinged upon humoral theory rather than microbiology, defined infection and contagion in loose and interchangeable terms that embraced ideas about pollution and putrefaction as well as personal contact.[194] Drawing no distinction, as we would today, between the hereditary (genetic) and congenital transmission of disease, practitioners deemed both processes to be contagious. In the words of one fifteenth-century surgeon: 'leproues amonge all syknes ys moste contage & seknes lykly to passe by in herytaunce as fro fadyr to sone'.[195] He did *not* mean that it spread rapidly through casual contact.

The same vocabulary might be employed to convey the inexorable process of internal decomposition so characteristic of *lepra* in its advanced stages. Writing in the late twelfth-century, Giles of Corbeil described the spread of purulent humours round the body in terms of *contagio*, as one organ after another succumbed to contamination.[196] Since, according to this aetiological system, each case of leprosy developed according to the unique physiology of the individual patient, we can readily appreciate that his understanding of contagion had little in common with our own. It may still be found in a late medieval English translation of Lanfrank's *Science of Cirurgie*, which provides the type of succinct and accessible explanation that a busy surgeon (who trained through apprenticeship rather than at university) would have valued:

> Lepra is a foul sijknes that cometh of malancolie corrupt, outhir of humouris that ben brought to the forme of malancolye corrupt. & it goith into al the bodi, right as a cancre is in oon lyme of a mannes bodi. For whanne malancolie multiplieth, & a mannes guttis ben not strong for to putte it out, & the weies bitwixe the splene

192   Liveing, *Elephantiasis Graecorum*, p. 16.
193   As, for example, 'The whole Middle Ages believed that Leprosy was extremely contagious . . . those who did not flee the person on whom God had let fall his wrath would meet with the same punishment': Jacquart and Thomasset, *Sexuality and Medicine*, p. 185.
194   Nutton, 'Did the Greeks Have a Word', p. 158.
195   BL, MS Harley 1736, fo. 135r. Likewise, Bartholomew Anglicus argued that, at conception, 'contagioun passith into the childe': Seymour, *On the Properties of Things*, i, p. 426.
196   Touati, 'Contagion', pp. 188–9.

ben stoppid & the poris of the skyn closid, than malancolious blood wole rote withinne, & rotith complexiouns of the lymes . . . & this is oon of the syknessis that ben contagious.[197]

By then, however, an awareness that leprosy might well be passed more directly from one person to another, albeit after prolonged periods of association, had found its way into the medical literature. Significantly, authors who described this mode of transmission felt it necessary to qualify their choice of words by noting that leprosy was 'a contagiouse sekenesse *and* infectynge', as if to introduce their readers to a new idea.[198]

One of the most enduring legacies of Greek medicine was its holistic view of mankind as part of an all-embracing cosmological system. Since it shared the same basic components (heat, moisture, coldness and aridity) as the rest of the universe, the human body naturally appeared vulnerable to external environmental factors. From the time of Hippocrates, if not earlier, physicians were expected to understand how the climate, location and natural resources of a particular place would affect the health and fertility of its inhabitants. Hippocratic texts such as *Airs, Waters, Places* shaped the outlook not only of medieval physicians but of the population in general, providing the rationale behind most measures for late medieval urban improvement and sanitary reform. The quality of the air seemed especially important, since it had the most immediate and potentially deleterious impact upon the natural, vital and animal spirits.[199] This was because all odours were regarded as corporeal entities, or 'smoky vapours', somewhere between water and air, which transported the 'prynte and likenes' of the thing from whence they came into the human body. They might be used medicinally, to strengthen the patient, but could, on the other hand, cause irretrievable damage. As we have seen, air from the lungs helped to create the body's life force, or *pneuma*, while that inhaled through the nose mixed with the animal spirits to generate movement and thought.[200] It could also pass through the open pores directly into the venous system, thereby affecting the production, distribution and digestion of humoral matter. Whereas clean and bracing air invigorated the entire body, promoting a sense of happiness and equilibrium, noxious vapours (of the sort absorbed during sex with a contaminated prostitute) had the opposite effect.

---

197  R. von Fleischhacker, ed., *Lanfrank's 'Science of Cirurgie'* (EETS, cii, 1894), p. 196.
198  Ogden, *Cyrurgie of Guy de Chauliac*, p. 381. See also Bartholomaeus Anglicus, who notes that 'the yuel is contagious *and* infectith othir men': Seymour, *On the Properties of Things*, i, p. 426; BL, MS Sloane 282, fo. 129v; Touati, 'Contagion', p. 196.
199  G.E.R. Lloyd, ed., *Hippocratic Writings* (Harmondsworth, 1983), pp. 148–69. Climatic factors were rarely advanced as a prime cause of leprosy, although John of Gaddesden suggested that a sudden change in air quality, as experienced in autumn, could promote adustion: *Rosa Anglica*, fo. 56r. A Hanseatic merchant in the 1460s blamed his condition upon protracted hard work and exposure to the cold: F. Bergman, 'Hoping against Hope? A Marital Dispute about the Medical Treatment of Leprosy in the Fifteenth-Century Hanseatic Town of Kampen', in H. Marland and M. Pelling, eds, *The Task of Healing: Medicine, Religion and Gender in England and the Netherlands 1450–1800* (Rotterdam, 1996), p. 36.
200  Seymour, *On the Properties of Things*, ii, pp. 1296–7, 301; C. Classen, D. Howes and A. Synnott, *The Cultural History of Smell* (London, 1994), pp. 61–4; R. Palmer, 'In Bad Odour: Smell and its Significance in Medicine from Antiquity to the Seventeenth Century', in W.F. Bynum and R. Porter, eds, *Medicine and the Five Senses* (Cambridge, 1993), pp. 61–8.

The exhalations of the sick seemed especially dangerous. Galen advised his colleagues not to linger at the bedside of patients whose breath had become so putrid that their houses reeked,[201] a warning which assumed particular significance where newly observed cases of *elephantia* were concerned. Several of the Classical and early Christian authors who first described and discussed this disease at any length either considered it prudent to avoid unnecessary contact with sufferers, or cited the opinions of others to this effect. Aetius believed that it was unsafe to speak with such people because the effluvia from their sores and respiration contaminated the atmosphere.[202] According to Caelius Aurelianus, some practitioners recommended the removal of suspects, especially if they were outsiders, although he himself expressed ethical reservations about more systematic segregation.[203] Claiming that patients would actually benefit from living in remote inland sites, where the air would be cooler and healthier, Paulus Aegineta felt that such an 'easily communicable' disease warranted firm measures. All, however, stressed that *discrasia*, which sprang from an inherent humoral imbalance, might be aggravated but could not itself be caused by exposure to the sick.[204] In short, the ultimate factor determining whether or not an individual would be predisposed to *elephantiasis* lay in his or her liver and spleen.

The Muslim scholars who inherited these ideas were torn by two conflicting religious traditions. One regarded the very concept of contagion as irreligious, since all disease came directly from God and could not be avoided, while the other claimed that Mohammed had urged his followers to 'flee the leper as you would flee from a lion'. In an attempt to reconcile these seemingly incompatible positions, scholars such as Ibn Qutayba (*c.* 870) argued that major epidemics were fated, while chronic conditions, including leprosy (*judhām*) and mange, could be communicated from one person to another. This, he maintained, was because 'the leper gives off an odour so strong that it causes anyone who long remains in his presence or eats with him to fall ill'.[205] Muslim physicians generally shared this opinion. The section on *lepra* in the *Practica* of the *Pantegni* makes only a vague reference to mephistic air as a potential cause, although the *Theorica* notes that some people contract the disease through association with its victims and by the inhalation of noxious fumes from their bodies.[206] The more disciplined and systematic Avicenna brought all this evidence together in book four of the *Canon*, where he proposed that, along with the other factors discussed above, 'the air corrupted by itself or because of the proximity of lepers' might significantly destabilise an already vulnerable patient.[207]

201  Palmer, 'Bad Odour', p. 65.
202  Adams, *Seven Books of Paulus Aegineta*, ii, p. 10.
203  Nutton, 'Did the Greeks Have a Word', pp. 149.
204  Adams, *Seven Books of Paulus Aegineta*, ii, p. 5; V. Nutton, 'The Seeds of Disease: An Explanation of Contagion and Infection from the Greeks to the Renaissance', *Medical History*, xxvii (1983), pp. 1–34. Aretaeus the Cappadocian (whose work was not widely known in the medieval West) paints an extremely bleak picture of responses to the disease: Adams, *Extant Works of Aretaeus*, pp. 366–73, 494–8.
205  L.I. Conrad, 'A Ninth-Century Muslim Scholar's Discussion of Contagion', in idem and Wujastyk, *Contagion*, pp. 163–77, quotation on p. 169; Dols, 'Leper in Medieval Islamic Society', pp. 895–8.
206  *Liber Pantegni, theorica*, liber VIII, cap. 15, fo. 39r; *practica*, liber IV, cap. 2, fo. 93r; Touati, *Maladie et société*, p. 146.
207  Avicenna, *Liber canonis*, liber IV, fen. iii, tractatus iii, cap. i, fo. 442v.

From the mid thirteenth century onwards, western physicians and surgeons, influenced by the 'bookes translatede out of Arabye tunge', regularly drew attention to the part played by foetid smells in triggering disease.[208] 'Infect and corrupt aier' in general figured among the ten or so 'diuers causes' of *lepra* itemised by Bartholomaeus Anglicus, who also advised against 'dwellynge . . . and ofte talkynge with leprous men'. His conviction that 'the breth is corrupt, and ofte hole [healthy] men beth infect with stench therof' underscored this point.[209] Although Bartholomew's encyclopaedia was not translated into English until the early fifteenth century, his opinions, along with those of respected physicians such as Gilbertus Anglicus and John of Gaddesden, circulated far beyond a narrow elite. Gaddesden, in particular, took a firm line. Recognising that pestilential vapours of any kind might spread the disease, he nevertheless regarded association and contact with the leprous as being particularly dangerous. Their eyes, nostrils, mouths, breath and, indeed, the skin of their entire bodies exuded miasmatic fumes which communicated a *morbus contagiosus* in the modern sense.[210] His concerns were rehearsed, in a sensationalised form, by Edward III in his ordinance of 1346 for the removal of lepers from the streets of London. Determined to crack down on rising levels of disorder and vagrancy in the city, he highlighted two potential hazards, warning that leprosy was not only spread 'by the contagion of . . . polluted breath' but also by 'carnal intercourse with women in stews and other secret places'.[211] The dissemination and impact of these ideas, especially in the years following the Black Death will be discussed at greater length in chapter six. Given the scale of the epidemic, later generations of practitioners could hardly ignore the redoubled threat posed by infected air. Guy de Chauliac, who lived through the first outbreak of pestilence, advocated a measure of isolation for lepers, recommending that advanced cases should be segregated 'fro[m] the peple with good counseillynge wordes and ledde into spitelles'.[212]

Close proximity brought other hazards besides polluted breath. Late medieval advice literature warned that the gaze of a menstruating woman spread poison like a basilisk and polluted whatever it fell upon. Having flooded the crystalline humour of the eye, which in a healthy person remained clean and pure, the corrupt vapours generated by menstrual blood would, according to Galenic theory, be projected outwards as 'visual *pneuma*' into the atmosphere.[213] Surprisingly, in view of the prevalence of such beliefs during the later Middle Ages, Gaddesden is one of the few practitioners to mention the potentially more

---

208  Ogden, *Cyrurgie of Guy de Chauliac*, p. 9; Bodleian Library, MS Ashmole 1505, fo. 30v; BL, MSS Sloane 5, fo. 153r; 2272 (part 1), fo. 91v.

209  Seymour, *On the Properties of Things*, i, pp. 424, 426. In the *Mirrour de l'omme*, John Gower compared lechery to leprosy because it was 'so virulent that it corrupts the air along with the wind that blows around it': Grigsby, *Pestilence*, pp. 80–81.

210  John of Gaddesden, *Rosa Anglica*, fo. 56r.

211  Riley, *Memorials*, pp. 230–31. It was initially believed that the pox spread on the breath: Fabricius, *Syphilis*, pp. 63, 259.

212  Ogden, *Cyrurgie of Guy de Chauliac*, p. 383. Suspect lepers were urged 'that thai come noght mykel among the peple'.

213  Lemay, *Women's Secrets*, pp. 48, 128, 130; S. Biernoff, *Sight and Embodiment in the Middle Ages* (London, 2002), pp. 51–2; S. Lobanov-Rostovsky, 'Taming the Basilisk', in Hillman and Mazzio, *Body in Parts*, p. 198.

serious risk posed by the toxic gaze of lepers. Since the long and detailed lists of symptoms recorded in the medical literature of the period generally include ocular damage, and descriptions of lepers in other contemporary sources frequently refer to their ulcerated and rheumy eyes, this lacuna is striking. An answer to one of the Salernitan questions recorded in the English manuscript discussed above does, however, refer to the vulnerability of small children. Anyone 'who has been corrupted since his conception and engendered by corrupt semen and nourished by corrupt humours', the author argues, must inevitably generate 'extremely corrupt spirits', which in turn will contaminate the surrounding air. Should this individual gaze intently upon a child, the latter will inhale the poisonous matter emanating directly from the eye and fall sick. Prolonged contact would compound the problem. 'Does one not become leprous through conversation (*ex collocutione*)?' he asks with a rhetorical flourish, adding that the only possible source of transmission in either event must be infected air (*non nisi ex infectione aeris*).[214] Concerns about ocular transmission may have been implicit in the loosely worded warnings about 'corrupcioun of the ayre and the touchinge of leprouse men' that appear in some fourteenth- and fifteenth-century medical literature, but are rarely spelt out.[215] Yet the general public was certainly aware of them. Describing an epidemic among poultry, which erupted in 1344, one Scottish chronicler noted 'that men utterly shrank from eating, *or even looking upon*, a cock or a hen, as though unclean and smitten with leprosy'.[216] In this instance, though, it was the *image* rather than the air that inspired fear.

Gilbertus Anglicus refers in passing to the breath and 'aspect' (*aspectus*) of lepers among many potential sources of transmission, subsequently explaining that the 'species' or image of leprosy will enter the eye of anyone who looks upon one of its victims. It will then pass to the animal spirits, and eventually suffuse the entire venous system.[217] As a reader of Avicenna, and perhaps also of the recently available Latin text of Alhacen's (Ibn al-Haytham, *fl.* 1030) *De aspectibus*, he was aware of a new approach to optics then commanding attention in the West. According to Aristotle and his Islamic followers, whose theories gained ground from the mid thirteenth century onwards, the eye (like the uterus) was a passive, rather than an active, organ. It received sensory impressions from the outside world and transmitted them along the optic nerve to the brain. These impressions travelled through the air as 'forms', 'virtues' or 'similitudes', which radiated outwards in a continuous sequence of multiple images from all visible objects and were regarded by some late medieval commentators as real, tangible entities. In view of the intimate relationship between the brain and the spirits,

---

214  Lawn, *Prose Salernitan Questions*, p. 98 (no. 179). Touati, 'Contagion', pp. 195–6, suggests that the author has misunderstood the concept of aerial transmission, but his views accord perfectly with Galenic theory. For wider fears about the association between lepers and children, see below, p. 281.

215  Ogden, *Cyrurgie of Guy de Chauliac*, p. 378. For the belief that an especially lethal 'air spirit' or 'diaphanous poison' would be transmitted through the gaze of a person dying of the plague, see Arrizabalaga, 'Facing the Black Death', pp. 263–4.

216  W.F. Skene, ed., *John of Fordun's Chronicle of the Scottish Nation* (Edinburgh, 1872), p. 358. Margaret of Anjou's words, 'What! Dost thou turn away and hide thy face? I am no loathsome leper; look on me', may recall this tradition: William Shakespeare, *Henry VI, Part 2*, act III, scene 2, vv. 73–4.

217  Gilbertus Anglicus, *Compendium medicine*, fos 337v, 339r.

the likelihood that such images would affect the body in direct and immediate ways seemed obvious.[218]

As we shall see, the *visibility* of the Eucharist during the Mass became a matter of pressing concern for the patrons and founders of *leprosaria*, not just for theological reasons, but because the body of Christ was believed to radiate substantive healing power. To look upon the Host at the moment of elevation was, for example, deemed sure protection against blindness.[219] Conversely, a distressing or frightening spectacle, such as that presented by a diseased beggar or leper, could have a malignant effect on susceptible individuals. For this reason, inordinate care was taken to protect pregnant women of high status from unpleasant sights, since, like hot wax, a developing embryo could easily retain whatever 'species' were impressed upon it from the mother's brain.[220]

The extent to which these beliefs informed and influenced daily reactions to the sick is harder to judge. A leper who was so deformed that people could not bear to look upon him (*tam deformis quod aspectus eum sustinere non posit*) was technically debarred from pleading in a thirteenth-century common law court. Similar criteria determined the point at which a leprous parish priest or abbot would have to appoint an assistant, and generally dictated whether or not suspects would finally be confirmed.[221] Yet they do not necessarily imply a fear of visual contamination, or, indeed, of any other form of infection, as we would understand the term today. Even in the plague-ridden years of the later Middle Ages, well informed men and women recognised that the humoral balance or temperament of the individual would, in the final resort, determine his or her vulnerability to external influences.[222] A reassuring degree of equilibrium could be maintained through the restraint and moderation advocated by Greek physicians and Christian theologians alike. But however assiduous one might be in pursuing the golden mean, a malignant conjunction of cosmic forces could still undermine the fragile edifice of human health.

## Murky and malicious planets

The relationship between medicine and astrology boasted a long history, which medieval scholars traced back to Hippocrates. What had, however, begun as a relatively loose and imprecise connection was transformed from the twelfth century onwards, as a number of key texts percolated through to the West. Skilled translators, such as Constantine the African and Gerard of Cremona, did not confine their attention to medical literature. The work of Ptolemy (d. *c.* AD 145), Albumasar (Abū Ma'šar, d. 887), Alcabitius (Al-Qabīsī, *fl.* 950) and other leading Greek and Islamic astronomers proved no less attractive.[223] And, as Latin

---

218 K.H. Tachau, *Vision and Certitude in the Age of Ockham: Optics, Epistemology and the Foundations of Semantics 1250–1345* (Leiden, 1988), pp. 8–10, 94–5; D.G. Denery, *Seeing and Being in the Later Medieval World* (Cambridge, 2005), pp. 82–9.

219 John Myrc, *Instructions for Parish Priests*, ed. E. Peacock (EETS, xxxi, 1868), pp. 10–11.

220 Cadden, *Meanings of Sex Difference*, pp. 243–53; J. Musacchio, *The Art and Ritual of Childbirth in Renaissance Italy* (New York, 1999), pp. 127–39.

221 Thorne, *Bracton*, p. 309; and below, pp. 194–5.

222 Horrox, *Black Death*, p. 185.

223 S.J. Tester, *A History of Western Astrology* (Woodbridge, 1987), chapter five; Rawcliffe, *Medicine and Society*, pp. 82–93.

versions began to circulate, their value to physicians and surgeons soon became apparent. As well as offering a coherent explanation for disease that rested upon the secure and rational foundations of humoral theory, astrological training enabled the practitioner to treat his patient more effectively and (in theory, at least) provide a more accurate prognosis. That it greatly enhanced his professional status in the eyes of impressionable laymen contributed not a little to the enthusiasm with which these ideas were embraced.[224]

Standing firmly at the centre of the Ptolemaic universe, the earth – or more properly mankind – was surrounded by a series of concentric spheres, each of which contained one of the seven planets visible to the naked eye. Beyond 'yuel and maliciouse' Saturn, the most distant and slow moving of them all, the signs of the zodiac shared a sphere of their own, which was divided into twelve partitions or houses, where each one dwelt. The outermost sphere, or *primum mobile*, kept the rest in a state of constant movement, watched over by God and his angels in the all-encompassing empyrean heaven [plate 10]. Whereas the sublunary world of earth, water, fire and air was vulnerable to change and decay, the stars and planets remained incorruptible.[225] They also exerted a profound influence upon this mutable environment, not least with regard to the health and sickness of each inhabitant. Their power was manifest in many ways. Every planet had its own gender, temperament and character, which rendered him or her malignant, benign or an ambivalent mixture of both. The two 'infortunes', Mars (choleric) and Saturn (melancholic), inspired the greatest fear, since their circuit around the firmament generally left a trail of war and disease in its wake.[226] Propitious and sanguine, Sol (the sun), by contrast, brought health and happiness to those who came under his sway, while Luna (the phlegmatic moon) was as slippery and unpredictable as her natural medium, water.[227]

The relative strength or weakness of each planet depended upon a complex combination of factors. An ascendant body acquired greater 'dignity' as it prepared to rise above the eastern horizon, becoming paramount at that time. Gradual decline set in as it moved westwards. As in life, however, additional status came through alliances with others. It was thus essential to determine the aspects, or geometrical relationships, between heavenly bodies. Like a great lord, whose might increased when he armed himself in his castle, a planet grew more powerful at home in (that is in alignment with) a house of the zodiac over which he or she ruled.[228] The twelve houses shared between them the characteristics of the four primary elements (earth, water, fire and air). It was thus appropriate

---

[224] R. French, 'Astrology in Medical Practice', in Garcia-Ballester et al., *Practical Medicine*, pp. 30–59, notably pp. 32–3; idem, 'Foretelling the Future: Arabic Astrology and English Medicine in the Late Twelfth Century', *Isis*, lxxxvii (1996), pp. 453–80.

[225] S. Page, *Astrology in Medieval Manuscripts* (London, 2002), pp. 14–60.

[226] French, 'Astrology', pp. 53–4; BL, MS Egerton 2572, fo. 64r; Trinity College, Cambridge, MS O.I.77, fos 124v–126v.

[227] See, for example, 'a rewle to know whiche be good plenettis and whiche be evylle and which be indifferent or meane': Bodleian Library, MS Ashmole 340, fos 1r–22v.

[228] 'Ilke planete in his awne house is as a kynge in his heyght of his glory blise & ioye, and he ys as a kynge when he ys crounede': BL, MS Egerton 2572, fos, 58r, 64v–65r; C. Burnett, K. Yamamoto and M. Yano, eds, *Al-Qabīsī (Alcabitius) The Introduction to Astrology* (Warburg Institute Studies and Texts, ii, 2004), p. 240.

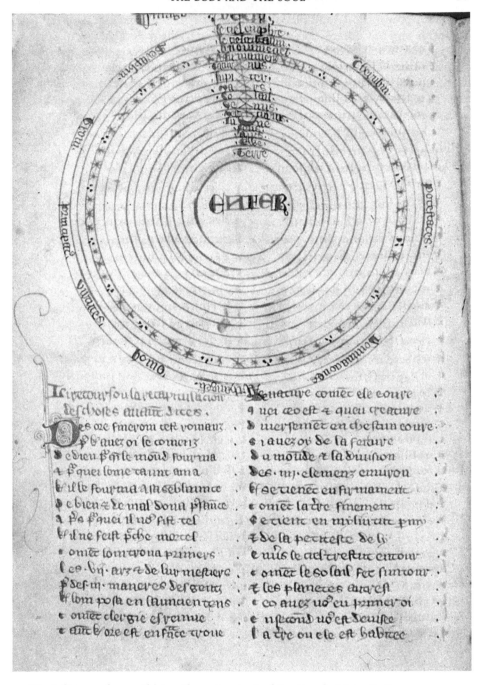

10. A diagram from a thirteenth-century text of Gautier de Metz, *Le Romaunce del ymage du monde*, owned by an English scholar, depicts the concentric circles of the Ptolemaic universe, with hell (*enfer*) at the centre of the earth, around which the rest of the universe moves.

that Saturn, a melancholic planet, should flourish when aligned with the cold, dry earth sign of Capricorn and, to a lesser extent, the watery, frigid Aquarius.[229] Conversely, when he travelled through warmer, less sympathetic houses, his authority waned. A skilled astrologer could calculate the relative influence of each planet at any hour of the day by what might crudely be described as a points system. Marks were, for example, allocated according to the relationship between a planet and its 'triplicities'. These were groups of three signs that would likewise augment their master's forces as he (or she) lodged in their domain. Saturn's trio comprised Virgo, Capricorn and Taurus, the earth signs with which he enjoyed a natural affinity. In addition, every planet responded well or unfavourably to whichever sign of the zodiac happened to be in the ascendant. This might be a friend or foe. Saturn was exalted in Libra but diminished in Aries, a hot and dry sign associated with energy and youth, and thus his natural adversary.[230]

How could this knowledge help the physician? The position of the stars at the time of an individual's birth was clearly a matter of fundamental importance. Dividing the heavens into twelve segments (also called houses), astrologers assigned to each a specific aspect of human life, such as marriage, travel and family relationships. The sixth concerned health and the eighth mortality. By casting the natal horoscope of a child, it was possible to determine which of the planets then dominated these particular sections and thus assess with a remarkable degree of precision the type of medical problems likely to occur in later life.[231] The presence of Saturn in any house might well prove unfortunate, but his appearance in the sixth could presage a grim future, especially if a loyal sign had further augmented his powers. As the sworn 'enemy to mannes hele', he bestowed a malign gift of disfiguring and painful diseases.[232] According to the Muslim astronomer, Alcabitius, these included cancer, gout, *elephantia*, dropsy, hypochondria and other chronic illnesses that came from cold and dryness'.[233] Others spoke of 'the most varied pestilences in the body', while Leopold of Austria added *fistulae*, frostbite, quatrain fever and morphew to a list that began with leprosy and ended with 'fetid odours and bad breath from the mouth or nostrils'.[234]

The practice of commissioning a horoscope on one's birthday, in order to predict what lay ahead over the coming year, grew increasingly common. An individual who was already predisposed to leprosy from birth might be reassured – or alarmed – by the results, but would at least be forewarned to take preventative action. It was also possible to cast a horoscope, or assessment of 'annual revolutions', for the year itself. The astrologer-physician, Richard Trewythian, whom we shall meet in chapter five, customarily did this, fore-

229  Trinity College, Cambridge, MS R.15.21, fo. 41v.
230  BL, MS Sloane 3983, fos 32r–33v; Trinity College, Cambridge, MS O.I.77, fos 125v–126r.
231  Page, *Astrology*, p. 23.
232  G.C. MacCaulay, ed., *The English Works of John Gower* (2 vols, EETS, extra series, lxxxi, 1900, and lxxxii, 1901), ii, *Confessio Amantis*, book VII, line 943.
233  Burnett, Yamamoto and Yano, *Alcabitius*, pp. 257, 267–8; Klibansky, Panofsky and Saxl, *Saturn and Melancholy*, p. 131.
234  Page, *Astrology*, p. 54; Klibansky, Panofsky and Saxl, *Saturn and Melancholy*, pp. 130–31.

casting, for example, that 1452 (a year marked by extreme political instability) would witness an upsurge in 'chronic diseases . . . arising from coldness and dryness, such as insanity, epilepsy and leprosy'.[235]

A common assumption that men and women born when a specific planet was at its most powerful would share its characteristics spread from the pages of specialist text books into art, literature and popular culture. The children of Saturn limped sullenly at the rear of a procession headed by the blithe and handsome offspring of Sol and Jupiter. Although the Saturnine temperament was traditionally associated with scholarship and solitary contemplation, this positive image deteriorated dramatically as humoral theory and Ptolemaic astrology merged to create a far less attractive persona.[236] During the later Middle Ages, Saturn was transformed into a 'cold, dry, bitter, black, dark, violent and harsh' planet, who ruled over an ill-favoured crew of tanners, traitors, gravediggers, crooks, peasants and even phlebotomists [plate 11]. Their malformed bodies were further distinguished by 'foule and stinkinge clothinge' and a dark 'melancolik humour'.[237] Having been himself held captive, according to Greek myth, Saturn was also the patron of prisoners, whether in the literal sense or metaphorically with regard to those whose age, mental incapacity or illness chained them to a decaying body or failing mind. We may note, for example, that, as late as 1539, the dean of Norwich described the residents of a civic *leprosarium* as 'the prysoners of almyghty god', whose 'hatefull dysease and sykenes of leprye' restricted their mobility.[238]

The impact of celestial forces upon human physiology went far beyond these sweeping generalities. Each planet ruled over a particular organ, which, in the case of Saturn was the spleen, where black bile, and perhaps adust choler, seethed rebelliously in a fleshly prison.[239] He and the three acolytes who served him were regarded as *retentive* agents, whereas the watery triplicates of Cancer, Scorpio and Pisces promoted expulsion and excretion. Since leprosy was caused by the body's failure to eliminate poison, their precise alignment could assume life-threatening proportions.[240] The moon exerted particular influence over the blood, since it was believed to flow in sympathy with the waxing and waning of the lunar cycle. In his *Tetrabiblos*, Ptolemy suggested that, as she approached the vernal and autumnal equinoxes, Luna grew particularly malevolent, thereby creating an environment conducive to the onset of *lepra*.[241] As an ambivalent planet, easily swayed by others, she behaved just as badly when led astray by

---

[235] BL, MS Sloane 428, fo. 73r; S. Page, 'Richard Trewythian and the Uses of Astrology in Late Medieval England', *Journal of the Warburg and Courtauld Institutes*, lxiv (2001), pp. 193–228, at pp. 200–03.

[236] Klibansky, Panofsky and Saxl, *Saturn and Melancholy*, part 2, chapter one, passim; BL, MS Harley 4431, fo. 101v, a lavishly illuminated manuscript of the *Epitre d'Othea*, depicts the children of Saturn as scholars, although one has a disfiguring ulcer on the right side of his jaw.

[237] BL, MS Egerton 2572, fo. 62r–62v; MS Sloane 1315, fo. 36r; Klibansky, Panofsky and Saxl, *Saturn and Melancholy*, pp. 130–31; Seymour, *On the Properties of Things*, i, p. 479; and below, pp. 226–7. Alcabitius also associated the planet with the Jewish faith, thus strengthening the connection sometimes made between Jews and lepers: Burnett, Yamamoto and Yano, *Alcabitius*, p. 269.

[238] NRO, DCN 39/1; Klibansky, Panofsky and Saxl, *Saturn and Melancholy*, p. 144; and below, p. 288.

[239] The bladder, bones, teeth, right ear and memory also came under his jurisdiction: C.A. Mercier, *Astrology in Medicine* (London, 1914), pp. 40–43; BL, MS Sloane 282, fo. 18r.

[240] French, 'Astrology', pp. 54–5.

[241] Claudius Ptolemy, *Tetrabiblos*, ed. F.E. Robbins (Cambridge, 1980), book III, chapter 12, p. 327.

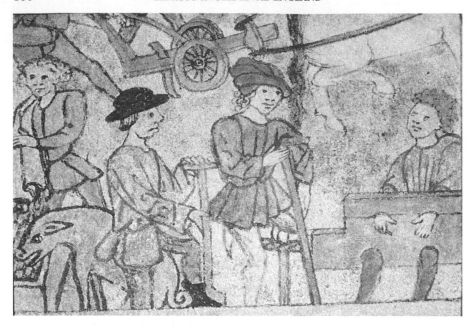

11. This detail from a fifteenth-century English astrological treatise illustrates
some of the characteristics of the children of Saturn, who are likely to be criminals
(hence the figure in the stocks), disabled or drawn to disreputable or dirty
activities, such as keeping pigs, themselves a potential source of diseased meat.

Saturn. Among other misfortunes, their partnership was said to promote 'the
fallen sicknesse [epilepsy], blacke chollere, leprosy and fistula . . . morphew,
goute and oftentimes sodaine panges', threatening not only to generate poison,
but also to hasten its spread through the vital organs. [242] Even worse, if no benign
planet were on hand to moderate its impact, an alignment of the heavens
whereby Luna took up residence in the house of Taurus while Saturn was in
Scorpio (or *vice versa*) could produce *elephantiasis*. [243] These linguistic distinctions, so clear to the Greeks, were lost on later generations of readers, who
regarded *lepra* and *elephantiasis* as synonymous.

    Since each sign of the zodiac dominated an area of the body, there was a
general consensus on the part of Muslim astronomers that the limbs or organs in
question would become particularly vulnerable to injury of any kind when the
moon entered that particular sign. It was, for example, extremely dangerous to
remove corrupt blood from the feet when the moon was in Pisces, or to attempt
surgery upon the hands when she passed through Gemini. As we shall see in
chapter four, the treatment of incipient *lepra* required a minutely calibrated
combination of surgical and medical remedies, which, in turn, demanded expert
astrological training, as well as the necessary mathematical skills to calculate

---

    Ptolemy observed that Saturn predisposed his subjects to *elephancia*, whereas the moon in the spring
    equinox would inflict 'white *lepra*' and in the autumn equinox '*lepra*'.

[242]  J. Parr, 'Cresseid's Leprosy Again', *Modern Language Notes*, lx (1945), pp. 487–91, at pp. 487–8.
[243]  J. Rhys Bram, ed., *Ancient Astrology: Theory and Practice* (Park Ridge, New Jersey, 1975), pp. 253–4.

exactly where each celestial body stood in relation to the others. Even the medicinal plants used to combat the disease were chosen because of their subservience to specific planets. A university-trained physician acquired this knowledge as part of the *quadrivium*, an essential component of the Arts degree he was expected to possess before reading medicine. Surgeons undertook a more pragmatic training through apprenticeship and private study.[244]

Already stimulated by the availability of texts from the Muslim world, the study of medical astrology received a further impetus from the late 1340s onwards, as plague became a recurrent fact of European life. A belief that the first outbreak was caused by a malignant conjunction of Mars, Jupiter and Saturn in the house of Aquarius in March 1345 led many governments and civic authorities to promote the academic discipline, and to insist upon the ownership of instruments and tables by medical practitioners.[245] Astrology did not, however, long remain the preserve of a narrow elite. Men and women with even a smattering of education sought to grasp the basic principles of a science that seemed to offer the means of preserving health. Thus, by the end of the century, the connection between Saturn, melancholy, plague and lepra had become an established literary *topos*. As 'the fader of pestilence', armed with a quiverful of 'maladyes cold' the malignant planet strikes down the hero of Chaucer's *Knight's Tale*, condemning him to a painful death beyond all medical help.[246] No doubt with these dramatic verses in mind, the Scottish poet, Robert Henryson, assigned a prominent role to Saturn in his *Testament of Cresseid* (*c.* 1492). Adding a novel twist to the familiar story of Cresseid, a beautiful but promiscuous young Trojan woman, Henryson describes how her pride, 'fleschelie lust' and blasphemy against the gods are punished.[247] Like most educated men of his day, he had acquired a good basic knowledge of medicine and astrology, which he used to telling effect. Having tried and condemned her in their heavenly court, the planets delegate Saturn to impose the sentence. With one touch he transforms her flesh into that of a cold, dry leper. Leaden in colour and swathed in a spotted gown, Luna accompanies him, to remove the last vestiges of warmth from Cresseid's body:

> Thy cristall ene mingit with blude I mak,
> Thy voice sa cleir vnplesand hoir and hace,

---

244 Rawcliffe, *Medicine and Society*, pp. 86–91.

245 Horrox, *Black Death*, pp. 158–72; Rawcliffe, *Medicine and Society*, pp. 82–3, 86. A similar conjunction in 1484 was blamed for the first outbreak of pox: Amundsen, *Medicine, Society and Faith*, p. 318; Arrizabalaga, Henderson and French, *Great Pox*, pp. 82, 109–11.

246 Geoffrey Chaucer, *Canterbury Tales*, p. 58; P. Brown and A. Butcher, *The Age of Saturn: Literature and History in the Canterbury Tales* (Oxford, 1991), pp. 212–23.

247 The sin of blasphemy aroused growing concern in the later Middle Ages, notably in France, where the practice of branding blasphemers on the lips until, in the case of frequent offenders, they were completely destroyed, mimicked the symptoms of *lepra*: Guenée, *Folie de Charles VI*, pp. 188–9. Thomas Gascoigne maintained that, in 1457, certain miscreants who had sworn oaths on parts of God's body had died bleeding from the same bodily parts: *Loci e libro veritatum*, p. 12. As English wall paintings of the period demonstrate, the verbal dismemberment of Christ fractured the social body, just as leprosy destroyed that of the individual: R. Marks, *Image and Devotion in Late Medieval England* (Stroud, 2004), pp. 134, 136. Not surprisingly, the pox was viewed in a similar light: Arrizabalaga, Henderson and French, *Great Pox*, pp. 88–9; Amundsen, *Medicine, Society and Faith*, pp. 312–13.

Thy lustie lyre ouirspred with spottis blak,
And lumpis haw appeirand in thy face:
Quhair thow cummis, ilk man sall fle the place.
This sall thow go begging fra hous to hous
With cop and clapper lyke ane lazarous.[248]

[I make your crystal eyes bloodshot, your clear voice grating, hoarse and rasping, your lovely countenance suffused with black spots and your face disfigured with leaden tumours. Wherever you go, everyone will flee the place. You shall go begging from house to house with a bowl and clapper like another Lazarus.]

However vindictive and capricious the stars and planets may sometimes have appeared, the underlying scientific validity of these beliefs went unchallenged. The medieval Church never questioned the power wielded by celestial forces over human affairs. Generations of theologians were, however, greatly exercised by the implications of any attempt to predict, and perhaps thereby depart from, God's plan for his creation. Judicial astrology, which sought to forecast future events, aroused grave suspicion, whereas the 'natural' variety, as practised by responsible physicians and surgeons, appeared more acceptable. Even so, the assumption that mankind lay at the mercy of remote and inexorable planetary forces raised some knotty moral issues. If Saturn, Luna or Mars had arbitrarily dealt him the cards of leprosy, madness or apoplexy, the patient could surely disclaim any personal responsibility for his condition. Indeed, it might even be argued that there was little point in following a sound physical and spiritual regimen at all. Here the practitioner was obliged to tread carefully, emphasising the importance of free will and human agency.[249] Allowing, of course, for the fact that God might well use the planets as instruments of retribution, the writers of medical textbooks went out of their way to stress that prayer, penitence and clean living could overturn the most inauspicious horoscope. By the same token, no planet, however benign, could protect its child against the destructive consequences of a 'wykede wyll and sinfull life'.[250]

From the cold hand of Saturn to the consumption of rotten meat, the physical and environmental factors likely to provoke the onset of leprosy in a vulnerable individual were sufficiently diverse to provide a logical explanation in almost all eventualities. They reflect a coherent, sophisticated idea of the body as a complex network of veins, nerves and arteries, whose proper function depended upon the cultivation of a precarious balance. Concern about the risks of infection (in the modern sense), which first became apparent in mid-thirteenth-century England, increased significantly after the Black Death, while, at the same time, the steady dissemination of ideas about sexual transmission provided another cudgel with which to beat the urban underclass. On the other hand, members of the medical profession (whose patients invariably came from the more reputable strata of society) were reluctant to moralise, especially when

248 Henryson, *Testament of Cresseid*, p. 73, and pp. 30–34, for a discussion of the poet's knowledge of astrology.
249 Tester, *History of Western Astrology*, pp. 176–8; L. Thorndike, *A History of Magic and Experimental Science* (8 vols, New York, 1923–58), ii, pp. 584–5.
250 BL, MS Egerton 2572, fos 61v–62r; MS Sloane 1315, fo. 36r–36v.

the causes of *discrasia* lay, as in the case of heredity, beyond an individual's control. The steady refinement of Catholic teaching on purgatory meanwhile accorded every humble and penitent leper a crucial role in the economy of salvation. Through his Job-like suffering, he accumulated sufficient spiritual credit to purchase the release of others beside himself. Since his prayers thus became a desirable commodity, to be sought by the faithful and enlisted by sinners, it is hardly surprising that responses to his disease were just as varied as the explanations offered for it.

# 3

## The Sick and the Healthy: Reactions to Suffering

*But the service which the Christian leper is pre-eminently fitted for, is doubtless that of intercession. With heartfelt gratitude I acknowledge help thus received on several occasions through the prayers of leper Christians, whose help I always invoke when on any special mission. Perhaps some day we shall wake up to the fact that within our Asylums is a marvellous latent force ready for use, longing for employment; and some child of God will arise to the occasion and organise a band of praying lepers who will . . . give themselves continually to definite prayer and thus become a mighty force in the ranks of Christ's army.*

W.C. Irvine, Report on a Conference of Leper Asylum
Superintendents, *1920*[1]

As his name suggests, William le Gros, earl of Aumale (d. 1179), was a renowned heavyweight. So obese that, by middle age, he could not mount a horse (or undertake a penitential pilgrimage to Jerusalem), he cast a vast shadow over the north of England. In his more active youth he had successfully commanded an army against the Scots, being rewarded by King Stephen with the earldom of Yorkshire. Already a great landowner, he now ruled his kingdom beyond the Humber with an iron hand. He clearly brooked no opposition from either priest or layman, terrorising the bishop of Durham and his men into submission, and, in 1141, personally imposing Stephen's candidate for the newly vacant see of York upon the reluctant chapter. An excommunicate, who allegedly had his most trenchant ecclesiastical opponent castrated, he showed even less respect for the Church during the anarchy of Stephen's last years, when he attacked the estates of Whitby abbey and evicted the Augustinian canons of Bridlington. But once his former enemy, Henry II, mounted the throne he found ample leisure for repentance. It was, allegedly, in remorse for his profanity and pride that he embarked upon a spectacular programme of religious patronage, culminating in the foundation of two Cistercian monasteries at Meaux (Yorkshire) and Vaudey (Lincolnshire). The election of Roger de Pont l'Evêque as archbishop of York, in 1154, seems to have provided him with a mentor, through whose guidance his

---

[1]   Irvine, 'Christian Teaching', p. 134.

nascent piety and contrition were directed into productive channels.[2] They found perfect expression in the establishment of another, now long-forgotten house near his borough of Hedon in Holderness.

This deeply personal act of atonement was undertaken during the 1170s in a blaze of publicity. At York Minster, before the prior of Bridlington, the dean and assembled chapter (which, in earlier days he had cowed into submission) and a crowd of local notables, he humbly mounted the steps of the high altar to dedicate his offering to God, Saint Mary Magdalen and a community of lepers already living at Newton Garth. As his foundation charter reveals, it was a handsome endowment, comprising a substantial amount of land stocked with five hundred sheep, twenty-four oxen (three plough teams), six bulls, twelve cows, twenty pigs, a hundred hens and sixty geese. To this he added a neighbouring mill at Preston, then worth 66s. 8d. a year, as well as the right to hold an annual fair, recently confirmed by the crown, which took place in the last week of July around the feast of the Magdalen. The grant was to support a hospital for twenty lepers and a number of servants, along with two priests and two clerks to celebrate the divine office. Commemoration of the Christian departed loomed large in the lives of both clergy and patients. Specific provision was made for the salvation of Henry I, at whose court William had been raised. His first queen, Matilda, who, as we shall see, was celebrated for her devotion to the leprous, was also remembered. Other beneficiaries included the present king, Henry II, and his issue, as well as the family of the donor, whose own spiritual health was naturally a matter of considerable urgency. The endowment was to be managed by Archbishop Roger and his successors in conjunction with the dean and chapter, who would together ensure that the terms of the foundation charter were observed forever.[3]

Earl William's award reflects a combination of astute political calculation, aimed to win over an authoritarian monarch (many of his other endowments also made provision for the king's soul after death), anxiety about the afterlife and a desire to assist the needy. That such benevolence was more than a pious convention seems, however, to be confirmed by a chronicler of Whitby abbey, who had little reason to praise the earl's magnanimity. Noting his fearsome reputation and the havoc wrought by him on the monastic estates during Stephen's reign, he observed that, 'even so, he loved the poor, and especially lepers, and liberally distributed generous alms among them'. In response to an appeal from the abbot he left the *leprosarium* at Whitby unscathed, and allowed the inmates to collect their revenues in peace.[4]

Earl William was certainly not alone in his conspicuous regard for the leprous poor, or his recruitment of their services as intercessors for the redemption of a bruised and battered soul.[5] As we saw in the previous chapter, his contemporary,

2 B. English, *The Lords of Holderness 1086–1260* (Hull, 1991), pp. 16–28; J.C. Atkinson, ed., *Cartularium Abbathiae de Whitby* (2 vols, Surtees Society, lxix, 1878, and lxii, 1881), ii, pp. 517–19; E.A. Bond, ed., *Chronica Monasterii de Melsa* (3 vols, RS, 1866–67), i, pp. xiii–xvi, 76–7.
3 York Minster Library, MS B2 (3) a 4–5; W. Farrer, ed., *Early Yorkshire Charters* (3 vols, Edinburgh, 1914–16), iii, pp. 37–9. A brief history of the hospital may be found in W. Page, ed., *VCH Yorkshire III* (London, 1913), pp. 308–9.
4 Atkinson, *Cartularium Abbathiae de Whitby*, ii, pp. 517–19.
5 Ranulph, earl of Chester, offers a similar example of a warlord whose later life was marked by a desire

Abbot Walter de Lucy of Reading (d. 1171), another 'hard and haughty man' noted for his ruthless defence of monastic liberties, was much given to acts of self-abasement before malodorous and ulcerated paupers. Lepers, in particular, earned his compassion. 'Not only did he not shrink from them', one chronicler reports, but 'frequently ministering to them himself, he would wash their hands and feet and kiss them gently in deep sympathy of his charity and piety'.[6] Admirable as they seem, however, the abbot's actions, and the very words used to record them, had by then become commonplace. The charitable works of Robert the Pious, king of France (d. 1031), and Theobald the Great, count of Blois and Champagne (d. 1152), are, for example, described in almost identical terms.[7] Like their kinsfolk across the Channel, leading members of the Anglo-Norman nobility had learned to venerate *Christus quasi leprosus*. Members of the elite who could not actually bring themselves to tend the sick in person did so vicariously as founders and benefactors of the countless *leprosaria* and hospitals that became such a prominent feature of the medieval landscape.

Having imposed their awesome military presence upon a conquered nation, the new Norman overlords of England set about a comprehensive programme of religious reform. The twelfth century witnessed an unparalleled rise in the number of monastic foundations. Over 200 abbeys and priories, mostly for new orders such as the Cistercians and Augustinians, appeared between 1066 and 1135 alone, playing a notable part in the ongoing process of colonisation.[8] But these fortresses of prayer represented more than a crude desire to cow a subject population. Hand in hand with respect for the increasing number of men and women who felt drawn 'to live the life of Christ' went a quest for personal salvation, which might be achieved through their intercession.[9] And if the endowment of a monastery brought manifold spiritual benefits, that of a hospital was hardly less commendable. Whereas the largest and richest barely differed from monastic houses, and were often run by canons or monks, even the smallest constituted a work of charity for Christ's poor. In catering for the material and spiritual wants of the sick and destitute, the hospital patron not only fulfilled an important social need, but also guaranteed his or her speedy passage through the fires of purgatory.

Although numbers are notoriously hard to determine, and foundation dates remain even more elusive, a bare minimum of 320 *leprosaria* were established in England between the close of the eleventh century and the Dissolution, most being in existence well before 1350 [map 1].[10] This means that between one

---

for 'repentance and reparation', and whose many endowments included a *leprosarium* at Chester: J.A. Green, *The Aristocracy of Norman England* (Cambridge, 1997), p. 419, and chapter twelve, passim.

6    Searle, *Chronicle of Battle Abbey*, pp. 260–61, and for Lucy's character, p. 12.

7    Helgaud de Fleury, *Vie de Robert le pieux*, eds R.H. Bautier and G. Labory (Paris, 1965), pp. 126–7; Walter Map, *De nugis curialium*, ed. M.R. James, revised C.N.L. Brooke and R.A.B. Mynors (Oxford, 1983), pp. 462–5. As the concept of *Christus quasi leprosus* became more popular, the leper tended by Theobald was transformed from an ordinary mortal into Christ: Caesarius of Heisterbach, *Dialogue of Miracles*, ii, pp. 30–31.

8    E. Cownie, *Religious Patronage in Anglo-Norman England 1066–1135* (London, 1998), pp. 173, 187.

9    Green, *Aristocracy of Norman England*, p. 412.

10   Satchell, 'Emergence of Leper-Houses', pp. 69–112, 250–399, offers the most reliable list of 299 *leprosaria*, fourteen of which cannot now be documented before 1350 at the earliest. He counts Yarmouth's hospital (which had separate quarters for men and women) twice, and omits eight

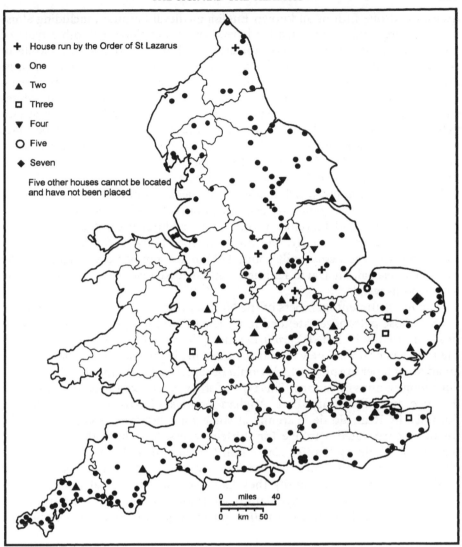

1. English leper houses founded before *c.* 1350 (Phillip Judge)

pre-1350 foundations: St Katherine's, Rochester, Kent, 1316 (S. Sweetinburgh, *The Role of the Hospital in Medieval England* (Dublin, 2004), p. 79 n. 49); St Mary Magdalen, Luton, Bedfordshire, by 1271 (*CPR, 1266–1272*, p. 537); Brichtiu's, by *c.* 1170, and St Benedict's, by 1305, both Norwich, an unnamed leper house at New Buckenham, *c.* 1140, and St Lazarus, Wormegay, 1166 x 75, all in Norfolk (C. Rawcliffe, *The Hospitals of Medieval Norwich* (Norwich, 1995), pp. 48–50; and notes 15 and 188, below); St Petronilla's, Bury St Edmunds, and a house at Wentford in Poslingford, Suffolk, both twelfth-century (C. Harper-Bill, ed., *Charters of the Medieval Hospitals of Bury St Edmunds* (Suffolk Records Society, Charter Series, xiv, 1994), pp. 3–9, 98–9; idem and R. Mortimer, eds, *Stoke by Clare Cartulary* (3 vols, ibid., iv–vi, 1982–84), ii, no. 436). To this total should be added Burton Lazars, Leicestershire, *c.* 1157, and up to seven daughter houses run as *leprosaria* (sometimes for only a short time) by the Order of St Lazarus (Marcombe, *Leper Knights*, pp. 154–61). At least six more were founded after 1350 (below, pp. 351–2), which gives us a working total of 320, subject to constant revision as more evidence comes to light.

quarter and one fifth of all known English medieval hospitals, including alms-houses, were initially intended for lepers, sometimes along with other types of patient. In Scotland the proportion also stood at around one fifth, while in Ireland *leprosaria* may possibly have comprised well over half a total which is, however, far from certain.[11] Some endowments constituted a pragmatic response to an immediate domestic problem. Claims and anecdotes surrounding the foundation of specific institutions can rarely be taken at face value, but it appears that several were set up, or at least supported, by benefactors whose friends, servants and relatives had contracted leprosy. Thus, for example, Hugh, earl of Chester (d. 1181), is said to have established the hospital of St Mary Magdalen, at Spon, near Coventry, as a refuge for one of his household knights. His grant, which included a chapel and sufficient land to pay for a priest, was, however, generous enough to provide for any local people who became leprous, and therefore promised the additional spiritual credit he so devoutly sought.[12] Similarly, the borough leper house at Cashel, in County Tipperary, was reputedly built about 1230 to accommodate a daughter of the English seneschal, Sir David Latimer, but provided a welcome resource for the townsfolk as well.[13]

The more affluent members of the Norman elite, such as Roger Mowbray (d. 1188), whose patronage extended to no fewer than twenty-two separate institutions, invariably included *leprosaria* among their many endowments.[14] Indeed, the founders of several new monastic houses made provision from the outset for an adjacent leper hospital, which would be supervised and supported by the resident monks, nuns or canons. This type of arrangement obtained, for example, at the two twelfth-century East Anglian priories of Wormegay and Butley. Founded by Reginald de Warenne at some point between 1166 and 1175, the former incorporated a refuge for thirteen lepers, for whom the canons were responsible.[15] Henry II's justiciar Ralph Glanville (d. 1190) and his wife Berta likewise entrusted their new *leprosarium* at West Somerton to the pastoral care of the Augustinian community they had established nearby at Butley. In this instance, as we shall see, their lambs fell among wolves.[16] Lesser barons and landowners lacked the means for such grandiose gestures, but still possessed the

---

11  Gilchrist, *Contemplation and Action*, pp. 10–11. A. Gwynn and R.N. Hadcock, *Medieval Religious Houses in Ireland* (London, 1970), pp. 346–57, list fifty-four *leprosaria*, one being very dubious. See Orme and Webster, *English Hospital*, pp. 10–11, on the difficulty of counting medieval hospitals.
12  William Dugdale, *The Antiquities of Warwickshire* (2 vols, London, 1730), i, p. 197.
13  Lee, *Leper Hospitals*, p. 40.
14  Green, *Aristocracy of Norman England*, pp. 419–20. Mowbray's various endowments are itemised in Gibbs, *Complete Peerage*, ix, p. 372; and his generosity to the English Order of St Lazarus is discussed in Marcombe, *Leper Knights*, pp. 35–9.
15  N. Vincent, 'The Foundation of Wormegay Priory', *Norfolk Archaeology*, xliii (1999), pp. 307–12. William de Warenne (d. 1088), Reginald's grandfather, may well have set an example at Lewes, Sussex, where the Cluniac priory which he endowed was closely linked to the *leprosarium* of St Nicholas: W. Page, ed., *VCH Sussex II* (London, 1907), pp. 64–5, 104; J. Caley and J. Hunter, eds, *Valor Ecclesiasticus* (6 vols, London, 1810–34), i, p. 331. Eudo Dapifer (d. by 1120), steward to Henry I, likewise founded both a monastery and a leper house at Colchester: W. Page and J.H. Round, eds, *VCH Essex II* (London, 1907), pp. 93, 184.
16  BL, Harley Roll N 20; R. Mortimer, 'The Prior of Butley and the Lepers of West Somerton', *BIHR*, liii (1980), pp. 99–103; below, pp. 317–18.

resources necessary for the foundation of a small hospital or leper house, perhaps for just a handful of people. Friends, retainers, relatives and tenants could, moreover, be relied upon to augment what might have been an initially modest endowment, often centred upon a church or chapel.

The few surviving cartularies of medieval English *leprosaria* confirm that individual gifts were often small and scattered equivalents of the widow's mite. William le Mercer's grant of one and a half pence rent a year to illuminate the daily Mass at St Peter's, Bury St Edmunds, in about 1220 seems far more typical than the ostentatious philanthropy of William le Gros.[17] Most of the settlements made upon the hospital of St James at Thanington, outside Canterbury, which accommodated twenty-five leprous women under the guardianship of the cathedral monks, fell into this category. Although by the fourteenth century the hospital owned well over 170 acres of land, its holdings had been acquired piecemeal, through gifts and exchanges averaging no more than two or three acres at a time made by local people in the hope of redemption.[18] Run under the patronage of the de Mauley family (which eventually entrusted it to the wealthy London hospital of St Thomas Acon), St James's, Doncaster, depended upon an equally supportive network of kindred and neighbours. The largest of the forty-four endowments recorded in its cartulary comprised just twelve acres of reclaimed land 'to dig and dyke' given by the relatives of Peter de Mauley's late wife, while annual rents from other pious donors ranged from one penny to a shilling.[19] We can rarely penetrate below the tip of the iceberg to the scores of suburban *leprosaria* whose origins are so tantalisingly obscure. But a pattern of acquisitions similar to that found at St Bartholomew's, near Oxford, and St Nicholas's, Royston, must have been common. Between them, these two hospitals attracted at least sixty-six donations of rents and property, mostly from smallholders, farmers and burgesses of middling stature.[20]

More surprisingly, although the great wave of foundations ended well before the Black Death, when many *leprosaria* had already either disappeared or ceased to accommodate the sick in significant numbers, the display of philanthropy continued. The testators of fourteenth- and fifteenth-century Norwich were far from unusual in earmarking local leper houses as their preferred recipients of charity, while in nearby Yarmouth the threat of *mors improvisa* during the Black Death prompted a dramatic and hitherto unprecedented increase in the size of legacies settled upon such communities.[21] Fear of miasma and the threat posed by the proximity of lepers had established a powerful hold by this date, but it was

---

17 W.H. Turner and H.O. Coxe, eds, *Calendar of Charters and Rolls Preserved in the Bodleian Library* (Oxford, 1878), p. 436.

18 BL, MS Add. 32098, fos 1r–21v. See also, W. Somer, *The Antiquities of Canterbury* (London, 1703), part 1, pp. 41–2.

19 BL, MS Cotton Tiberius C V, fos 233r–286r.

20 Satchell, 'Emergence of Leper-Houses', pp. 176–89.

21 Two out of every five Norwich testators, between 1370 and 1532, whose wills survive remembered the city's *leprosaria*, usually leaving at least a few pence to each of the five, or else to each inmate: N. Tanner, *The Church in Late Medieval Norwich* (Toronto, 1984), p. 133. For Yarmouth, see NRO, Y/C4/70, rots 1v–7r. Around 80 per cent of late medieval testators in Beverley and 40 per cent of those in Scarborough made bequests to *leprosaria*: P. Cullum, 'Hospitals and Charitable Provision in Medieval Yorkshire 936–1547' (University of York, DPhil, 1990), p. 293.

certainly not the only explanation for generosity to extramural hospitals. Even if the image of *Christus quasi leprosus* had grown somewhat tarnished, the intercessionary prayers of their inmates could still be traded as valuable currency in the purchase of paradise.

This chapter will explore the symbiotic, but often deeply ambivalent, relationship between the sick and the healthy in medieval England. Having first examined the very different attitudes to *lepra* reflected in the Old and New Testaments, we turn to the saints, whose lives and legends exercised such a powerful influence upon the residents and benefactors of leper houses. Personifying the qualities of penitence, humility and compassion, Mary Magdalen, in particular, presented a role model for the leprous. The sacrament of confession offered a unique opportunity for them, like her, to repent and embark upon a new vocation. But it was, in some respects, a double-edged sword. As we shall see, the intimate connection between sin and disease fostered in the 'confessional society' of the thirteenth century did not always work to their disadvantage. This was because generosity to the poor of Christ offered a hope of salvation to men and women who had scant reason for optimism about the life to come. Yet a growing preoccupation with the torments and stench of hell, along with widespread fears of bodily and political disintegration, had less positive connotations. A society that both despised and admired physical beauty would inevitably regard extreme disfigurement with mixed feelings. The hospitalised leper was, none the less, far too useful ever to forfeit his or her pre-eminent role as a vehicle for redemption, although, as the final part of this chapter reveals, the exchange could sometimes become crudely mechanical. It is hardly surprising that the examples presented here convey a disjointed, even contradictory, picture of medieval reactions to *lepra*. Attitudes to the sick in any society are rarely monolithic, nor do they change at a uniform rate, however persuasive the arguments of the Church, the state or the medical profession may be. Even a study of the Bible, to which we first turn, furnished instances of both ostracism and inclusion, and thus served to justify conduct ranging from overt vilification to ostentatious reverence.

## 'Bothe fowlle and fayer': saints and sinners

The thirteenth and fourteenth books of Leviticus specified in great detail how and by whom *sāra'ath* was to be diagnosed, the ceremonial form of exclusion and the rites of purification to be observed by those who had apparently recovered and might be readmitted into the community.[22] The overriding concern of Mosaic Law was with pollution rather than infection, which meant that the priest played a crucial role at all stages. In the words of the Wycliffe Bible:

> The Lord spak to Moyses and Aaron, and seide, A man in whos skyn and fleisch rysith dyuerse colour, ether whelke, ethir as sum schynynge thing, that is, a wounde of lepre, he schal be brought to Aaron preest, ether to oon who euer of

---

[22] For a full exposition of the 'eight commandments' concerning leprosy, see H. Danby, ed., *The Code of Maimonides: Book Ten, The Book of Cleanness* (New Haven and London, 1954), pp. 147–204.

hise sones; and whanne he seeth lepre in the skyn, and the heeris chaungide in to whijte colour, and that spice of lepre lowere than the t'other skyn and fleisch, it is a wounde of lepre, and he schal be departed at the doom of the preest.[23]

Uncertain cases were subject to a brief period of segregation to see if the disease developed. But once it had been confirmed there was only one possible outcome:

> Therfor whoeuer is defoulid with lepre, and is departid at the doom of the preest, he schal haue hise clothis vnsewid, bareheed, the mouth hilid [covered] with a cloth, he schal crye hym silf defoulid, and viyl [vile]; in al tyme in which he is lepre and vnclene, he schal dwelle aloone without the castels.[24]

Just as individuals, such as Miriam and Gehazi, personified particular vices, so the various manifestations of *sāra'ath* minutely catalogued in Leviticus might be read in a more general way as analogies for sin in its infinite variety. Both Gregory the Great and Isidore of Seville, for example, regarded the coloured spots and lesions, itemised in Mosaic Law, as 'a figure' or metaphor for the manifold blotches of heresy that defiled the body of the Church.[25] Such an approach provided fertile ground for a range of metaphors that embraced every part of the body and every conceivable act of transgression, from laziness to apostasy. Tertullian (d. 220), for example, compared the reappearance of *lepra* in a house that had previously been cleansed by the priest to a lapsed sinner who reoffended after baptism, thereby resuming 'the scabs and stains of the flesh'.[26] This type of commentary reached its apogee in works such as the *De morali lepra* (*c.* 1470) of the Dominican theologian Johannes Nider, which took the reader systematically through each of the seven deadly sins (and their offspring), added accidie as an eighth for good measure, and then itemised the spiritual conse- quences of ignoring the Ten Commandments.[27]

Comparisons between different symptoms of *lepra* and breaches of the Decalogue, such as murder, covetousness, idolatry and Sabbath-breaking, fitted into the general pattern established by commentators on Leviticus, although they tended to focus upon the New Testament rather than the Old. As Hugh of St Victor (d. 1142) observed in his *Allegoriae in Novum Testamentum*, this was because the ten lepers miraculously healed by Christ [Luke 17, vv. 12–19] together offered a perfect analogy for all those men and women who had disobeyed the precepts given by God to Moses. They were, as a result, defiled by the leprosy of 'diverse and damnable' sins, which might only be absolved

---

23  J. Forshall and F. Madden, eds, *The Holy Bible . . . by John Wycliffe* (4 vols, Oxford, 1850), i, p. 319.
24  Forshall and Madden, *Holy Bible*, i, p. 322.
25  Bliss, *Morals in the Book of Job*, i, p. 262; Isidore of Seville, *Opera omnia: Quaestiones in Vetus Testamentum*, PL, lxxxiii, cols 328–30; Brody, *Disease of the Soul*, pp. 124–6.
26  A. Roberts and J. Donaldson, eds, *The Writings of Quintus Sept. Flor. Tertullianus* (3 vols, Edinburgh, 1895), iii, p. 115–16.
27  Johannes Nider, *De morali lepra* (Nuremberg, *c.* 1470), unpaginated. Accidie, or spiritual sloth, was a particular vice of men and women in religious orders, including the inmates of *leprosaria*: A. Murray, 'Religion among the Poor in Thirteenth-Century France: The Testimony of Humbert de Romans', *Traditio*, xxx (1974), pp. 285–324, at pp. 112–13.

through divine grace [plate 12].[28] Writing at greater length about the cleansing of the solitary leper after the Sermon on the Mount [Matthew 8, vv. 1–4], Hugh explained how this single individual might likewise be taken as a representative of all mankind, whose sins had been washed away by Christ's sacrifice on the cross.

> This leper is the human race, which, while it was leprous, was separated and far distant from God and the City of God, that is to say Jerusalem (which on high is our mother). But the Lord . . . has healed the leper, and made him a citizen of his city. Nor does the Lord disdain to perform this miracle every day through His grace. For there are, indeed, many within the body of Holy Church who are befouled by the leprosy of vice and polluted by the contagion of sins, as by leprosy. All the impure, fornicators, concubines, the incestuous, adulterers, the avaricious, usurers, false witnesses, perjurers, those who call a brother 'fool', and who look lustfully upon a woman, and even those who do not perform wicked acts, but harbour wicked desires: all such people, who are isolated from God because of their faults, are deemed to be leprous by the priests, who know and keep the law of God, and they are therefore separated from the company of the faithful in a *spiritual*, but not physical, sense.[29]

Those who had committed venial but not mortal sins, would be afflicted by scabies rather than leprosy, and could thus continue to live among their Christian brothers, but most, at some point in their lives, contracted *lepra* and thus remained in urgent need of the divine physician. From such a standpoint, the real, suffering leper stood for Everyman, his diseased body personifying both human sin and the potential for redemption. It was a truly comprehensive image.

We should also bear in mind the emphasis placed by theologians, from St Jerome onwards, upon Christ's *rejection* of the old Jewish law, especially with regard to lepers and other social outcasts, whom He welcomed into the community of the faithful.[30] At the very time that Anselm of Laon (d. 1117) and other scholars were developing this theme of inclusiveness, a remarkable legend about the consecration of the great basilica of Saint-Denis almost five centuries earlier began circulating throughout northern France. It told how a poor leper, fearing that he might not be allowed inside to watch the service, hid in the church overnight to be sure of a place. To his consternation, as darkness fell, Christ, accompanied by his saints and a host of angels, entered through one of the windows in a blaze of light and performed the ceremony in private. His eye fell upon the leper, whom He ordered to announce what had happened to King Dagobert and his bishops. Not surprisingly the leper demurred, on the grounds of his vile appearance. With a sweep of his hand, Christ removed the ulcerated and suppu-

---

28  Hugh of St Victor, *Opera omnia*, PL, clxxv, *Allegoriae in Novum Testamentum*, iv, cap. xxv, col. 823.
29  *Allegoriae in Novum Testamentum*, iv, cap. xvi, cols 789–91. For unexplained reasons, this text (which the editors consider 'questionable') is attributed by Brody, *Disease of the Soul*, p. 127, to Richard of St Victor (d. 1173). Bériac, *Histoire des lépreux*, pp. 101–2, follows suit.
30  Touati, 'Contagion', p. 183. According to the Apocrypha, Christ's sympathy for lepers began in childhood, for he reputedly effected cures during his infancy: R. McL. Wilson and W. Schneemelcher, eds, *New Testament Apocrypha, I* (SCM Press, 1973), p. 410.

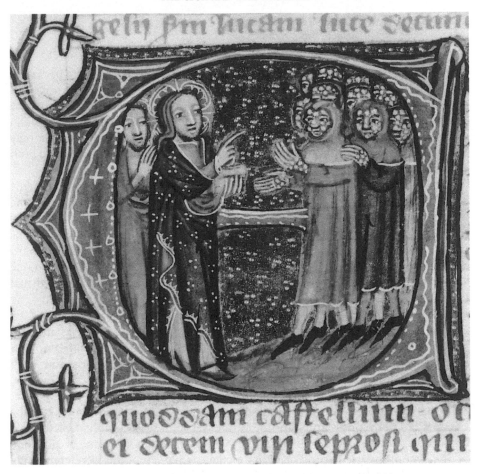

12. Christ heals the ten lepers [Luke 17, vv. 12–19], who are depicted in this particular illumination from a late fourteenth-century English gospel with the tuberous hands and faces that the artist would have associated with advanced cases of the disease.

rating flesh from his face, placing it, like a stone death mask, upon one of the pillars, where it provided eloquent proof of a miracle.[31]

Assiduously propagated by the clergy of Saint-Denis, the cult of 'Saint Ladre' or 'Saint Pérégrin', as he was known, flourished until the French Revolution. Successive versions of the tale, in both prose and verse, reflect the spread of the medical ideas described in the previous chapter. Whereas the first account is silent, as one would expect, on the topic of infection, a thirteenth-century verse reports the leper's protest that:

> Nobody will want to look at me,
> Nobody will dare to speak to me,
> Because I have polluted breath [*infeitueuse alainne*].[32]

But, at all stages, the power of this foundation myth hinges upon the person of the leper, whose piety and faith were so generously rewarded by a merciful Christ, and whose macerated features, now welded into the very fabric of the basilica, bore witness to His presence. The fact that a bemused local fisherman was said to have witnessed St Peter's consecration of Westminster Abbey may have been entirely fitting in light of the saint's original calling, but it lacked both the sheer drama and pathos of this remarkable encounter.[33]

Christ's love for the despised and leprous outcast remained a constant theme of devotional writing throughout the Middle Ages. Thus, for instance, the author of the Middle English poem *Cleanness* contrasted the courtesy invariably extended by Christ to 'lazares', and others whom Mosaic Law then treated as pariahs, with His loathing for the foul pollution of sin. Whatever one's outward appearance, *inner* purity was the sole prerequisite for salvation.[34] Nor could one aspire to spiritual health while rejecting those to whom the Son of God had extended His hand. 'Grucche noght to uisite the seke', warned one fifteenth-century tract, prompting the reader to follow the example set by Christ. 'For it is write in the gospel that He touched bare the meseles and thei were made hole, wherfore the seruaunt schulde noght haue disdeyn to doo that his lord dede'.[35] The horrific fate awaiting those who failed to show such compassion was spelt out unambiguously in the parable of Dives and Lazarus, which, as we saw in chapter one, greatly exercised the medieval imagination. Although he appears in Luke's gospel as a beggar 'full of sores' [16, v. 20], the Lazarus of later iconography and literature was almost invariably depicted as a leper. So close was his identification with the disease that his name became one of the synonyms used to describe its victims, while *leprosaria* were commonly known as lazar houses. Like Job, he ranked high among the intercessors to whom the victims of skin diseases (and later syphilitics) most often had recourse, one of his principal attractions being the divine favour which he so demonstrably inspired.

The story of Lazarus was both dramatic and powerful [**plate 2**]. Near to death, he was carried to the house of Dives, a man of great wealth, where he begged crumbs from his groaning table. Yet only the dogs came to help him, gently licking his sores with their tongues before he expired outside the gates. At this very moment, though, in the words of one medieval homilist, 'the dice were changed'.[36] For Lazarus was transported directly to heaven by angels, while Dives was condemned to roast in the eternal flames of hell as a punishment for

---

[32] Lombard-Jourdan, *Saint-Denis*, p. 199. The leper is, significantly, described as *elephantiosus* in the first account.

[33] Lombard-Jourdan, *Saint-Denis*, p. 197.

[34] R.J. Menner, ed., *Purity, A Middle English Poem* (Yale Studies in English, lxi, 1970), p. 42; B. Stone, ed. and trans., *The Owl and the Nightingale, Cleanness and St Erkenwald* (Harmondsworth, 1971), p. 123.

[35] BL, MS Harley 45, fo. 84v.

[36] W. Nelson Francis, ed., *The Book of Vices and Virtues* (EETS, ccxvii, 1942), p. 204.

his refusal to share the gifts that had been lavished upon him. It is interesting to note that, as well as being the archetypical 'riche glotoun', Dives personifies greed, pride and avarice, sins punished in the Old Testament *with* leprosy, but in the New redeemable *through* the person of Lazarus, the abused beggar.[37] Not surprisingly, the benefactors of leper houses were as anxious as the patients to enlist his support. Bishop Richard Poore's charter of 1228 to the leprous sisters of Maiden Bradley evoked the poignant image of Lazarus seeking crumbs from the rich man's table. Destined for a life outside the camp and tormented by their physical sufferings, the nuns were, however, assured of succour from their bishop, who, as guardian of the Lord's flock, compared himself, with becoming humility, to one of Dives's dogs.[38] Unusually for an English *leprosarium*, the house may have fostered the cult of St Lazarus, for at least one undated endowment was made upon it specifically in his honour.[39] By and large, though, he was far more popular as a dedicatee and patron in continental Europe, where many hospitals bore his name. Still surviving in the nineteenth century, the banner of one Flemish leper house depicted Lazarus, crowned with a halo but still displaying his sores, beside the infant Christ, his mother and a dog. Transformed into a heraldic device, his beggar's rattle provided an appropriate border, interspersed with the arms of the patrons, the lords of Gruthuyse. Further to advertise their identification with the supreme representative of Christ's poor, the lord and lady appear in miniature kneeling in supplication at his ulcerated feet [plate 13].[40]

Employed in medieval England as a means of instruction in the Christian virtues of compassion, humility and submissiveness, 'debates' or 'disputations' between the two protagonists of the parable – one in heaven the other in hell – stressed the potentially corrosive effects of health and riches upon the soul.[41] Aside from teaching an obvious lesson about the merits of institutional charity, which the ruling elite earnestly took to heart, the tale of Lazarus offered yet another example of suffering rewarded. One book of vernacular remedies for 'pore folk that falleth into sekenes' (a version of the *Liber pauperum de medicinis* of Pope John XXI) advised that:

> God sendeth also good men syknes here for they shuld haue the more blysse herafftir yf they taketh her syknes in *pacience* and without gruchyng [complaint]. And in this wise lazer was syke that lay ful of buyles [boils] at the riche mannys yate. And aftirward he lay in Abrahames bosom when the riche man was buyried in helle. And god punyssheth good men with seknes for . . . profite of other men.

---

37  Significantly, in some homilies, Dives is also associated with 'sins of the mouth': Diekstra, *Book for a Simple and Devout Woman*, p. 175.

38  B.R. Kemp, ed., *EEA, 19, Salisbury 1217–1228* (Oxford, 2000), no. 319.

39  BL, MS Add. 37503, fo. 21r. With the exception of Sherburn (see note 55 below), Radford, near Stafford (M.W. Greenslade, ed., *VCH Stafford III* (London, 1970), pp. 289–90), and Wormegay (see note 15 above), very few English *leprosaria* besides those run by the Order were dedicated to St Lazarus.

40  The banner of 1502 was painted on cloth, and would have been used in religious processions: P. Lacroix, *Vie militaire et religieuse au moyen âge* (Paris, 1873), p. 389, fig. 271.

41  See, for example, Trinity College, Cambridge, MS 0.9.28, fos 188v–189r, which possibly belonged to the collegiate church of St Mary, Warwick; C. Davidson, 'The Fate of the Damned in English Art and Drama', in idem and T.H. Seiler, eds, *The Iconography of Hell* (Kalamazoo, 1992), pp. 41–66.

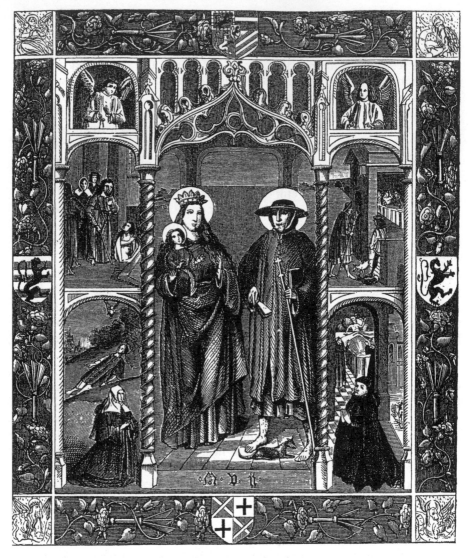

13. A banner of 1502 from a Flemish leper house dedicated to St Lazarus reflects the desire of patrons to advertise their compassion for the leprous poor of Christ and thereby secure their own salvation (the leper's rattle displayed in the border has assumed the status of a heraldic device). The contrast with Dives, whose soul is borne away by a demon on his deathbed (bottom right), is striking. The Lazarus whom Christ raised from the dead (top left hand) was by this date widely assumed to be the poor beggar, which further strengthened his cult. Symbols of the evangelists appear in the corners. The drawing was made in *c.* 1870, when interest in medieval *leprosaria* was reviving.

And thus Job and Toby [Tobias] were syke to yeue other men ensample of hou *pacient* they shuld be.[42]

We shall return to the Church's expectations of how lepers and other victims of disease should behave later in this chapter, but it is important to note here that, for most medieval men and women, Lazarus was a composite character derived from two very different biblical figures.

Lord Gruthuyse's banner depicts a series of incidents from the saint's life, one of which shows him rising from the grave, with Christ at his side. The picture actually refers to another Lazarus, the brother of Martha and Mary of Bethany, in whose home Christ often stayed. When this Lazarus suddenly fell ill, the two women sent for their Lord, but He arrived four days too late to find the young man already entombed. The raising of Lazarus from the dead was the greatest of all Christ's miracles, which led the Pharisees to demand His arrest and, indeed, prefigured His own resurrection [John 11, vv. 1–45]. Following the conventional (but clearly erroneous) assumption that Lazarus of Bethany had contracted leprosy, Hugh of Lincoln made much of his remarkable history when visiting *leprosaria*.[43] Guy de Chauliac likewise consoled his patients with the thought that Christ had 'loued Lazer, the leprouse man, more than other men'.[44] Indeed, as we saw in the previous chapter, he also assured them that, like Lazarus, they would survive what must have seemed a living death. Certainly, the cult of a holy leper who rose from the grave flourished widely. Part beggar and part revenant, he became the patron of a crusading order initially composed of leprous knights, which in England established its headquarters with generous support from Mowbrays and their retainers at Burton Lazars in Leicestershire. Here, in the hospital chapel, his image (which did not survive the Reformation) attracted the offerings of the faithful.[45] His legendary status helps to explain the popularity of another saint, who also extended her protection to lepers.

The N-Town cycle of mystery plays, which were performed in East Anglia during the fifteenth century, includes a version of *The Last Supper*, set in the house of Simon the leper. This humble man, clad 'in sympyl aray', enthusiastically welcomes the disciples into his home, where Christ promises him the gift of eternal life:

> There joye of all joyis to the is sewre [sure]
> (Symon, I knowe thi trewe intent),
> The blysse of hefne thu xalt recure;
> This rewarde I xal the grawnt present.[46]

This compassionate gesture leads Mary Magdalen, another outcast, who plies her trade as a prostitute, to bewail the fact that she will know neither peace nor

[42] BL, MS Sloane 3489, fo. 29r–29v.

[43] Douie and Farmer, *Life of St Hugh*, ii, p. 14.

[44] Ogden, *Cyrurgie of Guy de Chauliac*, p. 381. This, and much other English evidence, renders untenable Marcia Kupfer's assertion that 'by the late thirteenth century the medicalised stereotype of the irascible leper, derelict, foul and lascivious, drowned out the competing paradigm of the poor Lazarus': Kupfer, *Art of Healing*, p. 142.

[45] Marcombe, *Leper Knights*, pp. 3–6, 194, 196, 258.

[46] S. Spector, ed., *The N-Town Play, I* (EETS, supplementary series, xi, 1991), p. 267.

salvation because of her evil life. Tearfully begging Christ to cleanse her soul from sin, she washes His feet with costly ointment, and dries them with her hair. He, in turn, acknowledges the true contrition of a 'sorwefful hert', and casts out the seven devils that have been tormenting her.[47] Pronounced free at last from her spiritual burden, she joins the company of the apostles and proceeds to play a major role in the momentous events of Holy Week. Medieval audiences had no reason to question the historical veracity of this lachrymose penitent, who was, in fact, the subject of an even more complex case of mistaken identity than that concerning St Lazarus.

The morally ambiguous Magdalen of stage and legend represented a *melange* of at least four, if not more, biblical figures. Her reputation for piety derived from Mary of Bethany, the sister of Lazarus, who was hailed as a model of the contemplative life.[48] Luke's gospel describes her deep devotion to Christ, while John records how she bathed His feet with 'a pound of ointment of spikenard, very costly', as he sat at her table [12, vv. 3–7]. In accordance with established tradition, however, the author of the N-town play of *The Raising of Lazarus* calls her 'Magdalyn', thereby perpetuating the confusion that had long since arisen between her and a second Mary, who came from Magdala on the Sea of Galilee.[49] The latter was a witness to both the crucifixion and resurrection, having joined Christ's band of female followers after he released her from seven devils [Luke 8, vv. 2–3]. There is no evidence to connect either her or Mary of Bethany with the unnamed woman of bad repute who washed Christ's feet with tears and costly unguents in the home of Simon the Pharisee. Even so, tradition soon turned this loyal, and apparently blameless, acolyte into a repentant prostitute, whose heartfelt remorse contrasted so sharply with the Pharisee's priggish self-righteousness, and whose many sins were freely forgiven 'for she loved much' [Luke 7, v. 47].

Two of the gospels report that another anonymous, but not ostensibly penitent, woman interrupted the meal hosted by Simon the leper, bearing a 'box of ointment of spikenard, very precious', which she poured over Christ's head [Mark 14, v. 3; Matthew 26, v. 7]. This extravagant gesture prompted some of the guests to protest that so much money should have gone to the poor, a view for which Christ had little sympathy. His rejoinder that the woman had come to anoint him for burial clearly forged another link with Mary of Magdala, because it was indeed she who subsequently brought 'sweet spices' to his tomb [Luke 16, v. 1]. Since, as we have seen, in St John's gospel this particular incident features Mary of Bethany, a degree of misunderstanding on the part of medieval commentators may easily be forgiven.[50]

---

47   Spector, *N-Town Play*, p. 270. See also the roughly contemporary play of *Mary Magdalene* in F.J. Furnivall, ed., *The Digby Plays* (EETS, extra series, lxx, 1896, reprinted 1967), pp. 55–136. 'Woman, in contrysson thou art expert', says Christ before the exorcism of her demons: ibid., p. 81.

48   S. Haskins, *Mary Magdalen: Myth and Metaphor* (London, 1994), chapter one; G. Constable, *Three Studies in Medieval Religious and Social Thought* (Cambridge, 1995), pp. 3–22; and K.L. Jansen, *The Making of the Magdalen* (Princeton, 2000), chapter one, trace the development of the 'composite' Magdalen in greater detail.

49   Spector, *N-Town Play*, pp. 230–45. See also the Digby play of *Mary Magdalene*, in which she is likewise portrayed as Lazarus's sister: Furnivall, *Digby Plays*, pp. 83–90.

50   The confusion did not stop at Mary and Lazarus. Simon the leper and his namesake the Pharisee are, for example, combined into a single character in the Digby play of *Mary Magdalene*: Furnivall, *Digby*

Even so, it was their search for a deeper symbolic meaning and moral symmetry that really consolidated the Magdalen's association with physical as well as spiritual pollution. Since she was both a penitent and a prophetess, Miriam the sister of Moses ranked as Mary's Old Testament precursor, just as Job seemed to prefigure Christ. The two women often appeared together in late medieval iconography, Miriam's punishment with leprosy and her ensuing remorse serving as a companion piece for the Magdalen's prostration at the feet of her Saviour.[51] Indeed, since the Augustinian canon, Osbern Bokenham, described Mary as a sinner 'wyth spottys defoulyd ful horrybylly', it might be argued that her soul seemed as leprous as Miriam's body.[52] Other equally tenuous links bound her to the ritually impure. St Ambrose and many others after him identified Mary of Bethany's sister, Martha, with the woman whose issue of blood was healed by Christ.[53] Like leprosy, her apparently unceasing menstrual flow rendered her a permanent outcast until she touched the hem of His robe and was miraculously cleansed [Matthew 9, vv. 20–22]. Although none of the Evangelists even hint at a shared identity, this assumption enabled medieval theologians to depict the three siblings, Mary, Martha and Lazarus, as individuals defiled, respectively, by sin, blood and leprosy/death. Each of them found redemption through the agency of divine grace earned by the Magdalen's exemplary penitence.[54] Significantly, one of the largest and most generously endowed English leper hospitals, founded at Sherburn by Bishop le Puiset of Durham in about 1181, was dedicated jointly to this powerful trio.[55] A celebrated cycle of wall paintings dating from c. 1200, which still survives at Aignan-sur-Cher in central France, includes depictions of the raising of Lazarus, the penitent Magdalen and Martha as *haemhorrissa*.[56] The church was a focus of pilgrimage and stood at the centre of a network of hospitals. It is easy to imagine the deployment of similar iconography in the chapels of English *leprosaria*, which, as we shall see, were often profusely decorated with religious imagery.

Yet the Magdalen above all others commanded the devotion of benefactors, nurses and patients throughout England. William le Gros was but one of many Anglo-Norman noblemen and prelates to commit his foundation to her protection and, implicitly, to enlist her assistance in his own quest for salvation. One of the earliest hospitals in England, the *leprosarium* of St Mary Magdalen at Sprowston, outside Norwich [plate 28], was reputedly the work of Bishop

*Plays*, pp. 78–80. See also, E.H. Weatherby, ed., *Speculum sacerdotale* (EETS, cc, 1936), p. 170; and Osbern Bokenham, *Legendys of Hooly Wummen*, ed. M.J. Serjeantson (EETS, ccvi, 1938, reprinted 1971), whose *Life of Mary Magdalen* refers to 'oon symon leprous', p. 148.

51  Haskins, *Mary Magdalen*, pp. 47–8; Jansen, *Making of the Magdalen*, pp. 21, 63, 174; J.Ph. Berjeau, ed., *Biblia pauperum* (London, 1859), p. 29 and plate XIII.

52  Bokenham, *Legendys*, p. 149.

53  Constable, *Three Studies*, pp. 1–141; Bokenham, *Legendys*, p. 151; J.P. Albert, *Odeurs de sainteté: La mythologie Chrétienne des aromates* (Paris, 1990), pp. 215–22. Another tradition associated the woman with St Veronica: see below, pp. 244–5.

54  A point specifically made by Jacobus de Voragine, *The Golden Legend*, eds G. Ryan and H. Ripperger (London, 1941), p. 356.

55  G. Allan, ed., *Collections Relating [to] Sherburn Hospital* (Durham, 1771), unpaginated, foundation charter. See Jansen, *Making of the Magdalen*, pp. 82–3, for the three siblings as exemplars of charitable giving.

56  Kupfer, *Art of Healing*, pp. 4, 13, 36–7, 104–7, 109, 124–5, figs. 19–27.

Herbert de Losinga (d. 1119), who also began the cathedral. Such an act of piety seems fitting in light of his simoniacal purchase of the see of Norwich, which, as a latter-day Gehazi, he is said bitterly to have repented. It certainly accords with his eloquent preaching on the obligations of the rich to the sick and destitute.[57] Allegedly on the orders of his royal master, Henry I, Eudo Dapifer founded a leper hospital of St Mary Magdalen at Colchester, possibly intending to place it under the aegis of the Benedictine abbey he had also built there.[58] Soon after the conquest of Ireland, in 1169, Richard 'Strongbow', earl of Pembroke, endowed another *leprosarium* bearing her name on his newly colonised estates at Wexford.[59] The prior of Bath, whose monastery had been given a chapel dedicated to the Magdalen outside the city during the late eleventh century, regarded it as the obvious site for a leper house. Tradition maintained that Archbishop Thurstan of York (d. 1140) was the founder of a once substantial refuge at Ripon for the support of blind priests and local lepers, both resident and in search of temporary shelter. It, too, honoured St Mary, and promised additional doles of food to all comers on her feast day.[60] Were other, less eminent individuals, whose lives – and transgressions – are now cloaked in obscurity, also attracted to this burgeoning cult?

Because so little information survives about the smaller *leprosaria* that sprang up in England during the twelfth and thirteenth centuries, it is impossible to determine the relative popularity of patron saints with any degree of accuracy. The dedications of about 220 of the 300 or so institutions whose existence has been documented before the early fourteenth century are, however, known, no fewer than sixty-nine (just under a third) being to Mary Magdalen.[61] In medieval Ireland the proportion seems to have been even higher. The existence of many of the ninety-odd leper houses listed by A.G. Lee is at best conjectural, although the Magdalen accounts for no fewer than half of the forty dedications noted by him.[62]

This was because her appeal as the patron and protector of lepers and those who cared for them went far beyond mere association with the ritually impure to embrace some of the most important developments in medieval spirituality. Commonly depicted with a jar of ointment in her hand, she was seen as one of the chosen few who had been healed by *Christus medicus* 'of many ailments', both in body and soul, and who could herself assist in the process of cleansing

---

57   J.W. Alexander, 'Herbert of Norwich, 1091–1119: Studies in the History of Norman England', *Studies in Medieval and Renaissance History*, vi (1969), pp. 119–232, at pp. 124–5, 216–17; Rawcliffe, *Hospitals of Medieval Norwich*, pp. 13, 41–7. The bishop's obit was held on 22 July, the feast of the Magdalen: E.M. Goulburn and H. Symonds, eds, *The Life, Letters and Sermons of Bishop Herbert de Losinga* (2 vols, Oxford, 1878), i, pp. 334–45, which suggests that the hospital may have been dedicated soon after his death.

58   King Henry took this step after Eudo's death: Page and Round, *VCH Essex II*, p. 184.

59   Lee, *Leper Hospitals*, p. 59.

60   J. Manco, *The Spirit of Care* (Bath, 1998), pp. 22–3; J. Raine, ed., *Memorials of the Church of SS Peter and Wilfrid, Ripon I* (Surtees Society, lxxiv, 1881), p. 228.

61   Satchell, 'Emergence of Leper-Houses', gazetteer, pp. 250–399, offers a comprehensive list of hospital dedications, to which should be added St Mary Magdalen and St Lazarus, Wormegay, Norfolk (above, note 15). Jansen, *Making of the Magdalen*, pp. 111–12, is less reliable.

62   Lee, *Leper Hospitals*, pp. 27–64. Gwynn and Hadcock, *Medieval Religious Houses in Ireland*, pp. 346–57, record a more modest total of fifteen out of twenty-nine known dedications.

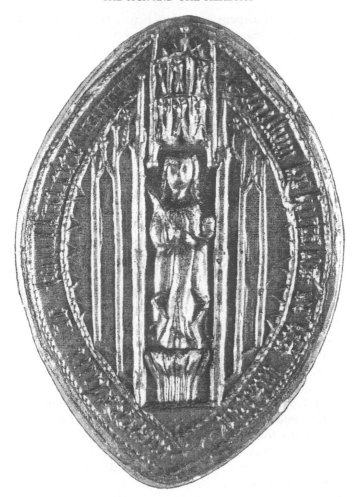

14. The fifteenth-century seal of the leper hospital of St Mary Magdalen,
Tavistock, depicts the patron saint bearing the jar of costly ointment with which,
according to medieval legend, she washed Christ's feet and prepared his body for
burial. In this context, the image underscores her connection with healing and
spiritual regeneration.

through which all repentant sinners had to pass [**plate 14**]. The profusion of
legends about Mary's life after the crucifixion further augmented her appeal as a
saint whose devotees not only included prostitutes and apothecaries, but also
hermits, the mentally ill, mendicants, prisoners and academics. Significantly, the
sister order of Knights Hospitallers of St John bore her name.[63] The belief that
she had travelled to Marseilles with her brother, preaching the word of God,

---

[63] Haskins, *Mary Magdalen*, pp. 217, 444 n. 9, 449 n. 52. Seals of hospitals dedicated to the Magdalen
often depict her with a jar of ointment: *Catalogue of Seals in the Department of Manuscripts of the
British Museum I* (London, 1887), xlv.24–5, xlvii.714, lxi.85, lxii.7.

performing miracles and dispensing charity before eventually withdrawing into the wilderness for thirty years of solitary introspection, crowned her reputation as the *apostola apostolorum,* who had combined in her ministry both the active and contemplative lives.[64] This long period of isolation, during which she had ample time to reflect upon the misdeeds of a colourful past, struck an immediate chord with those leprous men and women who felt drawn to the religious life. Following her lead, they embraced a calling that combined pious contemplation and penitence in equal measure, buoyed up by the promise of a celestial reward. 'I wyll ever abyte me with humelyte, & put me in pacyens, my lord for to love', declares the *beata peccatrix,* before her soul ascends to heaven.[65] This too was the Church's message to the leper, who might also have much to repent.

The Magdalen's seven devils were commonly taken to represent the seven deadly sins, which, as we saw in the previous chapter, not only followed inevitably from the Fall, but also constituted the direct or indirect cause of all human suffering. Given her life as a prostitute, lust invariably headed the list. The *Speculum sacerdotale,* a fifteenth-century preachers' handbook, described Mary as 'the synneful woman' who initially succumbed to 'hure fleschely desires', but who secured complete forgiveness by virtue of her abject penitence.[66] Since sexual misconduct, notably with an infected prostitute, ranked among the many presumed causes of *lepra,* the assumption that some (but by no means all) hospital inmates had probably succumbed to the lure of illicit sex may have been widespread. Other vulnerable individuals might have developed the disease by ignoring the Church's rules about coitus during menstruation, or have tipped their humoral balance over the edge through simple excess.[67] The belief that, once established, leprosy (or more accurately an overabundance of black bile) was likely to stimulate the sexual appetite of its male victims was, however, a more immediate cause for concern on the part of hospital authorities.[68]

From the outset, benefactors such as Archbishop Lanfranc (d. 1089), who endowed one of England's first *leprosaria* at Harbledown, near Canterbury, were anxious to preserve a monastic atmosphere conducive to prayer, contemplation and spiritual regeneration. It was for this reason that he insisted upon the strict segregation of the sexes, who were housed in separate buildings and forbidden to mix.[69] Hospitals tended to exaggerate the antiquity of their regulations, often attributing to the presumed founder statutes that were considerably later in date. Those for the leper house of St Mary Magdalen at Dudston, near Gloucester, spuriously credited to Odo of Chartres (d. 1115), survive only in a four-teenth-century copy. Even so, we can assume that here, and in other hospitals subject to ecclesiastical supervision, the insistence placed upon absolute chastity had obtained from the outset. Vigilance was particularly important because, like

---

[64]  Voragine, *Golden Legend,* pp. 357–62; Bokenham, *Legendys,* pp. 157–72.
[65]  Furnivall, *Digby Plays,* p. 130.
[66]  Wetherby, *Speculum sacerdotale,* p. 170. Her connection with *luxuria* and *vanitas* is considered at length in Jansen, *Making of the Magdalen,* chapters five and six.
[67]  See above, pp. 81–5.
[68]  Gilbertus Anglicus observed that 'lepers search for sexual pleasure more than they ought; they are ardent in the act; yet find themselves weaker than usual': *Compendium medicine,* fo. 339v.
[69]  Eadmer, *Historia novorum in Anglia,* ed. M. Rule (RS, 1884), pp. 15–16.

Harbledown, St Mary's accommodated both men and women. Any patients of the opposite sex who associated without the master's prior approval were subject to forty days' harsh penance, while acts of fornication incurred immediate and automatic expulsion.[70] The Benedictines of St Albans actually moved their female lepers to another site in order to avoid the 'detestable excesses' that had previously defamed the mixed community.[71] And as late as 1525–26, the married couple who ran the *leprosarium* at Cambridge on behalf of the borough authorities stood liable for a fine of ten marks should they fail to prevent 'the leprous men and women' from committing acts of fornication or adultery.[72]

It is important to stress that many general hospitals and almshouses employed similar measures to preserve their sacred spaces from sexual sin, notably by restricting the movements of nursing sisters and laundrywomen.[73] Yet, insidiously, the belief that lepers probably needed tighter controls and greater protection appears to have taken root. The thirteenth-century cardinal-bishop of Tusculum, Eudes de Châteauroux, who often preached in *leprosaria*, delivered one sermon in honour of the Magdalen on the theme of *luxuria* as a virulently contagious disease (in the modern sense) which polluted all who touched it.[74] By the same token, Bishop Hugh of Lincoln frequently visited the lepers in his diocese, 'refreshing them with the word of God' in the hope of strengthening their moral resolve. 'Grievous to say', one of his biographers reports, 'calamitous pleasure used to sway them with its colourable lure, because the itch of leprosy kindled the sparks of libido.'[75] And who better than Mary Magdalen, herself a former prostitute, to deliver her charges from the snares of lust? Even so, Mary's sins, just like the potential causes of human misery, were many and various. Before her portentous visit to the home of Simon the leper, she had been vain, proud, gluttonous and slothful, envious of others and prone to fits of temper. In short, like the leper touched by Christ, she personified all the imperfections that, in the eyes of the Church, exposed mankind to diseases of both the body and the soul. Her appeal was universal.

It was not, however, exclusive, for many other saints offered support to the sick and their benefactors in adversity. Whatever the complaint, from toothache (St Apollonia) to cancer of the breast (St Agatha), a celestial helper, whose exploits, miracles or earthly torments equipped him or her for this specialist

---

70 PRO, C115/K2/6683 I, fo. 75r, edited in E.J. Kealey, *Medieval Medicus* (Baltimore, 1981), pp. 108–9. Walter, constable of Gloucester (d. 1128), allegedly founded the hospital, entrusting it to the care of Llanthony priory, where he ended his days. When confirming a grant made to St Mary's by his father, Roger, earl of Hereford, insisted in the early 1150s that 'contumacious and incorrigible offenders' should be expelled. Among his own generous endowments, he provided support for a priest to improve the quality of religious observance: D. Walker, ed., 'Charters of the Earldom of Hereford, 1095–1201', *Miscellany XXII* (CS, fourth series, i, 1964), pp. 24–5.

71 Thomas Walsingham, *Gesta abbatum monasterii Sancti Albani*, ed. H.T. Riley (3 vols, RS, 1867–69), i, p. 202.

72 W.M. Palmer, ed., *Cambridge Borough Documents, I* (Cambridge, 1931), p. 55. Some may, by then, have been suffering from the pox.

73 C. Rawcliffe, 'Hospital Nurses and their Work', in R. Britnell, ed., *Daily Life in the Later Middle Ages* (Stroud, 1998), pp. 43–64; Bériac, 'Fraternités des lépreux', pp. 207–8; and below, pp. 264, 280.

74 Jansen, *Making of the Magdalen*, p. 173.

75 C. Garton, ed., *The Metrical Life of Hugh of Lincoln* (Lincoln, 1986), p. 65.

role, might be found.[76] We have already seen that lepers shared their dubious status as children of Saturn with prisoners, so it is not surprising to find St Leonard, the protector of men and women held in captivity, among their patrons. A Frank, born at the very beginning of the sixth century, Leonard declined the offer of a bishopric, preferring instead to follow the solitary life. But he also spent time preaching the word of God, healing the sick and freeing those who languished in chains. Most of his posthumous miracles fall into the last category, but one concerned a wealthy burgess named Rampnaldus, who lived near the abbey of Noblac where Leonard's relics were kept. According to the saint's *vita*, Rampnaldus was struck by God with leprosy and retired to a cell outside the abbey. Realising that, in spiritual terms, his riches had been suffocating, he gave everything away as an act of penance, thus permitting his soul to breathe freely even though his wretched body could not. Religious enlightenment eased the tragic process of physical decline, although, as his extremities fell away, it proved impossible for him to continue with the nightly vigils during which he had been consoled by a vision of a ladder, full of angels, extending from heaven to the saint's altar. Yet all was far from lost, for, as he lay dying, Leonard himself, accompanied by this heavenly host and a blaze of light, restored him to health.[77] Some sceptics questioned this famous miracle, the author dryly observes, although it still found its way as far as Beccles, in Suffolk, where legend had it that Rampnaldus had founded a hospital.[78] At least thirty-eight English *leprosaria* (and several other institutions besides) were dedicated to St Leonard, which accounts for about a fifth of those whose names are known to us.

Because of the ordeals that they had patiently endured at the hands of their tormentors, Christian martyrs were especially qualified to offer consolation to the sick.[79] Having been flayed alive, St Bartholomew seemed an obvious patron of men and women with dermatological disorders. Pieces of his skin were certainly among the most ubiquitous of medieval hospital relics. One was acquired by the *leprosarium* dedicated to him outside Oxford, where it attracted welcome donations until the fellows of Oriel College made off with it.[80] The 'longe and manyfolde passion and peyne' borne by St Laurence involved even greater brutality. After being 'spoylid and cruelly bete with scorpiones', as well as whips and cudgels, he was imprisoned in a cage, and then slowly roasted, one side after another, on a gridiron, until his flesh turned completely black.[81] Such

---

76  Rawcliffe, *Medicine and Society*, pp. 96–7, 178–80.

77  *Acta Sanctorum*, lxvii, November III (6 November), pp. 172–3; Voragine, *Golden Legend*, pp. 657–61.

78  BL, MSS Add. 8195, fo. 46r; 19112, fo. 58r. This Rampnaldus was, however, cured by bathing in a healing spring and his hospital was dedicated to the Magdalen: see below, pp. 228–9.

79  St George's brutal martyrdom made him a popular dedicatee of leper hospitals in northern Europe, whereas the English regarded him as a *miles Christi*, triumphing over the dragon of temptation: S. Riches, *Saint George: Hero, Martyr and Myth* (Stroud, 2000), pp. 36–57.

80  *CIM, 1387–1393*, no. 313.

81  Weatherby, *Speculum sacerdotale*, pp. 179–82. Blackness might be spiritual as well as physical. In another of many sermons he preached on the Magdalen, Eudes de Châteauroux described her as 'blackened and deformed by a multitude of sins' but remade and adorned by God with beauty and grace. Others observed that she had been suffering from leprosy of the soul: Jansen, *Making of the Magdalen*, pp. 211, 254.

acute physical suffering, often replicated on the body of the leper, may in part account for Laurence's popularity as a dedicatee of English *leprosaria*, for around a dozen in England and several in Ireland bore his name.[82] But he had other important attributes, too. The *Golden Legend*, which served in the later Middle Ages as a principal source of information about saints and their cults, records that, while in prison, he not only performed healing miracles but also confessed and baptised Christian converts.[83] As might be expected, the hearing of confession and granting of absolution were the hallmarks of many saints associated with hospital foundations, both for the sick poor and lepers.

John the Baptist, whose life was notable for its humility and extreme asceticism, as well as a long sojourn in the wilderness, naturally exercised a powerful appeal in this respect. 'And thefor was Seynt John sent for to preche penaunce', explained the *Speculum sacerdotale*, 'to make fayre of fowle . . . for grace of regeneracion to be hadde'.[84] About half a dozen *leprosaria* and many medieval hospitals for the sick poor invoked his protection, as, significantly, did English guilds of surgeons and barber surgeons.[85] Prefigured in the Old Testament by the cleansing of Naaman the leper in the Jordan [II Kings 5], his baptism of Christ not only signified the conquest of original sin (from which all believers might benefit) but also the laundering of each individual soul through the bitter tears of repentance.[86] The frequent analogies drawn between Naaman and the remorseful medieval penitent were reinforced by the fact that, at the behest of the prophet Elisha, he had immersed himself *seven times*, once for each sin [**plate 15**]:

> The flum Iordan [river Jordan] is as moche to seie as a litle ryuere of jugement that bitokeneth schrifte [confession], wher euery man and womman schal jugge hymself with grete sorwe of herte and grete repentaunce, so that a litle ryuere of teres mowe renne bi the coundight of ieghen [may run from the conduit of the eyes], and thus schal the mesel be clensed and be heled, that is the sinful, yif he wascheth hym seuene tymes, that is yif he ariseth out of alle the seuene dedly synnes.[87]

That the healing unguent of tears might not flow easily was a constant source of anxiety to those who invoked the Magdalen's help in prompting a heartfelt

---

82  Satchell, 'Emergence of Leper-Houses', pp. 250–399; Lee, *Leper Hospitals*, pp. 27–64.

83  Voragine, *Golden Legend*, pp. 437–45.

84  Weatherby, *Speculum sacerdotale*, p. 167; R. Morris, ed., *Old English Homilies of the Twelfth Century* (EETS, liii, 1873), pp. 136–41; Jansen, *Making of the Magdalen*, p. 134.

85  Satchell, 'Emergence of Leper-Houses', pp. 250–399; Rawcliffe, *Medicine and Society*, pp. 131, 134–5, 200.

86  Hugh of St Victor considered the immersions of Naaman in terms of 'the seven-fold leprosy of human pride . . . in the possession of goods, vanity in dress, physical voluptuousness, twice in the things of the mouth and twice in those of the heart'. These he contrasted with 'the seven-fold humility of Christ': *Opera omnia*, PL, clxxvii, *Miscellanea*, lib. III, cols 639–40. Significantly, Protestant authors continued to explore the theme of Naaman as a paradigm of human frailty. 'We are all Naamans leprous, but more foule', asserted Joseph Fletcher (d. 1637), 'till in his bloody sweat [Christ] purge our soule': *Christes Bloodie Sweat, or the Sonne of God in His Agonie*, by I.F. (London, 1613), sig. D2.

87  Nelson Francis, *Book of Vices and Virtues*, p. 224. This English text, based on the *Somme le roi*, an instruction manual by a thirteenth-century French Dominican, describes the Holy Ghost as a 'goode phisicion' able to restore humoral balance through confession: ibid., p. 127. See also, A. Henry, ed., *The Mirour of Mans Saluacioun* (Aldershot, 1986), pp. 87–9.

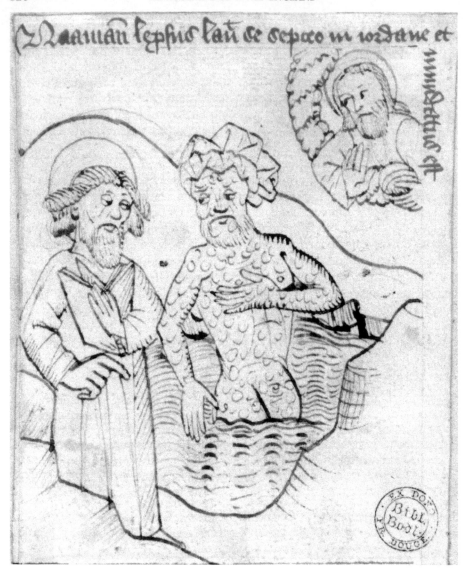

15. As instructed by the prophet Elijah, Naaman, the leprous Syrian general,
bathes seven times in the Jordan under the benign gaze of God. He is thus
cleansed (*mundatus est*), like all remorseful sinners who repent their misdeeds.
The depiction of his symptoms in this fifteenth-century English text of the
*Speculum humanae salvationis* goes beyond the conventional use of random spots,
to suggest the disfiguring nodules and lesions described in contemporary medical
literature.

display of contrition.[88] Others, who feared even to confront their misdeeds, needed additional support.

Hugh of St Victor's *Allegoriae in Novum Testamentum* described the ten lepers who had humbly displayed their afflictions to Christ as repentant sinners. Yet only one of them had obeyed His injunction that they should show themselves at once to the priest: in other words, that they should confess their misdeeds at the first opportunity. And he alone, who personified the universal Church, had benefited from an everlasting flow of divine grace.[89] In a powerful sermon preached on this theme in about 1170, Maurice de Sully likewise warned members of his French congregation to hasten to confession as soon as they detected the first symptoms of spiritual leprosy. Only 'the supreme judge and physician' could diagnose and treat them effectively, but he, in turn, demanded complete honesty from his patients.[90] Famed in medieval legend for his miraculous intercession on behalf of the incestuous emperor, Charlemagne, for whom he secured celestial absolution, St Giles (d. *c.* 710) offered hope to the most hardened and reticent sinner. His reputation as 'medicine to the sick in their distress' hinged largely upon these intercessionary powers, which promised the elusive panacea of spiritual health to all who called upon him. He was, for example, believed to assist those who died contrite but unconfessed. The many *vitae* and images that both reflected and increased his popularity also stressed his voluntary renunciation of wealth, the long years he spent in the wilderness as a hermit and his many acts of charity to the poor. A history of physical suffering and a clutch of miraculous cures further enhanced his qualifications as a guardian of lepers. Not surprisingly, more than a dozen English *leprosaria* were dedicated to him.[91]

The naming of hospitals might also reflect the impact of a recent canonisation (a few dedications to Thomas Becket occurred after 1170), local sentiment and the devotional practices of the founder. The Cambridge burgess, Henry Tangmere (d. 1361), may well have been prompted by an uneasy conscience to found the hospital of St Eloy and St Anthony, just outside the town. Guilt over some shady business deal would certainly explain his attachment to Eloy, an unusual dedicatee for an English lazar house, whose patronage customarily extended to goldsmiths and financiers.[92] We shall, on the other hand, never know why one Norwich *leprosarium* promoted the cult of Brichtiu, a destitute French leper who was cured by the relics of three obscure Christian martyrs.[93] It was, none the less, an appropriate, if unique, dedication, that once again underscores the priority accorded to spiritual care and celestial help in hospitals of all sizes, large and small. Through their humble acceptance of suffering and their

---

88  P. Nagy, *Le don des larmes au moyen âge* (Paris, 2000), pp. 256–67.
89  Hugh of St Victor, *Allegoriae in Novum Testamentum*, iv, cap. xxv, col. 823.
90  Bériou and Touati, *Voluntate Dei leprosus*, p. 59; R. Morris, ed., *An Old English Miscellany* (EETS, xlix, 1872), p. 31.
91  Voragine, *Golden Legend*, pp. 516–19; Kupfer, *Art of Healing*, pp. 92–102; Rawcliffe, *Medicine for the Soul*, pp. 24–5; Satchell, 'Emergence of Leper-Houses', pp. 250–399.
92  M. Rubin, *Charity and Community in Medieval Cambridge* (Cambridge, 1987), pp. 122–3. The St Anthony in question was almost certainly the hermit, who protected sufferers from ergotism.
93  *Acta Sanctorum*, xxxiii, July VI (27 July), p. 463; Thomas of Monmouth, *Life and Miracles of St William*, p. 148.

close association with the penitential process, the patron saints of *leprosaria* were ideally placed to set both patient *and* patron upon the road to recovery.

### 'For loue of her lowe hertis': humility, penitence and confession

The early fathers of the Christian Church regarded pride, the downfall of Uzziah, as the first and most lethal of the seven deadly sins, whose cure demanded extreme remedies. Developing the theme of Christ as the *medicus humilis*, St Augustine of Hippo (d. 403) stressed that such a malignant tumour could only be excised with the burning cautery of abjection.[94] St Gregory the Great, who also used medical metaphors to enliven and illustrate key doctrinal points, explained how Christ had given mankind a sovereign remedy for the terminal wound first inflicted upon Adam and Eve in paradise. It would, however, only benefit the meek.[95] This caveat was reiterated and embellished throughout the Middle Ages, reappearing, for instance, in the aptly named *Summa virtutum de remediis anime*, a thirteenth-century work on spiritual medicine which inspired the Parson's homily in Chaucer's *Canterbury Tales*. Here, as in so many other texts, the lowly and patient leper serves as an exemplar, whose readiness to swallow his or her spiritual medication stands as a model to others:

> It is reported of a virgin in Wales that, when she was so much infected with severe leprosy that she lost her nose and eyes and her whole body swelled up with pustules like a tree with knotty bark, she said that she was much afraid that she might be unworthy of God's love because he did not inflict as much pain on her as she was able to bear with her last breath.[96]

Here, then, was a coin by which the sick might exchange their earthly torments for spiritual goods.[97] Yet, if it seemed more meritorious to suffer without complaint 'than to laboure in other gud werkes ryght bysily', those who grumbled about their lot had less cause for optimism. Such people, one homilist warned, squandered their celestial capital, turning 'golde in-to copur, preciose stonys in-to fen [dirt], corn in-to chaffe, wynne in-to water, hony in-to galle, day in-to nyghte [and] ioye into sorowe'.[98]

The mute acceptance of divine will was an ideal to which few could aspire. But it found expression in the rules that governed many of the larger, quasi-monastic leper houses and hospitals of medieval England, where patients freely submitted to the quotidian rod of the religious life as well as the lash of disease. At the *leprosarium* of St Mary Magdalen, founded 'out of devotion' by Abbot Ancher of Reading in about 1135, for example, displays of wrath, arro-

---

94  R. Arbesmann, 'The Concept of "*Christus Medicus*" in Saint Augustine', *Traditio*, x (1954), pp. 1–28, at pp. 10–16.

95  Bliss, *Morals in the Book of Job*, iii, p. 424.

96  S. Wenzel, ed., *Summa virtutum de remediis anime* (Athens, Georgia, 1984), pp. 198–9.

97  The commercial metaphors are striking. As one fourteenth-century saint observed, 'If people realised how useful diseases are for detaching the soul from earthly things, they would go out and purchase them in the market': R. Kieckhefer, *Unquiet Souls: Fourteenth-Century Saints and their Religious Milieu* (Chicago, 1984), p. 57.

98  G. Holmstedt, ed., *Speculum Christiani* (EETS, clxxxii, 1933), pp. 196–8.

gance and mendacity were subject to humiliating public correction in order to achieve that atmosphere of perfect *caritas* in which prayer and penitence could flourish.[99] The mid twelfth-century foundation statues of another hospital dedicated to the Magdalen, at Gaywood, near King's Lynn, likewise warned the inmates to behave peacefully, charitably, soberly, chastely, modestly and quietly. Applying themselves with diligence to the service of God, they were to set aside all earthly pride, comporting themselves with due humility and meekness. Needless to say, there should be no muttering against the Lord, or any other displays of anger or irritation.[100] It was quite probably in this hospital that the fifteenth-century mystic, Margery Kempe, bent on her own *imitatio Magdalenae*, followed in the steps of a legion of pious Christians by embracing and comforting the female lepers 'for the lofe of Ihesu'. Here, she explains in her spiritual autobiography, she sank to her knees and kissed two sick women 'with many an holy thowt & many a deuowt teer . . . & telde hem ful many good wordys & steryd hem to mekenes & pacyens that thei xulde not grutchyn wyth her sekenes but hyly thankyn God therfor & thei xulde han gret blysse in Heuyn'.[101]

In a similar vein, new regulations drawn up in 1344 for the hospital run by the Benedictine monks of St Albans required the leprous to comport themselves 'in their manner and their dress more contemptible and humble than other men'. Quoting the passage from Leviticus which required them to live 'without the camp', the ordinances none the less warned against the temptation to blasphemy or despair, cubs spawned by the lion Pride. On the contrary, because Christ had voluntarily assumed the guise of a leper they should give thanks for their good fortune and cultivate the patience of Job in adversity.[102] Being thoroughly versed in recent medical literature, the ecclesiastical authorities who devised and implemented the statutes of *leprosaria* recognised that, as the balance of their humours grew increasingly unstable, the residents would become suspicious, irritable and depressed. Warning of the dangers posed by 'grucchynge', the fourteenth-century *Visitatio infirmorum* observed that 'nothyng is wers to a seek man than to be malencolious'. To make matters worse, the author adds, 'thou greuest thi fadir the whiche coueiteth [desires] to be thi leche, and thus as a fool thou harmest thi-self in double manere'.[103] It might be

---

99 These rules have been dated to 1165 x 73, with fourteenth-century additions: BL, MS Cotton Vespasian E V, fo. 39r; B.R. Kemp, ed., *Reading Abbey Cartularies* (2 vols, CS, fourth series, xxxi, 1986, and xxxxii, 1987), i, pp. 183–4.

100 Archbishop Winchelsey's revised statutes of c. 1304 provide the first surviving text, which may have been significantly amended by him: Owen, *Making of King's Lynn*, pp. 106–7.

101 Meech, *Book of Margery Kempe*, p. 177. Significantly, this visit follows an imagined discussion between Christ and Margery about His regard for her in relation to the Magdalen, another fallen woman. Margery was greatly influenced by the writings of St Bridget of Sweden, and may have recalled her warning that 'some are withouten disese, and that is, for thai cannot bere disese withouten gruchyng, and that suld be cause of the harder dome to thame; and some are not worthi to be disesed': R. Ellis, ed., *The Liber Celestis of St Bridget of Sweden: Volume I Text* (EETS, ccxci, 1987), p. 385.

102 Richards, *Medieval Leper*, pp. 131–2. Any patient who defied the rules about footwear and adopted 'low shoes' rather than laced sandals was to go barefoot until the master excused him, 'in consideration of his humility': Walsingham, *Gesta*, ii, p. 504.

103 C. Horstmann, ed., *Yorkshire Writers: Richard Rolle and his Followers* (2 vols in 1, Woodbridge, 1999),

argued that, in attempting to contain such behaviour, hospitals performed an important therapeutic function for the body as well as the soul.

In this environment, sickness served as the companion and spur to repentance. Prominent among the allegorical figures that populated man's pilgrimage towards the city of God, Infirmity was Nature's messenger sent to remind the healthy of the omnipresence of Death, while Penitence, the laundrywoman, ensured that their souls were 'porged and wel wasshen' in preparation for this last, momentous encounter.[104] That many victims of *lepra* dwelt upon their past misdeeds and sought, where possible, to make due atonement, seems more than likely. Such was evidently the experience of Gilbert de Sanderville, who attempted to recover the site of a chapel in Flitwick, Bedfordshire, which his father had conveyed to the canons there. Having evicted the priest in charge, he fell victim to leprosy, and thus, in the eyes of the archdeacon of Bedford, at least, suffered his just deserts. According to a report made in the late 1170s Gilbert appeared in person before the entire synod, and, in a tearful voice confessed that God had justly chastised him for his misdeeds. It was thus as a repentant sinner that he confirmed the original grant and restored all the property, along with two churches and a mill as further atonement.[105] We do not know if Gilbert had already entered a monastic *leprosarium*, although his remorseful behaviour suggests that he was certainly contemplating such a step.

The practice of entry *ad succurrendum* into religious life enjoyed widespread popularity in the twelfth and thirteenth centuries. Aged, sick and disabled individuals who could afford to do so elected in increasing numbers to retire from the world into the peaceful environment of the cloister or hospital. Not all were driven by vocation, but many sought the assurance of salvation that membership of an order seemed to offer. As 'a talisman powerful enough to forgive sins and to ease the transition into the next world', the religious habit exercised a particular appeal for the leprous, who were taught to regard their disease as both a calling and a unique opportunity for repentance.[106] We have no means of telling how many individuals took this step, but the circumstantial evidence is striking. A few examples will here suffice, beginning with Brian de Insula (d. *c.* 1149), lord of Abergavenny, who reputedly settled a substantial estate upon the priory that his uncle had founded there on the understanding that it would receive and support his two leprous sons for life.[107] It was also during the mid twelfth century that Elinald the sheriff conveyed tithes, ten acres of land and a mill to the Suffolk priory of Stoke-by-Clare, 'along with Adam the leper, his son, whom

---

ii, p. 451. Theoderic, for instance, noted that lepers 'grow angry very easily, and more easily than was customary. Evil, crafty habits appear; patients suspect everyone of wanting to hurt them': Campbell and Colton, *Surgery of Theoderic*, ii, p. 171. Discussion of these '*mores mali*', to which most authorities refer, was, however, generally free of censure. As Luke Demaitre points out, they were regarded as 'behavioural concomitants of bodily illness', and thus did not prompt the value judgements a modern reader might be disposed to make: 'Description and Diagnosis', pp. 337–8.

[104]  A. Henry, ed., *The Pilgrimage of the Lyfe of the Manhode* (EETS, cclxxxviii, 1985), p. 170.

[105]  C.T. Clay, ed., *Early Yorkshire Charters, VII: The Honour of Skipton* (Yorkshire Archaeological Society, Record Series, extra series, v, 1947), pp. 101–3.

[106]  J.H. Lynch, *Simoniacal Entry into the Religious Life from 1000 to 1260* (Columbus, Ohio, 1976), pp. 27, 31, 34–6; Green, *Aristocracy of Norman England*, pp. 421–2.

[107]  William Dugdale, *Monasticon Anglicanum*, eds J. Caley et al. (6 vols, London, 1817–30), iv, p. 616.

he made a monk'.[108] Depending upon their age, the sick children of such influential men may have had little choice but to comply with parental wishes, but
others were clearly anxious to end their days in a monastic *leprosarium*. In 1174,
for instance, the Northamptonshire landowner, Robert de Torpel, 'infirm and
afflicted with leprosy', settled the two manors of Cotterstock and Glapthorne
upon Peterborough abbey. Before a large crowd of monks, retainers and relatives in the chapel of St Leonard's hospital, which had been founded by Abbot
John de Séez (d. 1125), he dedicated himself 'body and soul' to God and St Peter.
The chapter, in turn agreed to support him and four of his knights for life, and
to clothe him after death in the Benedictine habit.[109]

Hospitals like St Leonard's, which followed a monastic rule from the outset,
may already have insisted upon a full confession upon entry, and then at fairly
regular intervals. By the mid thirteenth century, if not well before, most of the
larger English hospitals and *leprosaria* had taken this step, often at the behest of
patrons who were anxious about the quality as well as the quantity of commendatory prayers said on their behalf.[110] Patients, too, welcomed the opportunity
to shed their spiritual burdens, although refusal was hardly an option. St Elizabeth of Hungary (d. 1231) allegedly took a whip to one obdurate old woman in
her hospital at Marburg, forcing her to comply. [111] This incident, so shocking to
modern sensibilities, would have elicited a very different response at the time,
since confession promised to disperse the miasmas of sin which otherwise
threatened both the individual and the institution. The reforms of Pope Innocent III were clearly making themselves felt.

The canon *Omnis utriusque sexus* of the fourth Lateran Council of 1215 is
widely believed to mark a turning point in the history of Western Europe,
greatly consolidating the authority of the Church and prompting a decisive shift
in the devotional life of the laity. It made annual confession before one's parish
priest or another appropriately qualified *medicus animarum* compulsory, and
forbade anyone who did not do so to enter a church, take communion or receive
a Christian burial. The wording is, significantly, replete with medical imagery:

> The priest shall be discerning and prudent, so that like a skilled doctor (*more periti
> medici*) he may pour wine and oil over the wounds of the injured one. Let him
> carefully inquire about the circumstances of both the sinner and the sin, so that he
> may prudently discern what sort of advice he ought to give and what remedy to
> apply, using various means to heal the sick person.[112]

On the ground that the physically ill 'should provide for the soul before the
body', the Council also insisted that confession ought henceforward to precede

---

[108] Harper-Bill and Mortimer, *Stoke-by-Clare Cartulary*, i, nos 37, 136–7.
[109] E. King, *Peterborough Abbey 1086–1310* (Cambridge, 1973), pp. 27–8, 38; Serjeantson and Adkins, *VCH Northampton II*, p. 162.
[110] See below, pp. 338–9.
[111] Voragine, *Golden Legend*, p. 685.
[112] N. Tanner, ed., *Decrees of the Ecumenical Councils* (2 vols, Georgetown, 1990), i, Decrees of the Fourth Lateran Council, 1215, cap. 21. See also, A. Murray, 'Counselling in Medieval Confession', in P. Biller and A.J. Minnis, eds, *Handling Sin: Confession in the Middle Ages* (Woodbridge, 1998), pp. 63–77.

medical or surgical treatment, any practitioner who ignored the ruling being threatened with excommunication. Once again, the terminology reflects the intimate relationship between body and soul:

> As sickness of the body may sometimes be the result of sin . . . so we by this present decree order and strictly command physicians of the body, when they are called to the sick, to warn and persuade them first of all to call in physicians of the soul so that after their spiritual health has been seen to they may respond better to medicine for their bodies; for when the cause ceases so does the effect.[113]

Many scholars have argued that such measures, which effectively institutionalised the connection between transgression and disease, must have fostered discrimination against a variety of 'excluded and persecuted groups', including lepers. Some, such as R.I. Moore, regard Lateran IV as the last refinement of a 'comprehensive apparatus of persecution' created in the previous century. Others, including F.O. Touati, suggest more plausibly that an already discernible hardening of attitude actually gained momentum around this time.[114] The extent of the change and the type of individual who might (or might not) be stigmatised are, however, still open to debate. Sweeping assertions to the effect that 'the leper' henceforward became 'a malignant, noxious entity to be excised or spewed forth from the cohesive body of the "whole" ' do scant justice to the sheer complexity of medieval responses to men and women whose personal circumstances and behaviour inevitably shaped reactions to their disease. Indeed, although the pogroms of 1320–21 might be cited in support of Marcia Kupfer's argument that leprosy came to be seen by the French as 'nothing but the living embodiment of the continuity between moral corruption and carnal degradation', it is important to reiterate that no such atrocities ever occurred in England.[115]

As we shall see in the next chapter, diagnosis might well take place in the confessional, where priests enquired closely into the moral as well as the physical symptoms of suspect lepers. But the changes introduced by Pope Innocent did not *inevitably* mark a worsening of the leper's position. Firstly, Lateran IV imposed a degree of uniformity on existing practice, which for many people already involved confession, sometimes up to three times a year.[116] Several leprous pilgrims who travelled to Becket's shrine in the 1170s, for example, had confessed before setting out and received appropriate advice about their behaviour.[117] Moreover, the disclosure of sinful conduct was only part of an exercise that also demanded contrition, satisfaction and absolution before the sinner could be released from his or her spiritual burden.[118] Repentance and the

---

[113] Tanner, *Decrees*, i, Decrees of the Fourth Lateran Council, 1215, cap. 22; Amundsen, *Medicine, Society and Faith*, pp. 199–203, 273–7.

[114] Moore, *Formation of a Persecuting Society*, p. 66; Touati, *Maladie et société*, pp. 23, 764–7.

[115] Kupfer, *Art of Healing*, pp. 135–6.

[116] P. Biller, 'Introduction', in idem and Minnis, *Handling Sin*, pp. 3–33, examines the question of continuity in penitential practice.

[117] See below, p. 181.

[118] The *Sentences* of Peter Lombard (1151–57) distinguished three elements in perfect penance: heartfelt compunction, confession and satisfaction: *Opera omnia, PL*, cxcii, *Sententiarum libri quator*, lib. IV, distinctio xvi, cols 877–8.

expiation of sin through penance were thus essential parts of a cumulative process, at which it might be argued the sick excelled above all others. If Dysmas, the good thief who hung beside Christ at the crucifixion, could be hailed as a model penitent, his soul transported, like that of Lazarus, by angels to heaven, the repentant leper might surely play an even more inspiring role.[119]

Hospital patients performed other useful functions, too. The voluminous literature produced for the guidance of confessors and penitents during the later Middle Ages stressed that charity and humility were twin keys to the gates of paradise. As preachers so often exhorted their healthy congregations, almsdeeds, especially when performed in person, were like a phlebotomy or a purge, which cleansed the soul of sin. Anyone who visited and relieved the residents of the *leprosarium* of St Mary Magdalen and St James, Chichester, might, for instance, claim fifteen days' remission of enjoined penance, rising to forty in 1362. The first of these indulgences was, significantly, awarded in the late twelfth century by Bishop Seffrid to the 'truly confessed and penitent' in the name of the Magdalen, 'whose sins were forgiven because she loved much'.[120] Ironically, though, where lepers were concerned, the effectiveness of many such activities depended upon the extent to which the donor's initial nausea or revulsion had been overcome. There was, after all, little to be gained by dwelling among the fragrant. It would be hard to find a more effective gesture of contrition than washing the feet of the ulcerated poor (although some repentant sinners went even further and drank the water too).[121] As their biographers recognised, the merits of saints such as Elizabeth and Hugh of Lincoln shone forth so brightly because the recipients of their ministrations appeared so physically repugnant. Literature of this kind consequently transmitted an ambivalent message, for in stressing the monstrous, rather than the human or Christ-like aspect of the medieval leper, hagiographers and homilists exploited deep-seated fears as well as aspirations.

## 'Thou art a foule lepre': conflicting responses

In an age before antibiotics and disinfectants, the odour of physical decay had a powerful effect on responses to the sick, most notably in advanced cases of *lepra*. Although, as we shall discover in chapter six, bathing constituted an important aspect of palliative care, not even the best treatment then available could effectively mitigate the nauseous stench of ulcerated flesh.[122] When searching for words to convey the horrors of Malebolge, the eighth circle of hell, Dante could find no better comparison than with the sick of countless hospitals, tipped in a

---

119 M.B. Merback, *The Thief, the Cross and the Wheel: Pain and the Spectacle of Punishment in Medieval and Renaissance Europe* (London, 1999), chapter seven.
120 Rawcliffe, *Medicine and Society*, p. 58; BL, MS Add. 24828, fos 137r–137v, 139r–140v; H. Mayr-Harting, ed., *Acta of the Bishops of Chichester, 1075–1207* (Canterbury and York Society, 1964), no. 107.
121 Walker Bynum, *Fragmentation and Redemption*, p. 132. True penitents, who overcame their revulsion, reputedly found the water 'delicious and swete of sauour, as it had be ful of good spicerie': BL, MS Harley 45, fo. 84r.
122 The unpleasant smell (*fetor*) of breath, flesh and sweat ranked among the 'general' symptoms of *lepra*: Gilbertus Anglicus, *Compendium medicine*, fo. 339r.

ditch during the height of summer, 'plus that stink that usually comes from ill bodies'.[123] Long before fears of miasmatic infection took hold in the later thirteenth century, the unpleasant smell associated with confirmed lepers prompted some predictable reactions. These were exacerbated by contemporary beliefs about scent, which, as Dante's image suggests, drew a close connection between sanctity and sweetness, while conversely associating evil with physical decomposition. Like paradise before the Fall, heaven was a place of clean and ordered perfection, heady with the smoke of incense and more subtle floral delights. 'There lilies and roses always bloom for you, smell sweet and never wither', rhapsodised one ecstatic monk at the prospect of odours 'breathing eternal bliss into the soul'.[124]

Christ's body, in particular, was regarded as a repository of the finest perfume, his blood exuding an ambrosial blend of myrrh, balsam and incense.[125] When describing Theobald of Blois' penchant for washing the feet of lepers, which was done in memory of 'the great Magdalen', Walter Map observed that because Christ invariably emitted 'an odour of sweetness that drew the heart to it' her task was infinitely more agreeable than his.[126] Medieval saints, too, were frequently praised for their fragrance, which in many cases lingered about their persons long after death. Not only did the bodies of holy men and women often defy the process of decomposition, remaining intact in the grave for years, but they also continued to perfume the surrounding air.[127] Mary Magdalen, the bearer of costly unguents, was predictably blessed, but many others, such as St Edmund of Abingdon (d. 1240), offered similar proofs of sanctity. When his body was exhumed for translation in 1247, it appeared quite unscathed, 'redolent with a heavenly scent surpassing that of any balsam or thyme'.[128] The physical incorruptibility of Saints Edmund (the king and martyr), Etheldreda and Cuthbert led one leprous nobleman to choose their shrines as preferred places of pilgrimage, since it apparently enhanced their powers to halt the march of disease.[129]

Jews, on the other hand, who had no place in the Christian heaven, allegedly reeked of filth and corruption, their malignant odour acquired in part through

---

[123] Dante Alighieri, *Hell*, trans S. Ellis (London, 1994), p. 174.

[124] C. McDannell and B. Lang, *Heaven: A History* (New Haven and London, 1988), pp. 70, 72. The many versions of the twelfth-century *Tractatus de purgatorio Sancti Patricii* contrast the stench of purgatory with the luscious scent of paradise, 'swetter of sauour than of al the spicers shoppes that ever were': R. Easting, ed., *St Patrick's Purgatory* (EETS, ccxcviii, 1991), pp. 110–11, 23–4, 102–5, 64–5. See also J.T. Rhodes and C. Davidson, 'The Garden of Paradise', in C. Davidson, ed., *The Iconography of Heaven* (Kalamazoo, 1994), pp. 69–109; and C. Davidson, 'Heaven's Fragrance', ibid., pp. 110–27.

[125] Albert, *Odeurs de sainteté*, pp. 145–6, 174–7. Richard Rolle, the mystic, described Christ's body as 'lyk to a medow ful of swete flours and holsome herbes': H.E. Allen, ed., *English Writings of Richard Rolle* (Oxford, 1963), p. 36.

[126] Map, *De nugis curialium*, pp. 462–3.

[127] P. Camporesi, *The Incorruptible Flesh: Bodily Mutilation and Mortification in Religion and Folklore* (Cambridge, 1988), pp. 3, 8–12, 179–207; Classen, Howes and Synnott, *Cultural History of Smell*, pp. 53–4.

[128] Albert, *Odeurs de sainteté*, p. 222; Matthew Paris, *The Life of St Edmund*, ed. C.H. Lawrence (Stroud, 1996), p. 167.

[129] J. Raine, ed., *Reginaldi monachi Dunelmensis libellus de admirandis beati Cuthberti* (Surtees Society, i, 1835), pp. 38–9.

unsavoury habits but also because of a notorious association with usury.[130] Both
hell, the destination of unscrupulous money lenders, and purgatory were
noxious places, notable for the miasmas of evil that clung like a blanket to each
wretched sinner. The twelfth-century *Vision of the Monk of Eynsham*, which was
translated into English during the fifteenth century, dwells upon the 'ful
horrable clowde' of poison hovering above the icy lakes and furnaces of purgatory. Here was 'myxte and medylde to-gedir a fume of brymstone wyth a myste,
a gret stenche and a flame blak as pycche'.[131] Misshapen and terrifying, the residents of this nether world breathed fire through their noses and (like lepers)
exhaled mephistic air from gaping mouths.[132] It is easy to see how fear of
miasma took root among men and woman already saturated in the olfactory
imagery of sin and damnation.

Some saints, such as Hugh of Lincoln, who carried with them 'the sweet
perfume of Christ', remained impervious to the vile odours that made others
retch, and thus experienced few problems in burying the dead or visiting
lepers.[133] But squeamishness was no excuse in lesser mortals. The sense of smell,
as all good Christians knew, could be profoundly deceptive. It offered a seduc-
tive pathway to temptation, precipitating the unwary into acts of gluttony,
vanity and lust. It also bred fastidiousness and distaste for the unwashed, ailing
poor. Preaching on the theme of spiritual health (and the need for patience in
infirmity), Jacques de Vitry cited the famous *exemplum* of the angel who gagged
at the scent of an elegant young man but was unaffected by the stench of a
rotting corpse. The sins of the arrogant youth reeked to high heaven, he
explained, whereas the dead body was nothing more than a disposable envelope
of flesh that had once contained a noble soul.[134] 'Why should a man who generally overindulges himself in the use of sweet perfumes not sometimes be obliged
to endure a noxious smell, especially when comforting sick folk?' asked William
Lichfield (d. 1447), a London rector.[135] This was a rhetorical question, which
permitted only one response.

Those who were able to overcome their natural delicacy in such matters were
promised an appropriate reward. One of many tales on the theme of *Christus
quasi leprosus* recounts how a pious noblewoman defied her husband by offering
their bed to a wretched, noisome leper. Forcing open the chamber door on his
return, her angry lord encountered a blissful aroma of 'gude spicis' so powerful
that he thought he had been transported to paradise. Henceforward, he 'waxe
meke as a lambe, and . . . luffid God and lepere men better', a moral from which

---

130  The Jewish temperament was believed to be strikingly similar to that conventionally associated with
     the leper, namely solitary, melancholic and corrupted by 'gross blood': R.I. Moore, 'Anti-Semitism
     and the Birth of Europe', in D. Wood, ed., *Christianity and Judaism* (Studies in Church History, xxix,
     1992), pp. 33–57.
131  R. Easting, ed., *The Revelation of the Monk of Eynsham* (EETS, cccxviii, 2002), pp. 45, 49.
132  Easting, *Revelation of the Monk of Eynsham*, p. 77. See also, Le Goff, *Birth of Purgatory*, pp. 94–5;
     Bede, *Ecclesiastical History*, pp. 489–99; Davidson, 'Fate of the Damned', pp. 41–66, for further
     examples.
133  Douie and Farmer, *Life of St Hugh*, ii, pp. 82–3.
134  Beriou and Touati, *Voluntate Dei leprosus*, pp. 123–4.
135  BL, MS Royal 8 C I, fo. 130. See also Brandeis, *Jacob's Well*, pp. 242–3.

the wrathful as well as the unduly pampered might benefit.[136] The harsh reality of caring for patients in the advanced stages of *lepra* on a daily basis was, however, another matter, as senior clergy such as Jacques de Vitry and Humbert de Romans, who often visited and preached in hospitals, frankly admitted. Both stressed the unusual degree of dedication necessary to work in such places, a fact that, paradoxically, increased their attractions for the men, and especially the women, who regarded nursing as a religious vocation or penitential exercise.[137] According to the Augustinian canon, Osbern Bokenham, Elizabeth of Hungary's daily visits to the lepers and other sick folk in her hospital at Marburg not only provided an ideal opportunity to encourage others, but also to test her own endurance of the miasmas that contaminated such places:

> She hem yaf many an exhortacyoun
> That thei from *pacyence* shuld not falle.
> And how she euery stynkyng exalacyoun
> Of the eyr bare alwey heuyly,
> Yet for goddys loue seke mennys corrupcyoun
> She not abhorryd, but ful *pacyently*
> It suffryd euyr, & eek [also] ful dylygently
> Hyr besyid [she worked hard] hem for to helpe & cure
> Whan hyr maydyns wych stodyn by
> Vnneth [none] of hem myght the breth endur.[138]

Other distressing symptoms associated with the disease provoked equally ambivalent responses, in part because of the terror of physical dismemberment entrenched within the medieval psyche.

Fear of the *corps morcelé*, or fragmented body, has excited the interest of many historians, who have come to regard the person of the leper as the embodiment of society's most deep-seated anxieties.[139] Both S.N. Brody and R.I. Moore, for example, suggest that suspect lepers were increasingly 'scapegoated' during the thirteenth century because of a tendency to conceptualise their disease as 'living decay' in its ultimate form.[140] 'It was', Caroline Walker Bynum maintains, 'because parts broke off the leper's body, because it fragmented and putrefied and became insensate when alive, in other words because it was a living death,

---

136  M.M. Banks, ed., *An Alphabet of Tales, I, A–H* (EETS, cxxvi, 1904), pp. 117–18. For the use of this *exemplum* as an exhortation to married hospital workers, see S. Farmer, 'The Leper in the Master Bedroom: Thinking through a Thirteenth-Century Exemplum', in R. Voader and D. Wolfthal, eds, *Framing the Family: Narrative and Representation in the Medieval and Early Modern Periods* (Arizona Center for Medieval and Renaissance Studies, 2005), pp. 79–100. I am most grateful to Professor Farmer for providing me with a copy of this essay.

137  Murray, 'Religion among the Poor', pp. 295–7; Rawcliffe, 'Hospital Nurses', pp. 49–50; Bird, 'Medicine for Body and Soul', p. 110.

138  Bokenham, *Legendys*, p. 272. Osbern's tale is based on Voragine, *Golden Legend*, pp. 675–89, at p. 681.

139  The work of the post-Freudian, Jacques Lacan (d. 1981), has had a notable impact in this regard: idem, *Ecrits*, ed. and trans. A. Sheridan (London, 1977), pp. 4–5; D. Luepnitz, 'Beyond the Phallus: Lacan and Feminism', in J.M. Rebate, ed., *The Cambridge Companion to Lacan* (Cambridge, 2003), pp. 225–6. See also, J. Kristeva, *Powers of Horror: An Essay on Abjection* (Columbia, 1982), pp. 101–2, who interprets fear of the leprous body in terms of anxieties about birth and 'the devouring mother'.

140  Brody, *Disease of the Soul*, pp. 79–80; Moore, *Formation of a Persecuting Society*, pp. 58–63.

that it was used as a common metaphor for sin.'[141] Although only the most advanced cases of *lepra* would appear so mutilated, there can be little doubt that serious disfigurement was bound to invite – if not always incur – a degree of moral censure. Diseased souls, infected with evil, were certainly described as 'deformed', in the sense that wickedness, like cancer or leprosy, had gnawed away at the divinity within, leaving them hideous and misshapen. Observing, with no little satisfaction, the results of his handiwork, Satan reflected that each sinner had corrupted 'the figure that God hath set in hym in his owne resemblaunce and likenes withoute slyme or fylthe, conformynge hymselfe wilfully and counterfetynge in hymself the fasone of *my* foule figure'.[142]

The process of decomposition was, moreover, only just beginning. As we saw in the previous chapter, malignant diseases might be visited as a specific punishment or purgation in the next life. In addition, souls in torment were routinely forced to endure the type of physical mutilation that characterised *lepra* in its final stages. A revelation of purgatory, allegedly vouchsafed to a female visionary in 1422, is typical of the *genre*, itemising in lurid detail the various tortures inflicted upon negligent or corrupt religious. She describes, for example, how devils attacked a gluttonous nun, cutting away the flesh and lips that had led her to abandon prayer for the pleasures of the table. Merrily slashing, burning, flaying and mutilating their victims, a host of little demons brandished 'strange hokes', designed to excoriate the flesh of sinners.[143] Embodying in his or her person a stark reminder of the ordeal to come, the leper cut a profoundly disturbing figure.

Although it assumed an extreme form in writing about the afterlife, the horror of physical collapse was no less marked in the work of political theorists, such as John of Salisbury, who adopted an organic view of the state. Like a physician, he traced the root cause of many ills to a malfunction of the digestive tract (the exchequer), but also stressed the vital role of the extremities. No doubt with the image of a leper or some other diseased pauper in mind, John reflected that, without its feet (the peasantry), the social body 'crawls shamefully, unseemly and offensively on its hands, or else is moved with the assistance of brute animals'.[144] The metaphor was not encouraging. A century later, one French polemicist castigated the clergy for failing to pay their taxes. 'Depraved is the part that does not conform with its whole', he warned, 'and useless and paralytic a limb that refuses to support its own body'.[145] Like the anaesthetised and

---

[141] Walker Bynum, *Fragmentation and Redemption*, p. 276.

[142] R. Potz McGerr, ed., *The Pilgrimage of the Soul: A Critical Edition of the Middle English Dream Vision* (New York, 1990), p. 14. Satan was conventionally described in the same language as that used to depict the leper. Julian of Norwich, for example, was tormented by a devil whose bright red skin was mottled with black spots, and whose hands were misshapen, without fingers: E. Colledge and J. Walsh, eds, *A Book of Showings to the Anchoress Julian of Norwich* (2 vols, Toronto, 1978), ii, pp. 635–6.

[143] M. Powell Harley, ed., *A Revelation of Purgatory by an Unknown Fifteenth-Century Woman Visionary* (Studies in Women and Religion, xviii, New York, c. 1985), pp. 59–86. In contrast to heaven and hell, souls in purgatory had not yet been reunited with their physical bodies, although visionaries still employed corporeal metaphors: Walker Bynum, *Fragmentation and Redemption*, p. 234.

[144] John of Salisbury, *Policraticus*, p. 67.

[145] E.H. Kantorowicz, *The King's Two Bodies: A Study in Medieval Political Theory* (Princeton, 1957), p. 258.

damaged hands and feet of the leper, such people seemed to threaten the rest of the body with gangrene.

The papal bull, *Detestande feritatis*, which in 1299 forbade the 'monstrous and detestable' practice of embalming, dividing and sometimes even boiling corpses before burial, has been seen as symptomatic of this growing revulsion against the fragmented body. For the best part of a century, successive popes had maintained a lively interest in medical literature, encouraging the production of *regimina* designed to preserve health and postpone physical decay.[146] Although the bull did not actually forbid the practice of dissection or the performance of autopsies, such events remained comparatively rare and, in the former instance, invariably involved the bodies of condemned criminals. Indeed, posthumous dismemberment seemed worse than the death sentence itself.[147] Nor was the papacy alone in its preoccupation with physical and moral integrity. Such considerations mattered, even where bricks and mortar were concerned. Every urban community had its own sinews, bones and organs, which were as vulnerable to the threat of physical collapse as the individuals who lived inside the walls. Like human skin, which protected the delicate mechanism within, the defences of English towns and cities offered protection against all manner of disruptive elements.[148] The worst of them might even end their days rotting on an extramural gibbet, or displayed, in disjointed parts, upon the gates.

Long before the arrival of the Normans in England, corporal mutilation was widely used to punish serious crimes, as the *vitae* of Anglo Saxon saints vividly attest. The removal of eyes, ears, tongues, noses, hands, feet and skin served to deter all but the most committed of recidivists, being employed, in extreme cases, serially as a means of prolonging the death agony and heaping shame upon persistent offenders. Such 'homoeopathic justice' demanded, for example, that a counterfeiter should lose his hand, while those found guilty of slander might have their tongues cut out.[149] Financial considerations rather than compassion led William the Conqueror and his successors to prefer heavy fines and outlawry to exemplary disfigurement, although the loss of eyes, testicles, hands and feet still lay at the monarch's discretion and was often enforced. Indeed, whereas most of the penalties listed in the *Leges Henrici Primi* were monetary, scalping, branding and the amputation of hands, feet and tongues remained in force for specific offences, including perjury and certain kinds of theft. The loss of an ear (frequently sustained by those who had been nailed to a post or pillory) constituted such a mark of shame that soldiers who suffered this type of injury in warfare reputedly asked for letters explaining their appearance, lest they be taken for criminals. Yet, whereas the law grew comparatively less

---

146  E.A.R. Brown, 'Death and the Human Body in the Later Middle Ages: The Legislation of Boniface VIII on the Division of the Corpse', *Viator*, xii (1981), pp. 221–70; A. Paravicini-Bagliana, *Le corps du pape* (Paris, 1995), pp. 199–233, 257.

147  M.N. Alston, 'The Attitude of the Church towards Dissection before 1500', *BHM*, xvi (1944), pp. 221–38.

148  G. Rosser, 'Urban Culture and the Church 1300–1540', in D. Palliser, ed., *The Cambridge Urban History of Britain* (Cambridge, 2000), pp. 339–41.

149  P. Wormald, *The Making of English Law: King Alfred to the Twelfth Century I* (Oxford, 1999), pp. 104, 125–6, 160, 282, 306, 363.

draconian in the matter of extreme physical punishment, the penalty for treason became increasingly brutal. At the time of the papal bull, for instance, the rebels Dafydd ap Gruffudd (d. 1283) and William Wallace (d. 1305) were sentenced to drawing on the hurdle, hanging, disembowelling, beheading, and quartering, their body parts being dispatched to disaffected outposts of the realm as a solemn warning to others. A similar fate awaited the royal favourite, Hugh Despenser (d. 1326), whose ordeal was compounded by its staging on a gallows fifty feet high.[150]

To function effectively, the body politic had not only to remain intact, productive and fit, but was expected to present a pleasing, symmetrical appearance. This emphasis upon what might be termed corporate aesthetics lingers on in the work of the Tudor polemicist, Thomas Starkey:

> Yet, though thys polytyke body be helthy & strong, yet yf hyt be not beutyful but foule deformyd hyt laketh a parte of hys wele & prosperouse state, thys beuty also stondyth in the dew proportion of the same partys togyddur, so that one parte ever be agreabul to a nother . . .[151]

Similar criteria applied to the human form. As Mary Magdalen discovered, physical attractiveness could pave the pathway to damnation, but when yoked to wisdom became a priceless commodity.[152] We shall see in the next chapter how much significance was placed upon the study of physiognomy during the later Middle Ages, but should note at this stage that facial features and deportment were widely regarded as a barometer of moral worth. The *Secreta secretorum*, an advice manual for kings and princes translated from Arabic in the twelfth century, offered a useful guide to the evaluation of character. Originally produced in Latin for elite use, it rapidly achieved widespread circulation in the vernacular. With his rheumy eye, rasping voice, collapsed nose, claw-like hands and distorted features, the leper – or at least the conventional image preserved in hagiography and literature – undermined every ideal of human beauty and thus apparently of reliability. By contrast, an individual of 'good disposicion', who might be trusted with affairs of state, appeared, at first glance, to be as agreeably proportioned and balanced in temperament as the body politic in its platonic form. Such a man was

> wele made in nature, that hath soft flessh and moist, meene betwix rovgh and smoth, not to longe neither to short, white declynyng to redenesse, plesaunt in looke, heres playn and meene, with grete eyen declynyng to roundnesse . . . of clere voice . . . with longe palmes and longe fyngres declynyng to sotilnesse.[153]

The onset of alopecia, a common symptom of *lepra*, constituted yet another

150  L.J. Downer, ed., *Leges Henrici Primi* (Oxford, 1972), pp. 110–11, 116–17, 180–81, 190–91, 214–15, 232–33, 246–7; F. Pollock and F.W. Maitland, *The History of English Law* (2 vols, Cambridge, 1911), ii, pp. 461, 498, 501; F.W.D. Brie, ed., *The Brut* (EETS, cxxxi, 1906), p. 240; N. Gonthier, *Le châtiment du crime au moyen âge* (Rennes, 1998), pp. 140–46, 191.
151  T. Starkey, *A Dialogue between Pole and Lupset*, ed. T.F. Mayer (CS, fourth series, xxxvii, 1989), p. 33.
152  Jansen, *Making of the Magdalen*, pp. 153–4.
153  M.A. Manzalaoui, ed., *Secreta secretorum: Nine English Versions* (EETS, cclxxvi, 1977), p. 113.

black mark. As the *Secreta* explained, 'the thynner the heeres ben the more gilefull, sharp, ferefull and of wynnyng covetous, it sheweth'.[154]

If, on the one hand, the ubiquity of skin diseases among the medieval population meant that, in practice, few people could aspire to such an ideal, it also placed a rare premium upon physical perfection, akin to that personified by Christ and His mother.[155] Sir Galahad, who alone possessed the virtue to succeed in the perilous quest for the Holy Grail, is repeatedly described as 'a youth so fair and so well made that it would be hard to find his peer'.[156] One would expect nothing less of such a chivalric hero. 'A man lame or ouer grete or ouer fatte, or that hath ony other euyl disposycion in his body . . . is not suffysaunt to be a knight' warned Ramon Lull (d. 1315), who regarded both physical and moral corruption as a bar to the profession of arms.[157] Conversely, when Tudor propagandists wished to emphasise the duplicity of Richard III, they created a monstrous cripple, whose physical appearance reflected his inner depravity. Although it was clearly impossible to follow the example of Henry IV's enemies and brand him as a leper, they, too, drew inspiration from Leviticus, which decreed that the 'crookbackt' might not make an offering to the Lord [21, vv. 16–23].[158]

The loss of the nose, in particular, was widely regarded as a sign of infamy, since it served to brand criminals and sexual miscreants. Such an obvious deformity, from which many lepers suffered, could not be hidden, and, indeed, ranked high among the unequivocal signs that the disease had entered its final phase. Henri de Mondeville and other medical authorities observed that lepers either talked through their noses (a further subversion of the natural order) or sustained so much nasal and maxillary damage as to render them virtually inaudible.[159] The *denasti*, or noseless, were deemed ineligible for the priesthood because of their blemish, and presented Albertus Magnus with a striking example of the connection between physical disfigurement and moral turpitude. That jealous husbands considered *abscissio nasi* a suitable punishment for an immodest or unfaithful wife underscored the connection between facial mutilation and lechery.[160] Yet, paradoxically, it might also betoken true repentance for past sins. Margaret of Cortona (d. 1297), whose biographer described her as 'as

154  Manzalaoui, *Secreta Secretorum*, p. 92.
155  I.M. Resnick, 'Ps.-Albert the Great on the Physiognomy of Jesus and Mary', *Medieval Studies*, lxiv (2002), pp. 217–40. For the intimate connection between goodness and beauty, see H. Kleinschmidt, *Perception and Action in Medieval Europe* (Woodbridge, 2005), pp. 131, 140.
156  P.M. Matarasso, ed., *The Quest of the Holy Grail* (Harmondsworth, 1969), p. 32.
157  Ramon Lull, *The Book of the Ordre of Chyvalry*, trans. William Caxton, ed. A.T.P. Byles (EETS, clxviii, 1926), p. 63.
158  A.J. Pollard, *Richard III and the Princes in the Tower* (Stroud, 1991), pp. 12–13. It was believed by some that the mark of Cain, placed upon him by God after the murder of Abel, was leprosy, although others maintained that he contracted palsy: R. Mellinkoff, *The Mark of Cain* (Berkeley, California, 1981), p. 57.
159  Nicaise, *Chirurgie de Henri de Mondeville*, pp. 616–17; Campbell and Colton, *Surgery of Theoderic*, ii, p. 171; BL, MS Harley 3, fo. 22r. 'The pacient haue a sor in the nose thyrls [nostrils] & fretynge and knawynge a way off the grystylles and grett stoppynge off the nose, the wyche may be parsayvyd by the voys off spkekynge': BL, MS Harley 1736, fo. 134v.
160  V. Groebner, 'Losing Face, Saving Face: Noses and Honour in the Late Medieval Town', *History Workshop Journal*, xl (1995), pp. 1–15.

second Magdalen', performed heroic penance for a misspent youth, even attempting to cut off her nose and upper lip in order to deface the beauty that had been her undoing.[161]

Eudes de Châteauroux clearly had both practices in mind when preaching to a congregation of lepers during the mid thirteenth century. In order to explain the reason for their suffering, he evoked the metaphor of a possessive rather than a vengeful spouse:

> By inflicting such a wound upon them, the Saviour has ensured that they are isolated from others and that they remain alone, almost alone, far from the company of healthy people. And this God does out of love, just as a man locks up his wife and jealously separates her from the company of other women who may corrupt her through their gossip and their suggestions. Still jealous, he sometimes shaves her hair and chops off her nose. But, if the woman loves her husband, she will bear all this with patience, and she will treasure such signs of a jealous love. Sometimes even, there are women who pretend to have been beaten. You therefore should rejoice, or at least bear with patience the fact that God has struck you thus. He does it to separate you from the love of the world.[162]

Standing nascent ideas about contagion upon their head, the bishop argued that the elect of God should flee from the moral miasmas of this world, which threatened the health of their immortal souls, and thus posed a far greater risk than their own decaying bodies ever could. Referring to the practice whereby housewives singed the glossy coats of their pet cats to prevent them being killed for fur, he congratulated his audience upon their narrow escape from the snares of vanity which invariably trapped the beautiful.[163]

It short, bodily fragmentation, mutilation or deformity carried an ambivalent, far from uniformly negative, message. If the butchered corpse of the traitor reinforced the shame of corporal punishment, that of the saint, whose remains might be scattered in countless reliquaries from Scandinavia to Byzantium, spoke a very different language. Widely distributed after his downfall and dismemberment at the battle of Evesham in 1265, the body parts of Simon de Montfort filled many reliquaries, becoming the focus of a cult that even flourished at the *leprosarium* of Burton Lazars.[164] Concerns about the reassembly of limbs and organs at the Last Judgement certainly did little to dissuade the aristocracy of late medieval Europe from the practices that Boniface VIII found so objectionable. Hearts and viscera were often removed for separate burial, sometimes in the hospitals that these men and women had founded in the hope of salvation.[165] In the final resort, the moral stature and conduct of the individual, rather than his or her physical condition, determined how the ravages of disease

---

[161] Haskins, *Mary Magdalen*, pp. 185–7; Jansen, *Making of the Magdalen*, p. 225.

[162] Beriou and Touati, *Voluntate Dei leprosus*, pp. 77, 98–9.

[163] Beriou and Touati, *Voluntate Dei leprosus*, p. 100.

[164] It was claimed that his relics possessed the power to heal a divided kingdom: S. Walker, 'Political Saints in Later Medieval England', in R.H. Britnell and A.J. Pollard, eds, *The MacFarlane Legacy: Studies in Late Medieval Politics and Society* (Stroud, 1995), pp. 82, 92, 96–7; Marcombe, *Leper Knights*, p. 97.

[165] Brown, 'Death and the Human Body', pp. 221–70.

would be perceived. For Alice of Schaerbeck and the other holy men and women who embraced – or even actively sought – leprosy, each additional torment offered a more perfect *imitatio Christi*.[166] Yet there was no room for complacency. Simply to be called by God was no longer enough. Delivered on the feast of the nativity of St John the Baptist, de Châteauroux's address dwelt, once again, upon the importance of *penitence* as a precursor to heavenly bliss.

## From *infirmitas* to *caritas*: the uses of leprosy

By fulfilling such weighty expectations the sick might overcome the prejudices and fears described above to acquire considerable reserves of spiritual authority. If, like Christ, the pious and repentant leper carried a disproportionate burden of suffering in this life, it seemed logical to assume that he or she would exert a corresponding degree of influence in the next.[167] During his sojourn in purgatory, the twelfth-century monk of Eynsham encountered an abbess whose torments there had been dramatically curtailed on account of the affection she had shown in her lifetime for two leprous nuns. Because their disease was so advanced, she explained,

> alle my systers of owre monasterye lothyd alle-moste to see or vysyte hem, or to toche hem, but to me, me thoughte and semyd full swete to haue . . . hem in my lappe or holde hem in my harmys, and furthermore alsoo to wesse [wash] hem in bathys, and also to wype her sores wyth my sleuys [sleeves]. And they ful wele and gladly sofryd that plage of lepur and tankyde God of that chastement and dyssese, and so delytyd hem yn hyt as they had resceyuyd of hym gracius gyftys of diuers ornamentys. And where a lytyl whyle agon they were peynyd yn the worlde by a longe martyrdome, now ful blessydly they folowyn the heuenly lambe, her spowse Ihesu Cryste, wythowtyn any spotte, wher-sum-euer He goo.[168]

Not only does the abbess's narration bring to mind the Virgin Mary, nursing the body of her crucified son, 'lyke a leprous man' [**plate 16**], but it also recalls the numerous female saints and holy women who had dedicated themselves to such uncongenial tasks out of devotion to Christ.

Given the aura of sanctity that regular association with lepers bestowed, it is easy to see how the *topos* of washing their ulcerated bodies came to figure so prominently in sermons, homilies and hagiography. Although it performed an important therapeutic function, the overwhelming purpose of the exercise was

---

166  Walker Bynum, *Fragmentation and Redemption*, pp. 133, 188 and chapter seven. Alice reflected that she had received the gift of leprosy in order to 'be free to rest with God alone, and linger in the room of her mind as in a marriage chamber and be intoxicated with the sweetness of his fragrance': *Acta Sanctorum*, xx, June II (11 June), pp. 473–4.

167  J. Agrimi and C. Crisciani, 'Charity and Aid in Medieval Christian Civilisation', in M.D. Grmek, ed., *Western Medical Thought from Antiquity to the Middle Ages* (Cambridge, Mass., and London, 1998), pp. 171–4. These sentiments are clearly expressed in grants to the lepers of Pont-Audemer: S.C. Mesmin, 'The Leper Hospital of Saint Gilles de Pont-Audemer: An Edition of the Cartulary and an Examination of the Problem of Leprosy in the Twelfth and early Thirteenth Century' (2 vols, University of Reading PhD, 1978), i, p. 117.

168  This quotation comes from the fifteenth-century translation: Easting, *Revelation of the Monk of Eynsham*, p. 137.

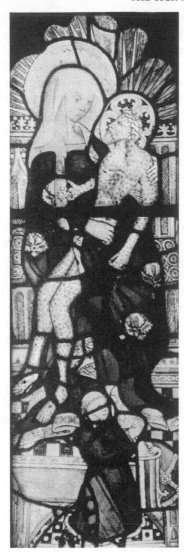

16. Late medieval congregations were familiar with images of the beaten Christ, whose torments resembled those of a leper. One such may be found in the stained glass at the church of The Holy Trinity, Long Melford, which depicts his lifeless body in the arms of the Virgin.

spiritual rather than hygienic. The legend of the Magdalen describes two occasions on which she bathed Christ's feet with her tears: the first during his life, and the second when he hung *quasi leprosus* on the cross, prompting a further outpouring of grief:

> To see his tendre fleshe thus rewfully arayed,
> On this wise so wofully displayed,
> Woundit withe nayll & spere!
> These blessite fete thus bludy to be-hold,
> Whom I weshid with teres manyfold![169]

[169] Furnivall, *Digby Plays*, p. 175.

The aristocrats, prelates and royalty who followed her example were also obeying and imitating Christ. His exhortation to the disciples that they should 'wash one another's feet', just as He had washed theirs at the Last Supper [John 13, vv. 4–15], was taken literally as well as figuratively. Many far exceeded His precept by kissing the recipients of their charity as well. The symbolism of this gesture is instructive, for as well as recognising Christ in the leper it constituted an even greater expression of humanity, respect and even deference.[170]

Saint Martin of Tours (d. 397) was apparently the first to go beyond Christ's simple touch and behave with such 'heroic compassion' towards a leprous beggar. Like the *haemhorrissa* in the Gospel, the leper is said to have accosted him at the gates of Paris by seizing the hem of his garment. In describing how the saint embraced and healed this terrifying creature, from whom everyone else shrank in horror, Martin's biographer, Sulpicius Severus, established a new and enduring literary *topos*.[171] It appears, for example, in two twelfth-century *vitae* of the Anglo Saxon princess, St Frideswide (d. 735). Substituting the streets of Oxford for the gates of Paris, her first biographer briefly describes how, on her entry into the city after a period of exile, she was approached by a young man 'full of leprosy'. He begged her to kiss him 'in the name of Jesus Christ', which she did after making the sign of the cross upon him. Miraculously, he was cleansed, while the townsfolk rejoiced at such an unambiguous display of sanctity. When retelling the story, a few decades later, the prior of St Frideswide's abbey, Robert of Cricklade, chose to emphasise the leper's raucous voice and monstrous, inhuman appearance, thereby throwing the saint's virginal purity into even sharper relief. Robert clearly knew his medical literature. Besides describing the youth's ulcerated, discoloured flesh, deformed body and reeking breath, he refers to the 'intolerable heat' of the disease. Unbalanced humours, rather than a crude display of male lust, prompted him to beg a kiss, and thus (he concludes) excused his presumption.[172]

The dramatic image of the 'triumphant thaumaturgical healer' was, however, soon destined to change. As Catherine Peyroux has demonstrated, saints such as Francis of Assisi seemed humbler, more overtly pious and, crucially, more concerned with their own spiritual health when they were dealing with the sick.[173] A cynic might reflect that this process of transition, vividly illustrated in the *vitae* of Hugh of Lincoln, coincided with the spread of medical information about leprosy and the imposition of more stringent criteria of proof where healing miracles were concerned. But this is, at best, a partial explanation. On his frequent visits to *leprosaria*, Hugh would first separate the sexes in order to

---

170  D. Damrosch, 'Non alia sed aliter: The Hermeneutics of Gender in Bernard of Clairvaux', in R. Blumenfeld-Kosinski and T. Szell, eds, *Images of Sainthood in Medieval Europe* (Ithaca and London, 1991), p. 191; J.C. Schmitt, *La raison des gestes dans l'occident médiéval* (Paris, 1990), pp. 297–8; Jansen, *Making of the Magdalen*, p. 86.

171  Sulpicius Severus, *Vie de Saint Martin*, ed. J. Fontaine (3 vols, Paris, 1967–69), i, pp. 292–3; ii, pp. 862–70.

172  J. Blair, 'Saint Frideswide Reconsidered', *Oxoniensia*, lii (1987), pp. 71–127, at pp. 78, 100, 113. Robert observes that Frideswide's kiss had the same effect as Naaman's ablutions in the Jordan. The Augustinian friar, John Capgrave (d. 1464), incorporated this tale almost verbatim in his own life of the saint: *Acta Sanctorum*, lvi, October VIII (10 October), p. 567.

173  Peyroux, 'Leper's Kiss', p. 181.

avoid any suggestion of impropriety. He would then 'kiss the men one by one, bending over each of them and giving a longer and more tender embrace to those whom he saw worse marked by the disease'.[174] His chancellor was naturally reminded of St Martin, and decided to test the bishop's motives by drawing attention to the similarities between them. Appalled by the very thought of such hubris, Hugh replied that 'Saint Martin's kisses healed a leper in the flesh, but the leper's kisses heal *me* of sickness of the spirit'.[175] From such a perspective, nurse and patient had effectively changed places, as Hugh sought to cleanse his soul through contact with Christ's representatives on earth.

Although the bishop's behaviour was far from unusual, having by then become part of the *cursus honorum* of many medieval saints, it may none the less have developed at a precocious age. The inspiration reputedly came at the knee of his mother, Anne, who

> used to wash the feet of veritable lepers. She was hope to the wretched, an eye to the blind, and a solace to the needy. She honoured Christ in them as the Head among the members of the body. Her completed work was given a fitting reward when the dying Anne was united to the living Lamb, and choosing wedlock with Christ over that with her husband, she left the one spouse and had the fortitude to hasten to the Other.[176]

This striking reversal of the customary anatomical metaphor of the social body, which equated leprosy with decay, disorder and the rot of heresy, reflects the reverence accorded to *Christus quasi leprosus* by pious men and high status women whose devotional practices focussed increasingly upon His humanity and suffering. This, in turn, had a significant impact upon responses to the sick.

One of Anne's undoubted models, Queen Matilda, the first wife of Henry I, certainly translated incarnational piety into action. Indeed, according to her earliest biographer, Aelred of Rievaulx, she constantly ministered to the abject and diseased poor. This is hardly surprising, for both she and her mother had been educated, along with many other noblewomen, at Wilton, a nunnery celebrated for its high scholastic achievements and intense spirituality.[177] A life of St Edith (d. 984) produced in about 1080 by Goscelin of Saint-Bertin, who spent some time as a chaplain there, preserves the stories that Matilda would have heard about the house's most celebrated royal pupil. Throughout her time at Wilton, we are told, Edith surrendered her life to communion with Christ. And, as a natural corollary,

> She devoted herself to the sick and destitute, she set the lepers of Christ before the sons of kings, she preferred to serve the lepers (*elephantiosis*) rather than have royal power; rather than ruling, she preferred to be beside ulcerated feet as if they were the footstool of Christ, and to tend them with bathing, and with her hair and

---

[174] Douie and Farmer, *Life of St Hugh*, ii, pp. 12–13.

[175] Garton, *Metrical Life of St Hugh*, p. 67. This incident provided late medieval preachers with a popular *exemplum*: BL, MS Royal 8 C I, fos 129v–130r.

[176] Garton, *Metrical Life of St Hugh*, p. 11.

[177] S. Hollis, 'Wilton as a Centre of Learning', in eadem, ed., *Writing the Wilton Women: Goscelin's Legend of Edith and liber confortatorius* (Turnhout, 2004), pp. 307–38.

kisses. The more anyone appeared to her deformed by disease, the more she offered herself to that person with empathy and kindness, full of service.[178]

An alb, reputedly made and embroidered by Edith herself, figured prominently among the relics listed by Goscelin. It depicted Christ and His apostles, with the princess 'in the place of Mary [Magdalen] the suppliant, kissing the Lord's footprints'.[179]

Matilda's mother, Margaret (d. 1093), who became queen of Scotland and was eventually canonised, enjoyed a similar reputation for extreme asceticism and selfless love of the poor.[180] It has been suggested that her *vita*, which Matilda commissioned in about 1106, served as a 'didactic tool', rather than a real biography, to provide the young English queen with a guide to royal deportment. Such an argument does not necessarily imply that the many instances of compassion it records were nothing more than abstract *exempla*, selected by the author from a library shelf.[181] Hagiographers must already have found it hard to describe the actual care of lepers in new and original ways. Aelred of Rievaulx did contrive, however, to inject a note of realism, even humour, when he came to describe Matilda's philanthropy. Although her brother, King David, was himself celebrated as a model of humility, he evidently lacked the stomach for intimate contact with noisome and deformed bodies. On entering the royal apartments one evening, he was shocked to find Matilda wrapped in an apron, washing and kissing the feet of leprous beggars. Her apparent indifference to their loathsome appearance prompted him to ask what King Henry would think if he knew his wife's mouth had touched such ulcerated flesh. 'Who does not know that the feet of the eternal king are preferable to the lips of a king who must die', she replied cheerfully, continuing with her task.[182] This story, which Matthew Paris incorporated into his *Chronica majora*, rapidly passed into vernacular literature, where it resurfaced in the late medieval legend of 'good queen Mold'.[183] But it, too, was far from original, having first appeared centuries

---

178  M. Wright and K. Loncar, eds, 'Goscelin's *Legend of Edith*', in Hollis, *Writing the Wilton Women*, p. 40.

179  Wright and Loncar, 'Goscelin's *Legend*', p. 48.

180  D. Baker, 'A Nursery of Saints: St Margaret of Scotland Reconsidered', in idem, ed., *Medieval Women* (Studies in Church History, Subsidia, i, 1978), pp. 119–41. Margaret was canonised in 1249–50, and at least one, probably more, of the fifteen English *leprosaria* dedicated to a St Margaret invoked her patronage: Satchell, 'Emergence of Leper-Houses', pp. 250–399. The gruesome fate of St Margaret of Antioch did, however, eminently qualify her to be a dedicatee of *leprosaria*: Bokenham, *Legendys*, pp. 15–24.

181  L.L. Huneycutt, 'The Idea of the Perfect Princess: The Life of Margaret in the Reign of Matilda II (1100–1118)', *Anglo-Norman Studies*, xii (1989), pp. 81–97; Hollis, 'Wilton as a Centre of Learning', p. 335 n. 137.

182  Aelred of Rievaulx, *Opera omnia*, PL, xcxv, *Genelogia regum Anglorum*, col. 736. John of Tynemouth was so impressed by the incident that he added it to his *vita* of Queen Margaret in the fourteenth century: Huneycutt, 'Perfect Princess', p. 92. Matilda narrowly missed canonisation, although her life was by no means as austere as might be supposed: C.W. Holister, *Henry I* (New Haven and London, 2001), p. 130.

183  Matthew Paris, *Chronica Majora*, ii, p. 130. The English verses attributed to Robert of Gloucester (*fl.* 1265) eulogise 'gode queen Mold': W.A. Wright, ed., *The Metrical Chronicle of Robert of Gloucester* (2 vols, RS, 1887), ii, pp. 638–41.

earlier in Venantius Fortunatus' near contemporary *vita* of the Frankish queen, Radegund (d. 587), yet another royal saint.[184]

Real or invented, such tales projected a powerful image of medieval queenship, which combined generosity and humility in equal measure. They also reflect the spiritual concerns and aspirations of Matilda's contemporaries. Herbert de Losinga, who may have been the queen's advisor, admired her greatly, reflecting that the odour of her devotion had spread like an exquisite perfume to 'the end of the earth'. He composed a prayer for her use, recommending that, just as the repentant Magdalen had bathed Christ's feet with her tears, so she, another sinner (who, like Mary, was no longer virginal), should abase herself before St John the Evangelist. 'Bowing down with her face towards the earth', she too should beg, weeping, for forgiveness at the foot of the cross. His prayer refers to the medieval legend that John, the most beloved of the apostles, had not only survived a bath of boiling oil but had also swallowed a draught of poison with no apparent effect, thus – by analogy – draining the bitter cup of confession. As the learned Matilda would have known, John was also said to have warned the citizens of Pergamum that they risked incurring the fate of Dives if they did not mend their ways and forgo the trappings of wealth. He was thus an ideal patron saint for any pious queen, although no more than a handful of English *leprosaria* were actually dedicated to him.[185] Strikingly, when Matilda founded a leper house of her own, in Holborn, on the outskirts of London, she named it after St Giles, the confessor saint *par excellence* [**plate 31**].[186]

Either out of genuine piety or a less commendable desire to bask in the adulation heaped upon her predecessor, Henry I's second queen, Adela of Louvain (d. 1151), followed Matilda's example by founding or enriching leper houses at Wilton in Wiltshire and Arundel in Sussex. She may well have been the moving spirit behind the establishment of another at Castle Rising, in Norfolk, where her next husband, William d'Albini, spared no expense in the creation of an impressive 'landscape of lordship'. Visitors to the new castle must have been overwhelmed by the vista of moats, deer parks and gardens, while noting with approval his concern for the leprous poor, who lived comfortably just outside the gates. Given his unenviable reputation as 'an arrogant and inordinately conceited' upstart, Earl William clearly needed all the moral authority and spiritual credit such a foundation could bestow.[187] A second d'Albini stronghold at New Buckenham, to the south of the county, seems also to have boasted a

---

184 J.A. McNamara and J.E. Halborg, eds, *Sainted Women of the Dark Ages* (Durham and London, 1992), pp. 78–9; Carrasco, 'Sanctity and Experience in Pictorial Hagiography', in Blumenfeld-Kosinski and Szell, *Images of Sainthood*, pp. 55–8, emphasises the differences between the *vita* and later iconography depicting Radegund in a pose similar to Christ washing the feet of His apostles.

185 Goulburn and Symonds, *Life, Letters and Sermons of Bishop Herbert de Losinga*, i, pp. 298–313. I am grateful to Mr T.A. Heslop for drawing my attention to this prayer. For leper hospitals dedicated to the fourth Evangelist, see Satchell, 'Emergence of Leper-Houses', pp. 250–399.

186 BL, MS Harley 4015, fo. 5r-5v; Honeybourne, 'Leper Hospitals of the London Area', pp. 20–31. Matilda reputedly founded the hospital of St Mary Magdalen and St James, Chichester, but there is no evidence to support this claim: W. Page, ed., *VCH Sussex II* (London, 1907), p. 99.

187 R.B. Pugh and E. Crittall, eds, *VCH Wiltshire III* (London, 1956), p. 362; Satchell, 'Emergence of Leper-Houses', pp. 134–5; R. Liddiard, 'Landscapes of Lordship: The Landscape Context of Castles in Norfolk 1066–1506' (University of East Anglia, PhD, 2000), pp. 177–8, 210; L. Watkiss and M. Chibnall, eds, *The Waltham Chronicles* (Oxford, 1994), pp. 76–9.

*leprosarium* as part of the planned layout: an arrangement which suggests that the lesson of Dives and Lazarus had struck home. Adela's role in the endowment of the last two hospitals (and a potential third at Wymondham) remains unclear,[188] as does the part played by women in general as providers of institutional care.

That it was far greater than the surviving records suggest seems almost certain. As many scholars of medieval literature have observed, the production, reworking and, indeed, invention, of hagiographical material satisfied the needs, as well as reflecting the changing values, of specific sectors of society. The Magdalen of later medieval legend was, for example, sufficiently versatile to draw women from the urban as well as the landowning elite into her orbit, offering them an exemplar of the *vita mixta*, which combined action and contemplation. Her voluntary embrace of poverty, good works and contemplation appealed to ascetics such as Elizabeth of Hungary. On the other hand, an increasing tendency to emphasise her wealth and status attracted women of means, whose circumstances obliged them to remain in the world.[189] But they had ample opportunity to divert land and money into *leprosaria*, several of which appear to have had female founders, or to have enjoyed generous patronage from women at an early stage.

Roger Mowbray's mother, Gundreda, who may well have fostered his charitable impulses, and who later married into the d'Albini family, was, for instance, a notable benefactor of St Michael's, Whitby.[190] The hospital of St Nicholas, Royston, appears to have been founded in about 1200 by Amphelise, a daughter of Robert Chamberlain, and subsequently endowed by one of her sisters.[191] At some point over the next fifty years Edith Bisset, who was apparently childless, used some of her landed wealth to establish a *leprosarium* at Cirencester.[192] The small and comparatively poor hospital of St Mary and St Clement, Norwich, boasted Margaret de Lungespee, countess of Lincoln (d. by 1310), as its founder, although this claim is harder to verify.[193] Such women clearly represented the tip of an iceberg. How often grants from married couples were, in fact, instigated and implemented by the wife cannot now be determined. Specific references to the use of dower lands and inherited properties are, none the less, suggestive. Eudo Arsic, a major benefactor of the leper house at Gaywood, near King's Lynn, may, for instance, have been acting on the wishes of his wife, Alice, who made even greater endowments upon it in her widowhood.[194]

Vanity and pride were widely seen as quintessentially feminine weaknesses. To religious women, in particular, the antidote to this terminal affliction lay not simply in supporting but in actually tending real, suffering lepers on a daily

---

188    Liddiard, 'Landscapes of Lordship', p. 179; Dugdale, *Monasticon*, vi, pp. 769–70.
189    T. Coletti, '*Paupertas est donum Dei*: Hagiography, Lay Religion and the Economics of Salvation in the Digby *Mary Magdalene*', *Speculum*, lxxvi (2001), pp. 337–78.
190    Atkinson, *Cartularium Abbathiue de Whitby*, i, p. 330.
191    L.F. Salzman, *VCH Cambridge and the Isle of Ely II* (London, 1948), pp. 310–11.
192    *CIM, 1399–1422*, no. 27.
193    Rawcliffe, *Hospitals of Medieval Norwich*, pp. 50, 59 n. 65.
194    King's Lynn Borough Archives, C56/2, 3. Satchell, 'Emergence of Leper-Houses', pp. 134–5, cites other examples.

basis. Hugh de Floreffe, the biographer of Jutta of Huy (d. 1228), reports that, through living intimately alongside her own patients in the *leprosarium* of the Grands Malades, she was able to overcome the flaws common to all her sex. Dwelling at length upon his subject's remarkable humility and her desire for the perfect *imitatio Christi*, he explains how her soul, if not her body, thereby became *viriliter*.[195] Few twelfth- and thirteenth-century English women sought to emulate the heroic feats of asceticism achieved by the *mulieres sanctae* of northern Europe, but many discovered an outlet for religious zeal and a sense of personal empowerment by nursing the sick. In his account of the alleged martyrdom of William of Norwich in 1144, Thomas of Monmouth describes the appearance of a 'fiery light' over the leper hospital that his fellow Benedictines ran at Sprowston.

> The Lady Legarda, formerly wife of William of Apulia, with her attendants saw it too, she who for the love of God has her dwelling hard by St Mary Magdalen's attending upon the sick, and engaged in such services lives as a beggar for the salvation of her soul. But the sick people of that place in the silence of the night as they were getting up for the midnight office, when Legarda showed it them, saw the brightness of that same light.[196]

The intercessionary powers of such women began to seem as valuable as those of the lepers they served, and prompted a generous response among patrons who found it easier to pay others to implement their charitable provisions. Many wealthy penitents none the less wished to perform conspicuous acts of self-abasement as well. It is easy to see how, in such a context, the leper became little more than a cipher or vehicle in the spiritual odyssey of his benefactor.

After his death, the body of the ascetic Robert d'Arbrissel (d. 1116) was taken to the leper hospital of St Lazare, which he had established as a mixed community near Fontevrault. Having made many penitential visits there in his lifetime, it seemed appropriate to include this final gesture of humility in his funeral rites.[197] Clearly aware of the importance of such gestures and the message they conveyed, Henry II halted his own remorseful journey to Canterbury cathedral, in 1174, at the Harbledown *leprosarium*, just outside town. Here he dismounted, entered the hospital to pray for forgiveness and made a handsome donation of twenty marks to the patients in memory of the recently martyred Thomas Becket. He then proceeded on foot to cleanse his soul with confession and submit *humblement* to a flogging at the hands of the monks.[198] The archbishop's warning that he would suffer the fate of Uzziah probably still rang in his ears. Adam of Charing, a Kentish landowner who had been excommunicated by Becket in 1169, felt a similar need to make fitting atonement by liberally endowing the *leprosarium* at New Romney, 'for the love of God and in honour of

---

195  *Acta Sanctorum*, ii, January II (13 January), p. 152; I. Cochelin, 'Sainteté laïque: l'example de Juette de Huy (1158–1228)', *Le Moyen Age*, xcv (1989), pp. 397–417, at pp. 405–10.
196  Thomas of Monmouth, *Life and Miracles of Saint William*, p. 31.
197  J. Dalarun, *L'impossible sainteté: La vie retrouvée de Robert d'Arbrissel* (Paris, 1985), pp. 194, 295.
198  Guernes de Pont Sainte Maxence, *La vie de saint Thomas le Martyr, poème historique du XIIe siècle*, ed. E. Walberg (London, 1922), pp. 200, 311; *Pipe Roll 21 Henry II, 1174–1175* (Pipe Roll Society, xxii, 1897), p. 213.

the reverend and glorious martyr, Thomas, and for the health of my soul and the souls of my ancestors'.[199]

Anxious Christians, who could already smell the pitch and sulphur of purgatory, certainly hoped that God would incline favourably to the commendatory prayers intoned, day after day, on their behalf by the sick. The first entry in the cartulary of the *leprosarium* founded by the counts of Champagne near Chartres records a gift of £10 a year made by an ostensibly penitent Henry I 'to God, St Mary Magdalen of the Grand-Beaulieu, and the lepers serving God there (*Deo servientibus*), for the souls of my father and family, and for the remission of my sins and the state and security of my kingdom of England and my duchy of Normandy'.[200] Following a profoundly disturbing dream, in 1131, Henry had consulted his physician, who addressed the root of the problem by advising him to purge his soul 'and redeem his sins by almsgiving'.[201] His donation calls to mind Robert Burton's celebrated remark that to endow a hospital under such circumstances was 'to steale a Goose and sticke downe a feather, rob a thousand and releeve ten', although it was, in fact, but one of many similar gifts.[202] Having provided a chaplain for the lepers at the *maladerie* in Lincoln, for example, Henry took the added precaution of funding two more to intercede there for his own spiritual health.[203]

We can only speculate about the personal history of Laurence the outlaw (*utlator*) of Lynn, who promised the leper house at Gaywood 'and the infirm brothers serving God there' one penny a year from his purse while he lived.[204] In comparative terms he was probably more generous than King Henry. Jacques de Vitry maintained that 'robbers and usurers' frequently gave alms to leper houses as a type of celestial insurance policy, observing that Marie d'Oignies (d. 1213), another of the holy women who dedicated herself to the service of *Christus quasi leprosus*, was so concerned about the provenance of the gifts made to her hospital at Willambroux, in the diocese of Liège, that she adopted a vegetarian diet rather than risk eating flesh from stolen animals.[205] Right across the social spectrum, from royalty to humble shopkeepers, from bishops to petty – and not so petty – criminals, men and women supported *leprosaria* as they supported other religious institutions, in the hope of redemption.

---

[199] C.R. Cheyney and B.E.A. Jones, eds, *EEA, II, Canterbury 1162–1190* (Oxford. 1986), no. 306; A.F. Butcher, 'The Hospital of St Stephen and St Thomas New Romney: The Documentary Evidence', *Archaeologia Cantiana*, xcvi (1981), pp. 17–26, at pp. 18–19.

[200] R. Merlet and M. Jusselin, eds, *Cartulaire de la léproserie du Grand-Beaulieu, Chartres* (Chartres, 1909), p. 1; C. Johnson and H.A. Cronne, eds, *Regesta Regum Anglo-Normannorum II* (Oxford, 1956), no. 1917. Henry's sister, Adela, the wife of count Stephen, was a notable patron of the hospital and may have solicited the gift: K.A. LoPrete, 'Adela of Blois and Ivo of Chartres: Piety, Politics and Peace in the Diocese of Chartres', *Anglo-Norman Studies*, xiv (1992), pp. 131–52, at pp. 144–5.

[201] P. McGurk, ed., *The Chronicle of John of Worcester, III* (Oxford, 1998), pp. 199–203.

[202] Robert Burton, *The Anatomy of Melancholy*, eds T.C. Faulkener et al. (6 vols, Oxford, 1989–2000), i, p. 87.

[203] Dugdale, *Monasticon*, vi, pp. 627–8. For some of Henry's other grants to *leprosaria*, see: Johnson and Cronne, *Regesta*, ii, nos 1260 (Harbledown), 1918 (Pont-Audemer, but assigned by Mesmin, 'Saint Gilles de Pont-Audemer', ii, pp. 97–100, to Henry II); iii, no. 730 (Rouen); Satchell, 'Emergence of Leper-Houses', pp. 176–84 (Oxford). Kealey, *Medieval Medicus*, p. 96, overestimates the scale of his largesse.

[204] King's Lynn Borough Archives, KL/C56/5 (undated).

[205] Jacques de Vitry, *The Life of Marie d'Oignies*, eds M.H. King and M. Marsolais (Toronto, 1993), p. 76.

Nor, as we saw at the start of this chapter, did the flow of charity run dry. As late as 1399, Richard II left an implausible sum of five or six thousand marks (£4,000) in his will for the lepers and chaplains celebrating for the salvation of his soul at Westminster and Bermondsey.[206] Covering some twenty-one closely written pages, the obit roll begun at some point before 1296 by the Gaywood leper house, outside Lynn, continued to record the names of beneficiaries until the sixteenth century. Men and women throughout East Anglia and beyond regularly sought membership of the fraternity, paying handsomely for a share in the commemorative prayers and spiritual merits of the hospital's few remaining lepers.[207] On the very eve of the Reformation, the *leprosarium* in Cambridge, founded almost two hundred years earlier by Henry Tangmere, listed among its recent acquisitions a 'steyned' altar frontal and four images 'new painted' which a local testator had recently bestowed upon the hospital chapel. The daily prayers still said there by 'the leprous men and women' for the mayor and burgesses clearly merited appropriate and continuous investment.[208]

Long before this date, and in parallel with the increased quantification of both intercessionary and penitential practices, the larger leper houses of medieval England bowed to a strong current of market forces. The provision of a more comprehensive range of spiritual services, performed around the clock by the residents and their priests, was, at its most basic, a commercial exchange of commendatory prayer for hard cash. It also constituted a response to changes in the common law, which demanded that tenurial relationships should be defined in clearer and more specific language. Put crudely, each acre of land and penny of rent could now be commuted into *Aves* and *Pater Nosters*.[209] Yet, in theological terms, the relationship between patron and patient was considerably more complex.

To understand the basis of this reciprocal arrangement, it is worth returning briefly to the legend of Mary Magdalen. Having shed her seven devils, the repentant sinner became a notable exponent of the Seven Comfortable Works, through which all Christians might achieve salvation. Feeding, clothing and housing the poor, visiting them in prison or when they were sick, giving drink to the thirsty and providing a decent burial were all deeds of compassion from which the leper derived immediate benefit. It was, indeed, upon such charitable foundations that all medieval hospitals were built. Even more important, however, were the Seven Spiritual Works, which provided equivalent solace for the soul rather than the body, and of which the Magdalen proved a no less formidable exponent. The sick stood in particular need of instruction, counsel, comfort, forgiveness, forbearance and, when necessary, reproof, but, in return,

---

206  J. Strachey et al., eds, *Rotuli Parliamentorum* (6 vols, London, 1783), iii, p. 421.
207  NRO, Bradfer Lawrence MS IX d. An extract appears in Owen, *Making of King's Lynn*, pp. 108–16. Both St James's, Doncaster (BL, MS Cotton Tiberius C V, fos 263v–264r), and St Bartholomew's, Dover (Bodleian Library, MS Rawl. B.335, fo. 37r), also kept obit rolls, now lost. So apparently did the nuns of Maiden Bradley (BL, Add. Charter 19137; MS Add. 37503, fos 16r–16v, 27r).
208  Palmer, *Cambridge Borough Documents*, i, p. 56; Rubin, *Charity and Community*, pp. 124–5.
209  B. Thompson, 'From "Alms" to "Spiritual Services": The Function and Status of Monastic Property in Medieval England', in J. Loades, ed., *Monastic Studies II* (Bangor, 1991), pp. 227–61.

they could offer the seventh and most valuable gift of commendatory prayer.[210] In short, the grateful patient, duly confessed and cleansed of sin, would render thanks to his or her benefactors in the most effective means possible: by petitioning God for the welfare of their immortal souls.[211]

Preaching on the text 'whosever will come after me, let him deny himself, and take up his cross, and follow me' [Matthew 11, v. 38], one twelfth-century priest described the three crosses that every member of his congregation would have to carry to achieve salvation. It was, he stressed, essential to share the bodily pain of Christ, through *carnis maceratio*, or the mortification of the flesh. Each Christian must learn to endure hunger, thirst, cold, painful garments, sleeplessness, heavy labour and the lash in order to secure forgiveness for his or her sins. Then came *contricio*, or heartfelt remorse, and lastly *proximi compassio*, or pity for the plight of others.[212] However reluctantly, the leper had already assumed the first of these burdens. There was no need for him or her to submit, like St Nicholas (the dedicatee of over a dozen English leper hospitals), to a battery of physical austerities.[213] As William Langland observed, 'penaunce and purgatorie here on erthe' was the reward for the poor, sick and crippled folk 'that taketh this myschief mekelych, as meseles and othere'.[214] Having rendered full physical atonement, the leper had none the less still to show contrition and, through the medium of prayer, demonstrate his or her sympathy for those who lagged behind him or her on the road to Calvary. A tendency to regard the hospital patient as little more than a 'liturgical appendage', whose remaining years were spent in an unremitting and essentially mechanical round of intercession, tends to obscure what was, in theory, a mutually beneficial activity. The practice may have seemed more one-sided.

We shall explore the religious life of the medieval *leprosarium* in chapter seven, but it is important to stress here that, in common with all hospitals of any size, the larger leper houses had always demanded a strict regimen of observance. This derived its structure from the seven canonical hours of the *opus Dei*, which regulated the life of all monastic foundations. On the assumption that few lay residents would be conversant with the Latin liturgy, the recitation of familiar prayers might be required instead. Concern with both the frequency and quality of intercession was, therefore, far from new and explains why founders such as William le Gros were so anxious to entrust their hospitals to the care of senior ecclesiastics. In about 1181, the lepers of Pont-Audemer enumerated the 'manifold benefits of the house in the form of hymns, psalms, vigils and prayers . . . which the brethren and sisters chant daily from dawn to dusk for the sake of their own souls and the souls of their benefactors' in the

---

210   The Spiritual Works are itemised by Thomas Aquinas, *Summa Theologica* (6 vols, Rome, 1894), iii, II, part 2, question 32, articles 2–4. See Rawcliffe, *Medicine for the Soul*, pp. 4–6, for a discussion of the Comfortable Works in the context of the medieval hospital.

211   This requirement was actually spelt out as a precondition of entry in the rules of some *leprosaria*, such as St Lazare, Montpellier (1129 x 58), and Amiens (1305): L. Le Grand, ed., *Statuts d'hôtels Dieu et de léproseries* (Paris, 1901), pp. 183, 224–5.

212   Morris, *Old English Homilies*, pp. 206–7.

213   Voragine, *Golden Legend*, p. 18.

214   William Langland, *Piers Plowman Text B*, ed. W.W. Skeat (EETS, xxxviii, 1869, reprinted 1898), pp. 114–15.

hope of attracting further patronage. The exercise was clearly successful, prompting Bishop Herbert Poore of Salisbury (d. 1217) to commended those who 'in the anguish of bodily affliction offer daily thanks to the Lord for their benefactors with a joyous mind'.[215]

English hospitals employed similar tactics. From at least 1200 onwards, the *leprosarium* of St Margaret and the Holy Sepulchre, Gloucester, expected a daily minimum of about 300 *Aves* and *Pater Nosters* from each resident. Although they rarely came cheap, special arrangements for personal commendation were also on offer. Thomas Toli's gift of money to feed the patients and provide a lamp to illuminate their church was, for example, conditional upon additional prayers being said daily on his behalf during Mass. A similar endowment, also made to the house in 1230, demanded weekly Masses for the donor and his family.[216] As a further inducement to charity, monastic patrons sometimes promised to augment the power of such prayers. From the 1170s, if not earlier, the Augustinian canons at Taunton offered patrons of the local *leprosarium* membership of their own fraternity. Shortly afterwards, the Benedictines of Christ Church, Canterbury, dug into their coffers to fund a priest 'professed in the form and habit of religion' to sing requiem Masses daily at the hospital of St James for the souls of benefactors.[217]

The *minutiae* of the liturgical round assumed even greater importance as the release of captive souls from purgatory became a matter of such obsessive calculation. Bishop Stratford's revised rules of 1346 for the hospital of St Mary the Virgin at Ilford, in Essex, offer a typical example:

> We also command that the said lepers do not omit attendance at their church to hear the divine office unless they are prevented by grievous bodily infirmity. They are to preserve silence there; they are to hear matins and mass throughout, if they are able; and, while they are there, to be intent on prayer and devotion, as far as their infirmity allows. We also desire and command that, as it was ordained of old in the said hospital, every leprous brother shall say every day for the morning office a *Pater Noster* and an *Ave Maria* thirteen times; and for each of the other hours of the day, that is to say prime, terce, sext, nones, vespers and compline, a *Pater Noster* and an *Ave Maria* seven times; and, in addition to the aforesaid prayers, each one of them shall say a *Pater* and an *Ave* thirty times every single day for his founders and the bishop of the place and all of his benefactors and all other faithful, living or dead.[218]

Although a good deal of laxity obtained in many houses, those patients who still seemed capable of shouldering even a modest burden of suffrages were formally

215  Mesmin, 'Saint Gilles de Pont-Audemer', ii, pp. 172–4, 224–7.
216  *HMC, Twelfth Report, Appendix IX* (London, 1891), pp. 426–7; W.H. Stevenson, ed., *Calendar of Records of the Corporation of Gloucester* (Gloucester, 1893), no. 241.
217  Robertson, *Materials*, i, pp. 428–9; Somer, *Antiquities of Canterbury*, p. 41; J. Brigstocke Sheppard, ed., *Literae Cantuarienses* (3 vols, RS, 1887–89), iii, p. 77. The hospital of St Mary Magdalen, Liskeard, also belonged to a network of religious houses that pooled their spiritual resources: Orme and Webster, *English Hospital*, pp. 206–7.
218  Dugdale, *Monasticon*, vi, p. 629. Matins, the morning office, took place during the night in this period; prime was at sunrise, terce at about nine, sext at noon, nones at three in the afternoon, vespers in the early evening and compline at the end of the day.

required to do so. Indeed, at St Bartholomew's, Dover, the leprous brothers and sisters (who swore on admission to intercede devoutly for their patrons) had to say half their daily round of prayers in the middle of the night, seated upright in bed. In this way all but the most incapacitated could play some part in the religious life of the house.[219]

It is easy to see why many suspect lepers opted for the less regimented, if more Spartan, life of a modest suburban *leprosarium*, where the liturgical round was less demanding and fewer restrictions were imposed upon personal freedom. Others, as we shall see, either preferred, or were obliged, to congregate in informal settlements or take to the open road as beggars. Although they had been welcomed into the households of the great and the royal chambers at Westminster during the twelfth and thirteenth centuries, the vagrant, leprous poor exercised a less secure claim upon the philanthropy of late medieval benefactors. While continuing to pay lip service to the concept of *Christus quasi leprosus*, the latter were more likely to acknowledge His presence in reputable men and women who played by the rules. Neither penitent nor docile, the indigent also began to inspire more immediate concerns about contagion. But before we examine this shift in attitudes to segregation, it is important to determine exactly who might be considered leprous and how this definition was achieved. For although the *concept* of leprosy, with its heavy freight of theological baggage, was ubiquitous in medieval England, lepers themselves were fewer in number than the evidence of this chapter might suggest. After all, even during the early wave of foundations, only a comparatively small number of hospitals accommodated over a dozen patients. Moreover, increasingly complex and refined theories about diagnosis and treatment meant that the gap between suspicion and confirmation grew steadily wider.

---

[219] Bodleian Library, MS Rawl. B.335, fos 1v, 2v. The rules (of an allegedly earlier date) were recorded in 1372–73, and demanded 400 *Aves* and 400 *Pater Nosters* a day. An indulgence of 1375 promised that 4,000 daily *Pater Nosters*, *Aves* and Creeds might be purchased from the residents of Harbledown for just one half penny: J. Duncombe and N. Battely, *The History and Antiquities of the Three Archiepiscopal Hospitals at and near Canterbury* (London, 1785), p. 203.

# 4

## Priests and Physicians:
## The Business of Diagnosis

*These misfortunes having no cure, the priesthood assumed authority for controlling leprosy, and of making it a religious issue. This has led certain thoughtless individuals to assume that the Jews were veritable savages, led by mountebanks. To be sure, their priests did not cure leprosy, but they separated anybody with scabies from society, and thus acquired prodigious power. Everyone stricken with this evil was imprisoned like a thief; to such an extent that any woman who wished to be rid of her husband simply had to find a priest; the husband was shut away: it was a kind of lettre de cachet of those days.*

*Voltaire*, Dictionnaire Philosophique, *1765* [1]

The ecclesiastical career of William Mustardere, the newly installed rector of Sparham, a parish some fourteen miles north-west of Norwich, seemed to be progressing well during the late 1460s. After several years of relative obscurity spent tending his first flock, in the neighbouring hamlet of Foxley, he was able, through the good graces of an aristocratic patron, to augment his initially modest stipend. Having secured the necessary papal approval, in 1467 he combined the more lucrative living of Sparham with Bawdeswell, which suggests that, although he was not apparently a university graduate, he must have been relatively well educated.[2] That, like most of his peers, he possessed at least a smattering of medical knowledge also seems more than likely, for he soon felt sufficiently confident of his diagnostic abilities to pronounce one of his parishioners 'gretely infect with the sekenes of lepre'. In the privacy of the confessional, Mustardere repeatedly urged the unfortunate John Folkard to 'withdrawe hym from the compayne of other men'. This, he later explained, was a pastoral duty incumbent upon any 'gostely fader . . . for very affeccion and love that he ought to his seid parissen[er]s'. In short, the priest 'secretly councelled' Folkard 'that

1    L. Moland, ed., *Oeuvres complètes de Voltaire*, 19, *Dictionnaire philosophique, III* (Paris 1879, reprinted 1967), p. 574.
2    NRO, DN, reg. 6, book 11, pp. 49, 151, 158, 164, 291.

his sekenes was contagious, and might hurte moche people, and so dyvers tymes advertised hym to departe and kepe hym selfe oute of felawship'.[3]

It was at this point that things began to go badly wrong. Whatever spiritual authority he might have possessed, Mustardere had taken a considerable risk in antagonising such a potentially dangerous adversary. Folkard was the son of a Norwich alderman who had prospered in the grocery trade, although it was from his mother that he inherited a modest country estate.[4] Like many such *arrivistes*, he thus had his foot poised on the bottom rung of the ladder of gentility, which must have made the imputation of leprosy even harder to bear. Far from accepting the rector's advice, Folkard allegedly 'manassed' him, and warned 'that he shuld repent that ever he made any such noyse'. In desperation, Mustardere alerted the rest of his congregation to the threat lurking in their midst, whereupon 'dyvers of the meniall servants of the seid John, undrestandyng that he was infect with the seid sekenes, wold no legger [longer] abyde with hym, but they and all other men, seyng the seid sekenes shewe upon hym so evidently, wold not be accompanied with hym, but eschewed to come nygh hym'. Folkard sought his revenge in Norwich, suing out a writ of trespass against the rector in the sheriffs' court, where the influence of his 'dyvers kynnesmen and grete frendez' could be mobilised to telling effect. Having been thrown into gaol, Mustardere petitioned the court of Chancery for assistance. The outcome of the case remains unknown, although he eventually returned to Sparham, where his long life passed without further incident. This was partly because Folkard died soon afterwards, in April 1469, leaving a will notable for its remarkable brevity. He set aside a derisory 20*d.* for unpaid tithes but otherwise bequeathed nothing to his parish church. His seemingly innocent request for burial in the adjacent cemetery none the less constituted a provocative challenge to Mustardere, who must have been well aware that confirmed lepers would customarily be interred in the graveyard of a *leprosarium*.[5] As we shall see, these regulations were frequently breached (not least in Norwich), but Folkard was establishing a final point of principle.

Allowing for its obvious bias, Mustardere's petition casts a fascinating light upon the nature of diagnosis in late medieval rural England. The important role of the priest and his use of the confessional for the transmission of medical advice are as striking as his apparent influence upon men and women who seem previously to have been untroubled by any risks of infection. Either they looked upon Folkard with new eyes, or his condition took a dramatic turn for the worse. We may note, on the other hand, that the latter's 'kynnesmen and grete frendez' in Norwich remained staunchly supportive, albeit, perhaps, from a distance. The imputation of leprosy was clearly a contentious issue for all concerned.

In a society consumed with fears of disease-bearing miasmas, the consequences of a positive diagnosis could be profoundly serious, even for a man of

---

3    PRO, C1/46/158.
4    C. Rawcliffe, 'A Case of Imputed Leprosy at Sparham, Norfolk', in R. Horrox and M. Aston, eds, *Much Heaving and Shoving: Late-Medieval Gentry and their Concerns* (Lavenham, 2005), pp. 145–56.
5    NRO, NCC, reg. Jekkys, fo. 134. For the burial of lepers, see below, pp. 259–63.

Folkard's status. Medical practitioners, such as the eminent French surgeon, Guy de Chauliac (whose work then circulated widely in translation), understandably advised careful deliberation:

> . . . it is mykel [much] to be taken hede aboute the examynynge and the dome [judgement] of leprouse men, that is the moste iniurie [wrong] to sequestre or withdrawe tho men that schulde not be sequestred or withdrawen and leue leprouse men with the peple, for-whye [because] it is a contagiouse sekenesse and infectynge. And therfore a leche that schal deme ham, he schall ofte byholde ham and turne and vnturne the tokenes [symptoms] with hymself, and he schall see the tokenes of one voyce [unequivocal] and whiche that ben of even voys [equivocal], and that he deme noght by one tokene but by concourse of many tokens, and specially of tokenes of one voyce.[6]

However laudable it may have been, concern about the psychological consequences of misdiagnosis or the risks it might pose to the wider community was not the only consideration behind such a cautious approach. Experience taught that a disease as complex and polymorphous as *lepra* might develop in a variety of ways, and should thus be observed carefully over time until several unambiguous symptoms presented themselves. Medical students training at Montpellier during the early fourteenth century were advised to 'take a tablet and write the good signs on one side and the bad signs on the other, and you will not become confused'.[7] A growing propensity on the part of medieval patients, or their next of kin, to sue negligent practitioners for heavy damages must also have been a powerful disincentive against the rush to judgement.[8] As Mustardere discovered, his tonsure offered little in the way of protection.

The false or malicious imputation of leprosy might also result in a suit for defamation, especially if the individual in question was involved in the victualling trades and stood to lose his or her living as a result.[9] Certainly, anyone disposed to question the health of a senior official or prominent local worthy had to stand on very secure ground. Another unlucky cleric, John Colman, canon of Launceston priory, was heavily fined by the borough court in 1412 for calling the former mayor, Walter Skinner, 'a false traitor and lazar', and thereby bringing his office into disrepute.[10] Mistakes could thus inflict lasting damage on the person making as well as receiving the diagnosis, at least when they concerned suspects in a position to fight back. In some instances this may, indeed, have been literally the case. It is, for example, tempting to view a violent

---

6  Ogden, *Cyrurgie of Guy de Chauliac*, p. 381. Rarely disposed to speak well of the medieval practitioner, Brody, *Disease of the Soul*, pp. 24–5, asserts that 'he had no conception of a long incubation period, for he traced sources of infection with the confidence with which a food inspector today might attribute an infection to rotten meat'.

7  'The Symptoms of Lepers', in Grant, *Source Book*, p. 754. For a definitive attribution of this text, see L. Demaitre, 'The Relevance of Futility: Jordanus de Turre (*fl.* 1313–1335) on the Treatment of Leprosy', *BHM*, lxx (1996), pp. 25–61, at p. 26.

8  C. Rawcliffe, 'The Profits of Practice: The Wealth and Status of Medical Men in Later Medieval England', *SHM*, i (1988), pp. 61–78, at pp. 75–7.

9  R.H. Helmholz, ed., *Select Cases on Defamation to 1600* (Selden Society, ci, 1985), pp. liv, 5–6; and below, p. 196.

10  Cornwall RO, Launceston Borough Records, B/Laus/285, m. 2v. I am grateful to Dr Hannes Kleineke for bringing this reference to my attention.

assault made in 1392–93 by one John Eston of Yarmouth upon the son of a local *medicus* as retribution for an order demanding the removal of his wife, Beatrice, from the borough. Having ignored repeated complaints about her condition voiced over the previous decade, Eston was finally obliged to comply at this time on account of the new hazard she presented *propter fetorem*.[11] In common with the residents of other late medieval English towns and cities, the burgesses of Yarmouth were well aware of the problems caused by miasmic air and of the presumed risks lepers posed in this respect. There was no gainsaying such a verdict.

This chapter begins with a consideration of the differences between medieval and modern diagnosis. Far from languishing in a state of bewilderment and superstition, as some scholars have suggested, English practitioners deployed a complex range of tests and procedures to detect the humoral imbalances of *lepra*. Nor were they alone in enjoying access to a growing corpus of specialist literature, which was rapidly translated and adapted for a wide readership. Since the clergy were initially the principal users and disseminators of this knowledge, we turn first to their biblically sanctioned role as diagnosticians. This was exploited to telling effect at the shrines of healing saints, such as Thomas Becket, but it also played an increasingly important (and less subjective) part in the confessional, where spiritual and physical ailments merged seamlessly together. We then examine the activities of physicians and surgeons, most notably in the *judicium*, or formal examination for leprosy, before discussing the emergence of local juries and panels of lay 'experts' as agents for sanitary policing in rural and urban communities. Whatever their status, most assessors placed particular emphasis upon the facial symptoms of leprosy, a fact which underscores the impact of advice manuals composed for an expanding popular market.

## Applying science: the spread of information

The theory and practice of pre-modern diagnosis have provoked a lively debate among historians. Controversy surrounds such issues as the levels of expertise possessed by those involved and the changing criteria employed over time to determine who might or might not pose a threat to others. As Andrew Cunningham has recently argued, these considerations are fundamental to our understanding of responses to sickness and health in past societies. Yet there persists, in some quarters at least, a desire to judge them by the standards of modern, laboratory-based medicine.[12] This inevitably encourages a tendency to underestimate the sophistication and rationality of medieval assumptions about the body, while also propagating a mistaken belief that both the mechanics and purpose of diagnosis have remained immutable across the centuries. Before we

---

[11]   NRO, Y/C4/104, rot. 11r–11v. The Yarmouth evidence is discussed below, pp. 252–3, 269–70, 282–4. It is tempting to speculate that the authorities were familiar with the Latin text of Bartholomaeus Anglicus's influential encyclopaedia, which was translated not long after this incident. In the section dealing with *fetor* he specifically warns against the 'stinking breath' of lepers and its dire effects on healthy men: Seymour, *On the Properties of Things*, ii, pp. 1296–1304.

[12]   A. Cunningham, 'Identifying Disease in the Past: Cutting the Gordian Knot', *Asclepio*, liv, fasc. 1 (2002), pp. 13–34.

examine the wider social and religious aspects of these procedures, it is worth exploring a few fundamental differences in approach.

The distinction now made between the causes and symptoms of a disease – between, say, the presence of *Mycobacterium leprae* in a tissue sample and the neural damage observed in that patient – was less pronounced in an age before the microscope. Simply to describe a case of vulpine leprosy (*alopecia*) was axiomatically to identify the excess of adust sanguine humour (blood) that had given the sufferer his or her characteristically red and distended features:

> ... al the here of the iyeliddes and of the browis falleth, and the iyen swelleth hugeliche and beth ful *rede*. In the face beth *rede* pimples and whelks, out of the which oft renneth *blode* and quyttir [matter]. In such the nose swelleth and is grete, the vertue of smellinge failleth, and the breth stynketh right foule, and in the gomes is ful grete infeccioun and corrupcioun.[13]

The Classical medical tradition, which had such a powerful impact upon both theory and practice in the Middle Ages, relied heavily upon the careful observation of outward signs likely to reveal the delicate humoral balance unique to each individual patient.[14] Since it was impossible to open the living body for investigative purposes, the physical appearance (complexion) came under intense clinical scrutiny. In a healthy individual, the red, yellow, black and white of 'the thermochromatic palette' were sufficiently well mixed to produce a pleasing and uniform skin tone, which seemed neither too ruddy nor too jaundiced. Nor was it excessively saturnine or pallid. Once that enviable equilibrium had been lost, however, telltale eruptions and discolorations became apparent, revealing the turmoil within. To a trained eye or hand, each lesion, spot and swelling reflected some internal disturbance, as the body tried to eliminate excessive quantities of blood, choler, black bile or phlegm before they proved toxic. The skin, which both absorbed and excreted matter, was thus prime diagnostic material, to be read by scent and touch as much as visual appearance.[15]

But there were other, less superficial, ways of evaluating levels of physiological dysfunction. As we have already seen, the humours were generated, or 'digested', from a mixture of water and chyle in the liver, and transported as nourishment throughout the body by the venous system. Excess liquid, which had served to dilute and convey the chyle (originally 'as thick as sodden barley') from the stomach through the intestines to the liver, was diverted via the kidneys to the bladder. It was then secreted as urine. The science of uroscopy, or diagnosis by means of urine samples, thus enabled a practitioner to ascertain the exact state of humoral equipoise at this crucial stage in production, thereby detecting any

---

13 Seymour, *On the Properties of Things*, i , p. 425. Bernard Gordon's translator similarly observes 'yif that lepre comyth of blode the colour of hys face wole be *rede & derke* and some dele sewllynge with many *rede* whelys and his eyghen *rede* & hys eyghledys tourned in & out . . . and for lytel enchesoun [reason] he wole *blede* at nose & the sauour of hym is greuous & stinkynge in al the body. His vryne wole be *reed* & thicke . . .': Bodleian Library, MS Ashmole 1505, fo. 31r.

14 Siraisi, *Medieval and Early Renaissance Medicine*, pp. 123–8.

15 S. Connor, *The Book of Skin* (Ithaca, NY, 2004), pp. 19–20, 24, 163–4. Noting the extent to which diseases, such as cholera, glaucoma and porphyria, derive their names from physical discoloration, Connor describes the pre-modern body as 'predominantly chromatic'.

current or potential problems.[16] The ubiquity of the jordan (the glass phial used to examine samples) in medieval iconography underscores the importance of this procedure, which played a similar part in the physician's professional armoury to the stethoscope or white coat [plate 18].[17] Since the immediate physiological cause of *lepra* lay in the malfunction of the liver and its failure to deliver nourishment to the rest of the body, the patient's urine offered a particular insight into his or her condition.

An even better appreciation of humoral interaction might, however, be gained from the venous blood itself. Because of the popularity of phlebotomy as both a prophylactic and curative measure from Anglo Saxon times onwards, supplies were readily available for scrutiny. The twelfth-century *Ancrene Riwle* refers to the practice of letting blood cool before routine testing, and before long a significant corpus of literature was available – as it was for uroscopy – on the methodology involved.[18] Much of this was culled from the works of Galen as transmitted by Arab commentators to the West. Bernard Gordon's *De flebotomia* (1308), for example, contains five chapters on haematoscopy, which he regarded as an essential means of gaining knowledge about 'the disposition of the whole body'.[19] At about the same time, John of Gaddesden recommended three blood tests to provide infallible proof of *lepra*, however equivocal the other symptoms might still be.[20] Surgeons were naturally expected to possess these skills. 'Gode blode', observed Guy de Chauliac, 'is that that is noght to[o] grete in substaunce ne thenne, but it is able to breke [blend] and wel temperate, in colour rede and bright and louesome in smelle and in sauour . . . that forsothe that is fulle of greynes and of asshen bytokeneth the lepre'.[21]

As we shall see in the course of this chapter, clinical tests to determine leprosy ranged across a wide spectrum of potential symptoms, usually beginning with those held to be 'general' or common to all of the four humoral types. Loss of facial hair, coldness, prickling and lack of sensation in the extremities, claw-like hands, the spread of *maculae* and nodules, constriction or collapse of the nostrils, distortion of the eyes and mouth, decay of the gums, foetid breath and hoarsening of the voice were 'manifest' signs that ordinary men and women could easily recognise. Late medieval English physicians and surgeons, on the other hand, armed themselves with a far longer catalogue of twenty or more indicators of *lepra*, both 'manifest' and 'occult'. Otherwise concealed from the

---

16  Cameron Gruner, *Treatise on the Canon of Medicine of Avicenna*, pp. 88–9, 323–50.
17  M.R. McVaugh, 'Bedside Manners in the Middle Ages', *BHM*, lxxi (1997), pp. 201–23; Rawcliffe, *Medicine and Society*, pp. 46–50, and plate 5.
18  Salu, *Ancrene Riwle*, p. 53. P.M. Jones, *Medieval Medicine in Illuminated Manuscripts* (London and Milan, revised edn, 1998), p. 49, figure 43.
19  This treatise is part of a more extensive work *De conservatione vitae humanae*, later printed together with his *Opus lilium medicine* (Lyon, 1574), pp. 667–727. See P. Gil-Sotres, 'Derivation and Revulsion: The Theory and Practice of Medieval Phlebotomy', in L. García-Ballester et al., *Practical Medicine*, pp. 151–2; and Demaitre, *Doctor Bernard de Gordon*, pp. 61–3.
20  H.P. Cholmeley, *John of Gaddesden and the Rosa Medicinae* (Oxford, 1912), pp. 47–8. They involved dissolving salt in the blood; testing it with the fingers for stickiness; and placing a sample in clear water to see if it sank.
21  Ogden, *Cyrurgie of Guy de Chauliac*, pp. 544–5. This text and its 'termes of Latyn' were translated into English 'beste to be vnderstonden . . . and most esy, namely to men that can [know] but the comune langage': ibid., p. 290.

untrained eye, the latter came to light through scrutiny of the blood, urine, pulse and inner recesses of the nostrils. Once they had identified the disease, medical experts worked through a second checklist of up to forty or fifty 'tokenes' relating to its four specific forms [tabulated on p. 75] in order to reach a more precise diagnosis.[22] They would generally expect to find over half of the common signs and at least some of the others before recommending that the patient withdraw from society. To a greater or lesser degree, depending upon individual circumstances, the suspect's sexual conduct and his or her lifestyle would also be taken into account. Any hereditary predisposition towards leprosy, or evidence of protracted contact with its victims, was also closely monitored.[23]

Historians vary in their assessments of such criteria, largely because of a continuing preoccupation with the question of 'clinical accuracy'. S.N. Brody, a particular advocate of the comparative approach, weighs Theoderic of Cervia (d. 1298) in the balance against R.G. Cochrane and other leprologists writing during the middle years of the twentieth century and finds him sadly wanting. His diagnostic methods are disparaged because of their brevity, vagueness, inclusion of symptoms not associated with Hansen's disease and reliance on 'the authority of tradition' rather than empirical observation. Nor, in the harsh light of scientific progress, do authorities such as Bernard Gordon or Guy de Chauliac escape censure:

> The explanation for the frequent unreliability of medieval medical accounts is clearly the rudimentary level of medical knowledge in the Middle Ages. Physicians were unskilled and untrained, and their theories were usually faulty; they could not help but be unreliable. Medieval doctors could not properly describe leprosy because they could not tell it apart from scabies, psoriasis, eczema, and a host of other skin conditions.[24]

As both Luke Demaitre and S.R. Ell have persuasively argued, this negative view of pre-modern diagnosis is largely unfounded. The blood tests recommended by practitioners such as Gilbertus Anglicus and John of Gaddesden to determine abnormal levels of coagulation and adhesion were, for example, not only based upon clinical experimentation, but may actually have helped to identify cases of Hansen's disease.[25]

Moreover, although their assumptions about aetiology seem very different from our own, medieval physicians and surgeons differentiated minutely between a remarkable number of dermatological conditions. Some, indeed, felt that the bewildering range of terminology used to describe such disorders was counterproductive, and sought to rationalise it on the basis of personal experi-

---

[22] See, for example, Gilbertus Anglicus, *Compendium medicine*, fos 139r–140v. An English translation of part of this section appears in Grant, *Source Book*, pp. 752–4.

[23] Ogden, *Cyrurgie of Guy de Chauliac*, pp. 379–83.

[24] Brody, *Disease of the Soul*, p. 41. F.C. Finucane likewise maintains that 'practically nothing was known about health or sickness in the "scientific" sense' during this period: 'The Use and Abuse of Medieval Miracles', *History*, lx (1975), pp. 1–10, at p. 6. A similar point was made much earlier by Creighton, *History of Epidemics in Britain*, i, pp. 72–8.

[25] Ell, 'Blood and Sexuality', pp. 157–8. See also, Demaitre, 'Description and Diagnosis', pp. 327–42. The clinical value of Gaddesden's tests was recognised as early as 1912: Cholmeley, *John of Gaddesden*, p. 48.

ence.[26] Their observations were duly transmitted to the owners of domestic remedy books and medical advice literature. Bartholomaeus Anglicus' popular encyclopaedia, *De proprietatibus rerum* (*c.* 1245), contains lengthy sections on apostumes or swellings, ulcers, pustules, scabies, impetigo and morphew, each of which was further subdivided by humoral type and clearly distinguished from *lepra* [**plate 17**].[27] Even so, to judge the theory and practice of medieval physicians solely by the standards of modern biomedicine is, in the last resort, as unproductive as it is predictable. At the root of the comparative approach lies a series of assumptions which, to quote the early modernist, Mark Jenner, 'beautifully exemplify the abiding condescension of posterity'.[28] We can be reasonably certain that some – perhaps many – of the individuals described in the following pages were indeed suffering from Hansen's disease, as we define it today. Yet such a conviction brings us no nearer to understanding how medieval men and women came to grips with the realities of chronic sickness before the microscope.

Nor is competence the only issue. The motives of medieval diagnosticians also appear questionable to many historians, notably those who see *leprosaria* as little more than penal colonies. Sheldon Watts has argued that, so long as the detection of lepers remained largely an ecclesiastical matter, the disease served as a convenient means of policing social undesirables. The burgeoning of a 'humanitarian' medical profession, which he dates from the appearance of Guy de Chauliac's *Chirurgia*, in 1363, broke the Church's hegemony and brought an end to what he has called 'the great leper hunt'. Henceforward diagnosis became a clinical rather than a moral issue. 'For religio-political authorities *circa* 1090 who hit upon the leprosy Construct as a felicitous way of ridding themselves of troublemakers', he maintains, 'the last people they wanted meddling about were medically informed experts.'[29] Given that the most prominent 'medically informed experts' of twelfth- and thirteenth-century England were either monks or members of the secular clergy, and that the majority of graduate physicians remained in higher orders until the Reformation, the idea of such an extreme polarity between medicine and the Church seems largely untenable. Chauliac himself was a chaplain at the papal court in Avignon; and the curia in Rome already boasted a long and impressive tradition of scientific and medical inquiry.[30] Indeed, despite the rise of a confident and articulate *cadre* of British surgeons, empirics and well-informed laymen and women during the later Middle Ages, priests, friars and even hermits continued to play a notable part in the dissemination of medical knowledge, not least through the written word. In marked contrast to the nervousness displayed both by ecclesiastical and secular

26  M.R. McVaugh, 'Surface Meanings: The Identification of Apostemes in Medieval Surgery', in W. Bracke and H. Deumens, eds, *Medical Latin from the Late Middle Ages to the Eighteenth Century* (Brussels, 2000), pp. 13–29. For the complexity of later medieval writing about the skin, see D. Jacquart, 'A la recherche de la peau dans le discours médical de la fin du moyen âge', in *La pelle umana* (Micrologus' Library, xiii, Turnhout, 2005), pp. 493–510.

27  Seymour, *On the Properties of Things*, i, pp. 415–30.

28  M.S.R. Jenner, 'Underground, Overground: Pollution and Place in Urban History', *Journal of Urban History*, xxiv (1997), pp. 97–110, quotation at p. 101.

29  Watts, *Epidemics and History*, p. 49.

30  Paravicini Bagliani, *Corps du Pape*, pp. 199–257.

e puis si pinez fort le frunt. E de ceo q̃ d̃ cel frument ist chaut
oignez la maladie suuent. i cest oignement uaut ensemēt
a saure fleume. por oster serpigo.

Or oster une maladie q̃ e apele serpigo e en franceais
dirre fairef uel oingnemir pnez litargire. e blanc uer-
te e plū art. e les conce de la brornne arse e uuf en pul-
dre. e un po de lasiue uelerir unce une. e confizez iffi od le
ius dun herbe q̃ est apele ciclanus. e od oile merlez les de-
uant d̃tes puldrus e merrant ore del un ore del autre e par-
tiez les merlez ensemble q̃ bein se sorent pus en un. e pus
les metez en salf. e quant mestier serra si en oignez la
maladie e par trois iorz le ringe sur sei. e uel lune par
en uele. E en apres le teiz si faites bain gnier. e ce face iesq̃

Or phe une e morphe blanche e neire. il sort sein.

blanche. e l'autre e neire si est une espece de lepre de cel
dont une puit estre sanee si cū la blanche. e la neire nun.
O cele q̃ doit estre curee: d̃ nez iffi esprouerit. pnez une agul-
le e poiniez d̃ d̃nz le q̃r del malad̃ si sanc en ist si pot estre
garri si. e lbe blanche en ist ne pot estre sanee. A la blanc
che morphe faires uel oingnemir pnez tartariū e sulfre uif.
e or prenir sil buuilliez cristal uerre sauon. sarazin argē

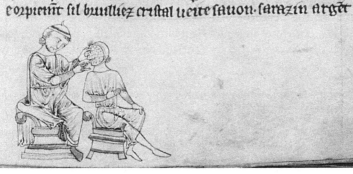

17. A marginal illustration in this Anglo-Norman text of the *Chirurgia* of Roger
Frugard and his pupils (*c.* 1250) depicts an examination for morphew, one of
many skin conditions that might, if untreated, degenerate into *lepra*. By pricking
the nose with a needle, and observing the matter that escapes, the practitioner can
judge if the condition is curable.

authorities where translations of the Bible and other key theological texts were concerned, every encouragement was given to the production of accessible vernacular guides to practical medicine and basic theory.

By the third quarter of the fourteenth century, a significant number of clergy had begun translating medical literature, often in an abridged or simplified form as a charitable work for the common good.[31] Their efforts initially focused upon self-help manuals for diagnosis and treatment. John Trevisa (d. 1412), Oxford graduate and vicar of Berkeley in Gloucestershire, whose translation of Bartholomaeus Anglicus' *De proprietatibus rerum* is quoted above, was but one of many priests with a mission to educate.[32] During the early 1370s, John Lelamour, who taught grammar at Hereford, translated a *Liber de iudiciis urinarum* as well as Macer's *De viribus herbarum* into English.[33] Soon afterwards the Dominican friar and celebrated herbalist, Henry Daniel, produced a longer and more detailed *Liber uricrisiarum* at the request of Walter Turnour of Ketton, who wanted a guide to uroscopy in the 'vulgare comune langage' he could understand.[34] The book contains a great deal of diagnostic advice based on physical symptoms as, for example, the warning that evidence of *gutta rosacea* in women 'is comunly a tokne of disposicion toward a lepre'.[35] A product of 'gleymy and bloody and colerik humours', the condition had to be closely monitored for signs of deterioration into leonine or vulpine leprosy.[36]

A couple of decades later, the London barber, Thomas Plouden (d. 1413), persuaded one of his 'dere gossips' among the clergy to translate a Latin work on phlebotomy, 'nought to clerkys', but evidently for personal use. This simplified Middle English version, which is geared to the needs of a busy practitioner, refers, significantly, to the current dearth of 'wise fysicians'.[37] In the meantime, a Franciscan named Bartholomew began rendering Walter Agilon's *Commentarium urinarium* 'briefly in the mother tongue' for the specific benefit of the laity, reputedly at the behest of Richard II and Queen Anne. Bartholomew also warned of the shortcomings of 'uncunnyng leches and negligent', and consciously set out to demystify potentially complex subjects. Aware that they

---

31   F.M. Getz, 'Charity, Translation and the Language of Medical Learning in Medieval England', *BHM*, lxiv (1990), pp. 1–15.

32   Bartholomaeus, a Franciscan friar, produced the most popular encyclopaedia of the Middle Ages in *c.* 1245, and in translating it Trevisa 'helped to make English a capable instrument for conveying technical information to the average educated man': T. Lawler, 'On the Properties of John Trevisa's Major Translations', *Viator*, xiv (1983), pp. 267–88, at p. 288.

33   Wellcome Institute Library, Western MS 784, fos 13r–32v; BL, MS Sloane 5, fo. 57v. See also S.A.J. Moorat, *Catalogue of Western Manuscripts on Medicine and Science in the Wellcome Historical Medical Library, I, Mss. Written before 1650 A.D.* (London, 1962), pp. 578–9.

34   BL, MS Royal 17 D I. The genesis of the work is explained on fo. 4r (pencil foliation). See also, J. Norri, 'Entrances and Exits in English Medical Vocabulary, 1400–1550', in Taavitsainen and Pahata, *Medical and Scientific Writing*, p. 102.

35   BL, MS Royal 17 D 1, fo. 105r (pencil foliation). Significantly, the author observes that, in women, this condition is sometimes called 'the lepre'. It was generally regarded as a type of 'red morphew' and thus one of the many 'equivocal' signs of emergent leprosy: Cholmeley, *John of Gaddesden*, p. 45; BL, MS Harley 1736, fo. 141r.

36   The reader had only to turn to Trevisa's translation of *De proprietatibus rerum* to find a useful account of *gutta rosacea* and allied facial conditions: Seymour, *On the Properties of Things*, i, p. 427.

37   L.E. Voigts and M.R. McVaugh, eds, 'A Latin Technical Phlebotomy and its Middle English Translation', *Transactions of the American Philosophical Society*, lxxiv, part 2 (1984), pp. 1–69.

might lack specialist knowledge, he reassured his readers that he would explain any 'harde wordes', such as 'adustion', which he concisely defined as 'brennyng of kinde [nature] for to moch hete'.[38] As we have seen, the generation of adust (that is burnt) black bile or melancholia through an excess of choler was regarded as a prime cause of leprosy. Thanks to a lively and appropriate use of metaphor, the dangers of humoral imbalance – and, of course, how to spot it through the examination of urine – became immediately intelligible.

The proliferation of textbooks on diagnosis and humoral management was but one aspect of the rapidly expanding market for accessible vernacular guides to health, collections of remedies and, notably, advice about the avoidance of pestilence.[39] This, in turn, reflects the rising number of men and women with at least rudimentary reading skills. Michael Clanchy has shown how rapidly these skills spread during the twelfth and thirteenth centuries.[40] By the accession of Henry of Lancaster in 1399, the ability to read English, often along with some basic Latin and French, was widespread and came, increasingly, to be expected of apprentice barber surgeons and apothecaries. Some estimates suggest that up to a third of the population overall, and considerably more in major urban centres then knew their letters;[41] they, in turn, were able to explain what they read to the uninitiated. It is, for example, striking that a good deal of standard medical information was set down in verse, so that it could be more easily memorised and passed on to others. The Benedictine monk, John Lydgate, opted to write his popular tract on pestilence and the dangers of miasma in rhymed couplets; and similar poems on bloodletting, astrology, the medicinal properties of herbs, uroscopy and humoral management circulated widely.[42]

In many respects, therefore, the late medieval cleric, the medical practitioner and the educated layman shared a common pool of knowledge. The demand for

---

38  I. Taavitsainen, 'Transferring Classical Discourse Conventions', pp. 52–3. Almost certainly compiled by a priest, who combined morally uplifting advice along with remedies, BL, MS Sloane 3489, fos 29r–42r, lists 'a few medecynes that i-might help pore folk'. The author explains technical terms, because 'leches haue a queynt maner writing & hard for to rede in making of hir medicynes'. See also, Wellcome Institute Library, Western MS 784, fos 1v–7r.

39  Cohn, *Black Death Transformed*, chapter nine; P. Murray Jones, 'Medical Books before the Invention of Printing', in A. Besson, ed., *Thornton's Medical Books, Libraries and Collectors* (third edn, London, 1990), pp. 10–16; idem, 'Information and Science', in R. Horrox, ed., *Fifteenth-Century Attitudes* (Cambridge, 1994), pp. 97–111; idem, 'Medicine and Science', in L. Hellinga and J.B. Trapp, eds, *The Cambridge History of the Book in Britain, III, 1400–1557* (Cambridge, 1999), pp. 433–48; F. Getz, 'Gilbertus Anglicus Anglicised', *Medical History*, xxvi (1982), pp. 436–42; G. Keiser, 'Scientific, Medical and Utilitarian Prose', in A.S.G. Edwards, ed., *A Companion to Middle English Prose* (Woodbridge, 2004), pp. 231–47.

40  M. Clanchy, *From Memory to Written Record: England 1066–1307* (Oxford, 1993), chapter seven.

41  H.J. Graff, *The Legacies of Literacy: Communities and Contradictions in Western Culture and Society* (Bloomington and Indianapolis, 1987), pp. 95–106.

42  H.N. MacCracken, ed., *The Minor Poems of John Lydgate* (EETS, cxcii, 1934), pp. 702–7. See also, for example, C.F. Mayer, 'A Medieval English Leechbook and its Fourteenth-Century Poem on Bloodletting', *BHM*, vii (1939), pp. 381–91; L.R. Mooney, 'A Middle English Verse Compendium of Astrological Medicine', *Medical History*, xxviii (1984), pp. 406–9; BL, MS Egerton 1995, fos 65–80 (bloodletting); Trinity College, Cambridge, MS R.14.32, fos 135r–136r (betony), 147r–148r (rosemary). The use of verse in this context was common across Europe. A translation of Roger Frugard's *Chirurgia* was made into Occitan verse before 1209: T. Hunt, ed., *Anglo-Norman Medicine* (2 vols, Woodbridge, 1994–97), i, pp. 8–10. French rhyming couplets were also employed for the communication of medical information in thirteenth-century England: idem, ed., *Popular Medicine in Thirteenth-Century England* (Woodbridge, 1994), chapter four.

vernacular texts was certainly not confined to a lay readership, nor, on the other hand, were university-trained physicians and priests the only consumers of works in Latin. Recent research on the translation and transmission of scientific and medical literature has shown that very different 'discourse communities' used the same books, which, in any event, were rarely monolingual through-out.[43] Levels of complexity rather than language seem to have determined whether a work would appeal more to, say, a physician, a barber, an apothecary, an empiric or an interested member of the general public. Even here, however, it is unsafe to generalise. A Middle English translation of Bernard Gordon's *De flebotomia* and various staples of the Oxford medical syllabus appear, for example, to have been made into a single compendium for an ambitious barber surgeon who took seriously the recommendation that professional advancement lay through study.[44] In the section on colour as a guide to the diagnosis of blood samples, a marginal mark draws attention to the recommendation:

> We ow for to considere the disposicion of the body: for if the habitude of the body be lene, and fevre & labour and angrey haue gone afore, & the colour turneth to a maner citrynyte [interlineated: yelow] and the vrine is thinne, than sich a colour suld seme to be cause of brennyng [interlineated: adustion] and sich bene moste redy to lepre and manya [interlineated: frenesy] and sich other.[45]

There was, then, no monopoly on information about diagnosis. Nor, as this text shows, was careful attention to the lifestyle and temperament of a patient only to be found among the upper echelons of the medical profession.

Complex diagnostic tests were also widely deployed throughout society. The *Liber de morbis et medicinis* of the distinguished cleric, John Argentein, physician to Edward IV and his ill-fated sons, contains a brief account of three methods for determining the incidence and severity of leprosy. One involves placing a freshly laid egg in the patient's urine and then cracking it open within an hour to see if it has been corrupted or 'cooked' by adust humours.[46] A similar test, utilising newly phlebotomised blood, had already been described at greater length in a number of vernacular sources, including a book of medical charms and recipes compiled by, or for, one William Leech of Killingholme:

> If thou wilt haue verrey knowyng whether a man be lepre or no, take anne hen eye [egg] raw and hole and do [place] it in a dysshe and let the man or the woman blode on the veyn on the arme on that eye, til the eye be covered in blode. And

---

43  C. Jones, 'Discourse Entities and Medical Texts', in Taavitsainen and Pahata, *Medical and Scientific Writing*, pp. 23–36. For the persistent use of French, see Hunt, *Anglo-Norman Medicine*, ii, pp. 7–11.

44  BL, MS Sloane 6. This manuscript is discussed by F.M. Getz, 'Medical Education in Later Medieval England', in V. Nutton and R. Porter, eds, *The History of Medical Education in Britain* (Amsterdam, 1995), p. 81. See also P. Murray Jones, 'Harley MS 2558: A Fifteenth-Century Medical Commonplace Book', in M.R. Schleissner, ed., *Manuscript Sources of Medieval Medicine* (New York, 1995), pp. 35–54.

45  BL, MS Sloane 6, fo. 36r. The English translation of Bernard Gordon's *Lilye of Medicynes* warns 'colerike men that beth leene & hoot and adust and hauyth hoot lyuere be ham' to be careful because of their vulnerability to the disease: Bodleian Library, MS Ashmole 1505, fo. 30v.

46  Bodleian Library, MS Ashmole 1437, p. 62. John Bradmore (BL, MS Sloane 2272 (part 1), fo. 90v) and John Mirfield (BL, MS Harley 3, fo. 23v) also recommended this test, which also appears in a Latin medical compilation belonging to the schoolmaster at Middleham in 1484, along with various recom-mendations for the treatment of *lepra*: Trinity College, Cambridge, MS O.I.9, fo. 90v.

latte the ey ligge stil in the blode til it be cold and thenne take oute that eye and breke it on two; and yif thu ffynde it rawe then is that man hole and no lepre.[47]

Although the dissemination of this type of textual information is far easier to document from the fourteenth century onwards, the traditional involvement of laymen and women in legal processes, which made considerable demands upon their diagnostic abilities, suggests that such information had long been available.

Jurors and expert lay witnesses in the royal courts were accustomed to determining whether or not plaintiffs had been raped or mutilated, if they were pregnant, impotent, insane, senile or simply absent-minded, virginal, paralytic, blind, capable of trial by combat (despite fervent protestations to the contrary), or if their claims for damages because of physical injury had been grossly exaggerated.[48] Thirteenth-century coroners' juries did not simply pronounce upon death by violence, but were quite prepared to express medical opinions on the effects of miasmic air, the mental health of suicides, the debility of vagrants and, even, the risks of septicaemia if a wound was left untreated.[49] Nor did expertise pass in only one direction. If midwives were held to be better equipped than physicians or surgeons to diagnose gynaecological disorders, men and women who lived among leprosy sufferers felt themselves perfectly capable of distinguishing its symptoms. In continental Europe lepers themselves were often called on to make a diagnosis, having unique personal experience of the disease and its development. At Bethune in the Pas de Calais, for instance, juries drawn from *leprosaria* across the entire region met to examine suspects until the mid fifteenth century, when barber surgeons began gradually to replace them. Disagreements were not uncommon. A group of lepers overruled the findings of local medical practitioners at Aire in 1532 to pronounce an unequivocal verdict, while at St Omer a similar difference of opinion was, eventually, settled in favour of '*les ladres*'.[50]

Responsibility for the diagnosis of leprosy (or, indeed, of any other medieval malady) was thus far from clear-cut, and certainly extended beyond a narrow cadre of university-trained physicians and licensed surgeons. To a notable extent, factors of class, wealth and geography tended to dictate whether or not a suspect individual would ever encounter what we today might regard as a trained medical practitioner. This was certainly the case before the establishment of medical faculties at Oxford and Cambridge and the rise of urban guilds of surgeons and barber surgeons. As many twelfth- and thirteenth-century accounts of saints and their miracles clearly demonstrate, an assessment might in all probability be made by friends, family or neighbours, who would, just like

---

[47] York Minster Library, MS XVI.E.32, fo. 92r. See p. 209, below, for a similar experiment to determine the severity of the disease.

[48] *CRR, 1221–1222*, p. 37; *1223–1224*, nos 122, 602, 2761, 2768; *1225–1226*, no. 1579; *1227–1230*, no. 242; *1230–1232*, no. 897; *1233–1237*, no. 1929; *1242–1243*, no. 121; F.M. Getz, *Medicine in the English Middle Ages* (Princeton, 1998), p. 75.

[49] All these pronouncements were made by Norwich juries in cases of suspicious death between 1264 and 1282: NRO, NCR, 8A/1–2. See also R.F. Hunnisett, *The Medieval Coroner* (Cambridge, 1961), chapter two.

[50] Bourgeois, *Lépreux et maladreries*, pp. 27–31, 103, 115, 185–6, 237–8, 311–13; G.B. Risse, *Mending Bodies, Saving Souls: A History of Hospitals* (Oxford, 1999), pp. 168–9.

the physician, view the progress of the disease over time. They would eventually reach a decision based on a combination of medical knowledge and simple pragmatism, which inevitably varied from place to place. Suspicions would harden into certainties, but even then an element of doubt might linger on. Months, even years, could elapse before a predisposition towards *lepra* became indistinguishable from the real thing. In a world before the laboratory, diagnosis was a slow, deliberative process; and, just like the concept of a cure, it proved infinitely elastic.[51] But we can at least be confident that a member of the ecclesiastical establishment would almost certainly become involved at some stage in the procedure. Thus, for example, a Scottish knight living in the Auvergne was – like John Folkard – pronounced leprous in the early 1170s by members of the local clergy, and subsequently diagnosed as *percussus elephantia* by his bishop.[52] Folkard's experience was, however, in one respect untypical, since in the majority of cases clerical intervention seems to have been neither unwelcome nor unsolicited. How did the Church come to exercise such influence?

## Monks and miracles: the shrine

Like generations of clergy before him, William Mustardere based his freedom to examine and advise suspect lepers upon the unimpeachable authority of both the Old and New Testaments. The role of the priest in diagnosing *sāra'ath* and in pronouncing those who had recovered from it 'clean' was minutely described in the Book of Leviticus [13, vv. 1–46]. Once he detected 'the plague in the skin of the flesh', the priest could either declare that an individual was ritually defiled and thus unable to remain within the camp, or else arrange for him or her to be quarantined for up to a fortnight to see if further symptoms developed. Uncertain cases might, moreover, be called back and checked for incriminating signs of 'raw flesh'. Readmission into society likewise demanded a careful inspection, followed by a period of isolation and an elaborate ceremony of ritual cleansing again presided over by the priest. The fate of suspects thus lay in his hands alone.[53] Although Christ did not consider himself tainted by the touch of any outcast, however impure, he scrupulously upheld this aspect of Levitical law. Thus, 'the man full of leprosy' whom he healed with his hand was ordered to go at once, with an offering, to the priest [Matthew 8, vv. 2–4; Mark 1, vv. 40–44; Luke 5, vv. 12–14]; and the ten lepers who petitioned him from 'afar off' in Samaria to cleanse them were likewise dispatched to perform the necessary rituals [Luke 17, vv. 12–19].[54] That recovery from such an ill-defined skin condition as *sāra'ath* should often occur is unremarkable, but as *lepra* increasingly came to be identified with a far more serious, apparently incurable, disease the diagnostic responsibilities of the priest underwent a dramatic and fundamental change. His task was now also to authenticate and record miracles.

---

51  As was the case in French Colonial Mali: Silla, *People Are Not the Same*, p. 57.
52  Robertson, *Materials*, i, pp. 458–61. His family and neighbours also helped to reach this decision.
53  Lewis, 'Lesson from Leviticus', pp. 593–612.
54  J. Wilkinson, *The Bible and Healing: A Medical and Theological Commentary* (Grand Rapids, Michigan, 1998), pp. 46–8, 98–9, 113, 264–5. For the importance of these rituals see H. Danby, ed., *The Code of Maimonides, Book Nine: The Book of Offerings* (New Haven and London, 1950), pp. 166–71.

Christ had charged his apostles to 'heal the sick, cleanse the lepers [and] cast out devils' [Matthew 10, v. 8], a mission assumed during the Middle Ages by a rapidly expanding community of saints. Miracle-working shrines and relics served as potent propaganda in a battle initially waged to convert pagan populations, and then to keep them secure within the papal fold.[55] The prospect of divinely inspired healing offered a sure route to the hearts and minds of men and women beset by constant pain and the prospect of early death. It also generated a handsome income for those clergy who were fortunate enough to possess the remains of a saint or sacred artifact, such as the fragment of the True Cross, acquired after the sack of Constantinople (1204) by the monks of Bromholm on the Norfolk coast. Here, we are told, in a specific reference to Christ's own miracles, 'the dead came alive, the crippled recovered their mobility, the flesh of lepers was cleansed, the possessed were freed of their demons'.[56] Similar claims were made for shrines throughout England, notably in their early years, when they were fighting not only to gain recognition but, quite possibly, also to secure the canonisation of a local saint.[57] When describing the wonderful events that followed the discovery of St Milburga's remains at Much Wenlock priory, in 1101, William of Malmesbury observed that everyone who visited the shrine felt the touch of her healing hand. Even those suffering from *regius morbus* (his term for leprosy), 'which physicians cannot cure', experienced some relief.[58]

Save for raising the dead (a not uncommon phenomenon in cases of concussion and near-drowning), the cure of leprosy, especially as defined by the Greek and Arab commentators we met in chapter two, constituted the most dramatic and persuasive proof of sacred power, while also providing unimpeachable scriptural authentication for a cult or shrine. It offered evidence of an act performed *contra naturam*, or against the natural order of things, and thus conformed to the evolving theological definition of a true miracle.[59] Cardinal Odo of Ostia, who recorded St Milburga's five earliest *miracula*, and himself examined one young girl whom she had reputedly cleansed of *lepra*, frankly describes the scepticism not only of the local people but also of the Cluniacs themselves.[60] Before his arrival, he reports, 'certain people prating in utter fool-

55  B. Ward, *Miracles and the Medieval Mind* (Aldershot, 1987), pp. 100–01, 168. For the widespread appeal of pilgrimage, see R.C. Finucane, *Miracles and Pilgrims: Popular Beliefs in Medieval England* (New York, 1977); and D. Webb, *Pilgrimage in Medieval England* (London, 2000).

56  Roger of Wendover, *Flores Historiarum*, ed. H.G. Hewlett (3 vols, RS, London, 1886–89), ii, pp. 274–6. For the profitability of shrines, see B. Nilson, *Cathedral Shrines of Medieval England* (Woodbridge, 1998), chapter six.

57  While the body of St Edmund lay in London, in 1016, a number of 'biblical' miracles, including the cleansing of lepers, reputedly occurred: T. Arnold, ed., *Memorials of St Edmunds Abbey* (3 vols, RS, 1890–96), i, pp. 121–2. Likewise, at Glastonbury, on the translation of the remains of St Benignus, in 1091, crowds 'weighed down with the troubles of various diseases and infirmities', including *leprosi*, flocked to the altar and were healed: William of Malmesbury, *The Chronicle of Glastonbury Abbey*, ed. J.P. Carley (Woodbridge, 1985), pp. 161–3. Aelred of Rievaulx's life of St Ninian records a similar list of miracles: J. MacQueen, ed., *St Nynia* (Edinburgh, 1990), p. 113.

58  William of Malmesbury, *Gesta Regum Anglorum*, eds R.A.B. Mynors and others (2 vols, Oxford, 1998–99), i, pp. 400–01.

59  D. Wilkins. ed., *Concilia Magnae Britanniae et Hiberniae* (4 vols, London, 1737), iii, p. 637.

60  A.J.M. Edwards, ed., 'An Early Twelfth Century Account of the Translation of St Milburga of Much Wenlock', *Transactions of the Shropshire Archaeological Society*, lvii (1961–64), pp. 134–51, at pp. 150–51. Scepticism was, however, often used as a literary device to heighten the sense of drama.

ishness' had denied that so terrible a disease could ever be cured – even through divine intervention. Yet medical opinion was on their side.

As authorities from Aretaeus onwards unanimously agreed, once leprosy (*elephantia*) had taken hold it was implacable.[61] Echoing earlier generations of medical writers back to Haly Abbas (d. 994), the French surgeon, Henri de Mondeville (d. *c.* 1320), compared it to a cancer that could only be extirpated by something infinitely worse:

> Leprosy is a disease caused by melancholic matter, or by matter that has been converted into melancholia, tainted by an irreversible corruption, which has the same effect upon the entire body as a cancer in a cancerous member. So, just as the cancer can only be eliminated by gangrene of the entire member in which it is found, in the same way leprosy cannot be cured without the corruption or surgical removal of all the infected body. Now, that is impossible.[62]

An English translation of Guy de Chauliac's *Cyrurgie* graphically likened the disease to 'a cancrouse wolf', which gnawed remorselessly at the body of his victims.[63] Another vernacular work on surgery noted tersely that 'euery lepur confermyd . . . may not be helyd but in mirakyll off gode'.[64] Ecclesiastical authorities were equally dogmatic. In his confirmation of an early charter to the *leprosarium* of St Mary Magdalen, Exeter, in 1192, for example, Celestine III described the inmates as having been visited from on high with an incurable sickness.[65] Similarly, the early charters of the hospital of St Gilles at Pont-Audemer paint a sombre picture of men who 'carry the sins of the world in the pain of their bodies and yet are brought closer to God in their suffering'.[66] The cure of such hopeless cases lay far beyond human agency, however skilled.

It is thus easy to see why the chroniclers of Thomas Becket's early miracles were particularly anxious to record – and advertise – the martyr's ability to cleanse leprous flesh, since this was such a fundamental demonstration of sanctity. The blood of the lamb of Canterbury, like that of Christ, could wash away the most hideous diseases.[67] This point was tellingly made in the cathedral itself. A window of *c.* 1170–80 in the north-east transept contained roundels (now

---

61  Aretaeus observes that *elephantia* 'is mighty in power, for it is the most powerful of all in taking life . . . And from the disease there is no escape, for it originates in a deadly cause': Adams, *Extant Works of Aretaeus*, p. 368. Although he may not have known this text, Gilbertus Anglicus forcibly reiterates the same opinion: Grant, *Source Book*, p. 754.

62  Nicaise, *Chirurgie de Henri de Mondeville*, p. 616. Theoderic likewise describes leprosy as being 'like a general cancer of the whole body': Campbell and Colton, *Surgery of Theoderic*, ii, p. 167. For further examples of this simile, see Demaitre, 'Relevance of Futility', p. 29; idem, 'Medieval Notions of Cancer: Malignancy and Metaphor', *BHM*, lxxii (1998), pp. 609–37.

63  Ogden, *Cyrurgie of Guy de Chauliac*, p. 378.

64  BL, MS Harley 1736, fo. 135r, from the Latin MS Sloane 2272 (part 1), fo. 92r.

65  G. Oliver, ed., *Monasticon dioecesis Exoniensis* (London, 1846), p. 402.

66  Mesmin, 'Saint Gilles de Pont-Audemer', i, p. 117. See also, Bourgeois, *Lépreux et maladreries*, p. 267.

67  'On earth is God with us for love of the Martyr, and makes the dead to live, the dumb to speak, the deaf to hear, the deformed well-formed; He causes gout and fever to be cured; dropsied and leprous folk He restores; the blind He makes to see, and the mad return to their senses . . .': E.A. Abbott, ed., *St Thomas of Canterbury: His Death and Miracles* (2 vols, London, 1898), i, p. 244, and also pp. 231–2, 236. See also, Ward, *Miracles*, p. 102; N. Vincent, *The Holy Blood: Henry III and the Westminster Blood Relic* (Cambridge, 2001), p. 48. Pilgrim badges, purchased at the shrine, referred to Becket as 'the best physician of the worthy sick': C. Rawcliffe, 'Pilgrimage and the Sick in Medieval East Anglia', in C.

lost) depicting Naaman's immersion in the river Jordan and Christ's encounter with the leper after his sermon on the mount.[68] They provided a suitable context for the stained glass in the Trinity chapel ambulatory, which presented visitors with an account of the saint's most dramatic miracles, including three involving lepers.[69] There were many from which to choose. William of Canterbury, one of the martyr's first publicists, records no fewer than thirty-one, by far his largest single disease category, followed by twenty-four cures of paralysis and twenty-three relating to the blind. His fellow monk, Benedict of Peterborough, adopted a rather different scale of priorities, allocating the disease third place (nine cures), after the blind (thirty-eight) and paralytics (twenty-six).[70] But both writers followed the biblical model essential in the process of canonisation, and each stressed the limits of earthly medicine in the face of such intractable symptoms.

Remarking on the number of lepers drawn to the shrine of the *coelestus medicus* as news of such dramatic events spread, Benedict claimed that no saint in history could equal Thomas's record, while William described him as the Lord's 'high priest', entrusted with a special mission to heal the disease, 'not only in its serpentine or leonine forms, but elephantine and vulpine, and any other type of leprosy imagined by the physician'.[71] Raymonde Foreville has suggested that the two hagiographers were confused by the medical vocabulary and had little sense of the difference between Old Testament *lepra* and *elephantia*, but it is clear that each chose his specialist terminology with care.[72] William, in particular, considered it important to display a fund of medical knowledge, quite possibly because he was conscious that sceptics (of whom there were initially many) might question his diagnostic ability and thus belittle the martyr's power. When describing the case of a leper named Richard, whose condition was closely observed by several distinguished visitors to Canterbury, he refers to Galen's celebrated remark on the rarity of complete cures. Whereas, in the days of this great physician, theriac offered the only remote hope of recovery, visitors to Becket's shrine were now vouchsafed the more potent medicine of his holy blood.[73]

---

Morris and P. Roberts, eds, *Pilgrimage: The English Experience from Becket to Bunyan* (Cambridge, 2002), p. 211.

68  A third roundel bore the legend 'God clothed in flesh purifies the leprous and sin-laden human race': M.H. Caviness, *The Windows of Christ Church Cathedral Canterbury* (London, 1981), p. 113.

69  The identity of one of the lepers is problematic, although, since he is giving thanks for a cure on the way to Canterbury, he may be Cocubur, who was on the mend by the time he arrived (see n. 116 below). The other two are Richard Sunieve and Elias the monk from Reading: Caviness, *Windows of Christ Church*, pp. 189, 194–5, 212–13.

70  R. Foreville, *Thomas Becket dans la tradition historique et hagiographique* (Variorum, London, 1981), chapter seven, pp. 460–62. William was brought in to assist Benedict in about 1172, and it is at this point that cures of lepers begin to appear in the latter's notes.

71  Robertson, *Materials*, i, pp. 333–4; ii, pp. 183, 185. 'Great indeed is the number of people whose skin, roughened with the swellings of leprosy (*tuberibus leprae*), has been softened by the martyr': ibid., ii. p. 260.

72  Foreville, *Thomas Becket*, chapter seven, p. 464.

73  Robertson, *Materials*, i, pp. 332–4. Thorndike, *History of Magic*, i, p. 170, discusses Galen's *exemplum*, which involved the consumption of wine into which a viper had fallen. Becket is, of course, the true theriac, as Benedict points out in the case of a paralytic monk, whom no earthly medicaments could cure: *Materials*, ii, p. 42. For the significance of theriac, see below, pp. 220–22.

Like Jewish priests, William and his colleagues expected pilgrims whose cures happened elsewhere to report to them in person with supporting evidence from reliable witnesses.[74] Daniel, an Irish monk cleansed of leprosy, was reproved for his 'ignorance of the scriptures' and failure to observe these 'ceremonies of the Old Law', since he could produce no convincing testimonials.[75] More often, however, the parish priest, the head of a neighbouring religious house, or some other reputable cleric provided written corroborative evidence, which generally included an account of the original symptoms.[76] Since, at this date, there was no uniform approach to the documentation of *miracula*, such reports varied considerably. When, for instance, the prior of Taunton sent notice of the cure of John King, one of his monks, '*lepra gravi et manifesta percussum*', he concentrated in great circumstantial detail on the latter's journey to Canterbury from the *leprosarium* where he was then living. Dissatisfied by his correspondent's lack of clinical precision, Benedict himself observed that King had been allowed to remain within the monastic community for two years after his flesh became ulcerated and the hairs of his beard and eyebrows fell out. As his symptoms deteriorated, he had eventually been obliged to enter a hospital.[77] This concern for authenticity prompts us to ask exactly how Becket's hagiographers, their informants and competitors actually determined who might be suffering from the disease.

Despite the frequent jibes addressed by monastic chroniclers and theologians at medical practitioners, it is important to remember that some of the leading exponents of the healing arts in eleventh- and twelfth-century England might be found in monasteries. E.J. Kealey claims that about 13 per cent of the physicians he has identified in practice between 1100 and 1154 had taken the habit, while a further 25 per cent came from the ranks of the priesthood.[78] Statistics of this kind must inevitably remain impressionistic, although it is apparent that the monks in question enjoyed a distinction far greater than their numbers might suggest. The Benedictine abbey of Bury St Edmunds, for example, not only boasted an internationally famous shrine, but could also lay claim, in the person of Abbot Baldwin, to a *medicus* of corresponding celebrity who cared for two English kings.[79] To many observers, though, the growing popularity of monastic

---

[74] Benedict sent an embassy to Lisors in Calvados to discover the fate of a leper named Walter, who had been partially cured on his return home from Canterbury: Robertson, *Materials*, ii, p. 203.

[75] Robertson, *Materials*, i, pp. 217–19.

[76] Thus, for example, Humbald, prior of Wenlock, reported that the cure of one Mabel of Dudley had been authenticated by eight trustworthy monks and that a ninth, who cared for her on a regular basis, would send his own written testimony. He also described her symptoms, which included a raucous voice, tumorous lips, heavy blinking and squinting, cracked or fissured feet, swollen hands and a body covered in *maculae*: Robertson, *Materials*, i, pp. 338–9. Not all visitors to Canterbury were, however, happy to assist the process of documentation. A knight, who had spent six months at Becket's shrine and was cleansed of his *elephantia*, refused to testify before an ecclesiastical council at Bourges 'out of shame': ibid., pp. 458–61. Finucane, *Miracles*, pp. 149–50, suggests that this was a typical elite response to illness in general, but sufferers from leprosy must have been aware of its moral implications.

[77] Robertson, *Materials*, ii, pp. 429–31. King was cured on his way to the shrine.

[78] Kealey, *Medieval Medicus*, pp. 40, 121–51. See also E.A. Hammond, 'Physicians in Medieval English Religious Houses', *BHM*, xxxii (1958), pp. 105–20.

[79] C. Rawcliffe, 'On the Threshold of Eternity: Care for the Sick in East Anglian Monasteries', in C.

medicine, which often embraced surgery as well, threatened to undermine the
very foundations of the cloistered life. Fear that members of religious orders
would be tempted 'to promise health in return for detestable money' and thus
breach their oath of poverty, prompted a series of conciliar rulings in the 1130s.
These prohibited monks and canons regular from treating patients for crude
material gain, but did not forbid the study of medicine for charitable purposes.[80]
Ramelmus, a Cluniac canon and skilled *medicus* of Much Wenlock, who
dispensed advice and treatment among the local poor during the early twelfth
century, is typical of the kind of healer who escaped such regulations.[81] Others,
however, continued to cause unease, and in 1163 professed monks were specifically denied leave of absence 'for pondering medical concoctions under the
pretext of aiding the bodies of their sick brothers'.[82]

Even so, the study of medicine and science continued, perhaps with new
vigour, inside the precincts of communities with any pretensions to learning.
Men such as John of Cella (d. 1214), hailed as 'an outstanding physician and
incomparable judge of urine', read medicine in Paris *before* taking orders and
rising to become abbot of St Albans.[83] We do not know if Thomas of Northwick
(d. 1207), a monk of Evesham abbey, ever trained formally, although 'his
medical knowledge and practice attracted the favour and grace of the whole
surrounding countryside'.[84] As Faye Getz observes, these were eminent scholars,
whose appeal lay not only in their spiritual power but also in their command of
new scientific learning.[85] Few monasteries lacked access to the basic texts that
were to form the core of the English university medical syllabus for the best part
of three centuries, and some, such as the Cluniac house of Monk Bretton, in
Yorkshire, built up impressive collections to rival or even surpass those of
leading physicians.[86] That monastic libraries were, moreover, augmented by gifts
from secular practitioners is significant. At some point before 1153 the Durham
Benedictines took delivery from a local *medicus* of twenty-six, mostly specialist,
books, bound into at least five volumes. By 1331 the remarkable collection at
Becket's own cathedral priory included many similar offerings (including works
by Galen and Avicenna), although we do not, unfortunately, know what was
available at the time of his martyrdom.[87] It is, however, clear that the shrine

---

Harper-Bill, C. Rawcliffe and R.G. Wilson, eds, *East Anglia's History: Studies in Honour of Norman
Scarfe* (Woodbridge, 2002), pp. 43–5.

80  Amundsen, *Medicine, Society and Faith*, p. 206. See also, D.N. Bell, 'The English Cistercians and the
Practice of Medicine', *Cîteaux*, xl (1989), pp. 139–74.

81  Kealey, *Medieval Medicus*, p. 42; Edwards, 'St Milburga', p. 146.

82  Amundsen, *Medicine, Society and Faith*, pp. 230–1.

83  Getz, *Medicine*, pp. 14–15. He is actually depicted as a physician, with jordans, blood samples and
medicaments, in one illuminated monastic chronicle: BL, MS Cotton Claudius E IV, fo. 129v. Warin
(d. 1195), a previous abbot of St Albans, had reputedly trained at Salerno: *MPIME*, pp. 372–3.
William (d. 1242), a monk-physician who attended John on his deathbed, went on to become prior of
Worcester: *MPIME*, pp. 384–5.

84  *MPIME*, p. 353.

85  Getz, *Medicine*, p. 15.

86  The ongoing Corpus of British Medieval Library Catalogues reveals the extent of medical book
ownership in monastic houses. See, for example, R. Sharpe et al., eds, *English Benedictine Libraries:
The Shorter Catalogues* (Corpus, iv, 1996), and T. Webber and A.G. Watson, eds, *The Libraries of
Augustinian Canons* (Corpus, vi, 1998), both indices sub *medica*.

87  R.A.B. Mynors, *Durham Cathedral Manuscripts to the End of the Twelfth Century* (Durham, 1939), p.

keepers and other religious who encountered the sick on a regular basis were likely to command impressive reserves of practical and theoretical expertise. Did they apply their skills to the diagnosis (and palliative care) of leprous pilgrims? Or did they feel that a more circumspect approach would best serve the interests of ecclesiastical propaganda?

In some cases removal to, or imminent entry into, a *leprosarium* at the urging of priests and neighbours was alone deemed sufficient proof of advanced leprosy. Gerard of Lille, whose disease had affected his legs and feet, was just about to take this last halting step when Becket appeared to him in a vision, urging him to visit Canterbury, where he was cleansed.[88] As reported by the archdeacon of Coventry, a wretched creature named Humphrey had languished for three years, immobile and ulcerated, until his friends finally pronounced him *lepra precussus* and sent him off to hospital. Reluctant to accept what was, essentially, information garnered at second hand, William asked the erstwhile leper himself to report for examination, bringing a letter from his dean. Neither was, however, able to provide the kind of detailed evidence he would have wished.[89] Where possible, William sought to record specific symptoms of *lepra*, a disease which, more than any of the others cured by Becket, he describes with a careful eye for clinical detail.[90] Thus, for example, Agnes, another reputed leper whose condition necessitated removal from the community, is said (on close personal inspection) to have lost her eyebrows and to have been disfigured by a swollen nose and chin. Her flesh was ulcerated; her extremities rough and dry; her red, weeping and protuberant eyes virtually closed by eruptions on the lower lids.[91] Simon of Derby, the most extreme case described by William, presents so many of the characteristics associated with elephantine leprosy as to appear almost a textbook case. At the time of this very specific diagnosis, he was begging for money to enter a *leprosarium*. His symptoms, which seemed quite beyond medical help, then included the loss of hair, beard and fingernails, progressive and extensive ulceration, the inability to speak audibly (because of hoarseness and the collapse of his nose), inflamed eyes, changes of pigmentation and weeping sores. His condition deteriorated rapidly, as tumours and protuberances, scurf and scabs erupted over his body. His voice and cough grew raucous, compounding the horror he inspired in those who looked upon him. To add to his miseries, his hands, deformed by dilated veins and nodules, were further damaged by the retraction of his fingers into his palm, so that he could not feed himself.[92]

Notwithstanding an awareness that their audience might recoil from too

62 (and also p. 49 and plate 37); Kealey, *Medieval Medicus*, pp. 44–5; M.R. James, *The Ancient Libraries of Canterbury and Dover* (Cambridge, 1903), pp. 55–62, 138. See also, A.H. Sweet, 'The Library of St Radegund's Abbey', *EHR*, liii (1938), pp. 88–93, at pp. 91–2 (*de phisica*).

88  Robertson, *Materials*, ii, pp. 243–4.

89  Robertson, *Materials*, ii, pp. 183–5.

90  Foreville, *Thomas Becket*, chapter seven, p. 464.

91  Robertson, *Materials*, i, pp. 216–17. See Seymour, *On the Properties of Things*, i, p. 424, for a virtually identical list of the 'comyn signes' displayed by Agnes, who was not fully cured.

92  Robertson, *Materials*, i, pp. 334–6. Simon's ordeal throws into relief the shortcomings of the archbishop of York, who had been one of Becket's enemies: M. Lovatt, ed., *EEA, 20, York, 1154–1181* (Oxford, 2000), pp. xxx–xxxi, n. 14.

graphic a litany of human suffering, the chroniclers demonstrate a clear understanding of the need for proof. Had the disease really entered a terminal stage
beyond all hope of medical intervention? A royal foundling, whose condition
forced him to abandon his schooling at Abingdon abbey, certainly conforms to
the worst humoral type. Afflicted by a tuberous face, running eyes, limbs ulcerated to the bone, and a hoarse, barely audible voice, he is in every respect
'*elephantico morbo correptus*'.[93] Macerated, weeping flesh and loss of feeling in
the extremities are cited as signs of leprosy in a ten-year-old child, who, significantly, relapsed on his return home and grew worse than before. Unlike the rest
of his body, Benedict observes, the child's face was not covered with pustules,
but was tumorous, swollen and mottled with and red and white marks.[94] Equally
graphic are the accounts of Elias, the monk of Reading abbey, and Richard
Sunieve, both of whom were depicted in the great stained glass window near the
martyr's shrine. Diagnosed by many highly skilled – and very expensive – physicians, as *horrida lepra*, Elias's painful condition affected his eyes, 'dropping and
flowing with rheum' [plate 18]. It also left him covered in sores and scales, which
he shed profusely in bed during the night. A modern reader might suspect psoriasis, and Elias is, indeed, described in one of our sources as suffering from that
transient condition between leprosy and morphew, which permitted some hope
of recovery.[95] Sunieve, who fell asleep under a hedge and awoke with a swollen
and spotted face, deteriorated to such an extent over the following eight years
that 'not the space of an arrow's point was sound' throughout his body. The
inevitable stench of decaying flesh deterred all but his mother, who kept her
distance by feeding him at the end of a stick [plate 19].[96] As in the strikingly
similar case of Hugh de Ebblinghem of St Omer, the term *lepra* is here deployed
in a biblical sense, with little attempt at clinical precision, although it is apparent
that both men also had deformed and swollen features. Hugh's recovery began,
significantly, after confession, but he still lacked 'form or comeliness' [Isaiah 53,
v. 2] on arrival at Canterbury. His face was duly sprinkled with holy water, and,
on his next visit some months later, appeared miraculously cleansed.[97]

We shall return later to the importance placed by surgeons and physicians
upon the facial symptoms of *lepra*, but should note that both Benedict and
William often dwell upon them, as do many other hagiographers.[98] It was,
perhaps, because his restored features spoke so eloquently for themselves that
brother Daniel from Dublin felt it unnecessary to provide any further testi-

---

93  Robertson, *Materials*, i, pp. 213–14. The bishop of St Asaph had the boy examined by physicians after
his cure, and, having previously derided the cult of St Thomas, brought him personally to Canterbury
to give thanks. See also ibid., ii, p. 245, and below, pp. 278–9.

94  Robertson, *Materials*, ii, pp. 244–5.

95  Robertson, *Materials*, i, pp. 416–17; ii, pp. 242–3. Since it was believed that morphew might develop
into *lepra* if it was not properly treated, the two conditions seemed part of a continuum.

96  Robertson, *Materials*, ii, pp. 245–7.

97  Robertson, *Materials*, i, pp. 332–4; ii, pp. 259–60. For the therapeutic effects of bathing, see below, pp.
226–32.

98  See, for example, R.R. Dartington, ed., *The Vita Wulfstani of William of Malmesbury* (CS, third series,
xl, 1928), p. 121; Douie and Farmer, *Life of St Hugh*, pp. 12–13; Garton, *Metrical Life of St Hugh*, p. 67.
One of the stained glass images of Richard Sunieve shows his master feeling his face to check that all
signs of *lepra* have vanished: Caviness, *Windows of Christ Church*, fig. 299.

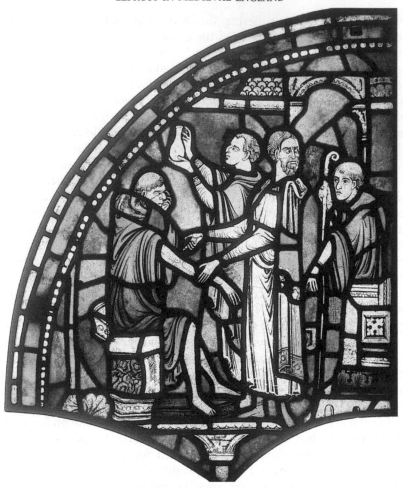

18. Powerful propaganda for the shrine of Thomas Becket may be found in this
stained glass panel of *c.* 1215 from the Trinity Chapel of Canterbury Cathedral.
For all their learning, the physicians consulted by Elias, the leprous monk of
Reading abbey, cannot cure him. One anxiously consults the patient's urine
sample in a glass flask, or jordan, while his abbot (who puts his faith in earthly
medicine rather than the saint) appears on the right.

monials. Conversely, a mottled or tumorous appearance automatically aroused
suspicion. The discoloured and distorted face of a once handsome young
Norman attracted far greater attention than his macerated hands and limbs.
Gerald the knight fled into exile because of his humiliating facial symptoms,
while the horrific aspect of an anonymous Welsh leper seemed to reflect the
spiritual corruption within. William Argentine's knotted hands and suppurating
legs contrasted sharply with his ashen complexion, although the saturnine
appearance of the count of Mellent's page proved even more distressing to the
assembled onlookers. Having enjoyed only temporary remission after a
pilgrimage – like Naaman – to the River Jordan, the young retainer deteriorated

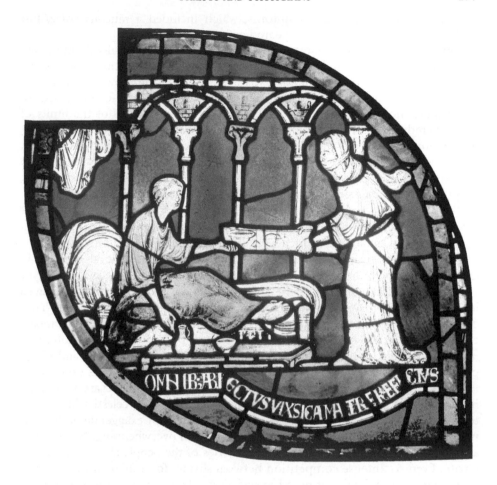

19. Another of the stained glass panels at Canterbury recounts the cure of Richard Sunieve, whose mother cared for him after leprosy spread throughout his body. But even she found the odour of disease so oppressive that she had to feed him from a distance (and in this image of *c.* 1215 has wrapped a cloth around her mouth because of the stench).

rapidly, his face erupting into a mass of dark swellings and tumours that would have ended all hope of employment in a baronial household. His nose, too, collapsed, this being the one remaining deformity that Becket in his wisdom declined to heal.[99] The saint often performed an incomplete cure, in order to keep his votaries in a state of abject repentance, to punish them for residual sins, or, more charitably, to leave behind some small proof of a greater miracle. In the case of a woman named Odelina, he assumed that earthly physicians could deal with such a routine matter as nasal damage (although he repaired the upper part

[99] Robertson, *Materials*, i, pp. 214–16, 337–8, 457–8, 541.

of the nostrils). Her other symptoms, which included a raucous voice, lost eyebrows and facial pallor, disappeared entirely.[100]

On the ground that the Gospel had provided no further details about the ten lepers healed by Christ in Samaria, William tells us little or nothing about some of those to whom Becket extended his mercy.[101] Mindful, however, that their readers might balk as much at bald statistics as they would at formulaic lists of symptoms, the two chroniclers displayed a shrewd awareness of the limits of human credulity. The case of Eilgar of Calne, a classic victim of *lepra*, led Benedict to ponder the exact nature of a cure. On returning home from Canterbury, Eilgar, whose symptoms ran the full gamut from claw-like hands and feet to widespread loss of physical sensation, ulceration, collapse of the nose and foetid, gasping breath, seemed much improved. Yet, although his flesh was healed, William felt that he had not been fully cleansed (*'arbitrio meo non plene mundatus'*). He now looked like man *disposed* to leprosy, rather than one caught in the throes of the disease, which, was, nevertheless, a miracle in itself.[102]

It is apparent from many of these examples, as from medieval *miracula* in general, that the concept of a cure was highly subjective. Often transitory or imperfect, such experiences might easily embrace cases of tuberculoid and even lepromatous leprosy as understood by twentieth-century physicians. They certainly allowed for that incipient or indeterminate stage of the disease apparently first described in the late thirteenth century by Theoderic, who notes that 'a common sign at the beginning of all *lepra* is that spots appear and disappear'.[103] In practice, one suspects that, despite their repeated stress upon accurate reportage, hagiographers were psychologically disposed to regard even slight improvements and periods of remission as evidence of a celestial hand. The temptation to deploy medical knowledge to embellish or exaggerate quite ordinary dermatological disorders must also have been overwhelming. Nor did our authors attempt to follow up the case histories of the people about whom they wrote. Even so, intense competition between shrines for a share of the lucrative pilgrim trade and the threat posed to ecclesiastical order by the mushrooming of local cults made proper authentication seem increasingly important. A papal monopoly over the process of canonisation, already asserted in the twelfth century, was incorporated into canon law by Innocent III, who characteristically tightened up procedures. Not only was the performance of posthumous miracles now deemed an essential prerequisite of sanctity, but far more stringent proofs were henceforth also demanded.[104] In the case of leprosy, such measures were reinforced by a growing familiarity with the newly translated texts, ideas and definitions discussed in chapter two.

---

[100]  Robertson, *Materials*, i, pp. 330–32.

[101]  Robertson, *Materials*, i, pp. 221–2. See also ibid., pp. 220, 339–40, 479–80.

[102]  Robertson, *Materials*, ii, p. 203. The chronicler is less compassionate in the case of Ralph Longton, who came to Canterbury as he was about to enter a leper house, and was cured. His hoarse voice, foetid breath, ulcerated limbs and weeping facial sores vanished, but on a pilgrimage to Jerusalem he relapsed, worse than before, because of his sins: ibid., pp. 182–3.

[103]  Campbell and Colton, *Surgery of Theoderic*, p. 168. See also Brody, *Disease of the Soul*, p. 34. This phenomenon was widely recognised by later generations of practitioners: BL, MS Sloane 2272 (part 1), fo. 90v.

[104]  Matthew Paris, *Life of St Edmund*, pp. 90–99.

Second-hand reports, however reputable the source, were now no longer sufficient, nor was much credence given to partial or uncertain cures. First person depositions taken under oath became mandatory, as, for example, in the case of Gilbert of Sempringham, whose canonisation in 1202 followed the new, more rigorous format. The relevant documents were brought together at this time by one of his canons, and include lists of both 'formal' (fully authenticated) and 'informal' miracles. A mere thirty in all, the former provide evidence of Gilbert's power over human suffering, but include only one case of leprosy. It concerns Juliana, a nun at Sempringham, who had displayed a number of blemishes and lesions since childhood. Eventually her entire body was affected, resulting in the loss of eyebrows, virtual paralysis, especially of the hands, and an inability to open her eyelids. According to the formal testimony of several sisters, including her nurse, after twelve years prostration in the infirmary she was cured, revealing skin 'as healthy as a child'.[105]

Attempts to secure the canonisation of politically controversial figures, such as Edmund of Abingdon, inevitably redoubled concerns about the reliability of depositions. A leper reputedly healed by the archbishop travelled reluctantly to the curia at Lyon, in 1246, for a compulsory examination before Innocent IV himself. 'The whole process', we are told, 'was prolonged with the most searching scrutiny', and, moreover, demonstrates the emphasis placed by the papal physicians on both facial symptoms and a uniform complexion:

> It was commanded that his garment should be rent in front of his breast, so that it might be plainly proved whether the grace of healing which appeared on his face corresponded with the colour of his breast, lest he might have altered the colour of his face by trickery, in which case it would differ from that of the breast. But without any deceit the colour was found to be the same, that is a healthy colour appeared both here and there. And it was found in like manner in the case of others. A trial was also made with his voice; for a certain hoarseness is wont to exist in the case of lepers . . . He proved that his body as well as his face was sound.[106]

Under such circumstances, it is hardly surprising to discover that miraculous recoveries from fully authenticated *lepra* experienced something of a decline.

## Physicians of the soul: the confessional

The diagnostic skills of the medieval clergy were not, however, confined to recording and attesting miracles. In a pre-Cartesian age, when the consequences of the Fall hung heavily upon all men and women, the health of the body seemed inseparable from that of the soul. The role of the priest was, indeed, often described in medical terminology, as, of course, was that of *Christus medicus* himself. As one fourteenth-century sermon explained:

> A doctor investigates the condition of the sick person and the nature of his sickness

---

[105] R. Foreville and G. Keir, eds, *The Book of St Gilbert* (Oxford, 1987), pp. lxii–lxiii, xcviii–xcix, 234–7.

[106] B. Ward, *St Edmund, Archbishop of Canterbury: His Life as Told by Old English Writers* (London, 1903), pp. 191–2. Mistrust of low-status deponents may also be detected here: S. Farmer, 'The Beggar's Body', in eadem and Rosenwein, *Monks and Nuns*, pp. 167–71.

by such methods as taking his pulse and inspecting his urine. Thus when Christ visits a sinner he first enlightens him with his grace to understand himself and his own sin, so that he may repent of his sins and shun them.[107]

Like pilgrimage, this diagnostic process often began in the confessional. Drawing upon the New Testament injunction that followers of Christ should 'confess your faults one to another and pray for one another, that ye may be healed' [James 5, v. 16], the early fathers of the Church regarded an untroubled conscience as the key to physical as well as spiritual health. Origen (d. 254) recommended confession for those who were 'choked by their peccant humours', while for St Augustine it opened body and soul to the investigative hand and lancet of God.[108] From their earliest appearance, penitentials (manuals for the guidance of confessors) stressed the priest's role as a spiritual physician, providing 'various sorts of treatment [for] the wounds, fevers, transgressions, sorrows, sicknesses and infirmities of souls'.[109] In this way, as earthly practitioners recognised, the body's natural, vital and animal spirits might be calmed and, free of anxiety, restored to a state of equilibrium.[110]

But first came a checklist of symptoms. Had the penitent escaped with a light case of impetigo, or was his soul already leprous? Robert Brunne's vernacular manual for parish clergy on *Handlyng Synne* (1303) tells the story of a priest to whom God granted miraculous powers. The face of each member of his flock changed as he or she approached the altar to reveal their ghostly diseases: some were suffused with the choler of wrath, others were blacked with lust, while those consumed with avarice 'hadde visages of meselrye'.[111] Although some theologians expressed concern that a scientific training might engender arrogance or complacency among the clergy, the majority, like Brunne, drew heavily on metaphors culled from the *regimen sanitatis* and other medical literature.[112] Comparing the process of confession to a surgical operation, one thirteenth-century manual warned against prudishness. 'Just as it is proper for a person to undress completely to show his bodily wounds to a doctor or a surgeon', the author urged, 'it is proper for someone to reveal his inner wounds to his spiritual doctor.'[113] Laymen and women responded to such compelling imagery, which drove home the symbiotic connection between sin, humoral

---

[107] S. Wenzel, ed., *Fasciculus Morum: A Fourteenth-Century Preacher's Handbook* (Pennsylvania, 1989), pp. 255–7.

[108] Hepworth and Turner, *Confession*, p. 43. The surgical aspects of the confessional are further explored in Brandeis, *Jacob's Well*, pp. 178–9.

[109] J. McNeill and H.M. Gamer, eds, *Medieval Handbooks of Penance* (New York, 1938, reprinted 1990), pp. 251–2, and passim; J.T. McNeill, 'Medicine for Sin as Prescribed in the Penitentials', *Church History*, i (1932), pp. 14–26. Such was the view of laymen as well as clergy. In his celebrated *Livre de Seyntz Medicines* (1354), Henry, duke of Lancaster, compared confession to the cleansing of a festering mouth, which is then healed by the grace of God: E.J. Arnould, ed., *Le Livre de Seyntz Medicines* (Oxford, 1940), p. 181.

[110] Harvey, *Inward Wits*, pp. 2–28.

[111] F.J. Furnivall, ed., *Robert of Brunne's 'Handlyng Synne'* (EETS, cxix, 1901, and ccxxiii, 1903, reprinted as one, 1973), pp. 317–19.

[112] J. Hughes, 'The Administration of Confession', in D.M. Smith, ed., *Studies in Clergy and Ministry in Medieval England* (Borthwick Studies in History, i, 1991), pp. 87–163.

[113] J. Shinners and W.J. Dohar, eds, *Pastors and the Care of Souls in Medieval England* (Notre Dame, Indiana, 1998), pp. 171, 178. See also, Murray, 'Counselling', pp. 69–70.

imbalance and disease. In about 1170, Maurice de Sully warned members of his French congregation to hasten to the confessional as soon as they detected the first symptoms of spiritual leprosy, for only 'the supreme judge and physician' was competent to diagnose them effectively.[114]

Yet God's houseman, the priest, could hardly confine himself to spiritual matters alone. As we have seen in the previous two chapters, some of the presumed causes of physical leprosy had their roots in behaviour of which the Church strongly disapproved, and whose detection lay as much in the province of the priest as the physician. It was often impossible to distinguish between them. Robert Grosseteste, bishop of Lincoln (d. 1235), who may have practised medicine, recommended that confessors should assess a sinner's humoral complexion by studying his or her external features before imposing penance. In this way, he argued, they would be able to spot any innate propensity towards specific vices and, by extension, each person's ability to resist temptation.[115] Before setting out on his pilgrimage to Canterbury, Cocubur, a leprous kinsman of the king of Connaught, consulted Abbot Marianus, who observed his symptoms and advised him to undertake a rigorous fast. According to Becket's hagiographer, the *elephantia* which had incapacitated his body, covering it with nauseating ulcers, could only be healed through repentance, humility and penance, and thus lay beyond the help of earthly medicine. Yet, as the abbot clearly recognised, a change of diet might bring immediate physical benefits, too.[116] The above-mentioned Hugh of Ebblinghem, whose disease was associated by the chronicler with commercial fraud, similarly 'confessed the unrighteousness that stood against him in the eyes of the Lord' and thereby began a process of physical and spiritual regeneration.[117]

At a basic physiological level, *lepra* might well spring from excessive indulgence in particular food or drink, itself a manifestation of gluttony, or, even worse, have been contracted from an infected prostitute and thus be condign punishment for lust. Robert Brunne itemised the principal risks presented by 'comoun wymmen':

> One ys, she may take thy brother,
> Fadyr, or sybkind [sibling], as well as another.
> Another, for cuntek [contention] and foul stryfe,
> Thou mayst, thrugh here, lese thy lyfe.
> The thredde ys the werste wem [one];
> Mesles, men seye, vsen hem;
> And, who taketh hem yn that hete,
> Clennesse of body he may sone lete [lose].
> Moche wo than, ys swyche to take,
> For these thre lakes [moral failings] sake . . .[118]

---

114 Bériou and Touati, *Voluntate Dei leprosus*, p. 59.
115 Resnick, 'Physiognomy of Jesus and Mary', p. 227.
116 Robertson, *Materials*, i, pp. 431–2. Cocubur may, perhaps, have been suffering from ergotism, which is caused by poisoned rye, or an intolerance to certain foodstuffs.
117 Robertson, *Materials*, ii, pp. 259–60.
118 Furnivall, *Robert of Brunne's 'Handlyng Synne'*, pp. 237–8; and above, pp. 82–5.

At times the roles of priest and practitioner must have seemed interchangeable, not least because the one consciously modelled himself upon the other. Guy de Chauliac actually advised the examining surgeon to adopt an approach similar to that of the confessor. The subject of the *judicium* was first 'to swere to saye the trowthe of thinges that schall be axed him', and then interrogated about his life. Were other members of his family afflicted with leprosy? Had he consorted with diseased persons? What were his habits, dreams and desires?[119]

Penitentials also warned against the dire risks to body and soul posed to a man by coitus during menstruation, in or out of marriage. Robert of Flamborough, for example, repeated the medical opinion that conception at this time would result in leprous issue and was thus to be avoided for physical as well as spiritual reasons.[120] Theologians disagreed over the gravity of the offence, which was regarded by some as a mortal sin (unless it prevented an act of adultery), and by others as a matter of 'counsel', and thus essentially venial. In either event, it was the priest's responsibility, just like the physician's, to scrutinise the conduct of his flock, and to observe anyone whose sexual activities occasioned concern.[121] This charge assumed even greater weight after the fourth Lateran Council of 1215, when Innocent III instigated a sweeping series of reforms designed to augment the status and authority of the clergy. As we saw in the previous chapter, the requirement that confession should not only be made annually as a matter of routine, but also at the outset of medical treatment, gave the priest, as well as the physician, an unrivalled opportunity to establish the causes of disease. Henceforward, manuals for the guidance of physicians at the bedside were assiduous in requiring them to ensure that their patients confessed on the first visit. If he was also a priest, as so often proved to be the case in England, the physician could assess the severity of spiritual and bodily symptoms at the same time, not least 'because many diseases arise from sins; and once a man has washed away his sins with the tears of a good conscience, he will often recover from these diseases through the mercy of the Sovereign Leech'.[122]

It is easy to see why Bishop Bronescombe of Exeter (d. 1280) should argue that the diagnosis of suspects was so demonstrably a sacerdotal function. 'It belongs to the office of the priest', he claimed, emphasising the message of Leviticus, 'to distinguish between one form of leprosy and another.'[123] Late medieval biblical dictionaries, such as that acquired by St John's hospital, Exeter, in the fifteenth century, reiterated his opinion in entries to be found for *lepra* and *leprosi*.[124] No doubt because of its usefulness, the Church's authority in this respect was formally upheld by the Scottish Parliament of 1427. 'The bishop's officials and deans' were then ordered to inquire diligently:

---

[119] Ogden, *Cyrurgie of Guy de Chauliac*, p. 381. English surgeons were required to be 'as priuie and as secrete as anye confessour of al thinges that they shall eyther heare or see in the house of their pacient': Thomas Vicary, *The Anatomie of the Bodie of Man*, eds F.J. Furnivall and P. Furnivall (EETS, extra series, liii, 1888, reprinted 1973), p. 16.

[120] Robert of Flamborough, *Liber poenitentialis*, p. 238; and above, pp. 80–82.

[121] Payer, *Bridling of Desire*, pp. 107–9.

[122] Hunt, *Anglo-Norman Medicine*, ii, pp. 21, 39–40; Grant, *Source Book*, pp. 742–5.

[123] Cartwright, *Social History of Medicine*, p. 24.

[124] Bodleian Library, MS Laud Misc. 156, fo. 37v.

in their visitations of each parish church if anyone is smitten with leprosy. And, if anyone so smitten shall be found, that they are reported to the king if they are lay people, and if they are clergy to their bishops. And that all burgesses must keep this statute under the penalty set out in the Statute of Beggars. And any leper who fails to observe this statute shall be permanently banished from that borough where he disobeys.[125]

The fact that expulsion was the punishment for *failing* to declare oneself to a priest and that the penalties imposed upon negligent boroughs were identical to those in force for the control of beggars should alert us to the underlying purpose of this decree. We shall return to the motives for segregation in chapter six, but for now the main point of interest lies in the close involvement of the priesthood in recording and reporting known lepers. This was occasionally a matter for English ecclesiastical visitors, such as those who inspected the Kentish parish of St Margaret-at-Cliffe in 1512, and discovered that 'a lepour' was being 'maynteigned contrary to the lawe' there.[126]

The medical expertise of clergy working in small communities, where they were familiar and trusted figures, was not confined to the detection of leprosy. Plague regulations drawn up for the city of Milan in 1374 ruled that 'parish priests shall examine the sick to see what the illness is and shall immediately notify the designated seneschal . . . under pain of being burnt alive'.[127] That many would have nursed and attempted to treat their parishioners, and even sometimes their clerical superiors, seems beyond doubt.[128] Their part in the diagnostic procedure was thus as much pragmatic as it was sacerdotal, a fact that further underscores the intimate union between body and soul characteristic of the period. For Master Guy, an Italian canon of the Cluniac house at Merton, physical and spiritual health merged seamlessly together. Having been ordained a priest after his arrival in about 1114, perhaps fresh from Salerno, he used his knowledge of medicine to augment a growing reputation as a true healer of wounded souls and suffering bodies through the medium of the confessional. It was in this way that he cured his own superior, who was seriously ill.[129] Not surprisingly, however, we know most about those clergy who abused their position. John Ottrington, a chaplain who came before the dean and chapter of York, in 1424, had not only breached canon law by practising as a 'common surgeon', but had compounded his offence by attempting various gynaecological procedures as well.[130] Far worse complaints were levelled at this time against the vicar of St Leonard's church in Fetter Lane, London, by a local jury, which accused him of gross immorality, adding, for good measure, that 'he presentit hym self a surgeon & a visicioun [physician] to disseve the peopl with is false connynge, that he scheuithe unto the peopl, by the whiche craft he hathe slayn

125  Thomson and Innes, *Acts of the Parliament of Scotland*, ii, p. 16.
126  K.L. Wood-Leigh, ed., *Kentish Visitations of Archbishop Warham and His Deputies 1511–1512* (Kent Archaeological Society, Kent Records, xxiv, 1984), pp. 115–16.
127  Horrox, *Black Death*, p. 203.
128  Rawcliffe, *Medicine and Society*, pp. 105–6.
129  Kealey, *Medieval Medicus*, pp. 34, 129; M.L. Colker, 'The Life of Guy of Merton by Rainald of Merton', *Medieval Studies*, xxxi (1969), pp. 250–61, at p. 259.
130  Borthwick Institute of Historical Research, Dean and Chapter Act Book, i, fo. 69r.

many a man'.[131] The sense of betrayal apparent from this presentment suggests that parishioners trusted their clergy to provide sound medical as well as spiritual advice. We can readily understand why the residents of Sparham placed such confidence in their priest's diagnostic ability.

As late as 1837 parish priests in Iceland were instructed to report to their bishop on the number of lepers living in rural communities, which were often remote and difficult of access. One medical practitioner dismissed their findings (a mere 128 individuals) as a serious underestimate based only on advanced cases, but his own criteria appear dangerously broad. Evidently the clergy followed a long medieval tradition of cautious deliberation founded on experience.[132] In this respect their figures may have been more reliable than those compiled by physicians with limited exposure to the disease. Half a century later, the Indian Leprosy Commission reported that almost 10 per cent of people considered suspect by doctors were suffering from entirely different illnesses, while the experience in French Colonial Africa seemed even less encouraging. 'How can one diagnose leprosy without a microscope?' asked one frustrated administrator, who felt that the statistics compiled by his professional colleagues were quite meaningless. It was then recommended that, in the interests of greater clinical accuracy, tests should include the pricking of discoloured patches of skin with a needle, to determine levels of sensitivity.[133] This technique had, in fact, been widely deployed, along with many others, in the medieval *judicium*.

## Practitioners at work: the *judicium*

In marked contrast to the practice in continental Europe, late medieval English towns and cities did not hire physicians and surgeons to provide free or subsidised treatment for the less affluent. Danielle Jacquart has estimated that, between 1288 and the end of the fifteenth century, almost 15 per cent of French physicians, a slightly higher percentage of surgeons and 8 per cent of barbers were retained on this basis. Prominent among their duties were the care of plague victims and the diagnosis of lepers. Not all of the 132 practitioners known to have taken part in these examinations were municipal employees, but many developed considerable expertise through their work in the community.[134] Contracts between north-European urban authorities and medical personnel, such as those surviving from the Hanseatic port of Kampen in the 1460s and 1470s, also record a specific obligation to examine suspects free of charge, which, in university towns might additionally fall upon members of the nearest faculty of medicine.[135] In Mainz and Cologne, for example, problem cases were referred to the resident academic bodies, thus further bolstering their authority. The

---

131  A.H. Thomas, ed., *Calendar of Plea and Memoranda Rolls Preserved among the Archives of the Corporation of the City of London, 1413–1437* (Cambridge, 1943), p. 127.
132  Ehlers, *On the Conditions under which Leprosy Has Declined*, p. 10.
133  Buckingham, *Leprosy in Colonial South India*, p. 20; Silla, *People Are not the Same*, p. 96. The experience in Hawaii was even worse: Gussow, *Leprosy, Racism and Public Health*, p. 95.
134  D. Jacquart, *Le milieu médical en France du XIIe au XVe siècle* (Haute Etudes Médiévales et Modernes, series 5, xlvi, 1981), pp. 121, 128, 133–5.
135  Bergman, 'Hoping against Hope', pp. 27–8, 43, 44.

papacy actively supported attempts by the aggressively monopolistic Parisian Faculty of Medicine to force anyone suffering from – or even suspected as having – a contagious disease to submit to its judgement.[136] English university-trained physicians, who were far fewer in number and lacked any coherent organisation, could only look on with envy.

There is no direct evidence that the examination of Nicholas Malesmains (a significant name) before the barons of the exchequer in the early thirteenth century to determine if he had leprosy was undertaken by medical experts. We are, however, told that the boy's guardian felt uncertain about his condition and needed proper guidance before entrusting him to a *leprosarium*, which suggests that some machinery may already have been in place for the assessment of difficult cases.[137] A similar inspection by unidentified individuals occurred shortly afterwards, in 1227, when the widowed Agnes de Westwick came into court to prove that she was not leprous and ought thus to recover her dower.[138] The formal scrutiny of suspects by physicians and surgeons along continental lines is certainly known to have occurred in late medieval England, albeit in response to specific circumstances rather than as a matter of routine. For this reason, the surviving evidence is, at best, patchy, often concerning members of the clergy whose health occasioned anxiety or speculation. In 1292, for instance, physicians assured Bishop Sutton of Lincoln that the vicar of Dalderby's unsightly and apparently leprous blemishes seemed curable. The verdict was, however, far less hopeful when, some eighteen years later, Sutton's successor selected a group of men 'skilled in the art of the practice of medicine' to examine another parish priest who vainly denied having the disease.[139] Although such scraps of information are often tantalisingly vague about the deliberations involved, it is clear that, as in mainland Europe, the *judicium* could be a long and meticulous business involving a comprehensive catalogue of tests and 'tokenes'.

As was also the case overseas, men and women who emerged free of any imputed leprosy were anxious to secure some form of certificate, which could be produced in the event of further trouble. These did not, however, come cheap, at least when issued by men whose fees might well amount to more than the annual income of a master craftsman, or even a chantry priest. Since the monks of Norwich cathedral priory enjoyed the best medical services then available in East Anglia, it is hardly surprising that they should make full use of professional advice when one of their number began to display incriminating symptoms. The case of Richard Walsham required careful handling, not least because administrative pressures had taken a heavy toll on his mental as well as physical health. His desire to retreat from the cloister to the peace of a hermitage may also have been prompted by speculation that he had contracted leprosy. It was in order to scotch such rumours that, shortly before January 1456, Prior John Molet called

---

136  Demaitre, 'Description and Diagnosis', p. 344; Risse, *Mending Bodies*, pp. 169–72; D. Jacquart, *La médecine médiévale dans le cadre Parisien* (Paris, 1998), p. 231.
137  *CRR, 1219–1220*, pp. 308–9.
138  *CRR, 1227–1230*, no. 247.
139  Satchell, 'Emergence of Leper-Houses', p. 50.

in a group of experienced practitioners.[140] Their verdict, reached after several visits, was recorded in a deed bearing his seal:

> Observing that, on account of the various illnesses from which he suffers, or because the levity of certain simple persons has taxed him with this, our said fellow monk has been suspected by some of bearing the signs of leprosy, we, taking steps for the discovery of the truth, have carefully arranged for many physicians and surgeons (*medicos plures et cirurgicos*) skilled in the knowledge and treatment of this disease to be summoned; and they, as a result of the evidence of his urine and other external tokens and proofs of his body and limbs, have on repeated occasions decided, agreed, and put down in their signed written statements, as a testimony to him and to our very great comfort, that this aforementioned beloved fellow monk of ours is wholly untouched by any infection of leprosy.[141]

Since, as we shall see in chapter six, many houses, including Norwich cathedral priory, ran their own *leprosaria* for infected brethren, incidents of this kind must have been a fairly regular feature of monastic life. Again, however, it seems that record keeping was far from systematic. Had brother Richard not wished to become a recluse, it is unlikely that his prior would have gone to such pains to provide the necessary documentation.

Two interesting cases of professional intervention followed appeals to the crown by individuals who felt that they had been misdiagnosed and faced removal from their communities as a result. The first, which bears all the hallmarks of local factionalism, involved Peter Nottleigh, sometime mayor of Winchester. He had been expelled from the city in 1312, soon after the promulgation of a royal order banning lepers from its streets. Concern about rootless beggars almost certainly lay behind the decree, which may have served as a useful pretext for the settlement of old scores. Nottleigh was duly examined before the royal council 'by physicians experienced in the knowledge of the disease' and given a clean bill of health. The result of this very public *judicium* was then communicated to the bailiffs of Winchester and sheriff of Hampshire, with orders that Nottleigh was to be molested no more.[142]

The examination of Joanna Nightingale of Brentwood, which took place 156 years later, is far better known, and is often described (with varying degrees of accuracy) in histories of medieval leprosy.[143] In July 1468, following complaints that Nightingale repeatedly refused to withdraw from public life despite her condition, the sheriff was ordered to summon 'discreet men of the county who have the best knowledge of Joanna's person and of the disease' to conduct a proper diagnosis. Should it prove positive, she was to leave home for 'a solitary

---

140  Details of Walsham's monastic career may be found in J. Greatrex, *Biographical Register of the English Cathedral Priories of the Province of Canterbury c. 1066–1540* (Oxford, 1997), pp. 568–9, although he is here mistakenly said to have been removed *because* of leprosy. For medical provision at Norwich cathedral priory, see Rawcliffe, 'Threshold of Eternity', pp. 41–72.

141  NRO, DCN 35/7.

142  *CCR, 1307–1313*, p. 559; *CPR, 1307–1313*, p. 534; D. Keene, *Survey of Medieval Winchester* (2 vols, Oxford, 1985), i, p. 80.

143  Sheldon Watts, *Epidemics and History*, p. 58, maintains that 'Considering the date of the incident . . . her accusers were as likely to have charged her with witchcraft.' It is, however, clear that Joanna manifested some symptoms likely to cause concern.

place, there to dwell as the manner is'. Before the sheriff could act, however, Joanna herself appeared in Chancery. Her powers of persuasion were such that she managed to arrange for a *judicium* by the king's three physicians, William Hattecliffe, Roger Marchall and Dominic de Sergio.[144] The trio of distinguished experts, who stood at the very peak of their profession, duly reported that they had begun with an examination of Joanna's body. They touched and handled her carefully for signs of the disease according to established principles devised by 'the older and most learned authorities on the subject'. A systematic assessment followed, whereby each of her symptoms was evaluated against an established checklist. Having explained that, 'according to medical science' (*ex scientia medicinali*), all types of leprosy shared certain common characteristics, they concluded that she did not manifest a sufficient number of the twenty-five best known ones to be pronounced leprous. 'And this is enough to free her from suspicion', they observed, 'since nobody can suffer from the disease unless they are afflicted by the greater part of these symptoms' (*multa pars huiusmodi signorum*). A more specific investigation, based on the forty or more signs associated with the four different humoral types (which the experts briefly identified) proved less equivocal, for Joanna displayed none of them.[145]

The duties of the king's physicians were carefully defined in the household ordinances of Edward IV, which required them 'to aspie if ony of this court be infected with leper or pestylence, and to warne the soueraynes of hym, till he be purged clene, [and] to kepe hym out of courte'.[146] Concern lest 'no perileous syk man . . . loge in the courte, but auoyd within iij dayes' clearly led to the removal of William Pole, one of Edward's yeomen, who was 'smitten with leprosy' and obliged to resign his position. Gratitude for his past service, as well as concern about the number of lepers reputedly 'walking at large within the realm', led the king to grant him a plot of land in Highgate, in 1473, so that he might build a *leprosarium*.[147] We may assume that he was just as carefully scrutinised for *signa infallibilia* before his departure, but there is no record of it. Indeed, since formal examinations were only mentioned if they had significant legal or administrative repercussions, we have no means of telling how common they may have been.[148] Royal physicians were certainly well informed about the manifold symptoms of

---

144  Brief biographies of these three men may be found in *MPIME*, pp. 36, 314–15, 398–9. Roger Marchall was a noted bibliophile, whose library contained many works on diagnostic procedures: L.E. Voigts, 'A Doctor and His Books: The Manuscripts of Roger Marchall (d. 1477)', in R. Beadle and A.J. Piper, eds, *New Science Out of Old Books* (Scolar Press, 1995), pp. 249–314.

145  *CPR, 1468–1476*, pp. 30–31. The Latin text appears in full in T. Rymer, ed., *Foedera, conventiones, literae et cuiuscunque generis acta publica*, V (The Hague, 1741), part 2, p. 166. Joanna's case shares many similarities with that of Pol Roze, a barber surgeon from Bethune, whose 'white morphew' was, in 1501, deemed to be an 'equivocal' sign of leprosy and thus, on its own, insufficient to condemn him. According to one of the examining physicians, he demonstrated eight 'unequivocal' signs out of a potential twenty-three or four: Bourgeois, *Lépreux et maladreries*, pp. 239–40.

146  A.R. Myers, ed., *The Household of Edward IV* (Manchester, 1959), p. 124.

147  *CPR, 1467–1477*, p. 373. In the previous year, Edward had complained about the number of lepers to be found begging on the streets of London: see below, pp. 281–2. Since Pole may already have been under scrutiny at this time, his case possibly sparked the king's anxiety.

148  The few documented instances of leprosy in the royal household generally involved the placement of valued servants in hospitals. In 1256, for example, one Walter Wastehus was sent to St Albans, presumably after a thorough examination: *CLR, 1251–1260*, p. 303.

*lepra* and, as the case of Joanna Nightingale shows, made much of a superior expertise acquired through years of study as well as practice. Joanna's examination was conducted with all the solemnity of the *collatio*, a formal consultation which drew upon the diagnostic and prognostic abilities of leading practitioners and was based upon the scholastic disputations held in faculties of medicine.[149] The emphasis placed by King Edward's medical advisers both upon their knowledge of theory – the *scientia medicinae* that dominated the first part of the north European medical syllabus – and their easy familiarity with ancient authors suggests vulnerability as well as pride.[150] Learning, honed by years of study of arts as well as medicine, set the graduate physician apart from the growing number of practitioners jostling for position in a crowded medical market place. But the gap was not as wide as he might have wished, and was closing fast.

Acting upon the advice of their eminent fourteenth-century colleague, John of Arderne, that 'the excercyse of bokes worshippeth a leche', many late medieval English surgeons zealously built up substantial libraries of their own. Although much of their training was acquired, like that of other craftsmen, through the highly pragmatic medium of apprenticeship, London surgeons, in particular, prided themselves upon their mastery of medical theory as well as 'manual operation'. Some, such as John Bradmore (d. 1412), who served at court and mixed on a regular basis with the king's physicians and apothecaries, were fluent in Latin and well versed in the basic university syllabus.[151] Indeed, Bradmore elected to compile his 'boke off surgery cald philomena' in Latin, drawing upon a range of established authorities, interspersed with occasional reflections upon his own wide experience.[152] His work contains a lengthy section on *lepra*, scabies and similar disorders that came under the surgeon's remit, and offers a comprehensive digest of information on aetiology, diagnosis and treatment. It begins, significantly, with instructions about the conduct of the *judicium*, recommending a comparison in bright moonlight between the faces of a healthy man and the suspect to reveal differences in colour. There follows a discussion of prophylactic measures, causation, common and specific symptoms and, at far greater length, a survey of the remedies which might be used to protect the vulnerable, arrest the disease in its early stages or, in the final resort, provide palliative care.[153]

---

149 Jacquart, *Médecine médiévale*, pp. 89–90.
150 C. Crisciani, 'Teachers and Learners in Scholastic Medicine: Some Images and Metaphors', *History of Universities*, xv (1997–99), pp. 75–101, at pp. 75–6. Professional rivalry may often have surfaced during the *judicium*: D. Jacquart, *Dictionnaire biographique des médecins en France au moyen âge* (Haute Etudes Médiévales et Modernes, series 5, xxxv, 1979), pp. 229, 238.
151 C. Rawcliffe, 'Master Surgeons at the Lancastrian Court', in Stratford, *Lancastrian Court*, pp. 192–210.
152 S.J. Lang, 'John Bradmore and his Book Philomena', *SHM*, v (1992), pp. 121–30.
153 BL, MS Sloane 2272 (part 1), fos 90v–100v. His accredited sources for the section on *lepra* include Haly Abbas, Gilbertus Anglicus, Avicenna, Guy de Chauliac, Roger Frugard, John of Gaddesden, Galen, Rhazes and Alexander of Tralles, although not all are quoted at first hand. The idea of conducting a moonlit examination comes from the Montpellier school: see *Le tresor des pauvres selon Maistre Arnoult de Ville Noue . . . et plusieurs aultre docteurs de medecine de Montpellier* (Lyon, 1512), fo. 37v; F.O. Touati, '*Facies leprosorum*: réflections sur le diagnostic facial de la lèpre au Moyen Age', *Histoire des Sciénces Médicales*, xx (1986), pp. 57–66, at p. 64. John Mirfield also recommended it: BL, MS Harley 3, fo. 23v.

Bradmore regarded the examination and care of lepers as a matter for both the physician and the surgeon,[154] but outside the privileged bastions of the aristocratic elite the task would, inevitably, have fallen more heavily upon the latter. Skilled practitioners of surgery were to be found in all the larger towns and cities of late medieval England. That they expected to play a full part in the *judicium* is, for example, apparent from an anonymous surgical work of 1446, which used Bradmore's book as one of its many sources. It, too, deals with *lepra*, on the grounds that 'yt ys nedfull ffor a surgene to haue knowlege ther off, ffor the wyche he may better do cur ther to, and also ffor to dysserne & deme [judge] trewly thes pepull that ar confermyd with lepur'. Anxious, like Edward IV's physicians, to establish his credentials in the face of ill-informed competition, the author explains that, because

> yt happons oft tymes to the surgens for to declar and [judge] lepurs, ther for wyll I spek off ther declaracion, schewynge schortly wych ar lepurs confermyd and wych ow to be dysseuered [separated] and partyd from the pepull with ther tokyns. It is to vndyrstond, after the comon pepull vndyr stondynge and beleuynge, that who so has any off thes tokyns schold be a lepur. That ys to say, rowndnes off eyne and the erys, lakynge off herys of the browes, spekynge in the nose, grettnese of lyppys, spekynge with a qwelpysch [hoarse] voice & a lowuysch, sik lokynge and horibull to the manur off a best cald a bauston.[155] And thow schall vndyrstond that any off thes for sayd tokyns alone aperand ar vnsekyr [insufficient] to deme a lepur by, ffor they may be causyd off odyr thynge than off lepurhod.[156]

Having carefully itemised a further fourteen signs of the disease in its various stages, he returns to the theme of popular ignorance, warning

> that non [no] lepours parsone be ryght wysse in demynge ow [ought] to be dysseuered [segregated] and partyd ffrom the comone pepull vnto [until] the fygur and the forme off [him] be corrupt & [he] haue sum rynnynge sores, *the wych myght infecte the eyr*. And yet, neuer the latter, now a daes ys done contrary, and specyally be demyng off them that has non vndyrstondynge ther in, the wyche ys contrary to reson.[157]

Given the intense competition that marked relations between the surgeons and barber surgeons of London during the fifteenth century, the author's strictures may have been directed as much against his commercial rivals as against 'amateur' diagnosticians, such as William Mustardere.

More numerous and readily available at prices to suit all pockets, the city's barbers would have played a notable part in the business of diagnosis at ward or

---

154 BL, MS Sloane 2272 (part 1), fo. 91v. The 'professional demarcation' observed by continental surgeons, such as Henri de Mondeville (Demaitre, 'Relevance of Futility', p. 37), did not obtain in England outside the royal court because so few university-trained physicians were practising medicine elsewhere.

155 A bausone or bawstone was a badger, piebald animal or beaver: *MED, B*, p. 674. The author is here attempting (at several removes) to translate Galen, who remarks that sufferers from *elephantia* looked like satyrs, or, as John Bradmore has it, a '*Saton in terra Arabica*': BL, MS Sloane 2272 (part 1), fo. 91v; *Claudii Galeni opera ominia*, vii, cap. XIV, pp. 727–8. See also above, p. 73.

156 BL, MS Harley 1736, fo.133v.

157 BL, MS Harley 1736, fos 134v–135r.

parish level.[158] Certainly, during periods of anxiety about pestilence and vagrancy, members of their guild were charged with the keepership of the city gates so that exclusion orders might be carried out more effectively. Thus, for example, in 1375, a barber named William Duerhurst swore, as porter at Aldgate, that he would prevent any lepers from entering London, if necessary confiscating their horses or outer garments or even placing them under arrest.[159] It would be surprising if other walled cities, such as York and Norwich, both of which boasted a sizeable guild of well-educated barber surgeons, did not occasionally follow suit.[160] Partly because of their ambivalent status, barbers rarely rose to occupy the upper ranks of the urban elite, but were often elected to minor office as ward constables, bailiffs and the like. Here, too, they were ideally placed to police their communities for dangerous symptoms. Richard Dod, a fifteenth-century London barber surgeon, was, for example, the proud owner of a book on the nature and cure of diseases, which contained a section on the identification, causes and treatment of leprosy. Translated into English, it provided all the basic information he would have required.[161]

## Popular perceptions: juries and presentments

Around 300 *leprosaria* have so far been identified in England before the early fourteenth century, about 85 per cent of which were modest suburban foundations, established to accommodate the residents of towns and cities.[162] Regarded as part of the 'obligatory landscape of urban development', which proclaimed the relative status and size of growing communities, these institutions reflect that striking combination of Christian compassion and growing concern about pollution discussed in the previous two chapters.[163] But they did not, as we shall see, offer places to everyone on an indiscriminate basis. In addition, an unknown, but significant, number of confirmed lepers elected either to remain in private quarters at home, to live in unstructured extramural groups or take to the road as beggars. The deliberations preceding their withdrawal or departure are rarely documented, and it is unlikely that more than a small proportion experienced the full scrutiny of the *judicium*. Many would have undergone what might best be described as an informal diagnostic review, conducted at parochial level by members of their immediate circle, but with the passage of time inspections by local 'experts' became the norm. Since these procedures were eventually administered and enforced by the courts, diagnosis thus became as much a

---

158   See T. Beck, *The Cutting Edge: Early History of the Surgeons of London* (London, 1974), chapters seven and eight; Rawcliffe, *Medicine and Society*, chapter six.

159   Riley, *Memorials*, p. 384. Gerard the Barber was made responsible for Newgate in 1310: R.R. Sharpe, ed., *Calendar of Letter-Books of the City of London, Letter-Book D* (London, 1902), p. 241. Another barber was appointed to report on 'disturbances of filth' and other health hazards in Langbourne ward (ibid., p. 312).

160   Rawcliffe, *Medicine and Society*, pp. 134–37.

161   BL, MS Sloane 5, fos 61r–157v, at fos 153r–155v.

162   Satchell, 'Emergence of Leper-Houses', p. 81.

163   Touati, *Archives*, pp. 73–4; P. Cullum, 'Leperhouses and Borough Status in the Thirteenth Century', in P. Coss and S.D. Lloyd, eds, *Thirteenth-Century England III* (Woodbridge, 1991), pp. 37–46.

matter for the law as it was for the family, the priesthood and the medical profession.

The manorial and borough courts of later medieval England functioned at two levels. On the one hand, they served to enforce the common law, as defined by the judiciary with regard to statute and precedent, and as interpreted in the numerous directives of an increasingly centralised royal bureaucracy.[164] On the other, their task was to ensure that local customs and regulations were observed. A significant, and growing, proportion of the latter related to environmental hazards, such as noxious dung heaps and sub-standard food, which impinged upon most aspects of communal life. Perceived threats to moral as well as physical health inspired particular vigilance, especially in a society fearful of the divine arrows of pestilence. As we shall see in chapter six, a growing hostility to unauthorised begging and prostitution, as well as fear of the miasmas of disease, meant that the Levitical ruling on lepers assumed greater urgency in periods of social upheaval. Save in exceptional circumstances, however, the crown recognised that the elimination or prevention of nuisances was a quotidian problem of urban or village life, and thus best tackled *in situ* by the appropriate authorities. Towns such as Launceston in Cornwall jealously guarded their liberties, which, in 1383, included the right 'from time immemorial' to remove any leper who 'entered within the gates of the borough'.[165] From Dublin to Yarmouth and Bristol to Berwick-on-Tweed, magistrates sought to prohibit anyone afflicted with *lepra* from living within the walls, although these regulations, like others concerning blocked drains, wandering animals and similar nuisances, tended to be applied sporadically in the aftermath of local or national epidemics.[166] Manorial courts responded in a similar fashion.

In theory, if not in practice, the legal processes involved in making complaints or 'presentments' about particular individuals or problems presupposed a considerable degree of unanimity. The headmen or capital pledges who made up the juries of manorial and borough courts spoke as representatives of smaller units known as tithings (originally of ten men each) and were expected to represent them at views of frankpledge, when communal problems were discussed. They served under oath and might be fined if they concealed public nuisances or made false accusations. The two Norwich juries that presented Thomas Fuystor and Isabel Lucas as lepers in 1390–91 must already have debated their condition at length, sounding out other members of the community, and perhaps approaching a parish priest, apothecary or barber surgeon for advice.[167] This system could, as we shall see, engender a culture of victimisation – Isabel's foul gutter and unpalatable ale cannot have won her many friends – but at best it made possible a degree of consensus about symptoms. How well informed might the tithingmen have been?

According to the late thirteenth-century *Mirror of Justices*, 'married women, deaf mutes, sick folk, idiots and lepers' were excluded from the view of

---

164  For the common law in relation to *lepra*, see below, pp. 271–4.
165  *CIM, 1377–1388*, no. 265.
166  See pp. 274–84, below.
167  Hudson, *Leet Jurisdiction*, pp. xxvi–xxxii, 71, 72 (lepers had also been presented in 1374–75, p. 68).

frankpledge, whilst those eligible to sit on a jury had, additionally, to be of free status.[168] But more subtle considerations were also involved. Studies of medieval village communities have revealed a system of local government that was more sophisticated and hierarchical than might at first be supposed. Wealthier residents with a larger share of customary land tended to dominate the juries of manorial courts, and to exercise a disproportionate influence in the matter of presentments. As the remit of local juries expanded in the thirteenth century to embrace a wide range of offences and nuisances, so too the expertise of these leading freeholders increased exponentially.[169] Although they might employ charges of leprosy to remove social undesirables, they were also more likely to have access to medical information. However modest their administrative status, minor manorial officials were not only familiar with basic diagnostic principles, but also knew how to apply them. The commonplace book (c. 1470) of Robert Reynes of Acle in Norfolk contains detailed instructions about bloodletting interleaved between a note of his duties as an officer of the watch and lists of taxes paid by members of his community.[170] His contemporary, John Crophill, of Wix on the Suffolk-Essex border, supplemented his income as bailiff for the local Benedictine nunnery by practising as a leech, herbalist and astrologer. Since his many skills extended to uroscopy, he would, in theory, have been able to perform some of the more complex tests for 'occult' signs required at a formal *judicium*.[171]

The case of Joanna Nightingale demonstrates that it was possible to challenge a presentment for leprosy by making an appeal to a higher legal authority. The best most ordinary men and women might hope for, though, was an examination by 'discreet men of the county' familiar with their symptoms and with the disease, or at least a stay of judgement, which many local authorities were prepared to offer. Given that suspects might attempt to prolong the process indefinitely, heavy financial securities could be demanded as an earnest of their readiness to accept a final diagnosis. Whether such unrealistic amounts were ever actually paid is another matter. At the Norfolk manor of Heacham, on 8 September 1310, twelve mainpernors, or guarantors, came forward to attest that a villein named John Hardy was, indeed, healthy, notwithstanding the sworn testimony of other 'good and lawful men, both workers and villeins of the lord' who made up the jury. The steward, William de Secheford, handed John over to his friends on the clear understanding that he would leave the manor before 1 November, should the jurors be proved right. Unfortunately, we know nothing

168  W.J. Whittaker, ed., *The Mirror of Justices* (Selden Society, vii, 1895), pp. 39–40. 'Open lepers' were among the substantial category of persons who might not be justices: ibid., p. 44.

169  R.M. Smith, 'Modernistation and the Corporate Medieval Village Community in England: Some Sceptical Reflections', in A.R.H. Baker and D. Gregory, eds, *Explorations in Historical Geography: Interpretative Essays* (Cambridge, 1984), pp. 173–4; P. Hyams, 'What Did Edwardian Villages Understand by "Law"?', in Z. Razi and R.M. Smith, eds, *Medieval Society and the Manor Court* (Oxford, 1966), p. 77.

170  C. Louis, ed., *The Commonplace Book of Robert Reynes of Acle: An Edition of Tanner MS 407* (New York, 1980), pp. 167–71.

171  L.J. Ayoub, 'John Crophill's Books: An Edition of British Library MS Harley 1735' (University of Toronto, PhD, 1994), corrects various misapprehensions in J.K. Mustain, 'A Rural Medical Practitioner in Fifteenth-Century England', *BHM*, xlvi (1972), pp. 469–76.

of the procedures then put into place, save that on 21 December John's goods, lands and tenement were confiscated and his mainpernors deemed collectively to have forfeited the sum of £40 to their lord. It is highly unlikely that the twelve individuals concerned were ever required to honour their pledges. Indeed, since all John's possessions were then granted to them, as his trustees, we may reasonably assume that they had in effect been bound over to manage the property for him in a responsible fashion as the law required.[172] Yet, whoever re-examined John Hardy clearly commanded sufficient authority to secure his prompt expulsion from the community. The steward may well have enlisted a local empiric, priest or itinerant *medicus* to provide an informed opinion.

When dealing with matters that required particular skills or knowledge, such as the assaying of sub-standard merchandise or tasting of ale, the courts could always call upon a reserve of expert help. At King's Lynn in 1376 a special jury of twelve leading townsmen, or jurats, was selected '*pro scrutino leprosorum*' after initial presentments had been made. This may have been a routine practice, for an entry in the town's first Assembly Book records that in March 1429 three people recently presented as lepers (*leprosi nominati*) had appeared before the authorities, so 'that their infirmity might be proved by discreet persons having knowledge in this respect'.[173] With its encircling ring of nine *leprosaria*, Lynn maintained the most impressive institutional provision for the disease in East Anglia, and evidently imposed strict controls upon suspects [**map 2**]. Were they, perhaps, unusually harsh? Françoise Bériac has suggested that, in France, qualified medical practitioners often resisted popular pressure to pronounce suspects leprous, offering them a more cautious, impartial and independent diagnosis than that proclaimed *vox populi*. This was evidently the experience of Peter Nottleigh and Joanna Nightingale, and also the view of our anonymous surgeon, although we cannot necessarily assume that all local communities rushed to judgement. In 1331, probably in response to the prompting of some concerned official, the bailiff of Beverley was ordered to send a list of lepers residing in the town to Chancery. He named five, two of whom had reputedly 'been afflicted' for three years, one for two years and the others for at least twelve months. The authorities seem to have been unconcerned about the risk to others.[174]

As nineteenth- and early twentieth-century colonial administrators discovered, native populations exposed to Hansen's disease were capable of diagnosing all but the most problematic cases without the benefit of Western medical expertise.[175] We may likewise assume that the residents of medieval English towns and villages could distinguish *lepra* in its advanced form, however rudimentary their knowledge of contemporary medical theory may have been. Yet, from a fairly early date, as we saw at the start of this chapter, they were exposed to a steady stream of increasingly specialist information, which, at the very least, provided a rationale for the decision to exclude certain individuals from the community,

---

172  NRO, Le Strange MS DA6, m. 2; E. Clark, 'Social Welfare and Mutual Aid in the Medieval Countryside', *Journal of British Studies*, xxxiii (1994), pp. 381–406, at p. 396.

173  R.F. Isaacson and H. Ingleby, eds, *The Red Register of King's Lynn* (2 vols, King's Lynn, n.d.), ii, p. 122; King's Lynn Borough Archives, KL/C7/2, p. 242.

174  Bériac, *Histoire des lépreux*, p. 62; *CIM*, 1307–1349, no. 1268, p. 310.

175  Silla, *People Are Not the Same*, pp. 96–7. See also, Watts, *Epidemics and History*, pp. 81–2.

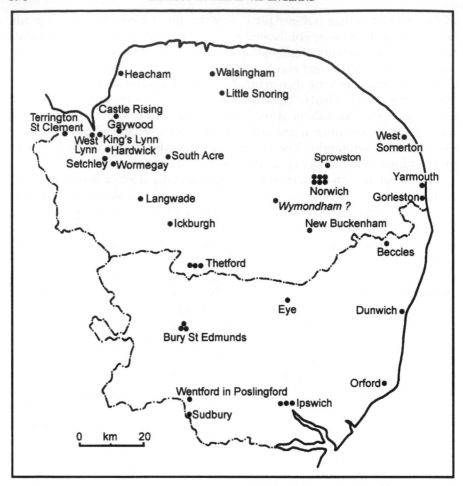

Map 2. The leper houses of medieval East Anglia (Phillip Judge)

while allowing others the benefit of the doubt. Ecclesiastical propaganda, such as that used to advertise Becket's miracles, provides a fairly consistent list of the signs commonly associated with the disease in its progressive state, the most obvious being easily discernible by sight and smell. Is it possible to gain a similar impression of the diagnostic criteria adopted as a rule of thumb by jurors, employers and officials? Did the same concerns about facial symptoms, miasma and vocal damage still obtain?

Disregarding for a moment the potentially self-fulfilling argument that medieval men and women would have encountered lepers on a regular basis, begging in the outskirts of towns or at the gates of extramural hospitals, and thus have grown familiar with their symptoms, we can identify a few other useful pointers. In his seminal text on *The Laws and Customs of England*, the jurist, Henry Bracton (d. 1268), ruled that the decision to exclude a leprous person from the community, and thus from the right to plead in a court of law, might be taken in cases of serious and visible deformity. As we saw in chapter two, the individual in question should appear horrifying to the beholder.[176] In practice, this graphic, but highly subjective, requirement presupposed extreme facial disfigurement, and reflects the assumptions of medical authorities from Aretaeus the Cappadocian onwards. Although his work was not widely known in the medieval West, it is worth quoting here what this observant physician has to say about *elephantia*:

> But the commencement of this disease gives no great indication of it; neither does it appear as if any unusual ailment had come upon the man; nor does it display itself upon the surface of the body, so that it might be immediately seen, and remedies applied at the commencement; but lurking among the bowels, like a concealed fire it smoulders there, and having prevailed over the internal parts, it afterwards blazes forth on the surface, for the most part beginning, like a bad signal fire, *on the face*, as it were a watch tower.[177]

No less an authority than Bernard Gordon confessed utter bewilderment at the appearance of one long-term patient, whose body seemed leprous, but whose face remained entirely unblemished for over twenty years. Perhaps, he conjectured, an unusual combination of diseases had produced this anomaly, which seemed to contradict all the great medical authorities, including Galen. Wishing to protect the man from the inevitable stigma of a positive diagnosis, he rather fudged the issue, but reported his deliberations at length to assist others. After all, as he observed, people took far better care of their faces and might thus be able to avoid detection.[178] Yet his guide to the diagnosis of *lepra*, as rendered into simple English during the second quarter of the fifteenth century, is unambiguous in describing facial deformity as a principal indicator of physical deterioration:

> Whan the heris fallith awey of the browys and they bycomyth grete, and his eighen bycomyth rounde, and his nostrell bycomyth grete with outforthe and strayte [narrow] with in, & strayte of brethe, and he spekith alle as it were with the nostrell, and the coloure of his face becometh ledy & ffusk [dark] & horrible byhaldynge, & with drawynge off the browys and of the nostrell. And by oon signe herof we schul not iugye hyt, saf by 2 other 3. These signes beth the most serteyne signys of alle, and there bith many othere, as pustule, & wexinges & wastynges awey of hys braun [flesh], & prinspaly that is bytwixe the thombe & the nexte fynger therto, & brekynge of the skyn, and whan his blode is y-wasch therbith blacke gobettes theron and as it were grauel, & many othere, but these signys sufficeth to me & *prinspaly signes that beth in the fface* . . . these thynges beth direct, & knowe in wham that they schewe he is sequestered.[179]

---

[176] Thorne, *Bracton*, iv, p. 309.

[177] Adams, *Extant Works of Aretaeus*, p. 368. His view that, once *elephantia* had reached this point, 'the patient is in a hopeless condition' (ibid., p. 494), was shared by many subsequent authors: Demaitre, 'Relevance of Futility', p. 30; Cholmeley, *John of Gaddesden*, p. 47.

[178] Demaitre, *Doctor Bernard de Gordon*, pp. 124–5. The problem of making an accurate diagnosis from the limbs alone emerges in the case of Henry Bounde, whose immobile arm was attributed variously by medical experts to paralysis, dropsy and *lepra* – the latter because of his scabies and tumours. He was miraculously cured by the controversial 'saint and martyr', Simon de Montfort (d. 1265), who had been dismembered on the battlefield: J.O. Halliwell, ed., *The Miracles of Simon de Montfort* (CS, old series, xv, 1840), p. 98.

[179] Bodleian Library, MS Ashmole 1505, fos 30v–31r. Guy de Chauliac agreed that 'the tokenes of the

Having itemised various other symptoms, including alopecia, corrupt breath, disturbed sleep and ulcerated flesh, Bernard reiterated his warning about the importance of close, long-term observation. Proof positive of the disease in its terminal stages was, once again, chiefly to be found in the face,

> whan that boon bytwix his twey nostrill that is clepyd *cartilago* ffretith & ffallith awey and whan hys hondys brekyth and hys fete fallith awey, and whan hys lippes bycomyth grete and hys body is glandulous . . . and he may noght wel drawe hys brethe, and his voyse sounyth as it were a cattis, & horrible lokynge, and the colour of hys face [is] blacke and his voys is rawe and hys pouse [pulse] lytel.[180]

The popular conviction that *lepra* had to affect the features before a firm diagnosis could be made is apparent from at least one successful suit for defamation, brought in 1413 by Christine Colmere, an alewife of Canterbury. Arguing that she was 'as *healthy and clean in the face* as she was accustomed to be, without disfigurement of leprosy', one witnesses for the prosecution maintained that she could not therefore be infected, as a commercial rival had claimed.[181] Conversely, the case of Margery Kempe's prodigal son, whose employer sacked him 'for no defawte he found with hym, but perauentur supposyng he had ben a lazer *as it schewyd be his vysage*', underscores how much appearances mattered.[182]

Understandably anxious to present a reassuring image to the public, the London barber surgeons ruled in 1482 that the master and wardens would henceforward 'duely examyne, oversee, serche and behold' every new apprentice and journeyman 'by the colour and complexion . . . if he be avexed or disposed to be lepur or gowty, maymed or disfigured'.[183] The city's grocers were likewise concerned that new recruits should be 'clen from lepur als fer as couth be consyderyd'.[184] As prime consumers of the burgeoning genre of advice literature, these wealthy entrepreneurs expected their servants and apprentices to be 'clenli clad', their 'handis & face waschen fayre' and their hair 'well kempt'.[185] Since facial blemishes were still regarded as the outward manifestation of a deformed soul in the sixteenth century, it is easy to see that nervousness extended far beyond the pages of medical literature.[186] Sensitivity on this score, as much as the contemporary obsession with deference, explains why one fifteenth-century Norwich merchant was fined the remarkable sum of £10 (a more than respect-

---

face ben moste certeyne': Ogden, *Cyrurgie of Guy de Chauliac*, p. 382, while John of Gaddesden advised that separation should not take place until 'the figure and form' of the face had changed: *Rosa Anglica*, fo. 57r.

[180] Bodleian Library, MS Ashmole 1505, fo. 31r.

[181] Helmholz, *Defamation*, pp. 5–6.

[182] See above, p. 85.

[183] T.A. Young, *Annals of the Barber-Surgeons of London* (London, 1890), p. 62.

[184] This ruling was made in 1429: J.A. Kingdon, ed., *Facsimile of First Volume of Ms Archives of the Wordshipful Company of Grocers of the City of London* (2 vols, London, 1886), ii, p. 180.

[185] F.J. Furnivall, ed., *The Babees Book* (EETS, xxxii, 1868), part 1, p. 176. See also pp. 29, 180–81, 309, and part 2, pp. 8–9, 16, 20.

[186] M. Pelling, 'Appearance and Reality: Barber-Surgeons, the Body and Disease', in A.L. Beier and R. Finlay, eds, *London, 1500–1700: The Making of the Metropolis* (New York and London, 1986), pp. 89–90.

able annual salary) for calling one of the city's aldermen 'gresii face and bocherfface'.[187]

Unless they were reduced to beggary and dressed in rags, medieval men and women displayed very little flesh in public. The face thus became a prime focus of attention, being widely regarded as a mirror of health, temperament and probity. We have already encountered the priest who could 'read' his parishioners' sins in their faces, a divine gift which less privileged mortals sought to acquire through the study of physiognomy. It is interesting to note that a compilation of important medical texts made at the turn of the fourteenth century for the infirmarer of St Mary's abbey, Coventry, included three short Latin works on this topic.[188] Vernacular versions already circulated widely at this time, often alongside guides to phlebotomy, uroscopy and other medical matters. Some were attributed to the great Classical authorities, Hippocrates and Aristotle, whose names lent credibility to an ideal of integrated physical and moral proportion. Whereas 'a long face & a croked' was believed to reflect a mendacious and 'gylefull' character, one could always rely upon a man whose smooth, pink-hued flesh, clear, round eyes and even features manifestly reflected his personal qualities.[189] The eye, in particular, as the organ projecting the very light of the soul, presented an unerring barometer of each person's physical and spiritual condition. The monastic chronicler, Jocelin of Brakelond (d. 1202), for example, need only observe that Abbot Samson's eyes were 'crystal clear, with a penetrating gaze' to assure us of his capacity for leadership. Conversely, physiognomies warned that swollen, discoloured or ulcerated eyes, of the kind described above, hinted at a far deeper malaise.[190]

It is hard to tell how far these beliefs influenced quotidian responses to *lepra* and other disfiguring skin diseases, but their evident popularity clearly underscored the significance accorded by medical writers to facial symptoms. Religious writing, of which the various legends surrounding the leprous pilgrim of St Denis furnish the most striking example, had long concentrated upon them. Indeed, the miraculous preservation of his mask-like features, 'in such a way that the subcutaneous humour still seemed to ooze from the ulcerated scars' speaks volumes about the way lepers were supposed to appear.[191] Devotional literature on the Passion, which, as we saw in chapter two, dwelt at length upon the deformity of *Christus quasi leprosus*, reveals a similar preoccupation. The harrowing imagery leaves little to the imagination:

> Our beloved Lord's holy *face* was as miserably transformed and disfigured as if He had been a leprous man; because the foul snot and the filthy yellow spittle of the

---

187   R. Frost, 'The Urban Elite', in C. Rawcliffe and R. Wilson, eds, *The History of Norwich* (2 vols, London, 2004), i, p. 240.

188   BL, MS Royal 12 G IV, fos 137r–140v. For the emphasis placed upon the quality of the skin (*subtilitas cutis*) in medieval physiognomies, see J. Ziegler, 'Skin and Character in Medieval and Early Renaissance Physiognomy', in *La pelle umana*, pp. 511–35.

189   Wellcome Institute Library, Western MS 510, fos 19r–22v. See also Western MSS 507, fos 49r–70r; 517, fos 115r–122r; 548, fos 151v–152v; 552, fos 20r–21v; above, pp. 139–40.

190   Jocelin of Brakelond, *Chronicles of the Abbey of Bury St Edmunds*, eds D. Greenway and J. Sayers (Oxford, 1989), p. 36; Wellcome Institute Library, Western MS 510, fo. 22r.

191   Lombard-Jourdan, *Saint-Denis*, pp. 199–200.

unclean malefactors lay baked and dried upon His holy *face*, and His sacred red
blood had thickly overflowed His *face*, hanging from it in congealed pieces, in such
a manner that the Lord appeared as if His *face* were covered in boils and sores.[192]

The proliferation of such relentless accounts of Christ's torments was matched
by an obsessive focus upon visual depictions of His macerated body. At the same
time, the icongraphy of *lepra* (and, indeed, of other diseases, including ergotism)
grew increasingly realistic.[193] The artistic convention whereby biblical lepers, in
particular, appeared semi-naked and spotted gave way to – or more accurately
continued alongside – an attempt to render specific symptoms in a more natu-
ralistic and recognisable fashion.[194]

Tracing this development from the arrival in the West of Avicenna's *Canon*,
which first emphasised the effects of *lepra* on the face, F.O. Touati detects a
striking correspondence between representations of the disease in art and medicine. The growing number of suburban *leprosaria* must also have influenced
these developments. It was easy enough to transport Job or the wretched Lazarus
to the gates of any late medieval city, where the artist could find a regular supply
of models. As Touati points out, most of the lepers who solicited alms and went
about their business in these places were decently covered, often by a copious
habit, and would reveal little more than their faces, hands and feet.[195] This, for
example, is the appearance presented by the female leper depicted in the margin
of the fourteenth-century Exeter Pontifical. Lacking her extremities, and
demonstrating characteristic facial symptoms, including a collapsed nose, she
personifies the many descriptions of 'lepur confyrmyd' listed in contemporary
medical works [**plate 20**]. Like Robert Henryson's Cresseid, she has good reason
to complain that 'now is deformit the figour of my face'.[196] A series of pen and
ink caricatures added at this time to the cartulary of the *leprosarium* of
Saint-Lazare at Meaux presents the inmates in profile, their foreheads, noses,
eyes and mouths grossly misshapen by disease.[197] Similar images may be found
in late medieval English woodcuts and drawings of the children of the planets, in
which Saturn's melancholy brood invariably includes at least one individual
whose facial features and limbs conform to type [**plate 11**].[198]

Partly because so much was lost at the Reformation, England possesses far
fewer examples of artistic representations of leprosy than survive in continental
Europe, although it is clear that some, at least, went far beyond the crude delin-
eation of symptoms. Perhaps in order to bring home a warning about the dire

[192] J.H. Marrow, *Passion Iconography in Northern European Art in the Late Middle Ages and Early Renaissance* (Kortrijk, 1979), pp. 53–4. Richard Rolle's influential *Meditations on the Passion* reiterate this
theme: 'thi lovely face so wan and so bolnyd with bofetynge and with betynge, with spyttynge, with
spowtynge . . . so lothly and so wlatsome [loathsome] the Jues han the mad, that a mysel art thou
lyckere than a clene man': Allen, *English Writings of Richard Rolle*, p. 21.

[193] A. Hayum, *The Isenheim Altarpiece: God's Medicine and the Painter's Vision* (Princeton, 1989).

[194] For a basic overview of the topic see W.B. Ober, 'Can the Leper Change his Spots? The Iconography
of Leprosy', *The American Journal of Dermatopathology*, v (1983), pp. 43–58, 173–85.

[195] Touati, '*Facies leprosorum*', pp. 58–64; and below, pp. 298, 305, 308–9, 311.

[196] Henryson, *Testament of Cresseid*, p. 77.

[197] Touati, '*Facies leprosorum*', fig. 3, p. 61.

[198] Brown and Butcher, *Age of Saturn*, plates 4–7. As we saw in chapter two, they were notoriously
'blacke, fowle, slotty & slowe . . . and the coloure of thir heddys ar wan': BL, MS Sloane, 1315, p. 36.

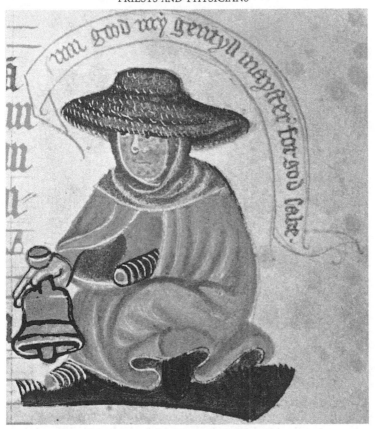

20. Begging at the wayside ('sum good my gentyll mayster for god sake'), this leper rings a bell to attract alms. The drawing appears in an English pontifical of *c.* 1425, and depicts the lost limbs and facial disfigurement associated with advanced cases of *lepra*. Since vocal damage would almost certainly have accompanied these more obvious symptoms, the bell would have been essential in order for the leper to make herself heard.

consequences of rapacity, the carved leper head in the angel choir of Lincoln cathedral (1255–80) presents a disturbing image of extreme facial distortion.[199] Although the subject still possesses a luxuriant beard and head of hair, the insidious destruction of the nasal cartilage, eyes, and mouth is clearly apparent, suggesting that the mason was personally familiar with *lepra* in its advanced state [**plate 21**]. There is good reason to believe that all but the very poorest leper hospitals would have been decorated with appropriate iconography, however rudimentary, while the richer foundations, such as Burton Lazars, enjoyed the

---

[199] Marcombe, *Leper Knights*, pp. 138–40, speculates that the head might be that of Robert FitzPernel, whose fate is discussed above, p. 52. Since the choir was constructed in honour of Hugh of Lincoln, the carving may have been intended to commemorate his celebrated love of lepers, however 'livid, diseased and deformed' their faces might be: Douie and Farmer, *Life of St Hugh*, ii, pp. 12–13.

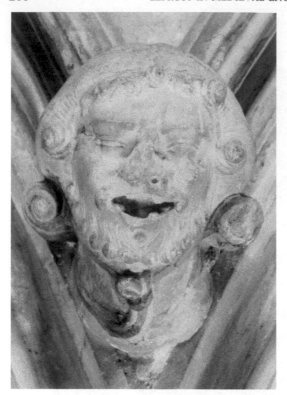

21. The thirteenth-century head of a leper, carved in stone in the angel choir of Lincoln Cathedral, which was constructed in memory of St Hugh of Lincoln, a notable patron of the leprous poor. It depicts in realistic detail the destruction of nasal cartilage, eyes and mouth, characteristic of *lepra* in its advanced state.

resources and patronage to aim far higher. Another carved leper head of *c.* 1250–1350, now in the local church, may originally have belonged to the nearby hospital of the knights of St Lazarus, who is perhaps the subject. Whatever its provenance, this, too, displays a clear understanding of the unequivocal signs which would have influenced jurors and practitioners alike.[200]

Even when their medium permitted the full-length depiction of a leprous beggar, pilgrim or patient, late medieval glaziers and illuminators tended increasingly to concentrate upon facial features that the viewer would immediately recognise. The artist who commemorated Abbot Richard Wallingford of St Albans in a list of benefactors had little choice but to focus upon the ulcerated, hairless and swollen face that emerges from the folds of his flowing habit [**plate 22**]. Yet he goes beyond a purely stylized rendition of *lepra* to record evidence of nasal and ocular damage in his portrait of the eminent scientist.[201] Rather more significant in this context is the portrayal of humbler lepers. Thus, for instance, the Norwich glass painter commissioned, in 1453, to produce a panel showing St Elizabeth of Hungary among the poor, paid unusual attention to the damaged profiles and leonine features of the supplicants at her feet [**plate 23**]. Likewise, the leprous woman who appears in the St William window of York Minster (*c.*

---

[200]  K. Manchester and D. Marcombe, 'The Melton Mowbray "Leper Head": An Historical and Medical Investigation', *Medical History*, xxxiv (1990), pp. 86–91.

[201]  See also BL, MS Cotton Claudius E IV, fo. 201r, which is more conventional in its depiction of the abbot's 'spots'.

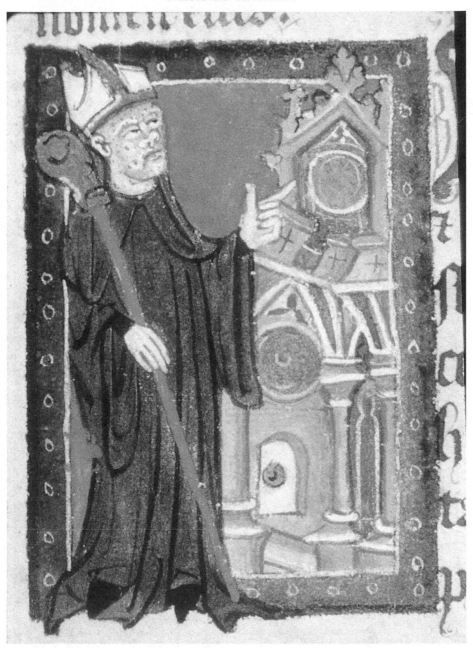

22. Abbot Richard Wallingford of St Albans (d. 1336) is portrayed in the abbey's Book of Benefactors of *c.* 1380 as both a leper and a distinguished scientist with a passion for clocks.

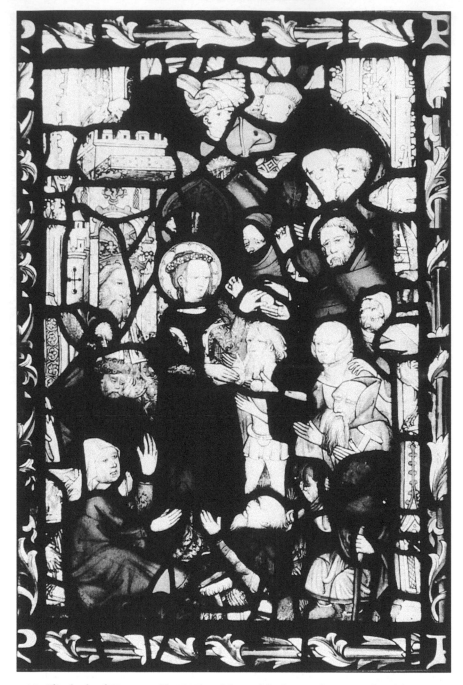

23. Elizabeth of Hungary (d. 1231), celebrated for her work among the sick poor and lepers, gives alms to the needy. This stained glass panel of *c.* 1453 from the church of St Peter Mancroft in Norwich depicts the facial and bodily disfigurements of the recipients with considerable realism. The face of the individual in the bottom right hand corner, in particular, is a mass of vivid sores.

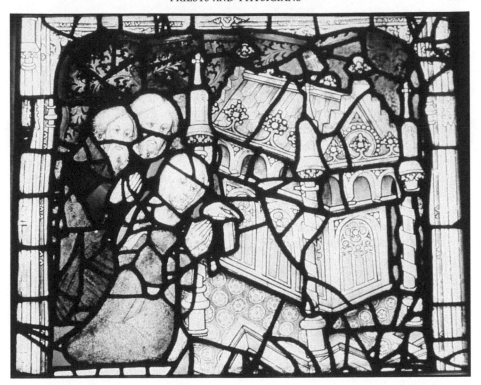

24.  A stained glass panel from the St William window of York Minster (*c.* 1423)
illustrates the miraculous cure of a female leper at the saint's shrine. Although the
original account of this miracle says nothing about her facial lesions, the artist has
added them in the interests of verisimilitude.

1423) may be identified by her misshapen nose and facial lesions as she
approaches the shrine. Significantly, the original account of this miracle does
not mention any specific symptoms, beyond observing that her face had
assumed a deathly pallor [**plate 24**].[202]

That suspect lepers should spend so much time and money upon the eradication of incriminating blemishes – and endure such acute physical discomfort in
the process – will surely not surprise. For after diagnosis came prognosis, which,
in the case of an equivocal judgement, would depend upon the patient's readiness to follow medical advice. If incipient *lepra* were caught in time, proper
humoral management might arrest its course, thus obviating the need for segregation. One old pauper from Bethune, in the Pas de Calais, was, for example,
examined in 1541 by four surgeons, who expressed alarm at the state of his body,
but were reassured that his head had so far escaped unscathed by any signs of
*lepra*. Hope remained. He was warned to keep a safe distance from healthy
people as he went about begging, and to behave circumspectly until the disease

202  J. Raine, ed., *Historians of the Church of York and its Archbishops* (3 vols, RS, 1879–94), ii, pp. 287–88;
J. Fowler, 'On a Window Representing the Life and Miracles of St William of York', *Yorkshire Archaeological and Topographical Journal*, iii (1873–74), pp. 198–348, at p. 318.

had been 'purged by a good regimen'.[203] Similar cases occurred in England, as men and women whose symptoms appeared uncertain awaited a final verdict, quite possibly dying before one was delivered. Some of them may well have been suffering from Hansen's disease, which, as we saw at the start of this book, takes many forms and often leaves the face unharmed. Charlotte Roberts has commented upon the unusually high proportion of leper burials excavated in urban and rural churchyards (thirty-three known sites) as opposed to those found in the cemeteries of *leprosaria* (a mere five sites at the time of writing).[204] As we shall see, the Church's efforts to provide leper hospitals with their own graveyards did not preclude the interment of patients elsewhere. On the other hand, many of the individuals whose skeletal remains present conclusive evidence of Hansen's disease to the trained palaeopathologist may well have displayed 'vnsekyr tokenes' of *lepra* to contemporaries. Living under the watchful eye of their communities, they took every possible step to halt any further physical deterioration. We shall now explore the ways in which this might be done.

[203] Bourgeois, *Lépreux et maladreries*, pp. 240–41, and also pp. 30, 239 n. 47, 314 n.108. See also Touati, '*Facies leprosorum*', p. 63, for a similar case of 1327 from Nîmes.
[204] Roberts, 'The Antiquity of Leprosy in Britain: The Skeletal Evidence', *PPL*, pp. 213–21.

# 5

## Medicine and Surgery:
## The Battle against Disease

*The treatment practised by the early physicians of this disease appears to have been founded on the principles of rational medicine, and to the present day we have made little progress beyond that point . . . our energies will be better employed in being devoted to the perfection of this plan than in seeking farther into the obscurity of experimental medicine. Aretaeus, who has left so excellent an account of elephantiasis in his writings, lays down as the proper plan for treatment the practice of venesection, followed by the use of purgatives, diluents, baths and inunction with fat, assisted by a plain, nutritious, and wholesome diet, accompanying the latter, if the powers of the constitution be reduced, with wine . . . amongst other medicinal substances employed, are decoctions of simples, particularly the plantain, and the flesh of serpents, which was held in high repute by the ancients; and when properly prepared, seems to have made a very agreeable article of diet, corresponding with the turtle-soup of the present day.*

Erasmus Wilson, The Lancet, 1856 [1]

In November 1408, a Flemish leech called John Luter delivered a sworn statement before the mayor and recorder of London. He was then being sued in Chancery by John Clotes, whom he had recently been treating, but who now sought to recover the substantial sum of £20 from him in lost goods and damages. Clotes alleged that some six weeks earlier he had surrendered fifteen semi-precious stones called 'serpentys' worth £6,[2] a gold tablet valued at 60s. and a sword, all of which the defendant was to keep should he succeed in curing him 'of a certain disease called *lepra*'.[3] His efforts had failed, yet the pledge had not been returned. Somewhat implausibly, Luter protested that he had undertaken the case on the strict understanding that Clotes was suffering from *salsefleume*[4]

---

1    E. Wilson, 'On the Nature and Treatment of Leprosy Ancient and Modern', *The Lancet*, lxvii, issue 1696 (1 March 1856), pp. 226–8, at p. 227.

2    Clotes may have acquired these stones for medical purposes, as they had considerable therapeutic value: Seymour, *On the Properties of Things*, ii, pp. 853–4.

3    CLRO, Plea and Memoranda Roll A40, m. 1; A.H. Thomas, ed., *Calendar of Select Plea and Memoranda Rolls Preserved among the Archives of the City of London, 1381–1412* (Cambridge, 1932), p. 289.

4    Caused by 'salt', or corrupt, phlegm, which gave rise to facial symptoms similar to *lepra*. It ranked

not leprosy, and that the plaintiff had, indeed, given him his word on this score. The mayor, however, knew a trickster when he saw one, and taxed Luter with promising what he clearly knew he could not perform. Nor did protestations that he had taught Clotes to make 'balsam and other medicines' cut much ice: he was found to have acted 'fraudulently, deceptively and injuriously' towards his vulnerable patient.

As this case reveals, substantial sums were to be made from the treatment of men and women afflicted with incipient *lepra* or the disfiguring skin conditions from which it apparently developed. There was, too, ample scope for the medieval equivalent of the snake oil salesman, with his ready patter and stock of miraculous remedies. Yet, as invariably happened where chronic diseases were concerned, the fees charged by a respectable practitioner could also be considerable. So dramatic – and potentially irreversible – an imbalance of humours required a complex and carefully calibrated course of therapy which mendacious opportunists, such as Luter, could easily exploit. Others were more scrupulous. Thirty-six years later, Richard Trewythian, a London-based astrologer and *medicus* of some repute and no little learning, attempted to cure the skinner, Nicholas of Ely. Following contemporary practice, the pair entered an agreement whereby Trewythian's fee of 66s. 8d. would be paid in instalments, depending partly upon the patient's rate of recovery. In August 1444 Ely made a deposit of 20s., promising to deliver a further 13s. 4d. at the end of September, but withholding the rest until such time as he could once again mix in public ('*quando honeste potest ambulare inter homines*'). This suggests that his condition was bad enough to keep him confined at home, where Trewythian presumably came at regular intervals with the medicaments either he or an apothecary made up at his own cost. His accounts record an outlay of 27s. 7d. on twenty-eight separate items, but we have no means of telling if he ever recovered the rest of the money and thus ended up in profit.[5] The list includes syrups and electuaries to aid the digestive process; purges, gargles and laxatives to expel corrupt humours; plasters, poultices and unguents to treat ulcerated skin; theriac to eliminate poison; fortified water (probably *aqua vitae*) to strengthen the vital spirits; and oil of violets and of dill to remove 'al scabe off the body'.[6] Trewythian did not practise surgery, and thus does not mention the phlebotomy, baths, clysters and other more aggressive remedies which might well have been administered during treatment. But even such a partial record of the measures adopted in these circumstances gives some idea of the battery of potential cures on offer. They, in turn, reflect the complexity and sophistication of medieval therapeutics, which offered the suspect leper a range of options from the searing pain of the lancet or cautery to the fragrant steam of a herbal bath.

Erasmus Wilson, the Victorian physician whose remarks introduce this

---

alongside morphew, scabies and other dermatological disorders which were deemed potentially leprous but curable: *MED, S–SL,* pp. 100–1.

5　BL, MS Sloane 428, fo. 18v; Page, 'Richard Trewythian', pp. 193–228. For contracts between patients and practitioners, see Rawcliffe, 'Profits of Practice', pp. 61–78.

6　A mixture of oil of violets, litharge (lead monoxide), white lead, mastic and frankincense was recommended for this purpose: see BL, MS Harley 1736, fo. 138r. Violets were widely used to perfume, moisturise and cool the skin: Nicaise, *Chirurgie de Henri de Mondeville,* p. 622.

chapter, adopted an unusually reflective approach to the topic. His contemporaries were more often inclined to dismiss medieval remedies, and especially those for serious chronic diseases such as *lepra*, as a benighted concoction of superstition, ignorance and debased Classical learning. A tendency to sensationalise the 'bizarre and fantastic', and to judge the efficacy of cures by the standards of modern medicine has further compounded the problem.[7] More recent work by Luke Demaitre and F.O. Touati offers a convincing and scholarly reassessment of the medical care available to medieval lepers, setting it firmly in the context of the period and suggesting new lines of inquiry.[8] However strange, even repugnant, some types of treatment may appear today, it is important to remember that they were devised and administered by men and women who worked within a very different, but entirely coherent, system of healing. Nor can we necessarily assume that practitioners actually *used* all the scores of different remedies described in the written record. Some of the more fanciful or macabre belong squarely in the realms of literature rather than medicine, while others were collected as curiosities by zealous encyclopaedists, who were reluctant to omit any fact or fallacy, whatever its provenance. It is hard to imagine any late medieval surgeon placing his trust in the liver of a unicorn mixed in egg yolk.[9] If we turn to the *practica* and casebooks of men such as Trewythian, who actually dealt with the disease, we can detect a more pragmatic approach, which appears both selective and adaptable.

It was also remarkably non-judgemental. With surprising candour, John of Gaddesden itemised the protective measures that a man might take after having sexual relations with a woman whom he believed to be leprous. These involved cleansing the penis with his own urine (or vinegar and water) at the first opportunity, and then seeking out a phlebotomist to expel any peccant matter already in the bloodstream. After intensive bleeding, a three months' course of purgation, unguents and medication seemed desirable. In advising the woman to expel her partner's semen by vigorous exercise or sneezing, and to douche the genital area, Gaddesden was offering contraceptive and prophylactic advice of which the Church could hardly approve.[10] Indeed, while accepting that *lepra* might constitute a divine punishment for sin, and thus lie beyond earthly help, medical authorities assumed that most cases sprang from natural causes. In this respect, at least, the disease appeared no different from any other.

Particular stress was, nevertheless, placed upon early treatment, before *lepra* had corrupted the vital organs. Aretaeus criticised the negligent practitioner,

---

7   A. van Ardsall, *Medieval Herbal Remedies* (London, 2002), chapter two, examines historical approaches to early medieval English therapeutics. Brody, *Disease of the Soul*, pp. 71–3, and Beriac, *Histoire des lépreux*, pp. 259–62, offer a less positive assessment of the care available to suspect and confirmed lepers.

8   Demaitre, 'Relevance of Futility', pp. 25–61; F.O. Touati, 'Pharmacopée et thérapeutic contre la lèpre au moyen age: quelques réflexions méthodologiques', *Actes du 113e Congrés National des Sociétes Savantes, Strasbourg, 1988* (Paris, CTHS, 1991), pp. 17–26.

9   P. Throop, ed., *Hildegard von Bingen's Physica* (Rochester, Vermont, 1998), p. 61.

10  John of Gaddesden, *Rosa Anglica*, fo. 61r–61v. The author of Bodleian Library, MS Ashmole 1505, fo. 30v, observes circumspectly that 'ther beth many othere maneres that we ne schulleth noght telle for to putte out the seede'. See also, Nicaise, *Chirurgie de Henri de Mondeville*, pp. 625–6. By cleansing the uterus this measure would have protected the woman's future sexual partners: above, pp. 82–5, 87, 181.

who, 'from inattention and ignorance of the patient's ailment, does not apply his art to the commencement when the disease is very feeble'.[11] As a surgeon, Lanfrank of Milan took such warnings very seriously indeed, being well aware that, once putrefying matter had begun to spread its poison, the choice of cures at his disposal would, perforce, dwindle and grow progressively more extreme.[12] The 'greet perel' occasioned by these 'stronge medicyns' was, moreover, compounded by the fact that they had to be 'ofte rehersid', a risk few late medieval surgeons wished to take.[13] They were justifiably exercised about the threat to their immortal souls posed by the death of a patient – however unavoidable – and more immediately worried about the consequences of failure upon their reputations. English surgeons were urged to be 'bold & hardy in sekyr [certain] thynges & fferfull & dowtfull in perelles' and 'to exchew from evyll currys' which might result in accidental homicide.[14] The London Fellowship of Surgeons went even further by insisting in its regulations of 1435 that 'ony cure desperate the which is lykli to falle into deeth' should only be undertaken after consultation with other colleagues.[15]

Few late medieval practitioners shared John of Gaddesden's concern about the physical dangers arising from professional contact with suspects, presumably because the patients whom they treated on a regular basis did not yet exude the insupportable miasmas associated with more advanced stages of the disease.[16] Indeed, however widespread they may have been, reservations about undertaking the care of truly hopeless cases seem to have focused more upon the potential loss of professional status and fee-paying patients than the likelihood of infection. Surgeons, such as Henri de Mondeville, whose involvement in a wide range of intimate manual procedures brought them into close physical proximity with the sick, risked most. It was, he felt, inadvisable for any practitioner to deal with individuals 'whose form and appearance is manifestly corrupt' unless

> they have been enlisted by the most urgent prayers and at a considerably higher fee, and after announcing their prognosis, since this is an extremely vile and contagious disease. And lastly, lepers greatly enjoy spending time with their physicians and making contact with them, and the physicians who care for them are vilified, once this becomes known, and considered to be corrupted and repulsive.[17]

---

11 Adams, *Extant Works of Aretaeus*, p. 369.
12 Lanfrank's *Chirurgia magna* of 1296 was the first surgical text to incorporate an *antidotarium*, or section on compound drugs: M. McVaugh, 'Surgery', in M.D. Grmek, ed., *Western Medical Thought from Antiquity to the Middle Ages* (Cambridge, Mass., 1998), pp. 283–4.
13 Fleischhaker, *Lanfrank's 'Science of Cirgurie'*, pp. 197–8. For the Church's belief that difficult cures should be avoided see Rawcliffe, *Medicine and Society*, p. 77.
14 BL, MS Harley 1736, fo. 7r.
15 Beck, *Cutting Edge*, p. 132.
16 John of Gaddesden, *Rosa Anglica*, fo. 58v. According to Demaitre, 'Description and Diagnosis', p. 333, only three late medieval medical treatises mention the dangers of infected breath in the *judicium*. Some authorities, such as Pierre de Saint-Flour, dismissed fears of contagion altogether: Jacquart, *Médecine médiévale*, p. 249.
17 Nicaise, *Chirurgie de Henri de Mondeville*, p. 618. The regulations of the barbers and surgeons of Gisors threatened any member of the guild with expulsion for a year and a day if he phlebotomised a [confirmed] leper or, significantly, kept a brothel or prostitute in his premises: L. Passy, ed., *Le livre*

Awareness of the need for an accurate prognosis, which would not raise the hopes of the patient, only to dash them later, redoubled this sense of caution among the less cynical.[18] Thomas Hoccleve's story of the leprous king, whose castle was surrounded by the heads of all those practitioners who had vainly promised to cure him, was, of course, pure − if salutary − fiction.[19] But, as John Clotes discovered, the risks of professional hubris could be real enough.

In their efforts to establish 'levels of malignancy and severity', and thereby determine what the practitioner might realistically hope to achieve, writers on *lepra* identified successive stages of progression. These were generally believed to move from predisposition to the insidious development of occult symptoms, and thence to outward manifestation, confirmation and terminal decline.[20] But other criteria might also be taken into account. Some authorities distinguished between 'natural' and 'accidental' causes, maintaining that *lepra* which had been inherited would be so entrenched as to prove ineradicable, whereas that which sprang from an ill-advised sexual encounter or negligence about one's diet could perhaps be healed.[21] Even alchemists, whose confidence in the efficacy of their elixirs generally knew no bounds, drew a clear line between the '*morbus hereditus*' and *lepra* 'that is causid oonly of rotun humouris'.[22] An Anglo-Irish collection of remedies, produced in about 1300, suggests an *experimentum* to determine which of these two types of leprosy a patient might have through the use of a blood sample. It also prescribes a herbal drink, of proven efficacy in 'accidental' cases, made of sage, mint, radish, wormwood, stinking camomile and nettles mixed with red wine. The draught was to be consumed from three vessels over a period of twelve days. The number three often occurs in medieval remedies, and was replete with religious symbolism, but the choice of herbs had a more scientific basis. As we shall see, these simples were noted for their capacity to purge corruption from the body, each possessing the requisite degree of warmth to restore the patient's lost equilibrium.[23]

   *des métiers de Gisors* (Pontoise, 1907), p. 14. English surgeons expressed no such concerns about treating lepers.

18  Prognostics played a notable part in the later medieval medical syllabus: L. Demaitre, 'The Art and Science of Prognostication in early University Medicine', *BHM*, lxxvii (2003), pp. 765–88. Its practical importance, in gaining the confidence of the patient and eventually helping him to prepare for death, was, however, never forgotten: Getz, *Medicine*, pp. 4, 13–15.

19  Furnivall, *Hoccleve's Works*, pp. 233–4.

20  Demaitre, 'Relevance of Futility', pp. 29–32; Ogden, *Cyrurgie of Guy de Chauliac*, p. 379.

21  Demaitre, 'Description and Diagnosis', pp. 331–2. A similar distinction was made between leprosy that resulted from conception *during* menstruation and the subsequent, less potentially harmful, damage inflicted *later* by contact between a growing embryo and corrupt menstrual blood: Fabre-Vassas, *Singular Beast*, p. 106. Hildegard of Bingen (d. 1179) argued that it was harder to cure *lepra* caused by 'gluttony and drunkenness' than that occasioned by 'unrestrained lust': Hildegard of Bingen, *On Natural Philosophy and Medicine: Selections from the Cause et Cure*, ed. M. Berger (Woodbridge, 1999), p. 103. Medical authorities likewise regarded 'idiocy' or 'natural folly' apparent from birth as untreatable, while maintaining that mental illness apparent later in life would respond to humoral management: Harper, *Insanity*, p. 33.

22  F.J. Furnivall, ed., *The Book of Quinte Essence* (EETS, xvi, 1866, reprinted 1965), p. 16; C. Crisciani and M. Periera, 'Black Death and Golden Remedies: Some Remarks on Alchemy and the Plague', in *The Regulation of Evil: Social and Cultural Attitudes to Epidemics in the late Middle Ages* (Micrologus' Library, ii, Turnhout, 1998), p. 21 n. 1.

23  Hunt, *Popular Medicine*, p. 250. In a variant of the test described above, pp. 166–7, the blood of the

Certain humoral types of *lepra* also seemed more amenable to treatment than others. Only a rash – or unscrupulous – healer would undertake to cure full-blown elephantine leprosy (*elephancia*), whereas victims of the vulpine type (*alopecia*) stood a good chance of recovery if it was caught 'atte the bygynnynge'. This was because the root cause sprang from a plethora of corrupt blood, whose inherent warmth and moisture made it 'lasse parylouse' than an over-abundance of adust black bile. Tyrian leprosy, being clammy and phlegmatic, lay somewhere in the middle, while views about the leonine type differed more sharply. On balance, most authorities adopted a gloomy prognosis because of the toxic effects of so much burnt choler. There was, however, a clear consensus that its characteristic speed and ferocity made early diagnosis imperative.[24]

The quest for diagnostic precision went beyond the identification of specific types of leprosy to embrace the shifting humoral balance and environment of each individual patient. By carefully monitoring any changes, the *medicus*, apothecary or surgeon could constantly modify the treatments he had prescribed, thereby rendering them more effective. 'Since not all lepers share the same complexion', Henri de Mondeville explained, 'and since each leper demonstrates some peculiarity not found in any other, and since, moreover, all leprosy is not of the same type . . . the quantity of remedies applied cannot be set in stone.' He went on to illustrate this point by advising his readers to use cool herbs in medicinal baths for lepers whose disease had a 'hot cause', and *vice versa*.[25] The financial circumstances of the patient posed another challenge to the practitioner, who was advised to provide cheaper preparations for the benefit of the less affluent.[26] Then, as now, though, poverty remained a relative concept. If surviving casebooks and treatises are any guide, cut-price treatment could still prove protracted and costly, often lasting for months, or even years.[27] There was, moreover, the added problem of 'accidents', or what we might call secondary complications, such as fever, ulceration, 'morphew, scabbe, icchynge and teter', all of which demanded attention.[28] Few, if any, medieval men or women can have experienced – let alone survived – the full repertory of cures described at length in medical texts, which were designed as an *omnium gatherum* to offer the widest possible range of options. Yet even a modest and relatively short course of treatment, such as that devised by Richard Trewythian for his patient, required a

---

patient was to be poured over a fresh egg, which would be more or less 'cooked' according to the severity of the disease.

24   'Allopicia is lasse parylouse & lighter for to cure ate the bygynnynge. And leonine is more light for to curye & his malice is more wexynge; and elefancia is longe or he come to his state & is most harde for to curye . . . and tyria is in the mene': Bodleian Library, MS Ashmole 1505, fo. 31v. John Bradmore, on the other hand, expressed the general view that leonine *lepra*, being occasioned by intense heat, was rarely or never healed: BL, MS Sloane 2272 (part 1), fo. 92r. John of Gaddesden, was slightly more optimistic: *Rosa Anglica*, fos 57v–58r. Andrew Boorde argued in 1552 that 'for as the Lyon is most fearcest of all the beastes, so is the kynde of leprousnes most worst of al other sykenesses, for it doth corrode and eate the fleshe to the bones': *Breuiary of Healthe*, fo. 69v.

25   Nicaise, *Chirurgie de Henri de Mondeville*, pp. 617, 619, 624. Many authorities maintained that *lepra* contracted through coitus would either be hot or cold, and should be treated accordingly: Campbell and Colton, *Surgery of Theoderic*, ii, pp. 178–9; John of Gaddesden, *Rosa Anglica*, fo. 61r–61v.

26   Bodleian Library, MS Ashmole 1505, fo. 32r.

27   BL, MS Sloane 2272 (part 1), fo. 91r.

28   Ogden, *Cyrurgie de Guy de Chauliac*, p. 389.

deep pocket, especially as surgical procedures and special foodstuffs cost extra. It was at this stage that anxious relatives, who saw their expectations diminish as medical bills soared, began to contemplate the advantages of prompt removal to a *leprosarium.*[29]

In the last resort, however, medieval therapeutics placed a considerable burden of responsibility upon the individual patient. As William of Canterbury pointed out, when describing Becket's miraculous cure of a young Norman pilgrim in the early 1170s, anyone who failed to seek medical advice about disturbing symptoms, or who clung to an unhealthy regimen, was asking for trouble. Having procrastinated for two years before attempting to deal with the blemishes that had appeared on his face, the youth felt too ashamed to seek help and withdrew from society.[30] Yet he could hardly claim ignorance. Already by this date, educated laymen and women were well aware that certain basic precepts about hygiene, encapsulated in *regimina sanitatis* (regimens of health), offered a comprehensive guide to survival in a dangerous world. They hinged upon the successful management of six 'non-naturals', or factors existing outside the body, which could be manipulated to achieve and then maintain an optimum state of humoral equilibrium and spiritual balance. In accordance with Classical, largely Galenic thought, diet took pride of place among the *res non naturales.*[31] The other five fell into the general categories of air and environment, physical exercise, sleep, the evacuation of waste matter and 'accidents of the soul' or psychological well being.[32] These rules were essentially prophylactic, in so far that they helped the reader to avoid disease,[33] but most curative procedures followed similar holistic principles. In a striking simile, Henri de Mondeville compared physicians and surgeons to dancers, who had to follow the tune played by Mother Nature.[34] The principles of the regimen guided their steps.

Initially introduced to the West through the translations of Islamic texts made by scholars such as Constantine the African and Gerard of Cremona, this type of literature soon took on a life of its own. Although *regimina* were at first tailored to the specific requirements of rich and powerful individuals, the genre rapidly expanded, attracting some of the best medical minds of the later thirteenth and early fourteenth centuries.[35] The rise of an articulate, increasingly literate and more affluent, urban class stimulated vernacular production, but it was successive outbreaks of plague from 1348–50 onwards that really galvanised

29 Bergman, 'Hoping against Hope', pp. 23, 28–9, 31–2.

30 Robertson, *Materials*, i, p. 215.

31 See M.W. Adamson, *Medieval Dietetics: Food and Drink in the Regimen Sanitatis Literature from 800 to 1400* (Frankfurt and New York, 1995), for a survey of texts.

32 L.J. Rather, 'The Six Things Non-Natural', *Clio Medica*, iii (1968), pp. 337–47; P.H. Niebyl, 'The Non-Naturals', *BHM*, xlv (1971), pp. 486–92.

33 As Guy de Chauliac pointed out, the prevention of leprosy was 'fulfilled with dewe admynistracioun of the sexe vnnatural thinges . . . and of soche othere that declynen or bowen to temperance': Ogden, *Cyrurgie de Guy de Chauliac*, pp. 383–4.

34 M.C. Pouchelle, *The Body and Surgery in the Middle Ages* (Oxford, 1990), pp. 38–40.

35 P. Gil Sotres, 'The Regimens of Health', in Grmek, *Western Medical Thought*, pp. 291–318; Getz, *Medicine*, pp. 53–63, 85–8; L. García-Ballester, 'Changes in the *Regimina Sanitatis*: The Role of the Jewish Physicians', in S. Campbell, B. Hall and D. Klausner, eds, *Health, Disease and Healing in Medieval Culture* (Toronto, 1992), pp. 119–31.

the demand for advice manuals.[36] As a result, brief, accessible *regimina*, often incorporating tracts about the avoidance of pestilence, a few basic remedies (including those for skin diseases) and information about *materia medica* became common currency throughout Europe.[37] The tenets and vocabulary of these tracts had, meanwhile, been absorbed into sermons, homilies and political propaganda, prompting the inevitable theological metaphors. Thus, for example, the role of the priest in the confessional was described in terms of a spiritual regimen:

> He gives us relief from our pain through contrition, and through confession we receive a purgative; he recommends a healthful diet through our keeping of fasts; he orders therapeutic baths through our outpouring of tears; he prescribes blood-letting through our recollection of Christ's passion. But what is this medicine? Penance.[38]

As this quotation indicates, medieval remedies were often administered serially, as part of a conventional sequence. The practitioner would generally begin his struggle against incipient *lepra* by addressing the patient's lifestyle, modifying his or her diet and attempting to purge the body of malign humours before they spread from the veins to the vital organs. Should he fail, it would be necessary to intensify the process of evacuation, while also administering medicaments to 'digest' or 'resolve' the corrupt matter before it solidified. The 'rectificacioun' of the liver (where the humours were engendered) and complexion now became a matter of some urgency. In more advanced cases the eradication, or at least concealment, of any obvious blemishes demanded increasingly aggressive cosmetic measures. By this stage, as palliative care assumed greater importance, a variety of unguents, oils, perfumed waters and other preparations would also be needed for external application.[39] Guy de Chauliac provides an interesting example of the successful use of carefully graded types of treatment, which he ascribes to the Muslim physician, Rhazes (d. 925).

> He helede a yong man that was lepre, in whos face the knottes bygonne to be made and the here [hair] felle of. The whiche he bygynneth to helpe with blode last [letting] and with lousynge of the wombe [purgation of the stomach] and with an appozyme of epithymum and of pillulis cochiis[40] in the purgacions. And he putte hym ofte in a bath, and he gaf hym moystinge metes. Afterwarde he ordeynede hym to be in quyte [rest] by some dayes. Afterward he goth ageyne to louse the

---

[36] Arrizabalaga, 'Facing the Black Death', pp. 273–85; Horrox, *Black Death*, pp. 173–94.

[37] R.H. Robbins, 'Medical Manuscripts in Middle English', *Speculum*, xlv (1970), pp. 393–415.

[38] Shinners and Dohar, *Pastors and the Care of Souls*, p. 171.

[39] Demaitre, 'Relevance of Futility', pp. 32–4; Ogden, *Cyrurgie of Guy de Chauliac*, pp. 383–4; John of Gaddesden, *Rosa Anglia*, fo. 61v. The section on *lepra* in the *Breviarium Bartholomaei* of John Mirfield is largely derivative, although he recommends a couple of plasters to render a contracted 'bear-claw' hand more malleable. He may have been shown how to make them by one of the staff of St Bartholomew's hospital, London, with which he maintained close connections: BL, MS Harley 3, fo. 23r; P. Horton-Smith Hartley and H.R. Aldridge, *Johannes de Mirfeld: His Life and Works* (Cambridge, 1936), pp. 8–9.

[40] That is a decoction of thyme and pills for purging adust humours. Like fumitory, thyme was warm and dry, and appears frequently in remedies for *lepra*: BL, MS Harley 1736, fo. 135r; Bodleian Library, MS Ashmole 1505, fo. 32r–32v; Campbell and Colton, *Surgery of Theoderic*, ii, pp. 173, 174.

wombe, and he doth it so ofte til that he haue lousede the wombe more than fourty tymes in fyue monthes. The whiche thinges done, the here bygan to sprynge ageyne, and the eyghen [eyes] and the colource and the face bygan to be amended.[41]

Bearing in mind that a ghostly physician would also be on hand to provide a similar range of spiritual cures, let us now examine these remedies more closely in the order they would have been applied.

## Diet and medication

Recommending a suitable diet for a suspect leper might be compared to shutting the stable door after a bolting horse, since he or she clearly required more than a change of food and drink to halt the spread of corrupt and adust humours. Even so, careful attention to such matters could help to restore a degree of balance, if the disease had not progressed too far, while also strengthening the body's natural and vital spirits, which constituted its frontline defences. As we saw in chapter two, men and women with a predisposition towards *lepra* could protect themselves by avoiding contaminated or dangerous foodstuffs likely to overheat the body or generate toxins. For those at a more perilous stage, it was essential

to abstayne from fryed mettes, salt mettes & sowr mettes and fro mettes that ar myche peparyd [peppered], and brennes to sor in the mowth, and from garleke, onions, watter fowle and fro venyson of buke and do[e], hart & hynd, & from harys [hares'] flesch and from myche nyght werke and surfett off mett and drynke . . . and frome all maner of quasy [unwholesome] mettes.[42]

Conversely, temperate foods of a mild and moist nature, such as poultry, newly baked bread, eggs, veal, good quality pork and fresh fish, along with light, aromatic wine, would pass more easily through the body, cooling the overheated digestive system.[43] Guy de Chauliac favoured a diet of fresh milk, which Avicenna had considered especially beneficial for the respiratory and vocal symptoms so often encountered in advanced cases.[44] Given the widespread assumption that medieval *leprosaria* offered little, if anything, in the way of

---

[41] Ogden, *Cyrurgie of Guy de Chauliac*, p. 386. See also BL, MS Sloane 2272 (part 1), fo. 92v.

[42] BL, MS Harley 1736, fo. 138r. Galen warned against the dangers of all these comestibles, notably beef, which, although nourishing, was indigestible and therefore likely to harm anyone of a melancholic temperament. It was, he thought, a potential cause of both *lepra* and cancer: M. Grant, ed., *Galen on Food and Diet* (London, 2000), p. 154; *Claudii Galeni opera omnia*, viii, lib. III, cap. X, pp. 183–4. For the impact of a diet high in saturated fatty acids upon the incidence of Hansen's disease today, see Ell, 'Diet and Leprosy', pp. 113–29, at pp. 114–17.

[43] John of Gaddesden, *Rosa Anglica*, fo. 59r; Campbell and Colton, *Surgery of Theoderic*, ii, p. 172; BL, MS Sloane 2272 (part 1), fo. 94r. A model regimen for the cure of leprosy may be found in Bodleian Library, MS Bodley e Mus 19, fo. 116v. As late as 1547, the physician, Andrew Boorde, offered 'a dyete for them the whiche haue any of the kyndes of lepored' in his *Compendyous Regyment or a Dyetary of Healthe* (London, 1547), sig. I verso–iir.

[44] Ogden, *Cyrurgie of Guy de Chauliac*, pp. 384–5; Avicenna, *Liber canonis*, fo. 444r. Aretaeus also praised the laxative qualities of milk: Adams, *Extant Works of Aretaeus*, p. 495. Fish and milk were not, however, to be consumed at the same time (above, p. 79). The monk, John Lydgate, warned in one verse regimen that such an ill-advised combination 'causith boody and fas [face] with lepre to be smet thorugh disposicion off vnkynde humours by inward corrupcioun': R. Steele, ed., *Lydgate and Burgh's Secrees of Old Philisoffres* (EETS, extra series, lxvi, 1894), p. 53.

physical care to their inmates, it is worth pausing at this point to observe that many institutions raised dairy cattle along with hens and pigs; and that some exercised fishing rights in well-stocked rivers. Thus, for example, the lepers of Boughton, outside Chester, claimed the ancient privilege of keeping a boat and tackle on the Dee, and of fishing on either side of the nearby bridge.[45] As we shall see in chapter seven, the larger leper hospitals, at least, were initially able to provide a regimen that accorded remarkably well with current medical advice on the management of the disease.

Even at its best, however, palliative care did not require the minute adjustments of diet which many physicians deemed essential when treating incipient cases of *lepra*. Lanfrank of Milan's recommendation that whey from goat's milk should be given instead of cow's milk in the early stages of leonine leprosy, because it was cooler, reflects the care taken to temper the patient's regimen.[46] The digestive and excretory processes could be further improved with syrups and semi-liquid pastes known as electuaries. These contained a wide variety of herbs and spices rendered palatable by the addition of a sweetening agent. Pioneered as a pharmaceutical product by Muslim practitioners, sugar ranked as a 'temperate' substance and was valued for its medicinal qualities. It also made possible the creation of new compound preparations for internal consumption. 'The evangelist of pharmacy', Masawaih al-Mardini, or Mesue (d. 1015), devoted twelve chapters of his medical formulary to the production of electuaries, and thus provided generations of European apothecaries with one of their essential texts. Known as the *Grabaddin*, versions of this guide circulated widely both in Latin and truncated vernacular forms.[47]

The idea of distinguishing between diet and medication was as alien to the medieval practitioner as that of separating body and soul, with the result that no clear line can, as today, be drawn between the two. The widespread demand for electuaries illustrates this point clearly, since the healthy as well as the sick drank them mixed in wine as a *digestif* after meals to settle the stomach. Essential in the treatment of *lepra*, they could either be taken alone or in combination with other *materia medica* at various stages of treatment. Some, such as diacyminum (an electuary made of cumin), which Richard Trewythian prescribed on four separate occasions for his patient, were so popular that recipes seemed unnecessary. Theoderic had, for example, advised its use, along with dianthos (one made of rosemary), for the 'digestion' of corrupt matter in cases of tyrian *lepra*.[48]

The opening of markets in the Middle East and the growth of the spice trade brought many exotic additions to the standard north European pharmacopoeia. Commodities such as cloves, cardamom, nutmeg and ginger, which we today

---

[45] G. Baraclough, ed., *The Charters of the Anglo Norman Earls of Chester c. 1071–1237* (Lancashire and Cheshire Record Society, cxxvi, 1988), no. 222; and below, pp. 313–14.

[46] Fleishhaker, *Lanfrank's 'Science of Cirurgie'*, p. 198. See also Bodleian Library, MS Bodley 484, fo. 176r.

[47] M. Levey, *Early Arabic Pharmacology* (Leiden, 1973), pp. 72–99; Rawcliffe, *Medicine and Society*, pp. 150–2.

[48] Trewythian also records six prescriptions of an unspecified syrup, which came to 11s. 4d.: BL, MS Sloane 428, fo. 18v; Campbell and Colton, *Surgery of Theoderic*, ii, p. 175. The lepers of St John's hospital, Brook Street (Essex), were allocated a tithe of cumin by the founder, who also made them a generous gift of meat, vegetables, fodder and grazing land: R.C. Fowler, ed., *Registrum Simonis de Sudbiria* (2 vols, Oxford, 1927–28), i, pp. 210–12.

relegate to the kitchen cupboard, figured prominently among the new medicines. Extreme caution was, however, required when prescribing them. Thus, for example, pepper, which became a staple in the treatment of disorders springing from excessive black bile or phlegm, might, on the face of things, have offered a useful specific against *lepra*. Yet, as Bartholomaeus Anglicus warned, such a hot substance would burn the blood, thereby generating rather than destroying the adust humours which 'bredeth atte laste meselrye'.[49] The qualities that made it dangerous for internal consumption by suspect lepers were, however, ideal for corrosive ointments to remove infected flesh, or as a means of purging the head through sneezing.[50] Accurate information consequently became a priority, and as the range of available plants, spices and minerals expanded so did the number of texts explaining their use.

Herbal lore was, to a notable extent, passed on from one generation to the next verbally and through apprenticeship without much need for written guidelines. The ability to identify and cultivate potentially dangerous herbal simples and prepare them for consumption was – and is – best acquired through a process of practical demonstration. Yet, alongside this oral tradition, there developed a notable corpus of textual material, which, in Europe, traced its origins to the *De materia medica* of Pedanius Dioscorides (d. AD 80). Listing some 600 plants and around 130 animal and mineral products, the truncated Latin version of this pioneering work provided a comprehensive survey, which was duly adapted to suit the needs of practitioners in cooler climates.[51] A process of revision and consolidation followed. The fourth-century Latin *Herbarium* of the Pseudo-Apuleius, which drew heavily upon Dioscorides, was, for example, translated into Old English at the turn of the tenth century, revealing the existence of a cosmopolitan and dynamic medical culture in the British Isles.[52] Some of the plants described in its pages were recommended for the treatment of itchy skin and other dermatological disorders, although the Anglo Saxon term, *hreofl/hreofla*, does not permit a more precise diagnosis.[53] Oswald Cockayne, who first edited the *Old English Herbarium* and other important near-contemporary vernacular medical texts in the 1860s, translated it as *lepra*, but others have been more cautious.[54] Even so, many of the plants, such as red dock, horsemint, calamint and nettles, listed in these cures were still being used in the treatment of leprosy and other acute skin conditions five centuries later. Indeed, the herbal baths described in the *Leechbook of Bald* (c. 1000)

---

49  Seymour, *On the Properties of Things*, ii, p. 1025.
50  Bodleian Library, MS Ashmole 1505, fos 32v–33r; John of Gaddesden, *Rosa Anglica*, fo. 60r–60v.
51  J. Stannard, 'Dioscorides and Renaissance Materia Medica', *Analecto Medica-Historica 1: Materia Medica in the XVI Century* (Oxford, 1966), pp. 1–21. Nigella, which drives away serpents, might, for example, be used to treat leprosy (p. 215).
52  Van Ardsall, *Medieval Herbal Remedies*, chapter two.
53  The word has multiple meanings, ranging from elephantine *lepra* to ulcers, pox and even sheep scab: J. de Vriend, ed., *The Old English herbarium and medicina de quadrupedibus* (EETS, cclxxxvi, 1984), p. 309.
54  Compare O. Cockayne, ed., *Leechdoms, Wortcunning and Starcraft in Early England* (3 vols, RS, 1864–66), i, pp. 203, 223, 271, with van Ardsall, *Medieval Herbal Remedies*, pp. 189, 197, 213–14; and M.L. Cameron, *Anglo-Saxon Medicine* (Cambridge, 1993), pp. 96–7.

differed little from those favoured by fifteenth-century physicians and surgeons.[55]

But herbals alone no longer sufficed. The arrival in the West of unfamiliar medical texts, drugs and methods of production and the emergence of a new breed of academically trained physician created a need for books which went beyond the description of largely – but not exclusively – indigenous botanical simples. The demand for an 'essential pharmacopoeia' was most effectively met by the *Antidotarium Nicolai*, which originated in twelfth-century Salerno and presented material from Islamic as well as older Greek texts in an accessible digest. Originally offering about 150 different remedies, it grew exponentially over the years to become the apothecary's bible.[56] Compound recipes from its pages reappeared in *regimina*, medical textbooks and vernacular collections, modified or expanded (sometimes beyond recognition) to suit local circumstances. A myriad of electuaries, fomentations, cataplasms, unguents, fumigants, pills, opiates, laxatives and diuretics provided the inventive practitioner with cures for every known malady.

To cite one of many examples from an Anglo-Norman remedy book, a recipe for syrup to cleanse the stomach, kidneys, liver and head in cases of scabies or leprosy took much of its inspiration from this source. The ingredients, which comprised dodder, wormwood, wild sage, borage seed, root of wild celery and fennel, liquorice, common polipody, oil of tamarind and cassia, grapes, mirobalans, roses, manna, violets, ginger, plums and the juice of fumitory and borage, represent an eclectic mixture of East and West.[57] They also reflect the increasingly sophisticated nature of late medieval therapeutics, since mirobalan fruit came in four different colours (red, white, yellow and black), each of which was believed to have a purgative action upon the appropriate humour. In this way remedies could be specifically customised to suit the individual patient, colour being one of many important considerations dictating the choice of ingredients.[58] The use of the *Antidotarium* was greatly facilitated by an explanatory commentary, *De simplici medicina*, written upon it at Salerno by Matthaeus Platearius (d. 1161). Generally known by its opening words as the *Circa instans*, it provided a guide to over 270 simple and compound medicines, and thus did much to spread information about developments in pharmacy.[59]

Many authors complained about the growing influence and greed of the men

---

55  Cockayne, *Leechdoms*, ii, pp. 76–9. Thus, for example, wallwort is described as a specific against *lepra* in the early eighth-century *Enigmata* of Aldheim of Malmesbury, and was still being used seven centuries later: Cameron, *Anglo-Saxon Medicine*, p. 26; and n. 99, below. Nettles were recommended in later herbals for the treatment of elephantine *lepra* because they purged venom. They were either to be mixed with wine and drunk, or rubbed directly on the skin: BL, MS Arundel 42, fo. 6v.

56  Hunt, *Popular Medicine*, p. 14; J. Stannard, 'The Herbal as a Medical Document', *BHM*, xliii (1969), pp. 212–20, at pp. 216–17.

57  Hunt, *Popular Medicine*, p. 333.

58  Roger Bacon, *De retardatione accidentium senectutis cum aliis opusculis de rebus medicinalibus*, eds A.G. Whittle and F. Withington (British Society of Franciscan Studies, xiv, 1928), pp. 52, 221. They were widely advocated by Avicenna, *Liber canonis*, fos 443r, 444r–444v. Potions and pills employed in the treatment of *lepra* were often coloured to match the humoral type: BL, MS Sloane 2272 (part 1), fo. 91r; Campbell and Colton, *Surgery of Theoderic*, ii, p. 171; Touati, 'Pharmacopée et thérapeutique', p. 21.

59  Grant, *Source Book*, pp. 787–9.

who now cornered the market in *materia medica*, making and even prescribing the new remedies.[60] According to the botanist, Henry Daniel, whose English herbal (*c.* 1385) lists various remedies for *lepra*, most apothecaries were 'wel lewyd [ignorant] in here craft . . . and wel defectif in her doynges'.[61] He was also highly critical of their unholy alliance with members of the medical profession, which served further to fleece the public. Yet apothecaries proliferated throughout the towns and cities of later medieval England, in response to a growing demand for spices, perfumes, fortified waters and compound medicines. Norwich had no fewer than thirty-four in the early fourteenth century, along with a *forum unguentorum* or *apothecaria* for the sale of their goods. The more successful were educated as well as affluent. Some, at least, owned copies of the Latin texts described above, while others appear, like surgeons and barbers, to have acquired them in translation. For instance, Robert Broke, the master of the stillatories at Henry VI's court, acquired an English version of Bernard Gordon's *Lilium medicine*, and may well have produced the fortified waters and electuaries recommended in the chapter on *lepra* for suspects at court.[62] Any urban practitioner or patient with the necessary funds would have found it easy to obtain all but the most recondite items recommended in his remedy books, and, indeed, to have experimented with new cures of his or her own.[63]

The classification of medicinal plants, minerals and animal products was now becoming an increasingly exact pharmacological science, at least in the hands of academically trained physicians. Following Galenic principles, they graded their *materia medica* according to a system of degrees. These ranged from one (mild) to four (extreme) and enabled the practitioner to achieve a precise combination of heat, cold, moisture and aridity to redress the humoral imbalance of each patient. Fumitory, for example, was deemed hot and dry in the second degree (moderate), and to possess the capacity to digest choler and eliminate 'all wykkyd humours', especially black bile. It thus figured prominently in cures for 'scab, lepyr and morfu', not least because its ruling planet, Saturn, was himself seen as the bearer of such diseases.[64] Should a more powerful agent be required in the struggle to eliminate 'lepir', black hellebore (one degree hotter and dryer)

---

60  Bacon, *De retardatione accidentium senectutis*, pp. 150, 163–4; Rawcliffe, *Medicine and Society*, pp. 155, 162.

61  BL, MS Arundel 42, fo. 49v. See J. Harvey, *Mediaeval Gardens* (London, 1981), pp. 118–19, 159–62, for an account of this important work. Daniel is here echoing Roger Bacon's *De erroribus medicorum*, which is even more hostile: *De retardatione accidentium senectutis*, p. 150.

62  Rawcliffe, *Medicine and Society*, chapter seven; eadem, 'Sickness and Health' in Rawcliffe and Wilson, *History of Norwich*, i, p. 320. For Broke, see above, p. 84 n. 162.

63  For the range of preparations available in one modest shop, see G.E. Trease and J.H. Hodson, 'The Inventory of John Hexham, a Fifteenth-Century Apothecary', *Medical History*, ix (1965), pp. 76–81. Such profusion contrasts sharply with the bishop of Winchester's complaint in 754 that the 'foreign' ingredients prescribed in his new remedy books were 'unknown to us and difficult to obtain': M.L. Cameron, 'The Sources of Medical Knowledge in Anglo-Saxon England', *Anglo-Saxon England*, xi (1982), pp. 135–55, at p. 137.

64  Its grey leaves and mottled flowers resembled bruised flesh: Risse, *Mending Bodies*, p. 189; Bodleian Library, MS Ashmole 1443, p. 114; BL, MSS Sloane 1315, p. 18; 2272 (part 1), fos. 91r, 92v–95r. Henry Daniel, who recommended fumitory for the cure of *lepra*, described it as 'on of the blissid medicyns . . . solutif of wik[ed] humours & comfortatif of kynde': BL, MS Arundel 42, fo. 90r. Because it caused 'swellynge and ventosite', fumitory was generally administered with fennel: Seymour, *On the Properties of Things*, ii, p. 959.

might be used, albeit with caution. Its capacity to purge the liver and stomach was offset by the potentially lethal effects of too large a dose upon the spleen and intestinal tract.[65] Scabious, a plant whose name and appearance testified to its occult power over a range of dermatological conditions, possessed similar qualities.[66]

Increasingly complicated mathematical rules for the production of compound medicines were developed by Islamic pharmacists and subsequently refined at Montpellier during the late thirteenth and early fourteenth centuries.[67] Although few practitioners can actually have attempted these difficult calculations when treating their patients, a working knowledge of the degrees, complexions, and qualities of plants circulated far beyond the groves of academe. Thanks to the process of translation and dissemination described in the previous chapter, such information was quickly absorbed into vernacular herbals, *regimina* and remedy books.[68] The reader could thus ascertain at a glance which warm, dry plants would best assuage 'the ewyl peyne of lepruse' and draw its 'venym out-warde'.[69] In many instances this system did little more than provide a scientific rationale for remedies that had been popular for centuries, while simultaneously distancing the physician yet further from the herbalist or empiric. Yet it also made available many new cures and treatments, which in turn offered a glimpse of hope to the victims of degenerative diseases.

Despite their ubiquity and usefulness, herbal simples alone or in combination were rarely enough to remove the disfiguring 'apostyms' and 'scabbes' that betokened incipient *lepra*. Nor did they possess the strength to eliminate the deep-seated poison that might already be creeping through the internal organs. The later medieval pharmacopoeia was, however, potentially limitless. This was because Nature, like the human body itself, functioned upon strict hierarchical principles, which bound minerals, plants, animals and human beings together in a great chain of being. Each component of this chain was reciprocally linked, and each – from the smallest lump of antimony upwards – possessed its own individual complexion, qualities and attributes. Any substance, from urine to pearls, might, therefore, be enlisted to fight the battle against sickness. Between the first and fourteenth centuries, the number of primary substances deployed in the

---

65  Bodleian Library, MSS Ashmole 1443, p. 110; 1505, fo. 32v; Nicaise, *Chirurgie de Henri de Mondeville*, pp. 618–19. Black was the colour of melancholia. White hellebore was used against an excess of phlegmatic humours: Seymour, *On the Properties of Things*, ii, pp. 946–7. An early awareness of these factors was demonstrated by the Byzantine physician, Alexander of Tralles (d. 605), whose work was well known in the West: F. Brunet, ed., *Oeuvres médicales d'Alexandre de Tralles* (2 vols, Paris, 1933–36), ii, pp. 76–7.

66  Bodelian Library, MS Ashmole 1443, pp. 164–5. So too did affodilus, a plant of Saturn, likewise prescribed for the treatment of *lepra*: BL, MS Arundel 42, fo. 12r; M.R. Best and F.H. Brightman, eds, *The Book of Secrets of Albertus Magnus* (Oxford, 1973), p. 18.

67  M.R. McVaugh, 'Quantified Medical Theory and Practice at Fourteenth-Century Montpellier', *BHM*, xliii (1969), pp. 397–413; J.M. Riddle, 'Theory and Practice in Medieval Medicine', *Viator*, v (1974), pp. 158–84.

68  Citing the *Circa instans*, one fifteenth-century vernacular text explains 'the special effectis of herbis and droggis that be the most comyne in use and her dyuers [de]grees of qualities, or of her complexions, and her propur and most special kind of worcheyng': Bodleian Library, MS Ashmole 1443, p. 190.

69  G. Brodin, ed., *Agnus Castus: A Middle English Herbal* (Upsala, 1950), pp. 139 (calamint), 187 (catmint).

treatment of *lepra* almost trebled, about a fifth of the new ones being of animal and mineral extraction.[70]

Animal products, including milk, faeces, testicles, fat and blood, had long been grist to the practitioner's mill. The unguents, lubricants and plasters used at all levels of the medical hierarchy, by housewives and physicians alike, required a base of wax or animal fats to bind the active ingredients and render them malleable. Clarified pork fat was generally recommended because of its availability. The 'medicinal ointments' with which the novice mistress at Sempringham massaged the leprous body of a young nun in the infirmary were almost certainly made of lard from the house's pigs and herbs from its garden. Recent research suggests that one of the patients in the *leprosarium* of St Mary Magdalen, Reading (who was suffering from osteomyelitis), had been treated with a similar poultice of dock leaves, applied to the inside of a copper-alloy leg brace.[71] A list of provisions to be supplied annually by the abbot of Peterborough to St Leonard's hospital included a stone of tallow (for lighting) and another of ointment or grease (*unctus*), which, appropriately, were due at the feast of St Martin.[72] Along with cows and poultry, many other English *leprosaria* either kept or were given pigs, which, despite their potential for causing disease, had considerable medicinal value. The seventy carcasses of pork presented by Henry III to five communities of lepers in 1246, and the two pigs assigned annually to each inmate at St Leonard's hospital, Northampton, were undoubtedly a source of unguents as well as food.[73]

Other animals were traditionally exploited for their perceived 'qualities', such as longevity, strength, fertility or speed. The possibility that, by consuming their flesh, blood or specific organs, the patient would absorb some of these characteristics seemed very real.[74] As might be expected, a wide variety of fauna was employed to combat leprosy, often in what we today might regard as a homoeopathic context. The flesh of hedgehogs (*hericii*) may have seemed effective as a palliative because it reputedly stimulated the regrowth of hair, or because the spines replicated the pricking sensation experienced by many patients.[75] The blood of the hare, whose Latin name, *lepus*, is clearly suggestive, was a staple ingredient in ointments and washes for serious dermatological complaints, although its flesh, as we have seen, figured high on the list of banned dietary substances. The corrosive, rich and heavy characteristics that made it so

70  Touati, 'Pharmacopée et thérapeutique', p. 24.
71  Foreville and Keir, *Book of St Gilbert*, pp. 282–5; R. Gilchrist and B. Sloane, *Requiem: The Medieval Monastic Cemetery in Britain* (London, 2005), p. 103.
72  BL, MS Cotton Vespasian E XXII, fo. 4r. He also presented three salted hogs and all their by-products.
73  *CCR, 1242–1247*, pp. 425–6 (the lepers were at Alkmonden, Derby, Chesterfield, Lichfield and Tutbury); C.A. Markham and J.C. Cox, eds, *The Records of the Borough of Northampton* (2 vols, Northampton, 1898), i, p. 404. The award of 'bacons' to *leprosaria* was a routine form of alms. See, for example, the bishop of Winchester's gift of seven to the lepers at Curbridge, Oxfordshire, in 1208, and Bishop Seffrid's grant of one every year to the hospital of St Mary Magdalen, Chichester, not long before: S. Townley, ed., *VCH Oxford XIV* (Woodbridge, 2004), p. 208; Mayr-Harting, *Acta of the Bishops of Chichester*, pp. 162–3; *CLR, 1245–1251*, p. 19.
74  That patients would be reluctant to swallow some of the toxic ingredients, such as poisonous beetles, deemed necessary to expel the corruption of *lepra* is apparent from one fifteenth-century text, which explains how to disguise them as harmless pills: Bodleian Library, MS Bodley 484, fo. 177r.
75  BL, MS Sloane 2272 (part 1), fo. 90v; MS Harley 3, fo. 23v; Demaitre, 'Relevance of Futility', p. 42.

dangerous for internal consumption were, however, ideal for treating ulcerated skin. Perhaps, too, the hare's speed and reputed gentleness promised to outrun and assuage the ferocity of leonine leprosy.[76] Conversely, the kite (*miluinus*), a rapacious bird of prey, seemed capable of dispatching *lepra*, at least in its early stages.[77]

Certain cures reverberated with occult power. As we shall see, some physicians stressed the medicinal qualities of distilled human blood, while the great majority prescribed the preparation known as theriac for their more affluent patients. The drug enjoyed a formidable reputation, largely because its most celebrated ingredient comprised *tyrus*, the flesh of vipers. A variety of theriacs had been used for medicinal purposes in the Classical world, most being entirely herbal in composition. It was the Emperor Nero's physician who added snakes to the recipe, in the hope of creating an antidote – or more accurately stimulating immunity – to poison. Created on the assumption that venom would drive out venom, the drug naturally appealed to nervous despots, as well as men and women whose putrefying humours were resistant to other forms of treatment. The sixty-four exotic ingredients used in its production, the length of time it took to mature, and the belief that it possessed curative powers far beyond the sum of its many parts, combined to make theriac a central pillar in the medieval pharmacopoeia. So too did the fact that Galen had himself extolled its versatility as 'a new substance, with a nature of its own'.[78] He had, significantly, prescribed it, with apparent success, in the treatment of otherwise incurable *elephantia*.[79]

Endorsed in the *Antidotarium Nicolai* as 'the chief of the Galenic medicines', theriac was recommended for 'the most serious afflictions of the entire human body', ranging from epilepsy to smallpox. It could allegedly expel a dead foetus, banish a migraine, cure the kidney stone, and heal all known respiratory diseases.[80] One celebrated medieval treatise on the postponement of old age through humoral management, the *De retardatione senectutis*, devoted a chapter to the production and use of this universal panacea, which might also be drunk with red wine as a remedy for *lepra*.[81] Although he did not write the book, as was once believed, the Franciscan, Roger Bacon (d. 1294), was a keen advocate of theriac, which he recommended in many of his medical works.[82] At Montpellier, too, physicians such as Arnald of Villanova, were intrigued by the drug's 'special form' which transcended its innate heat and dryness to achieve a unique

[76] Bodleian Library, MS Ashmole 1505, fo. 34r; Ogden, *Cyrurgie of Guy de Chauliac*, p. 387; John of Gaddesden, *Rosa Anglica*, fo. 60v; Throop, *Hildegard von Bingen's Physica*, p. 216. It has been suggested that the hare's long ears 'turned inside out' like the flesh of the leper: Gaignebet and Lajoux, *Art profane*, p. 113. But hares were also ritually unclean [Leviticus 11, v. 6], and thus promised to fight corruption with corruption.

[77] BL, MS Sloane 4, p. 72.

[78] G. Watson, *Theriac and Mithridatum: A Study in Therapeutics* (London, 1966), pp. 10–20, 49, 50, 68–9, 77–8, 81–2; M. Stein, 'La thériaque chez Galien: Sa preparation et son usage thérapeutique', in A. Debru, ed., *Galen on Pharmacology, Philosophy, History and Medicine* (Brill, 1997), pp. 199–209.

[79] *Claudii Galeni opera omnia*, xiv, *Galeni ad Pisonem de theriaca liber*, pp. 210–94, notably cap. xviii, p. 290. See also, Thorndike, *History of Magic*, i, pp. 170–72.

[80] Grant, *Source Book*, pp. 788–9.

[81] Bacon, *De retardatione accidentium senectutis*, p. 65. Old age, being cold and dry, was a melancholic stage of life, and thus many remedies for its postponement were applicable to *lepra*: above, p. 71.

[82] Getz, *Medicine*, p. 61.

property or essence.[83] We shall return to the search for elixirs of this type later, but should note that Arnald and his colleagues reiterated the value of theriac in treating *lepra*, both externally and internally.[84]

During the later Middle Ages, supplies were shipped to England from Genoa and Venice in sealed containers, and sold by specialist 'tryacle' vendors as well as apothecaries under stringent controls. The punishments for diluting, falsifying or otherwise tampering with theriac were severe, and reflect the heavy demand, which increased dramatically after the Black Death of 1348–50.[85] The plague tracts and *regimina* which flooded the popular market during the later fourteenth and fifteenth centuries set great store on theriac as both a prophylactic and therapeutic form of medication.[86] It assumed even greater prominence in remedies against potentially malign dermatological conditions, while acquiring a deeper spiritual significance in the writings of contemporary mystics. Comparisons between Christ, the divine physician, and spiritual 'tryacle' abounded, in part because of the aromatic spices and balsam which also went into the heady mixture.[87] Besides helping to prevent physical corruption (it was used in the embalming process), balsam was an aromatic, whose delicious scent revived the vital and animal spirits, strengthening the heart and generating warmth. Symbolically connected with the healing grace of Christ's sweet-smelling body and blood, it offered medicine for the soul as well as the body, augmenting in no small measure the drug's unique status.[88] Jacques de Vitry employed a telling simile when he compared Christ to an alabaster vase of ointment or 'a pharmacy cupboard' full of medicinal balsam. Indeed, by the close of the Middle Ages, the image of the celestial apothecary, prescribing a cure for original sin in a shop stocked with theriac, enjoyed widespread appeal.[89]

Theriac proper was sold in a tightly regulated market, but English practitioners followed their continental peers in confecting a bastardised version of it for the treatment of *lepra*.[90] As Luke Demaitre has pointed out, the method of production effectively removed any venomous elements, and thus vitiated the drug's avowed homoeopathic purpose. But any remedy involving snake's flesh must still have exercised a powerful psychosomatic effect.[91] Tryian, or serpentine, leprosy, which appeared 'ful of skales', took its name from the way in which snakes regularly sloughed off their skins; and it was assumed that some of their celebrated capacity for regeneration would be absorbed by whoever consumed

83  Arnald of Villanova, *De dosi tyriacalium medicinarum*, in M.R. McVaugh, ed., *Opera medica omnia, III* (Barcelona, 1985), pp. 57–73. Bernard Gordon composed a less complex work, *De tyriaca*, in c. 1305: Demaitre, *Doctor Bernard de Gordon*, p. 76.
84  For the use of theriac as an ointment, see Bodleian Library, MS Ashmole 1505, fo. 33r.
85  Rawcliffe, *Medicine and Society*, pp. 152–5.
86  For example, *A Litil Boke whiche Trayted and Reherced Many Gode Thinges Necessaries for the . . . Pestilence* (John Rylands Facsimiles, iii, 1910), p. 5; Horrox, *Black Death*, p. 187 (although its use is here circumscribed).
87  Rawcliffe, *Medicine and Society*, pp. 152–3.
88  Albert, *Odeurs de sainteté*, pp. 20–22, 108–11, 145, 174–5, 177, 203.
89  D. Alexandre-Bidon, 'Le coeur du Christ au pressoir mystique: le cas des céramiques du Beauvaisis au début du XVIe siècle', in eadem, ed., *Le pressoir mystique* (Paris, 1990), pp. 163–5. See also J. Ziegler, *Medicine and Religion c. 1300: The Case of Arnau de Vilanova* (Oxford, 1998), pp. 144–8, 195.
90  Many recipes are recorded in Arnald of Villanova, *Tresor des pouvres*, fos 38r–39v.
91  Demaitre, 'Relevance of Futility', p. 41. For myths and legends surrounding the longevity and power of snakes, see Albert, *Odeurs de sainteté*, pp. 37, 43, 202–3.

them.[92] There was, moreover, a pleasing irony in the use of snakes to expel corrupt humours, since they carried an ancestral burden of guilt for causing the initial problem. According to the *Causae et curae* of Hildegard of Bingen, black bile had 'first originated from Adam's semen through the breath of the serpent', for no sooner had he taken the apple than melancholia 'coagulated in his blood', with disastrous consequences for his descendants.[93]

For all these reasons, snake meat gave a tremendous boost to standard components of the pharmacopoeia. It was, for example, added to laxative preparations in the treatment of elephantine leprosy, the most intractable of the four humoral types:

> Take an edder [adder] the wyche fowndyd in the wodes, but no [harmless] snake, and kytt awey the hed & the tayll and bowel yt & culpyne [chop] yt and seth yt in a lytill whyt wyne to yt be sodyne tendyr inowghe & departe the flesch ther from the bones & to the weight ther off put as myche dyacene & dianthos[94] & menge [mix] all well togedyr . . . And euery iiijte [fourth] day do the pacient resaffe as mych as a walnut off this laxatyffe.[95]

Admitting that 'we haue non other waye in the helynge of leprouse men after the clensynge of the body but in serpentes', Guy de Chauliac followed Bernard Gordon and other practitioners in recommending a variety of foodstuffs and beverages containing their boiled, roasted or distilled flesh.[96] How far the average English practitioner availed himself of the more esoteric recipes is a moot point, although they were duly copied out and added to the pharmacopoeia, perhaps for their curiosity value. It is interesting to note that one late fifteenth-century Welsh remedy book refers to garlic as 'the poor man's treacle [theriac]' and, contrary to the advice given above, deploys it as a means of expelling the poison of *lepra*.[97]

Treatment began in earnest with the administration of purgatives to cleanse the entire system of impurities, a procedure that, in the case of elephantine leprosy, clearly demanded heroic measures. The conventional mixture of snake meat and senna described above might well be supplemented by a customised dose of 'oxymel' diuretic syrup in order to eliminate so much adust bile. This comprised a standard honey and vinegar base mixed with thyme, cinnamon, scammony and mastic gum, along with two compound preparations from the *Antidotarium*, known after their reputed creators as 'yeralogodion' and

---

92  Seymour, *On the Properties of Things*, i, pp. 423–4.
93  Hildegard of Bingen, *On Natural Philosophy*, pp. 39, 41. In one late medieval homily, Christ's passion is compared to the ordeal endured by a leper who has consumed snake's flesh in his wine, and must suffer before being cured: Oesterley, *Gesta Romanorum*, pp. 507–9. For the origins of this tale, see Thorndike, *History of Magic*, i, pp. 170–71.
94  Electuaries based on, respectively, senna and rosemary. Elsewhere these ingredients were recommended if the patient were 'a pore man' and could not afford the costlier drugs prescribed for 'a delicate man & riche': Bodleian Library, MS Ashmole 1505, fo. 32r.
95  BL, MS Harley 1736, fo. 135r. The water in which the snake had been cooked could be used for bathing: Bodleian Library, MS Ashmole 1505, fo. 33v.
96  Ogden, *Cyrurgie of Guy de Chauliac*, pp. 387–9; Avicenna, *Liber canonis*, fos 443r–444v. These recipes often included chicken fed on snakes: John of Gaddesden, *Rosa Anglica*, fo. 59v.
97  Cule, 'Diagnosis, Care and Treatment of Leprosy', p. 52. See also, Trinity College, Cambridge, MS O.I.13, fo. 153v.

'yerruffini'.[98] Following a similar four-day cycle to that recommended for purgation, the patient would also be 'stewed', or bathed, in a vat of hot water containing the leaves of dock, fennel, sage and scabious. It was assumed that the scented vapour would enter the body through the open pores, thereby intensifying the process of evacuation and encouraging perspiration.[99] To remove any deep-seated corruption, which could neither be sweated out nor reached by conventional laxatives, another stiff dose of theriac, administered with syrup of fumitory, seemed advisable. Before bedtime, moreover, the patient would be urged to spend half an hour bent over a steaming bowl of barley and oats to which a hot stew of borage and thyme leaves had been added. It was thus hoped to cleanse and moisturise the face, preparing it for the application of a series of unguents. We will return to the role of baths, and the surgical procedures that followed them, in the next sections of this chapter; of more immediate interest are the ointments prescribed for topical application, one of which was made of white lead mixed with powdered lily root and pork fat. Another, presumably intended for wealthier patients, called upon an exotic range of ingredients, including borax, camphor, frankincense, white coral and pulverised marble. It, too, relied on lead to camouflage discoloration and blemishes.[100]

Although they are now particularly associated with the rise of Paracelsian medicine in the sixteenth century, and with the aggressive remedies then used for treating the pox, mineral preparations enjoyed considerable vogue in the later Middle Ages.[101] They included gold, silver, copper, iron, cinnabar, mercury, antimony, alum and lead, along with medicinal salts and chemical products, such as zinc carbonate, zinc oxide, borax, lime, sulphur, arsenic, asphalt, ammonium chloride, potassium sulphate, potassium nitrate and lead monoxide.[102] On the basis that minerals, along with the rest of creation, could be ranked according to status, lead (a cold and dry subject of Saturn) glowered at the bottom of this *scala natura*, while gold (the king of all metals) shone forth as the most perfect, powerful and therapeutic. Sanguine and temperate in complexion, like its ruling planet, the sun, it was deployed by those who could afford it to 'clense superfluites ygendred in bodyes', and was thus widely used as a prophylactic 'agens lepre and mesellerie'. Citing Avicenna as his authority, the encyclopaedist, Bartholomaeus Anglicus, maintained that 'the fylyng of golde ytake in

---

98 A 'yera' or *hiera* was a type of antidote or purge, the two in question being attributed respectively to Logadios of Alexandria and the eminent physician, Rufus of Ephesus (*fl.* AD 200), whom we met in chapter two: Bacon, *De retardatione accidentium senectutis*, p. 221; Klibansky, Panofsky and Saxl, *Saturn and Melancholy*, pp. 48–55. Various *hierae* are listed in the *Antidotarium Nicolai*, logodion being described as a powerful weapon against black bile and phlegm, retention of menses, *lepra* and other 'cold' evils. Yerruffini was a cure for morphew and *elephantia*: W.S. van der Berg, ed., *Antidotarium Nicolai* (Leiden, 1917), pp. 183–7, 218. For another oxymel diuretic used in the treatment of scabies and leprosy, see Hunt, *Popular Medicine*, p. 333.
99 Baths for the treatment of leonine leprosy used leaves and stems of willow, borage and plantain. For tyrian leprosy dock, wallwort, lavender, elder, wild celery (smallage) and wormwood were recommended; and for vulpine leprosy borage and red dock: BL, MS Harley 1736, fos 136r–137v. The author relies largely on Theoderic here: Campbell and Colton, *Surgery of Theoderic*, ii, pp. 173–4.
100 BL, MS Sloane 1736, fos 136r, 157v–158r.
101 Arrizabalaga, Henderson and French, *Great Pox*, pp. 139–44.
102 For an assessment of the properties of minerals, see '*De lapidibus et metallis*' in Seymour, *On the Properties of Things*, ii, pp. 825–81; and, for their medical application, Getz, *Pharmaceutical Writings of Gilbertus Anglicus*, passim.

mete or in drynke or in medicyne preserueth and letteth [prevents] the bredyng of lepre or namelyche hideth it and maketh it vnknowen'.[103] Some considered it especially valuable for consuming and expelling the choleric humours of leonine *lepra*, while also recommending potable gold as a supplement to be taken with theriac for the treatment of all four types.[104]

Mercury (quick silver) possessed a cold, wet complexion, being valued for its regenerative and purgative qualities, most notably the capacity to destroy infected flesh and remove unsightly blemishes. Such a potentially toxic material could not, however, be used without risk. Galen had regarded it as too dangerous for inclusion in the standard pharmacopoeia, but several other Greek and Roman physicians extolled its virtues, as did a number of the influential Muslim authorities whose works became a staple of medical practice in the later medieval West. Al-Kindi (d. 870), 'the philosopher of Arabia', and Abu Mansur had, for example, listed mercurials among their *materia medica*. Thirteen of the seventy chapters of the *De aluminibus et salibus*, attributed to Rhazes and trans-lated in the twelfth century by Gerard of Cremona, were devoted to mercury and its compounds. Avicenna, the Holy Ghost of the medieval medical Trinity, had also prescribed them for external use.[105]

Drawing upon the 'Saracenic' authors who had so dramatically expanded the Classical pharmacopoeia, European surgeons and physicians eagerly incorpo-rated these new ingredients into their practice.[106] Notwithstanding an under-standable preference for cheaper, more accessible simples, the compilers of domestic remedy books also began to expand their range of pharmaceuticals. Anxiety about facial symptoms clearly ran deep. Even modest compilations of a few pages listed washes and ointments 'ffor a saucefleme face . . . a face that semyth lyk a lipyr . . . ffor rede pympyllys in the face . . . ffor blaynes in the face', and so forth.[107] Robert Thornton's *Liber de diversis medicinis* (1422–54) is typical in its recourse to excoriating chemical preparations for cosmetic purposes. The suspect leper is, for example, advised to mix the juice of cress and nettles[108] with the fat of a boar (as an unguent) and mercury, anointing his face with the prepa-ration twice a day. The recommendation that he should also wash the affected area would, hopefully, have mitigated the effects of such a potentially harmful procedure. A second recipe, employing two ounces of mercury and half a pound of powdered white lead (a compound of carbonate and hydroxide of lead), mixed with goose grease, virgin wax, honey, willow leaves and frankincense may have inflicted even more damage.[109]

---

103  Seymour, *On the Properties of Things*, ii, p. 829. So did Henry Daniel: BL, MS Arundel 42, fo. 37v. Chaucer plays humorously upon his Physician's love of gold in *The Canterbury Tales*: Benson, *River-side Chaucer*, p. 30.

104  Bacon, *De retardatione accidentium senectutis*, pp. 128, 134. John of Gaddesden, *Rosa Anglica*, fo. 59v, prescribed gold daily for rich patients with *lepra*, considering it 'the best medicine'. See also BL, MS Sloane 2272 (part 1), fo. 91r; MS Harley 3, fo. 23v; Avicenna, *Liber canonis*, fo. 444v.

105  L.J. Goldwater, *Mercury: A History of Quicksilver* (Baltimore, 1972), pp. 24, 88, 207–11.

106  Campbell and Colton, *Surgery of Theoderic*, ii, pp. 147–9. See also, John of Gaddesden, *Rosa Anglica*, fo. 60v; Nicaise, *Chirurgie de Henri de Mondeville*, p. 623; BL, MS Sloane 2272 (part 1), fo. 93v.

107  Bodleian Library, MS Ashmole 1443, pp. 6–8, 321–7. See also, BL, MS Arundel, fo. 34r–34v.

108  The nettle (hot and dry in three degrees: BL, MS Add. 19674, fo. 41v) was another powerful corro-sive, which 'brenneth the body that it toucheth': Seymour, *On the Properties of Things*, ii, p. 1088.

109  M.S. Ogden, ed., *The Liber de diversis medicinis* (EETS, ccvii, 1969), p. 39. See also, W.R. Dawson, ed.,

Medieval physicians recognised the need to modify the effect of strong corro-
sives by diluting them with gentler substances, and were well aware of the
hazards they posed to patient and practitioner alike. One remedy involving the
use of orpiment (yellow arsenic) mixed with chicken fat stressed the need for
thorough washing, 'be cause that hit wondyrly brennyth'.[110] Bartholomaeus
Anglicus observed that the vapours from mercury 'bredeth palsy and quakyng,
slakyng and neisshyng [softening] of the synewes', and offered an antidote for
anyone who accidentally swallowed it.[111] During the course of a long practice,
the sixteenth-century surgeon, John Banester, noted that barbers who applied
mercurials negligently when treating the pox experienced the same foul breath,
rotting gums, inflammation and ulcers as their patients.[112] Quite possibly some
suspect lepers (including the apprentice barber surgeons noted in the previous
chapter) may have been the victims of iatrogenic diseases caused by constant
exposure to dangerous chemicals.

The ubiquity of mineral preparations in medieval England is apparent – along
with their limitations – in Chaucer's brief but revealing description of the
Summoner in the Prologue to his *Canterbury Tales*. The latter's 'fyr-reed
cherabynnes face' testifies to years of self-indulgence, and suggests that a fatal
combination of gluttony, drink and sex will soon render him leprous:

> For saucefleem he was, with eyen narwe.
> As hoot he was and lecherous as a sparwe,
> With scalled browes blake and piled [hairless] berd.
> Of his visage children were aferd.
> Ther nas quyk-silver, lytarge, ne brymstoon,
> Boras, ceruce, ne oille of tarter noon,[113]
> Ne oynement that wolde clense and byte,
> That hym myghte helpen of his whelks white,
> Nor of the knobbes sittynge on his chekes.
> Wel loved he garleek,[114] onions, and eek lekes,
> And for to drynken strong wyn, reed as blood.[115]

---

*A Leechbook of the Fifteenth Century* (London, 1934), pp. 182–3; BL, MS Sloane 963, fo. 69r–69v. In
essence, these remedies barely differ from the type recommended in Latin texts. John Bradmore
favoured an ointment made of oil of laurel, frankincense, saltpetre (potassium nitrate), plantain,
pimpernel, fumitory, quicksilver and pork fat for the hands and feet: BL, MS Sloane 2272 (part 1), fo.
91r.

110  BL, MS Sloane 5, fo. 155r. See also, Getz, *Pharmaceutical Writings of Gilbertus Anglicus*, pp. 47–50.
White lead was a popular cosmetic, hence the name *alba dominarum* given to one ointment used by
English surgeons to treat *lepra*: BL, MS Harley 1736, fo. 136r.

111  Seymour, *On the Properties of Things*, ii, p. 832; BL, MS Arundel 42, fo. 34r–34v; Goldwater, *Mercury*,
pp. 89–92, 211.

112  John Banester's treatise on 'The Natvre & Propertie of Quick Siluer' appears as an appendix to
William Clowes, *Briefe and Necessarie Treatise Touching the Cure of the Disease called Morbus Gallicus*
(London, 1585), fos 47r–56r, and especially fos 53r, 56r.

113  That is mercury, lead monoxide, sulphur, borax, white lead and potassium hydrogen tartrate
(produced in fermentation): all were extensively used in the treatment of *lepra*.

114  Bartholomaeus Anglicus warned of the dangers of garlic, which 'bredeth lepra' and was 'cause of
madnesse and frenesye' in choleric men, such as the Summoner: *On the Properties of Things*, ii, pp.
909–10; and above, pp. 78–9.

115  Benson, *Riverside Chaucer*, p. 33. Attempts to diagnose the Summoner are discussed by E.M. Biebel,
'Pilgrims to Table: Food Consumption in Chaucer's *Canterbury Tales*', in M. Carlin and J. Rosenthal,

The despair of his confessor and physician alike, the Summoner offered a terrible warning to those who ignored the advice of the regimen.

## Baths

The belief that medieval Europe was beset by unremitting squalor is hard to dislodge. The picture of 'stagnant misery' painted by Victorian scholars, such as Augustus Jessopp, remains as vivid in some quarters as the image of the outcast leper. Indeed, Jessopp's depressing portrait of thirteenth-century urban life was cited at length by George Newman in his influential history of leprosy in the Middle Ages, which he blamed upon a combination of poor diet, 'uncleanness' and insalubrious surroundings.[116] The French historian, Jules Michelet, writing in 1862, was even more dogmatic:

> One imputes leprosy to the Crusades, to Asia. Europe had it within herself. The war which the Middle Ages declared upon the flesh and upon cleanliness bore its own fruit. More than one saint is praised for having never even washed her hands. And how much less the rest! The nudity of a moment had become a great sin. The laity followed these lessons of monasticism faithfully. This subtle and refined society, which denigrated marriage, and seems only to have loved the poetry of adultery, retained a singular scruple in such an innocent matter. It dreaded all cleansing as defilement. No bath for a thousand years! You may be sure that not one of these knights, these ethereal beauties, the Parsifals, the Tristans, the Iseults, ever washed themselves.[117]

Setting aside the fact that Tristan, and other heroes of chivalric romance, are known to have enjoyed the therapeutic (and erotic) pleasures of bathing, we should note how often the connection between personal cleanliness and health features in the pages of medieval advice manuals.[118] The children of Saturn, born under a murky sign, were not only associated with dirty and noisome trades, such as tanning and grave-digging, but also with a lamentable disregard for basic hygiene. All too often they wore 'fowle steynkande clothes' and were 'unclene as bestes', thus inviting the unpleasant skin conditions that also came under the planet's sway.[119] In his *Rosa Anglica*, John of Gaddesden drew a specific connection between vermin, filthy clothes and the onset of *lepra*, warning that extreme ascetic practices, such as the wearing of infested hair shirts, could engender skin

---

eds, *Food and Eating in Medieval Europe* (London, 1998), p. 18. Grigsby, *Pestilence*, pp. 84–9, assumes he is already leprous.

[116] Newman, *History of the Decline of Leprosy*, pp. 70, 84–5, 88–90; A. Jessopp, *The Coming of the Friars and other Historic Essays* (London, 1890), p. 21.

[117] J. Michelet, *La sorcière* (2 vols, Paris, 1952), i, p. 104. Farrow, *Damien the Leper*, p. 89, perpetuates this tradition, arguing that 'at least a quarter of northern Europe's population were lepers', and that England, being especially squalid, 'was the most sorely affected'.

[118] Rawcliffe, *Medicine and Society*, pp. 62–3, 181. Although the experience was more common in life than in literature: E. Archibald, 'Did Knights Have Baths? The Absence of Bathing in Middle English Romance', in C. Saunders, ed., *Cultural Encounters in the Romance of Medieval England* (Studies in Medieval Romance, ii, 2005), pp. 101–15. For bathing in general, see Kleinschmidt, *Perception and Action*, pp. 61–6.

[119] BL, MS Egerton 2572, fo. 64v. See also Klibansky, Panofsky and Saxl, *Saturn and Melancholy*, pp. 130–31, 195.

diseases.[120] Since melancholics were, reputedly, drawn to the solitary religious life, mortification of the body may have posed another threat to their precarious equilibrium. In view of the widespread assumption that lice, fleas and other parasites were actually engendered by the effluvia of 'sour' humours, lepers seemed especially vulnerable to infestation. They were therefore well advised to shun the rigours of monastic discipline. From a medical perspective, at least, the benefits of a freshly laundered shirt and herbal bath seemed incontestable.[121]

Bathing was, however, far more than a simple matter of hygiene. For those with sufficient resources, baths played an important part in the prevention and treatment of disease, in part because of a legacy from Roman times. They ranked, along with diet, as one of only two specific recommendations for the care of sick monks made in the Benedictine Rule, and were a staple of the *regimen sanitatis*. Sometimes they were included under the general heading of exercise, or, more often, that of evacuation, but in the context of *lepra* they merited a category of their own, since they were so widely employed as both a therapeutic and palliative measure.[122] A hot bath, or 'stew', was designed to make the patient sweat, and thus eliminate impurities. It also opened the pores, and therefore seemed extremely dangerous in plague time, since the miasmas of disease could more easily enter the body. But so too could the healing scent of medicinal herbs, whose fragrance would strengthen, nourish and restore the spirits. As we have already seen, odours were believed to possess a material substance, somewhere between air and water. Just as the stench of leprous sores threatened to infect those who inhaled it, so too the perfume of a herb or flower transmitted its therapeutic qualities in a more intense and immediate form, dispelling evil odours in its wake. Like the plants, animals and spices from which they came, all scents were graded according to their relative heat, coldness, aridity and moisture. Violets (which were appropriately ruled by the planet Saturn) produced a 'colde and moiste', humectant aroma, while that from calamint, another staple in the treatment of *lepra*, was considered 'hoot and drye'.[123] Baths thus constituted an important adjunct of humoral therapy, while also offering a measure of relief from pain. The experience cannot always have been entirely relaxing, or free from discomfort, however, since vigorous 'frotting' or scrubbing was also recommended. Having shaved his scalp and done his best to work up a good sweat 'for to put out alle superfluytes of hys body', the patient was to rub himself as hard as possible from head to foot with a rough cloth, perhaps using an agent such as powdered beans, burnt chestnut shells, meal or coarse herbs. Not only did this help to remove any scaly dead flesh or congealed matter – it was also believed to restore lost feeling to desensitised limbs.[124]

---

[120] John of Gaddesden, *Rosa Anglica*, fos 52r, 56v.

[121] G. Vigarello, *Concepts of Cleanliness: Changing Attitudes in France since the Middle Ages* (Cambridge, 1985), pp. 43–4. See below, p. 330, for the impact of these ideas on hospital regulations.

[122] M. Nicoud, 'Les médecins Italiens et le bain thermal à la fin du moyen âge', *Médiévales*, xliii (2002), pp. 13–40, at pp. 17–19; Gil-Sotres, 'Regimens of Health', p. 307.

[123] BL, MS Sloane 2948, fo. 56v; Palmer, 'Bad Odour', pp. 61–8.

[124] Bodleian Library, MS Ashmole 1505, fo. 33r; BL, MS Sloane 5, fo. 154v; Campbell and Colton, *Surgery of Theoderic*, ii, p. 172; John of Gaddesden, *Rosa Anglica*, fo. 60r; Arnald of Villanova, *Tresor des Pouvres*, fo. 38v. A fragrant moisturising agent, such as oil of violets, would be applied afterwards.

Medieval Christians naturally sought to exfoliate their souls as well as their bodies. All forms of medical treatment invited theological analogy, but the bath, with its overtones of baptism and confession, was especially rich in religious symbolism. The story of Naaman was taken literally as well as figuratively by some victims of *lepra*, who regarded immersion in the Jordan (especially at the reputed place of Christ's baptism) as a 'sovereign cure' for their disease.[125] Recent research suggests that the whirlpools in this stretch of river would, indeed, have had a beneficial, if temporary, effect upon disorders such as psoriasis, and that they attracted many visitors.[126] We have already encountered one young man who travelled for this reason to the Holy Land, although it was later, at Becket's tomb, that he regained almost complete health. William of Canterbury's proud assertion that his cathedral now boasted the source of 'the new Jordan . . . emerging from the head of the martyr' did not, however, dissuade some intrepid pilgrims from continuing to make the long and difficult expedition.[127] In 1236, for example, Henry III granted a house to St Nicholas's hospital, Portsmouth, in order to support one Philip the Clerk, a leper, or else to provide him with everything he needed to reach the Holy Land.[128]

The miraculous appearance of sacred springs, whose waters possessed the power to heal leprosy, is a recurrent theme of Irish and English legend. King Bladud, the mythical founder of Bath, was said to have been a leper, and to have been cured after immersing himself in its hot springs.[129] The miracle of Elias the leper monk, described in the previous chapter, confirms that suspect lepers had easy recourse to the facilities there. It is not clear from the two conflicting accounts of Elias's peregrinations whether or not he actually spent a symbolic forty days in the town, 'thinking the hot baths might do him good and that his pains might be relieved by the heat of the sulphur', or if he merely pretended to do so. In either event, his abbot, who remained sceptical about tales emanating from Canterbury, was far happier for him to seek relief through bathing and medication than by visiting 'the new Jordan'.[130]

Healing wells and springs were frequently associated with *leprosaria*, which needed a regular water supply, and were naturally drawn to sources rich in minerals. Having been cured by bathing in a nearby stream, a leper called Ramp [Rampnaldus] reputedly founded the hospital of St Mary Magdalen at Beccles,

---

[125]  See above, pp. 125–6.

[126]  Lieber, 'Old Testament "Leprosy", Contagion and Sin', pp. 112–13; M. Avi-Yonah, 'The Bath of the Lepers at Scythopolis', *Israel Exploration Journal*, xiii (1963), pp. 325–6.

[127]  Robertson, *Materials*, i, pp. 218–19, 337. A travel guide to pilgrimage sites in and around Jerusalem, which is part of a vernacular medical text produced in the 1450s, notes the continuing popularity of 'a lytyll watyr whyche is callyd *probatica piscine*, in the wyche many lepyrs are helyd by the vertu of a tre [beam] of the holy crosse that lay therin many yerys': Wellcome Institute Library, Western MS 8004, p. 155. Bathing was no less popular among Muslim visitors: Dols, 'Leper in Medieval Islamic Society', pp. 903–5.

[128]  *CPR, 1232–1247*, p. 134.

[129]  W. Bonser, *The Medical Background of Anglo Saxon England* (London, 1963), pp. 372–3. The leper hospital at Bath did not enjoy direct access to the hot spring, however, as some sources maintain: Manco, *Spirit of Care*, pp. 20–21.

[130]  Robertson, *Materials*, i, pp. 416–17; ii, pp. 242–3. Abbot, *St Thomas of Canterbury*, ii, pp. 170–79, provides parallel texts.

in Suffolk, 'for the benefit of all persons affected with the distemper'.[131] Quite possibly the lepers' well, which still bore his name in the nineteenth century, produced water with a high sulphur content, as did those next to *leprosaria* at Brewood in Staffordshire and Lyme Regis in Dorset. Another, dedicated to the Virgin Mary near the lazar house at Lubenham, Leicestershire, reputedly tapped into a chalybeate spring.[132] The lepers of a second Suffolk hospital, that of St James outside Dunwich, were said to enjoy the best water in the area, which they drew from a 'holy well' across the road from their chapel.[133] It is now hard to tell if the spring at Burton Lazars, which later became the site of a spa specialising in 'all sores, scorbutic and cutaneous disorders', actually lay within the hospital precinct. The residents clearly benefited from its availability, as they did from the 'uncommonly salubrious' environment.[134] Were sacred springs also a source of spiritual medicine? The recent discovery of immersion tanks in the chapel of the hospital of St John the Baptist, Oxford, for example, suggests that the healing powers of the patron saint were invoked there, appropriately enough, through the use of river water. St John's accommodated the sick poor rather than lepers, but it would be surprising if *leprosaria* on riparian sites did not observe similar rituals.[135]

The cleansing of hands and faces with holy water at shrines was certainly replete with religious symbolism. But it also served a hygienic purpose and may, in some cases, have contributed to the marked improvement in the appearance of pilgrims observed by shrine keepers and hagiographers, such as Benedict of Canterbury. The latter notes, for example, that shortly after washing his face in water from the martyr's shrine, Elias the leper monk acquired a bloodstained strip of Becket's clothing, which he squeezed into his bathwater and thereby 'cleansed away his leprosy'.[136] Faces and bodies stained with the dirt and dust of a long journey and congealed matter from suppurating sores would, inevitably, look better after a good soak. Historians have probably underestimated the extent to which bathing and other comparatively inexpensive forms of treatment may have been available to the poor pilgrims and beggars who congregated around shrines or sought out individuals with a reputation for sanctity.

An interesting example of such *ad hoc* medical care may be found in William of Malmesbury's twelfth-century life of Bishop Wulstan of Worcester (d. 1095). He recounts how a leper, who looked more like 'a living corpse' than a human being, approached the saint for help. Despite his pitiful entreaties, Wulstan felt it would be presumptuous to attempt a miracle cure and sent the wretched creature away with food and clothing. Convinced of his master's sanctity, a priest named Elmer 'took the sick man into his house and comforted him with kind words'. He then performed a holy theft, surreptitiously removing the water in

---

131  BL, MS Add. 19112, fo. 58r; above, p. 124.
132  Satchell, 'Emergence of Leper-Houses', pp. 146–7; J. Rattue, *The Living Stream: Holy Wells in Historical Context* (Woodbridge, 1995), p. 84. The hospital of St Leonard, Peterborough, also boasted a medicinal well: Serjeantson and Adkins, *VCH Northamptonshire II*, p. 162.
133  N. Comfort, *The Lost City of Dunwich* (Lavenham, 1994), p. 121.
134  Marcombe, *Leper Knights*, pp. 142–5.
135  Gilchrist, *Contemplation and Action*, pp. 37–8, 43.
136  Robertson, *Materials*, ii, pp. 242–3.

which Wulstan had washed his hands after celebrating Mass. This he handed to a servant,

> and had him pour it into the sick man's bath. The leper went to the water terrible to behold, his flesh covered in blemishes. But, miraculously, at once the swelling of the pustules went down, the deadly matter ran away, and, in short, all his flesh bloomed again with the purity of a little child's. Even the impetigo and scabs on his head were banished; his hair grew again as before.[137]

As we saw in chapter three, washing the feet of the sick poor, and especially of the leprous, was a hallmark of the medieval saint, demonstrating humility and compassion, as well as an obvious identification with Christ at the last supper. Some holy men and women went further. *The Little Flowers of St Francis*, a hagiographical text of *c.* 1330, tells how he cured a particularly cantankerous leper, whose irritability sprang, in part, from the filthy state in which he was obliged to live. Francis 'immediately had water boiled with many sweet scented herbs' and set about bathing the man from head to foot. The results were miraculous: 'as externally the water washed his body and the flesh began to heal . . . so too interiorly his soul began to be healed and cleansed', his tears of contrition dissolving the stains of sin while the perfume coursed over his ulcerated skin.[138] Elizabeth of Hungary, herself a Franciscan tertiary, was also famous for her willingness to tend the most despised and physically repugnant lepers, bathing them and dressing their sores with her own hands. She is depicted in one late medieval German altarpiece washing two female lepers in a wooden bath, while a servant brings nourishing food, including chicken, for them to eat [**plate 25**].[139] Ordinary sinners were urged to follow this example. The abbess who appears in *The Vision of the Monk of Eynsham* had personally helped to bathe her leprous sisters, thus shortening her time in purgatory through an act of Christian compassion.[140]

Unlike many of the measures described in late medieval medical literature, herbal baths were cheap and comparatively simple to prepare; they demanded little in the way of expertise; they provided considerable relief for a range of painful symptoms; and they must also have helped to curb the infection of open wounds and lesions. Although most authorities agreed that aggressive remedies were positively harmful once *lepra* had been confirmed, bathing remained a central element of palliative care. To dispel the stench associated with advanced cases, John of Gaddesden recommended the addition of rose petals and camomile to bath water, followed by the application of a perfumed wash, made of spice, mirobalans and roses.[141] Scented baths were certainly available in the larger French *leprosaria*. In 1448, for example, a priest from St Omer who appeared 'greatly inclined to leprosy' was advised 'to make himself comfortable

---

137 Darlington, *Vita Wulfstani of William of Malmesbury*, pp. 30–31. See also, E. Mason, *St Wulfstan of Worcester c. 1008–1095* (Oxford, 1990), pp. 178–9.
138 The improvement was, however, temporary, as the leper died a fortnight later 'of another illness': M.A. Habig, ed., *St Francis of Assisi: Writings and Early Biographies* (London, 1973), pp. 1356–9.
139 Habrich, Williams and Wolf, *Aussatz, Lepra, Hansen-Krankheit*, no. 7.3, p. 131.
140 See above, p. 142.
141 John of Gaddesden, *Rosa Anglica*, fo. 61v.

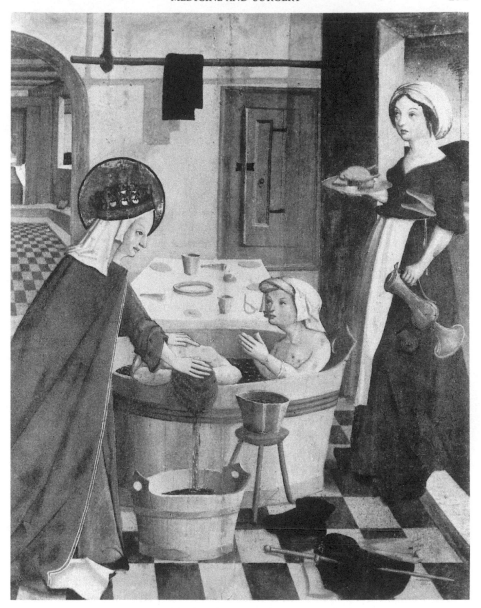

25. St Elizabeth of Hungary bathes two female lepers in a wooden tub, while a maid produces chicken for them to eat. This was the type of mild, moist food that was considered especially beneficial for the sick.

and to bathe'. Because of his poverty, the examining physicians recommended
that he should be allowed to enjoy the facilities at a local hospital free of charge.
These permitted complete immersion: in 1421 the house had acquired two
substantial tubs for the lepers, and a few years later one of the inmates left his
fellows 'a great pail' for their ablutions.[142] We know less about the facilities available in English hospitals, although some showed great concern about hygiene,
and it seems more than likely that their gardens produced herbs for use in baths
as well as in ointments and analgesic potions.[143]

## Surgical procedures

Never one to belittle his own achievements, Galen boasted of his ability to cure
*lepra* and other chronic diseases through the administration of purgatives alone,
although he rightly assumed that lesser physicians might lack such skills.[144] This
was not for want of information or *materia medica*. As we have already seen, by
the later Middle Ages the range of laxatives and diuretics available to the practitioner had increased dramatically, along with the choice of procedures for eliminating corruption in other parts of the system. Cleansing agents called
*caputpurgia* were, for instance, employed as an essential preliminary to any form
of surgery – such as cauterisation – upon the head or face, while also helping to
prevent the accumulation of peccant matter in the nasal area. An explosive
mixture of pepper, mace, oregano, celandine, agnus castus, pennyroyal and
nasturtium boiled in white wine might be dropped into the patient's nostrils
with a cloth or pipe before meals, or rolled into pills to 'make hym snese or pisse
and . . . purge the hede of watery humours'.[145] This type of remedy, along with
baths and the sudorific and cosmetic preparations that accompanied them, was
traditionally administered by a surgeon or barber surgeon, whose remit
extended well beyond the use of the phlebotomist's lancet. Venesection (bloodletting), the staple of his practice was, in fact, more circumspectly deployed, at
least in the later stages of *lepra*.

Ubiquitous as both a routine prophylactic and therapeutic measure, phlebotomy enabled the practitioner to remove superfluous amounts of venous
blood and humoral matter from his patient with comparative ease. In Bernard
Gordon's words, it was 'a universal medicine for all those ills caused by excess',
especially in men and women of a sanguine complexion.[146] Long before Galen's
principal work on venesection was translated into Latin in the first half of the
fourteenth century, a significant literature had developed on the subject. It dealt,
among other things, with the treatment of localised problems, such as lesions or

---

142  Bourgeois, *Lépreux et maladreries*, pp. 314, 312. Wooden tubs, made by a local cooper, were acquired
     by the *leprosarium* at Bethune in the early fifteenth century: ibid., p. 243.
143  See below, pp. 305–6, 316, 327.
144  A.Z. Iskander, ed., *Galeni de optimo medico cognoscendo* (Berlin, 1988), p. 123.
145  Bodleian Library, MS Ashmole 1505 fo. 32v; Ogden, *Cyrurgie of Guy de Chauliac*, p. 387; BL, MS
     Sloane 2272 (part 1), fo. 93r; Avicenna, *Liber canonis*, fo. 443v. White hellebore, which was deemed
     'more violent' than black, was also recommended. In the case of leprosy, the use of 'tents' or linen
     cloths soaked in medicinal oils offered a means of preventing the nasal passages from collapsing: BL,
     MS Sloane 5, fos 33r, 154v.
146  Gil-Sotres, 'Derivation and Revulsion', p. 119.

swellings caused by corrupt matter. Since knowledge of the circulation of the blood lay far into the future, it seemed logical to assume that it could be made to flow in the opposite direction from normal by opening a more distant vein on the 'other' side of the body. Through this process of revulsion or *antipasis*, the trained practitioner could not only prevent a dangerous concentration of putre-fying humours, but also inhibit heavy bleeding by diverting the flow elsewhere. The choice between revulsion and derivation (bleeding from the nearest vein) depended upon a variety of factors, including the perceived risk of disturbing congealed humoral matter once it had settled in a specific place.[147] *Lepra* posed an insuperable problem, however, for, once established, it was amenable to neither procedure. As 'a vniuersal corrupcioun of membres and of humours', it spread insidiously from the veins into the surrounding flesh. In short, the whole body was being 'inorischid and ifedde' by contaminated blood, every drop of which disseminated poison.[148] Prompt evacuation at the outset was therefore crucial, and explains why many of the most influential Islamic authorities and their successors placed phlebotomy first on the list of procedures to be attempted in cases of suspect *lepra*.

Because they suffered from an excess of adust sanguine humour, victims of the vulpine strain (*alopecia*) seemed especially responsive to venesection.[149] Female lepers who had failed to menstruate, and men whose haemorrhoids had stopped bleeding also appeared to benefit, since both conditions caused the retention of corrupt blood that would otherwise have found a natural outlet.[150] But in most cases a visit from the phlebotomist would simply weaken the leprous patient without doing any good, 'cooling and drying [the body], enfee-bling the vital spirits and setting corrupt matter in motion without eliminating it'.[151] Some authors did, however, recommend specifically localised bleeding from the 'lesser' rather than the 'greater' veins as a means of removing matter from troublesome areas, such as the nose.[152] Another exception to this rule, advocated by Avicenna and the eminent Muslim surgeon, Albucassis (d. 1013), concerned the respiratory problems so often encountered in advanced cases. The procedure, which was certainly not without danger, involved binding the patient's neck just below the jugular veins with a ligature, and removing a 'mod-erate' amount of blood by means of a longditudinal incision in each. Staunching

---

147 Gil-Sotres, 'Derivation and Revulsion', passim. For the general practice of phlebotomy, see Rawcliffe, *Medicine and Society*, pp. 64–8; Voigts and McVaugh, 'Latin Technical Phlebotomy', pp. 1–25.

148 Seymour, *On the Properties of Things*, i, p. 423.

149 Campbell and Colton, *Surgery of Theoderic*, ii, p. 171; BL, MS Sloane 2272 (part 1), fo. 92v. At this stage, blood was usually taken alternately from the cephalic vein on one side and the hepatic on the other.

150 John of Gaddesden, *Rosa Anglica*, fo. 58v; Bodleian Library, MS Ashmole 1505, fo. 31v. Moderate bleeding from haemorrhoids was regarded as a natural mechanism for the expulsion of 'malencolious blode', and thus of preserving the body from 'many sekenes aduste and corrupte, as is . . . lepre': John of Arderne, *Treatises of Fistula in Ano*, ed. D. Power (EETS, cxxxix, 1910), p. 57.

151 Nicaise, *Chirurgie de Henri de Mondeville*, p. 620. See also Demaitre, 'Relevance of Futility', pp. 38–9; Bodleian Library, MS Ashmole 1505, fos 31v–32r; Campbell and Colton, *Surgery of Theoderic*, ii, p. 171; John of Gaddesden, *Rosa Anglica*, fo. 58v; BL, MS Sloane 2272 (part 1), fo. 92v.

152 Theoderic favoured the application of leeches in cases of tyrian *lepra*: Campbell and Colton, *Surgery of Theoderic*, ii, p. 176.

the flow required considerable care, lest the patient suffocate under pressure.[153] Vernacular guides to phlebotomy, which, as we saw in the previous chapter, proliferated from the late fourteenth century onwards, conveyed this advice to their readers in a simpler format. For example, a fourteenth-century verse mnemonic, listing the principal points for venesection, noted that:

> At the hole of the throte ther ben too [two]
> That for lepor and streyte brest [breathlessness] must be vndo.[154]

Similar information was rendered diagrammatically in drawings known as 'vein men', which mapped these points on a sketch of the human body. Thus, among the nineteen depicted in a book owned by the York guild of barber surgeons, was 'the nek hole', where there were 'ij vayns that er gude to opyn for leper and for straytnes of wynde' [plate 26].[155]

Although venesection might no longer be viable, blood could still be drained from the capillaries by cupping or 'ventosyng'. This procedure, which was also deemed suitable for elderly, frail and pregnant patients, involved the scarification ('garsyng') of the skin, followed by the application of heated glass or metal vessels. The vacuum thus created stimulated a gentle flow of blood, drawing corrupt matter from beneath the surface of the skin and, indeed, from the adjacent internal organs themselves. Cupping on the lower back and buttocks was, for example, favoured as a treatment for malfunction of the liver and any 'scabbe of the body' resulting from it.[156] For obvious reasons, practitioners tended to prefer 'ventosyng' to the lancet, and prescribed it intensively, often after bathing, when the blood vessels were dilated. The experience must have been profoundly uncomfortable, as these recommendations for the treatment of *elephancia* suggest:

> Do the pacient be garsed in the nedyr parte of the raynes [kidneys] abowt the lenddes [lower back], and do ther on to be sett ventosse boxes & suffyr myche blod to be drawn owt ther at. And a bowt a fourtnyght after do the pacient to be garsed behind both legges agayns a fyer & strykeyt oftyn with a smale styke on the garsed place to make the blod to pase owt the lyghtlyar [more easily], & so contenew to the pacient haue bled well. And this maner of bledynge schall cause the mater to fall downe from the place.[157]

Whereas venesection required considerable expertise, cupping, like the preparation of herbal baths or ointments, could safely be left to a nurse or semi-skilled attendant.[158]

---

153  Avicenna, *Liber canonis*, fo. 443r; M.S. Spink and G.L. Lewis, eds, *Albucassis on Surgery and Instruments: A Definitive Edition of the Arabic Text with English Translation and Commentary* (London, 1973), pp. 632–3. Gil-Sotres, 'Derivation and Revulsion', p. 146, quotes Arnald of Villanova's account of this procedure.

154  Mayer, 'Medieval English Leechbook', p. 388. The verse additionally recommends bleeding from the forehead, as did Guy de Chauliac: Ogden, *Cyrurgie of Guy de Chauliac*, p. 385. See also, BL MS Egerton 2572, fo. 69v (pencil foliation).

155  BL, MS Egerton 2572, fo. 50r.

156  Ogden, *Cyrurgie of Guy de Chauliac*, pp. 545–50; Rawcliffe, *Medicine and Society*, pp. 68–9.

157  BL, MS Harley 1736, fo. 135v.

158  Murray Jones, *Medieval Medicine in Illuminated Manuscripts*, p. 97.

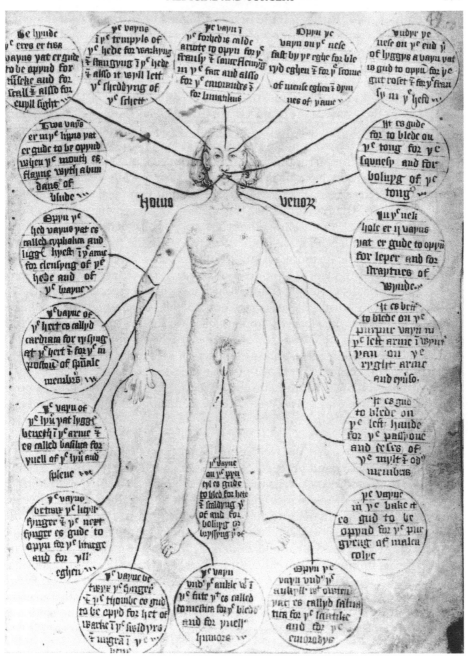

26. A vein man (*homo venorum*) from a late fifteenth-century book belonging to the barber surgeons of York recommends points for phlebotomy in a variety of chronic conditions and diseases. Bleeding at 'the nek hole' (third roundel down on the right) will ease the respiratory problems encountered in advanced cases of leprosy.

In common with bathing, these practices invited comparison with the spiritual benefits of confession. Among the *Gesta Romanorum* may, for example, be found the story of an ambitious knight, whose entire household became leprous through drinking poisoned water. Having taken medical advice, they embarked upon a regimen of phlebotomy, followed by baths and medication, which restored them all to health. Thus, the author explains, the contagion of sin may be purged 'by the vayne of the tunge', that is through confession, before cleansing in 'the teeris of compunccion and contricion'.[159] Blessed with an equally vivid imagination, one fourteenth-century preacher described charity as a cautery, which burns away the corruption of sin.[160] And, indeed, most patients faced with the red-hot iron would have given a good deal of their worldly wealth to the poor rather than endure one of the most notoriously painful of medieval treatments.

Developed by Islamic surgeons, this method of destroying diseased flesh, cleansing or sealing wounds, and eliminating the vapours generated by humoral corruption, was widely adopted in the West following the translation into Latin of Albucassis's classic textbook on surgical instruments. Although he was not, in the strict sense of the word, a pioneer in the use of cauteries for treating *lepra*, Albucassis rationalised the procedure, which he believed especially beneficial in cases arising from burnt phlegm (*tyria*) or black bile (*elephancia*). As the disease progressed, so the number of applications increased, on the ground that frequency promoted effectiveness.[161] Cauteries could also be applied topically, to deal with suppurating ulcers, and in conjunction with other forms of therapy as a means of combating the spread of poison within the body.

The irons, which varied in shape and size according to their specific purpose, were heated to maximum capacity on a brazier and applied with a precision that made them unusually responsive and versatile. (It was for this reason that Albucassis preferred iron to gold, which was less reliable.) Abbot Baldwin of Bury St Edmunds earned many plaudits for his expertise with them, being a master of both theory and practice. Not surprisingly, though, the fourth Lateran council of 1215 included cauterisation in the ban imposed upon the shedding of blood by members of the higher clergy, which meant that thenceforth surgeons generally performed this delicate operation.[162] Illustrations, along the lines of the vein men described above, depicted the best points for application in specific illnesses, and were especially useful as an *aide memoire* for men and women who learned the technique by apprenticeship. One set of fifteenth-century drawings illustrates (among others) the fifty-seven points for cauterisation in '*elephantia* or lepur', which, significantly, are far more numerous than for any other malady. The head is to be treated with a 'brod cauterie', but otherwise the choice of instrument is left to the practitioner, as Albucassis recommended [**plate 27**].[163]

---

159 Herrtage, *Gesta Romanorum*, pp. 263–8. For a variation on this theme, see Oesterley, *Gesta Romanorum*, pp. 420–21.
160 Wenzel, *Fasciculus Morum*, p. 257.
161 Spink and Lewis, *Albucassis on Surgery*, pp. 142–5. Albucassis itemised thirty-six cautery points, as well as every joint of the fingers and toes, for the treatment of advanced cases. For the general use of cauteries, see Rawcliffe, *Medicine and Society*, pp. 69–70.
162 Rawcliffe, 'Threshold of Eternity', pp. 43–4; D.W. Amundsen, 'Medieval Canon Law on Medical and Surgical Practice by the Clergy', *BHM*, lii (1978), pp. 22–43, at 39–43.
163 BL, MS Sloane 6, fo. 177r.

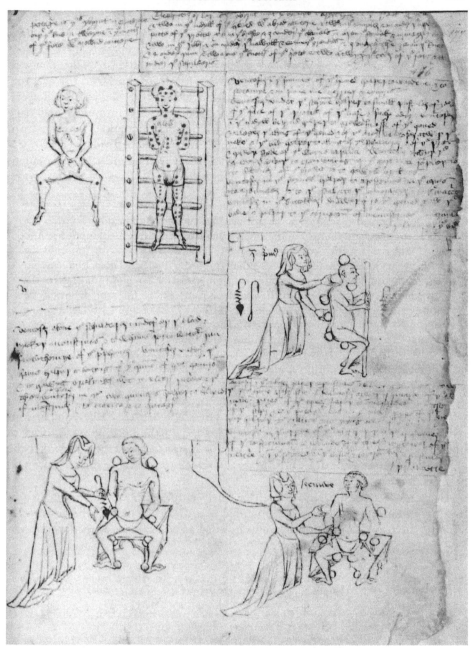

27. Multiple cautery points for the treatment of *lepra* are shown by dots on a human figure in a diagram from a fifteenth-century English vernacular surgical treatise. Below, the artist depicts the application of cups for the removal of blood (ventosing) and the use of a cautery. Both procedures are, significantly, undertaken by a female practitioner or nurse.

Some late medieval surgeons, such as Henri de Mondeville, followed Albucassis in his advocacy of repeated cauterisation in advanced cases, their enthusiasm being in part sustained by a significant awareness that the patient had grown anaesthetised to pain because of his or her disease.[164] St Francis of Assisi's capacity to endure extensive cauterisation from the ear to the eyebrow without apparently registering any sensation at all was regarded by his followers, but probably few surgeons, as a rare mark of sanctity. His immunity may have resulted from the neural damage characteristic of tuberculoid leprosy, from which he is now believed to have suffered.[165] Such a potentially dangerous operation could nevertheless cause serious trauma, as well as inflicting permanent damage. No less an authority than Guy de Chauliac advised his readers to be cautious and use it as a final resort:

> Aboute cauteries, it is to be vunderstonden that thai schal not be done but after alle the other cures, and namely in the roten lepre and that that is ful of humores. And thogh Albucasis putte [recommended] 70 cauteries for ham, for he saide the mo[re] that there be made the more thay conforten, neuerthelatter, I haue noght vsede ham, but the poynted cauterie or the rounde in the boghtes [branches] of the armes and of the legges and of the schares [groin] and of the arme holes, in the coppe [top] of the [head] and byhynde the nekke vnto setoun [to facilitate the insertion of a thread or bristle through a fold of skin for drainage].[166]

Corrosive ointments made of caustic substances, such as vitriol or arsenic, might be substituted for the cautery, although the risks to the patient were potentially even greater.[167] In either case, it was then necessary to dress the wound or ulcer with a styptic, to staunch any bleeding and dry out the residual matter, 'ellys it wolde rotyn & festryn agen'. The procedure invited predictable comparisons with the confessional, during which 'thi dedly synne be kut out, wyth sorwe of herte, fro the pyt of thi conscyens'. In this instance, contrition provided the cleansing agent, or 'drawyng salue of clene schryfte', which prevented re-infection.[168]

Even more extreme, and therefore rarely employed, was castration, which had, from antiquity, been recommended as a means of halting the advance of chronic disease.[169] Although it might be cited as an example of medieval medi-

---

164  Spink and Lewis, *Albucassis on Surgery*, pp. 144–5; Demaitre, 'Relevance of Futility', p. 37. Avicenna also favoured the early application of cauteries to prevent *lepra* from spreading: *Liber canonis*, fo. 444r.
165  R.B. Brooke, ed., *Scripta Leonis, Rufini et Angeli sociorum S. Francisci* (Oxford, 1990), pp. 174–5; Schatzlein and Sulmasy, 'Diagnosis of St Francis', pp. 190–91, 210–13.
166  Ogden, *Cyrurgie of Guy de Chauliac*, p. 389. The use of the cautery may have stimulated the body's production of endorphins, which would explain Albucassis's belief that they 'comforted' the patient.
167  BL, MS Harley 3, fo. 23r. John of Arderne, *Treatises of Fistula in Ano*, pp. 83–5, warned that only experienced surgeons should use these materials because of their 'distemperate violence'.
168  Brandeis, *Jacob's Well*, pp. 178–9.
169  Aulus Cornelius Celsus and Caelius Aurelianus observed that eunuchs were brarely troubled with such problems: Celsus, *De medicina*, ed. W.G. Spencer (3 vols, London, 1935–38), i, book iv, cap. 31.1; Caelius Aurelianus, *Tardarum passionum libri V*, ed. G. Bendz (Berlin, 1993), book v, cap. 2.29. Aetius maintained that castration could halt the progress of *elephantia*, noting that women rarely contracted the disease: Anonymous editorial, 'La lèpre et la castration', *Janus*, ii (1897–98), p. 289; Touati, *Maladie et société*, pp. 168–70.

cine at its most 'barbaric', the procedure did, in fact, accord perfectly with current ideas about human physiology. Since the testicles generated warmth, it followed naturally to authorities such as Theoderic that their removal would prove helpful in cases of leonine leprosy, which was caused by excessive levels of adust choler. As well as helping to cool the body, the operation might also raise levels of moisture, since the patient would subsequently assume the phlegmatic characteristics and soft skin of a woman.[170] Moreover, if, as we have seen, the retention of menstrual blood could render a woman leprous because of the putrefaction it might cause, so too an excess of semen (which was produced from venous blood in the testicles) could have a similar effect on men.[171] Under normal circumstances, as all celibates knew, a spare diet and regular sessions with the phlebotomist were deemed sufficient to keep any physical – and moral – problems under control, but in some cases more radical measures seemed necessary.

Faced with the prospect of rapidly deteriorating health and social rejection, some suspect or confirmed lepers apparently took this step out of desperation. Many years after the event, William of Malmesbury referred sneeringly to Hugh Orival, bishop of London (d. 1085), who underwent castration in the hope of curing his ulcerated body and was obliged to live on in shame as both a leper and a eunuch after the treatment failed.[172] If true, the tale is of considerable interest, since it confirms that clergy who threatened their errant congregations with the arrows of divine retribution from the pulpit were, in practice, generally disposed towards a scientific explanation of their own diseases. Like Elias of Reading and other religious, Orival turned to the medical profession for help when his own health was at risk. Few late medieval medical authorities do more than mention castration *en passant*, however, no doubt regarding it as an interesting curiosity rather than a useful remedy to be explained at length.[173] This no doubt offered some small crumb of reassurance to the patient, whose chances of recovery so demonstrably hinged upon his state of mind.

## Accidents of the soul

That fear and anxiety could themselves cause illness, while seriously undermining the body's resistance to miasmatic infections, was a commonplace of medieval and early modern therapeutics. The intimate relationship between

---

170  Demaitre, 'Relevance of Futility', p. 36; Jacquart, *Médecine médiévale*, p. 249; M.S. Kuefler, 'Castration and Eunuchism in the Middle Ages', in V.L. Bullough and J.A. Brundage, eds, *Handbook of Medieval Sexuality* (New York, 1996), p. 286.

171  Touati, 'Pharmacopée et thérapeutique', p. 25.

172  William of Malmesbury, *De gestis pontificum Anglorum*, ed. N.E.S.A. Hamilton (RS, 1870), p. 145. Since castration was then a punishment for serious crime, as well as a bar to the priesthood, the bishop's humiliation must have been great. Moreover, as Abū-Ma'šar pointed out, eunuchs appeared among the army of social misfits commanded by Saturn (another famous castrato): Klibansky, Panofsky and Saxl, *Saturn and Melancholy*, p. 129.

173  John Mirfield refers very briefly to it and recommends eating the testicles of asses (perhaps meaning mules, which were sterile) in this context: BL, MS Harley 3, fo. 23v. Unusually, the author or translator of a text belonging to the barber surgeon, Richard Dod, advised his readers 'that mony one ben preseruyd [from *lepra*] be puttyng a way of the ballokis': BL, MS Sloane 5, fo. 154r.

body, mind and soul meant that strong emotions would have a visible somatic effect. Bernard Gordon invariably questioned his patients about any sources of stress (such as noisy neighbours or urban crime) that might be preying upon their minds.[174] From the fourteenth century onwards, the authors of plague tracts reiterated the need for pleasant recreation, fresh air, and a positive outlook among those exposed to the disease, in part because of the calming influence this would have upon the vital spirits.[175] One had only to observe the pallor, chill and nervousness which followed their retreat from the extremities to appreciate the important role they played in fighting infection. To pursue the military analogy, their withdrawal left the body's defences open to attack by 'evil vapours', which could pass unhindered through the pores and thence to the citadel of the heart. 'Ye must beware of al thynges that shulde make you to be pensive, heavye, thoughtfull, angrye or melancholycke', advised the sixteenth-century physician, Thomas Phayer, 'for all such thynges are ynough to enfecte a man alone'.[176] These arguments, already centuries old, found their most eloquent expression in Robert Burton's *Anatomy of Melancholy*, which appeared in 1621. 'If the Imagination be very apprehensive, intent, and violent', he observes,

> It sends great store of spirits to, or from, the heart, and makes a deeper impression, and greater tumult, as the humours in the Body be likewise prepared, and the temperature it selfe ill or well disposed, the passions are longer and stronger. So that the first steppe and fountaine of all our grievances in this kinde is *laesa Imaginatio*, which misinforming the Heart, causeth all these distemperatures, alteration and confusion of spirits and humours.[177]

As we have already seen, wrath and fear, the allies of plague, also walked hand in hand with *lepra*. Another of the homilies in the *Gesta Romanorum* tells of three jealous physicians who concoct a devious plan to eliminate a successful rival by convincing him that he has become leprous. 'And when he seth vs alle accorde in oon', the ringleader explains, 'he shall trow [believe] in vs and then for drede he shal bycome lepre; for so a lepre may be made'. Their victim duly succumbs, although his equally dramatic recovery, after bathing in a vat of goats' blood, persuades him that his disease was induced by sheer terror.[178] Since men and women possessed of a melancholic disposition were naturally

---

174　Demaitre, *Doctor Bernard de Gordon*, pp. 47, 157; P. Horden, 'A Non-Natural Environment: Medicine without Doctors and the Medieval Hospital', in B. Bowers, ed., *The Medieval Hospital and Medical Practice* (Aldershot, forthcoming).

175　See, for example, John Lydgate's 'Dietary and Doctrine for Pestilence', in MacCracken, *Minor Poems of John Lydgate*, pp. 702–7, which advises that 'care a-way is a good medycyne'.

176　Thomas Phayer, *Treatyse of the Pestylence* (London, 1546), sig. N3v, cited by A. Wear, 'Fear, Anxiety and the Plague in Early Modern England', in J.R. Hinnells and R. Porter, eds, *Religion, Health and Suffering* (London, 1999), p. 349. He was here paraphrasing Haly Abbas: Harvey, *Inward Wits*, pp. 19, 27.

177　Burton, *Anatomy of Melancholy*, i, p. 249. A graphic example of this belief appears in the chronicle of Roger of Howden, who remarks that Thomas Becket's 'grave sickness' in 1165 was caused by 'wrath and indignation' following a heated confrontation with the king: Stubbs, *Chronica Rogeri de Houedene*, i, p. 225. John Mirfield specifically warned lepers against anger, as well as spending too long alone: BL, MS Harley 3, fo. 23r.

178　Herrtage, *Gesta Romanorum*, pp. 67–70. The moral hinges upon the importance of confession and the spiritual bath of good works.

predisposed to brooding introspection and misanthropy, it followed that anyone who seemed particularly susceptible to *lepra* or mental illness should endeavour to keep depression at bay.[179] Such advice carried even greater force once symptoms began to appear, since any activity likely to engender more black bile or adust choler could tip an already precarious balance towards morbidity. Even so, as John of Gaddesden recognised, the patient was trapped in a vicious circle. The corrupt humour that had caused his sickness would, in turn, exacerbate any existing tendency to irritability, deviousness and paranoia:

> His demeanour will appear morose, and shifty, and wretched, and anxious, and reclusive; and he will frequently imagine that he is leprous. Be vigilant here, for in one disposed to this disease the imagination often causes the real thing, through a failing in the regimen, such as overindulgence. And he will have many bad dreams and awake crying out in terror, so that he dare not sleep alone; and in his sleep he feels a great weight upon his body.[180]

It was asking a good deal of any suspect leper, whose future seemed so bleak, to remain positive.[181] Could anything be done to distract him?

Music and 'recreative spectacles' were widely recommended by physicians in the treatment of the mentally ill, 'to draw the mind back into healthful habits' and soothe the vital spirits.[182] Less is known about their deployment in cases of *lepra*, although it would be surprising if some type of music therapy were not enlisted as a means of restoring equilibrium and calming the nerves. The constant round of masses, prayers and canonical hours, which makes life in a medieval *leprosarium* appear so burdensome and oppressive to a modern reader, must have seemed extremely beneficial at the time. Aretaeus had prescribed 'vociferation' exercises to help his patients improve their breathing and revive their flagging spirits through the inhalation of fresh air. He and later generations of practitioners also favoured a combination of gentle exercise and diversion to quiet the passions, and – as Theoderic suggests – overcome insomnia. The fitter residents of the *leprosarium* of St Lazare at Falaise in Normandy were, for example, allowed to play *jeu de paume*, apparently with such enthusiasm that they damaged the church roof. Care had, of course, to be taken lest the body grew either too hot or cold, thereby undermining whatever progress had already

179 Klibansky, Panofsky and Saxl, *Saturn and Melancholy*, chapter two; Bodleian Library, MS Bodley e Mus 19, fo. 116v.
180 John of Gaddesden, *Rosa Anglica*, fo. 56v. See also, BL, MS Sloane 2272 (part 1), fo. 91v. In keeping with Classical traditions, medieval practitioners believed that dreams provided a valuable guide to the patient's physiological state: S.M. Oberhelman, 'Galen, On Diagnosis from Dreams', *Journal of the History of Medicine and Applied Sciences*, xxxviii (1983), pp. 36–47. Guy de Chauliac urged practitioners to inquire about them in the *judicium* (above, p. 182). In his 1542 *Questyonary of Cyrurgyens*, sig. Qiij r–v, which was based on this text, Robert Copeland elaborates further: 'Than enquyre hym of his dreames & yf his dremes be nat terryble and that he seeth blacke thynges and deuyls [devils]. Such dreames betoken the melancolyke humour to haue domynyon . . . Than aske yf he hath had great solyeytudes & chargeable thoughts that hath dried hym [and] made hym melancolyke.'
181 Demaitre, 'Relevance of Futility', p. 32.
182 P. Murray Jones, 'Music Therapy in the Later Middle Ages: The Case of Hugo van der Goes', in P. Horden, ed., *Music as Medicine: The History of Music Therapy since Antiquity* (Aldershot, 2000), pp. 120–44.

been made. Here was yet another reason for suspects to refrain from sexual activity, however legitimate, since it further upset the natural thermostat.[183]

Under the circumstances, religion seemed to offer the best hope of achieving a measure of tranquillity. Practitioners recognised the somatic benefits of confession, which, as we have already seen, was supposed to precede medical treatment.[184] The tears of repentance, a necessary precursor of spiritual healing, brought immediate physical relief to the phlegmatic, since they helped to rid the body of excessive moisture. Although black bile was cold and dry, some authorities believed that it, too, found a necessary outlet through the eyes, prompting 'grief for sin', as well as a corresponding improvement in the humoral balance.[185] But of far greater importance was the psychological effect of absolution in reducing levels of fear, anxiety and guilt. Hidden sins spread surreptitiously like *lepra*, corrupting first the veins and then the vital organs. Both had to be eradicated before it was too late:

> Yf the fylthynes of synne be ones conceyued in the soule, and long contynue ther by vnhappy custome, it maketh foule and infecteth it more and more, as we se by vryne [urine] or any other stynkynge lycour put in a vessell, the longer it be kepte in the same, so moche more it maketh foule the vessel and corrupteth it . . . As we se a byle [boil] or a botche [sore] full of matter and fylth the more and the lenger it be hyd, the more groweth the corrupcyon and venemouse infeccyon of it and also perceth to the bones and corrupteth them.[186]

Confession also marked the start of pilgrimage, which, as we saw in the previous chapter, ranked high among the therapeutic measures favoured by confirmed and suspect lepers alike. For some it was a last resort, to be undertaken when earthly medicine seemed powerless against the relentless march of disease. The prospect of a miraculous cure was, inevitably, the principal attraction, although the celestial benefits, in terms of medicine for the soul, should not be overlooked. The change of scene, the experience of the shrine and the ensuing sense of spiritual renewal must also have exerted a powerful physiological effect, which medieval physicians clearly recognised. Rationalist to the core, the sceptical

---

183  Adams, *Extant Works of Aretaeus*, p. 447; John of Gaddesden, *Rosa Anglica*, fo. 59r; D. Jeanne, 'Le group des lépreux à Saint-Lazare de Falaise aux XIVe et XVe siècles', in B. Tabuteau, ed., *Lépreux et sociabilité du moyen âge aux temps modernes* (Cahiers de GRHIS, xi, 2000), p. 52. See also Demaitre, 'Relevance of Futility', p. 32; Campbell and Colton, *Surgery of Theoderic*, p. 172; Nicaise, *Chirurgie de Henri de Mondeville*, p. 623.

184  R. Palmer, 'The Church, Leprosy and Plague in Medieval and Early Modern Europe', in W.J. Sheils, ed., *The Church and Healing* (Studies in Church History, xix, 1982), p. 86.

185  P. Brown, *The Body and Society: Men, Women and Sexual Renunciation in Early Christianity* (New York, 1988), p. 238; Klibansky, Panofsky and Saxl, *Saturn and Melancholy*, p. 109. William of Auvergne (b. 1180) described confession as the vomiting forth of 'the noxious humour of vices and detestable sins': L. Smith, 'William of Auvergne and Confession', in Biller and Minnis, *Handling Sin*, p. 96. See also, T.N. Tentler, *Sin and Confession on the Eve of the Reformation* (Princeton, 1977), p. 257; and, for the use of vomits to expel corrupt matter in the treatment of *lepra*, Avicenna, *Liber canonis*, fo. 443v.

186  J.E.B. Mayor, ed., *The English Works of John Fisher* (EETS, extra series, xxvii, 1876), p. 27. The climax of the story of the Emperor Jereslaus, retold by Thomas Hoccleve from the *Gesta Romanorum*, hinges upon the confession made by the Emperor's evil brother. Only when his last, terrible sin has been revealed through 'hoole schrift' is he cleansed of physical and spiritual *lepra*: Furnivall, *Hoccleve's Works*, pp. 166–73; above, p. 48.

Henri de Mondeville felt that most so-called miracles could be explained in purely medical terms, since travel would naturally affect the humoral balance.[187] Apparent failure was certainly no deterrent, for many reputedly leprous pilgrims proved doughty travellers, journeying from one shrine to another in search of healing and, no doubt, diversion.

Because they followed quasi-monastic rules, many hospitals and *leprosaria* were reluctant to allow their brethren and sisters unnecessary contact with secular society. In practice, this meant that long journeys involving one night or more outside the precinct required official approval and could never be undertaken alone.[188] Pilgrimage was, however, a legitimate – indeed desirable – activity, which in principle no master or warden could reasonably oppose. After all, the holy Peregrinus, eponymous protector of pilgrims, had been leprous until his momentous encounter with Christ at St Denis.[189] The *vita* of Godric of Finchale tells of a devoted mother, whose daughter lay, apparently incurable, in a leper house near Darlington. On hearing of the saint's posthumous miracles, she took the girl to his shrine, where, after three long visits, she was finally cured.[190] Frequent requests for leave of absence, or the choice of remote destinations may have proved more contentious. William de Malesmains apparently discharged himself altogether from a '*maladria apud Bidelington*' in 1218 in order to venture as a pilgrim to the Holy Land.[191] Perhaps he also hoped to bathe in the Jordan. The majority of lepers (like most English pilgrims) probably contented themselves with occasional visits to the nearest local shrine.

## Blood and alchemy

Medieval miracles often involved the consumption of holy water in which the bones or bloodstained clothing of saints had been dipped. That blood, the life force and nutrient of the human body, possessed the power to heal seemed axiomatic to medieval men and women, especially if it derived from a pure, untainted source. In the words of Bartholomaeus Anglicus,

> Kinde [natural] blood is pure, hoot and moist, sotile, and swete; and also it kepith the kinde vertu of fedinge. And blood is the sete of the soule and conteyneth hym, and maketh parfite youthe ... and kepith and saueth the herte and the spiritis and maketh hem glad, and waketh loue ... And if blood is wel and temperat, he kepith

---

187  S.C. Macdougall, 'The Surgeon and the Saints: Henri de Mondeville and Divine Healing', *Journal of Medieval History*, xxvi (2000), pp. 253–67, at p. 262.

188  See below, pp. 316–17.

189  See above, pp. 112–14.

190  J. Raine, ed., *Libellus de vita et miraculis S. Godrici, hermetiae de Finchale* (Surtees Society, xx, 1847), pp. 455–8. In 1342, new regulations for the pilgrim hospital at Eastbridge, Canterbury, excluded lepers, which suggests that they had previously been accommodated: Somer, *Antiquities of Canterbury*, part 1, appendix XVI.

191  *CRR, 1219–1220*, pp. 308–10; Page, *VCH Sussex II*, p. 98. Surprised by the modest number of miraculous cures of *lepra* reported in French – as opposed to English – sources, P.A. Sigal, *L'homme et le miracle dans la France médiévale* (Paris, 1985), pp. 251–2, speculates that there were far fewer *leprosaria* in England, with the result that lepers enjoyed greater freedom of movement. The evidence does not, however, support this hypothesis.

hele and helthe. And if he is corrupt, it bredeth corrupcion, as in *lepra* that is corrupt blood . . .[192]

The idea that good red blood would drive out bad was most fully realised in tales of innocent lives shed to overcome the horrors of leprosy.[193] The practice was, reputedly, an ancient one shared across time by many cultures. In his *Natural History*, Pliny the Elder (d. AD 79) noted that the rulers of Egypt had long employed this remedy, protecting themselves against infection by bathing in the warm blood of their subjects.[194] It was, however, the metaphorical implications of such anecdotes rather than any medical interest they may have possessed which attracted most medieval writers and their audiences. Exposure to the quotidian miracle of transubstantiation, whereby the Host changed into the macerated flesh of Christ before their very eyes, made them unusually receptive to the concept of sacrifice and redemption. Indeed, the blood He shed on the cross was commonly likened to healing syrup, or electuary, for use against the leprosies of sin.[195]

According to legend, the kerchief with which Saint Veronica allegedly wiped Jesus's bloodstained face on the *via dolorosa* cured the future Emperor Vespasian of '*une lepre si puant*' that he had been shut away in a tower. A brief glimpse of the cloth through a high window sufficed to purge him of all defilement and convert him to Christianity.[196] Just as Mary Magdalen came to represent a number of biblical characters fused into one, so Veronica was sometimes identi-fied as the woman whose issue of blood ceased when she grasped the hem of Christ's robe [Matthew 9, vv. 20–22]. She, like the leper cured by his touch, had been cast out from society because of physical pollution, which contaminated her entire body. Indeed, one early version of the Veronica story actually describes her as being 'so full of leprosy that she did not dare to mix with others'. Standing apart at the crucifixion, she gave her kerchief to the Virgin Mary, who used it to cleanse her son's face. Once transferred to the cloth, His miraculous image purified her and then the Emperor, both of whom became whole through faith.[197] Frequently retold, Veronica's legendary exploits provided the Church

192 Seymour, *On the Properties of Things*, i, p. 153.
193 Brody, *Disease of the Soul*, pp. 148–57, 159–70; P. McCracken, *The Curse of Eve, the Wound of the Hero: Blood, Gender and Medieval Literature* (Pennsylvania Press, 2003), pp. 1–9, 47–8; A. Berthelet, 'Sang et lèpre, sang et feu', in *Le sang au moyen âge: Actes du quatrième colloque international de Montpellier* (Cahiers du CRISIMA, iv, 1999), pp. 25–37.
194 Pliny, *Natural History, VII*, ed. W.H.S. Jones (London, 1956), Lib. XXVI, cap. 5, pp. 270–71. H.L. Strack, *Das Blut im Glauben und Aberglauben der Menschheit mit besonderer Berücksichtigung der "Volksmedizin" und des "jüdischen Blutritus"* (Munich, 1900), p. 37, refers to an early Jewish commentary on the book of Exodus, which describes the daily sacrifice of 300 Israelite children to cure the leprous king of Egypt. This is a possible source for many later legends, which added a perverse anti-Semitic twist.
195 *Speculum humanae salvationis: The Miroure of Mans Saluacionne* (London, for the Roxburghe Club, 1888), p. 75; Henry of Lancaster, *Livre de seyntz medicines*, pp. 170–88.
196 Robert de Boron, *Joseph d'Arimathie*, ed. R. O'Gorman (Toronto, 1995), pp. 120–83. In the Middle English *Siege of Jerusalem,* eds R. Hanna and D. Lawton (EETS, cccxx, 2003), p. 3, Vespasian not only 'lay laser at Rome', but was also afflicted by a nest of 'waspene bees' in the nose. In some versions the leprous Emperor is Tiberius. See also, E. Kuryluk, *Veronica and Her Cloth: History, Symbolism and Structure of a 'True' Image* (Oxford, 1991), pp. 120–22; and below, pp. 254–5.
197 A.E. Ford, ed., *La vengeance de Nostre-Seigneur* (Toronto, 1984), pp. 8, 58–80; Kuryluk, *Veronica*, p. 202.

with powerful propaganda, especially after the cult of the *sancta facies* attracted papal support in the early thirteenth century. By then many other accounts of the use of blood to heal the distorted features of lepers were in circulation, all, to a greater or lesser extent, developing the familiar themes of corruption, conversion, redemption and salvation.

English churchgoers were well acquainted with the history of Constantine, the pagan emperor who had allegedly been 'i-smyte with meselrie' after instigating a persecution of Christians. His priests, physicians and counsellors advised him to bathe in the 'hoot blood' of three thousand children, but the sight of their weeping mothers softened his heart. This display of clemency was followed by baptism at the hands of Pope Sylvester, which, predictably, restored him to physical and spiritual health.[198] It was thus through 'goddes cure' (mediated, as in the case of Vespasian, by the papacy), rather than heathen remedies, that 'the lepull felle away from hym, and he was as clene of skynne and hyde as any child that he delyuerd before'.[199]

The eleventh-century Latin poem of *Amis and Amiloun*, which passed through many versions and was eventually translated into both French and English, drew upon a similar topos. Struck down by *lepra* because of an act of deception committed (with the best intentions) on behalf of his dearest friend, Amiloun is forced to beg from door to door until they are joyfully reunited. An angel informs them that only one remedy is strong enough to overcome the disease, and that Amis must prepare a healing bath with the blood of his two young sons.[200] This he reluctantly agrees to do, sacrificing the boys on Christmas night out of love for his lifelong companion. The French text, known as *Ami et Amile*, dwells at some length upon the bath itself:

> Amile had a great vat brought,
> Had his friend climb into it,
> Yet he could barely lower himself because he was so sick.
> Once Ami had sunk into the bath,
> Count Amile grasped the round basin,
> With the red blood he rubbed his breast,
> His eyes, his mouth and all his limbs,
> Legs and belly – upwards over the whole body:

---

[198] J.R. Lumby, ed., *Polychronicon Ranulphi Higden* (9 vols, RS, 1865–86), v, pp. 123–9. This tale was immensely popular: it may be found in the *Legenda aurea*, and was retold in John Gower's *Confessio amantis*. Significantly, in the light of current medical knowledge, the poet has Constantine's 'clerkes' explain that his *lepra* springs from accidental rather than hereditary causes, and is therefore curable: Macaulay, *English Works of John Gower*, i, p. 216. Variants of the story sprang up across Europe. Icelandic legend tells of one Thorhal Knapp, 'a man of good and pure morals, though heathen and affected by leprosy'. Having destroyed his pagan temple to build a church, he began to recover, but it was baptism that cured him: Ehlers, *On the Conditions under which Leprosy Has Declined*, p. 6.

[199] T. Erbe, ed., *Mirk's Festial: A Collection of Homilies* (EETS, xcvi, 1905), p. 37. See also, M.M. Banks, ed., *An Alphabet of Tales, II, I–Z* (EETS, cxxvii, 1905), p. 478. The contrast with Herod, who denied Christ, massacred the Innocents and was struck down by God, is dramatic: Albert, *Odeurs de sainteté*, pp. 264–5.

[200] In the original Latin verse physicians convey this information, but over time the specifically Christian elements of the tale were embellished. Indeed, one version describes Amiloun's *lepra* as a mark of divine favour: M. Leach, ed., *Amis and Amiloun* (EETS, cciii, 1937), pp. ix–xxxii, lxii.

Feet, thighs, hands and the shoulders above them,
He wiped every spot with the blood.[201]

Purged of his sins, Ami[loun] is cured and the children are miraculously restored to their nursery.

Other tales deal with willing adult victims, whose sacrifice, like Christ's, is freely made to redeem human suffering. Implicit in some homilies, the analogy is spelt out in one of the *Gesta Romanorum*, which tells of a leprous girl who can only be healed by bathing in royal blood. Such is his love for her that a king freely empties his veins, '*usque ad mortem*', allowing her to live. And so, the preacher continues, Christ prepares a baptismal bath for all sinners, cleansing them with His blood.[202] The pages of medieval romance are populated with virgin martyrs, some of whom give – or at least offer – their lives for a similar cause.[203] In the thirteenth-century *Queste del saint graal*, for example, three of King Arthur's knights encounter the followers of a leprous noblewoman who demand a bowl 'brimful with blood' from the right arm of every young virgin entering her domain. Although she is too weak to survive this compulsory phlebotomy, Sir Perceval's sister, whose blood possesses particular qualities, insists on complying. The lady herself then appears, revealing a face 'so unsightly and pustulous and so disfigured that it was a wonder she could live in such affliction'. In a macabre parody of the grail itself, Perceval's sister fills the basin and expires, having first received the sacrament. The 'blackened and hideous flesh' of the lady is duly cleansed, although retribution follows fast in the shape of a divine thunderbolt. As Eve discovered before her, there can be no escape from the consequences of sin.[204]

The religious symbolism of these stories is as striking as their dramatic power and latent eroticism, which, in turn, exploits the conventional association between sin and disease. But can we assume, as some literary scholars are inclined to do, that the sacrificial blood of children or young virgins was a 'recognised specific' for the actual treatment of *lepra* throughout medieval Europe?[205] English legal records have yet to reveal a case similar to that of the Parisian midwife, Perrette de Rouen, who was imprisoned in 1408 for procuring the body of a stillborn child. The charge that she intended to use it in the manufacture of ointment for a leprous nobleman may perhaps have served an ulterior purpose, since Charles VI intervened personally to reduce her sentence.[206] Tales to the effect that Richard the Lionheart succumbed to leprosy while crusading,

---

201  P.F. Dembowski, ed., *Ami et Amile: Chanson de Geste* (Paris, 1969), lines 3057–67, p. 98.
202  Oesterley, *Gesta Romanorum*, p. 633.
203  See, for example, the German tale of *Die arme Heinrich*, discussed in Brody, *Disease of the Soul*, pp. 148–57.
204  Matarasso, *Quest of the Holy Grail*, pp. 245–49, 300 n. 67; Berthelet, 'Sang et lèpre', pp. 30–34.
205  Leach, *Amis and Amiloun*, p. lxii. As we saw in chapter one, Marcel Schwob dramatised this idea to considerable effect. But one did not have to be a French symbolist to derive a macabre fascination from it. The antiquary, W.W. Hodson, observed in 1891 that 'it was a current belief all through a great part of the Middle Ages that baths of human blood could cure the disease': 'John Colney's or S. Leonard's Hospital for Lepers at Sudbury', *Proceedings of the Suffolk Institute of Archaeology*, vii (1891), pp. 268–74, at p. 269. Strack, *Das Blut*, devotes a chapter ('Menschenblut heilt den Aussatz') to this practice, pp. 36–40, asserting that it was 'extraordinarily widespread' in the medieval period.
206  Jacquart, *Dictionnaire biographique*, p. 222.

and was advised by a Jewish physician to bathe in the blood of 'a newborn child', apparently circulated long after his death. Although his health often gave cause for concern, such fantasies clearly belong in the murky realm of anti-Semitic propaganda, where they were far from uncommon. True to his reputation as a beast in human form, Louis XI of France, 'the spider king' (d. 1483), was, also said to have drunk the blood of children in his last illness, again after a similar consultation.[207]

Beginning in the mid twelfth century and rising to a peak in early modern Germany, allegations concerning the ritual slaughter of children were periodically made against Jewish communities across Europe. They reputedly needed the blood as a prophylactic against the foul stench they shared with lepers, and, indeed, against the disease itself, to which some authorities believed they were especially vulnerable. (Jews were, paradoxically, also said to use sacrificial blood as a cure for haemorrhoids, which, by preventing the natural expulsion of corrupt matter, would actually have *increased* their chances of contracting *lepra*.)[208] Significantly, however, although the blood libel originated in England, no specific connection seems ever to have been made there between ritual murder and leprosy. Nor, after the expulsion of the Jews in 1290, were English lepers ever incriminated in such activities on their own account. There is certainly no hint that local, regional or ecclesiastical authorities felt the slightest anxiety on this score.[209] Occasional expressions of concern about confirmed lepers mixing with children sprang from specific, and clearly enunciated, fears of infection, not homicide.[210]

Yet human blood certainly figured on the long list of medieval *materia medica*, as did urine and faeces.[211] On the same homeopathic principle that prompted the use of theriac, namely of poison eliminating poison, the blood of the patient himself was regarded by some physicians as a powerful corrosive or cleansing agent. Bernard Gordon, who recommended the drastic measure of cutting away protuberant nodules 'clene with a rasour', instructed the practitioner to reserve any blood issuing from the incision. It was then to be mixed with powdered litharge (lead monoxide) and applied to the wound as a plaster.[212] In theory, menstrual blood, an equally toxic substance, seemed

---

[207] Richard was also to eat the child's heart 'quite warm and raw': Strack, *Das Blut*, pp. 38–9. See also J. Trachtenberg, *The Devil and the Jews: The Medieval Conception of the Jew and its Relation to Modern Antisemitism* (New Haven and London, 1945), p. 142. Posthumous rumours about Richard's health grew more sensational by the year. The chronicler, William of Newburgh, reports a common belief that he suffered from more than a hundred suppurating ulcers: *Historia rerum Anglicarum*, p. 306.

[208] Trachtenberg, *Devil and the Jews*, pp. 146–9; R. Po-Chia Hsia, *The Myth of Ritual Murder: Jews and Magic in Reformation Germany* (New Haven and London, 1988), pp. 2–4; P. Biller, 'Views of the Jews from Paris around 1300: Christian or "Scientific"?', in D. Wood, ed., *Christianity and Judaism* (Studies in Church History, xxix, 1992), pp. 187–207.

[209] Although Jews and wandering lepers were occasionally bracketed together as social undesirables in lists of civic ordinances: see below, p. 285 n. 162.

[210] See below, p. 281.

[211] The Renaissance physician, Coradino Gilino, referred as a matter of course to the use of blood in treating *lepra*, as did Paracelsus: Arrizabalaga, Henderson and French, *Great Pox*, p. 85; Strack, *Das Blut*, p. 40.

[212] Bodleian Library, MS Ashmole 1505, fo. 33v. See also, BL MS Sloane 2272 (part 1), fo. 93v; MS Harley 3, fo. 23r. Theoderic used blood removed with leeches or by phlebotomy from the patient's nose: Campbell and Colton, *Surgery of Theoderic*, ii, pp. 176–7.

powerful enough to contain the ravages of leprosy caused by 'lust or intemperance', although we have no means of telling if it was ever actually used.[213] Nor is it possible to determine how far assumptions about the invigorating effects of distilled blood, drawn from the body of a strong, healthy and temperate young man, were ever put into practice. The Catalan physician, Arnald of Villanova, produced a short treatise on the topic, arguing that such an elixir taken daily would prolong and enrich human life.[214] The circumstances of its production would, however, have been far less macabre than the above-mentioned stories might suggest, since copious supplies of blood were available for the asking from any barber's shop.[215] Like his numerical formulae for the prescription of drugs, Arnald's method was so complex and difficult that few practitioners are likely to have attempted it, although many had already mastered the necessary techniques for distillation. This was in part because of a growing interest in the theory and practice of alchemy, which exercised a powerful attraction upon many members of the medical profession.

In his efforts to transmute base metals, such as lead, into gold, the medieval alchemist was attempting to reverse a process of corruption that had begun at the gates of paradise. Through repeated sublimation in a still or alembic, he purged them of their impurities, until only an essential substance remained. As the Benedictine monk, John Lydgate, explained:

> Th'alknamystre tretythe of myneralles,
> And of metalles the alteracyouns,
> Of sulphur, mercury, of alomys, of sallies [salts],
> And of theire sundry generacyouns,
> And what is cause in there comixstyons,
> Why somme beo clene, some *leprous* and not able.[216]

The idea that metals, like bodies, were vulnerable to disease prompted some obvious analogies with *lepra*. Thus, for example, the *Gratarolus*, a work mistakenly attributed to Albertus Magnus, compared the decay of metals in the earth to the conception of a child in a 'corrupted womb'. Just as the human embryo would, inevitably, become 'leprous and unclean' in such an environment, so too base metal would grow tarnished and rusty.[217] Appropriately, given the nature of their crimes, the counterfeiters and alchemists in Dante's *Inferno* are 'dotted in scabs from head to toe', their bodies as foul and deformed as the metal they have

---

213 Throop, *Hildegard von Bingen's Physica*, p. 61.
214 BL Sloane 3124 fos 187v–191r; *Epistola Magistri Arnaldi Catalani de Villanova . . . de sanguine humano* (Basle, 1561), pp. 169–74. The consumption of human blood, along with that of semen, a blood product, merited three years' penance: F. Broomfield, ed. *Thomae de Chobham summa confessorum* (Louvain and Paris, 1968), p. 487. Thomas (d. *c.* 1236) bracketed this offence with forecasting the future and using a variety of suspect remedies, which suggests that the Church felt a particular need to eradicate such pagan practices. No reference is, however, made to their deployment in treating leprosy.
215 Furnivall, *Book of Quinte Essence*, p. 11. The disposal of blood collected by phlebotomists posed a serious health hazard in some cities: Gil-Sotres, 'Derivation and Revulsion', p. 120.
216 MacCracken, *Minor Poems*, p. 803.
217 G. Roberts, *The Mirror of Alchemy: Alchemical Ideas and Images in Manuscripts and Books* (London, 1994), p. 89.

passed off as gold.[218] At a more exalted level, the process of sublimation lent itself to comparisons with *Christus quasi leprosus*: 'After my Passion and manifold tormentes I am againe risen, beinge purified and clensed from alle spottes.'[219]

Justifiable concerns about counterfeiting and fraud, as well a perceived connection between transmutation and the black arts, led some rulers – including Henry IV – to ban such activities. Yet the dedicated alchemist, who regarded his work as akin to a religious calling (and had, indeed, often taken holy orders), followed a very different agenda. His search was for a 'fifth essence' that would restore *all* imperfect and corrupt bodies to a state of prelapsarian health. It would thus be possible to regain the balanced temperament and longevity enjoyed by Adam and Eve in paradise and thereby overcome most diseases. John of Rupescissa (*fl.* 1356), one of many Franciscan friars to pursue this goal, identified *aqua ardens*, a cordial produced by the repeated distillation of wine into virtually pure alcohol, as the key to success. He also explained how metals, plants and animal products – such as blood – might be sublimated to yield up their individual 'quintessence' or 'virtue', which could then be combined with *aqua ardens* in an alembic to create compounds powerful enough to vanquish even leprosy or pestilence.[220] Developed by the Arabs, and employed in the West from the twelfth century onwards, the use of the alembic had already facilitated the production of various fortified 'waters', such as *aqua vitae*, 'the parent and lord of all medicines'. The capacity of alcohol to absorb the essence of whatever animal, vegetable or mineral simples might be added to it, and thus to intensify their effect, was also understood.[221] Gold was, not surprisingly, a principal ingredient in these remedies, its healing qualities refined, preserved and concentrated through the power of strong liquor, which also rendered it potable.

Alchemy elevated this knowledge to a celestial plane. One fifteenth-century alchemical tract claimed that 'good brennynge watir', properly distilled, 'schal be a medicyn incorruptible almost as heuene aboue'.[222] Echoing John of Rupescissa, its author was careful to point out that certain strains of *lepra* lay beyond earthly help, but recommended an elixir of pearls, gold and pure alcohol as a certain cure for others. Not all his remedies were so exotic. Distilled strawberries or mulberries, preferably mixed with *aqua ardens*, would not only cleanse and restore leprous flesh but also prove a far safer (and more agreeable) alternative to the dangerous and painful cures favoured by 'summe lechis'.[223] Recipes for 'the precious potable licor [that] healethe bothe lepre & pestilence' circulated widely, in both Latin and English, not just among alchemists but medical practi-

---

218 Dante Alighieri, *Hell*, pp. 175–6.
219 BL, MS Add. 29895, fo. 133v, reproduced in Roberts, *Mirror of Alchemy*, plate XVI.
220 Thorndike *History of Magic*, iii, chapter twenty-two; Crisciani and Pereira, 'Black Death and Golden Remedies', pp. 7–39. Roger Bacon, another Franciscan, castigated physicians for their lack of alchemical knowledge, which he considered essential for both theory and practice: *De retardacione accidentum senectutis*, pp. 155–8.
221 Grant, *Source Book*, pp. 785–6.
222 Furnivall, *Book of Quinte Essence*, p. 16.
223 Furnivall, *Book of Quinte Essence*, p. 16.

tioners and educated laypeople whose concerns were more immediate.[224] Although the overwhelming demand for such cures arose during epidemics, there can be little doubt that a range of fortified waters was used both internally and externally in the treatment of *lepra*. Richard Trewythian prescribed an unspecified *aqua* costing 1s. for his patient in 1444;[225] and the royal physician, John Argentein, recorded the recipe for another in his case book. Apparently collected while he was studying in Italy during the early 1470s, it lists a potent combination of ingredients, which were largely dependent on the patient's budget. These included filings of gold, silver, copper, iron and lead, together with calamint, myrrh, gum, aloes, azalea and the urine of a virginal young boy (a useful substitute for blood). Over the next six days, white and red wine, the syrup of fumitory and fennel and the white of an egg were to be added, before distillation in an alembic. This 'precious water' was better than all the rest in treating eye problems and leprosy, he observed, while also helping to preserve youth. Storage in a gold or silver vessel would help to conserve its remarkable powers.[226]

As one of the leading practitioners of his day, Argentein demonstrated a lively interest in the collection of alchemical remedies, which, significantly, included the quintessence of human blood.[227] He had still been a scholar at Eton when an earlier generation of court physicians and alchemists had vainly sought an 'elixir of life', with which to cure the ailing Henry VI. The decline of his own royal patient, Edward IV, was hardly more encouraging, although the prospect of finding a universal panacea may still have exerted a powerful hold over his imagination.[228] His approach, like that of most medieval practitioners, was, however, essentially pragmatic and eclectic. Shorn of its elusive aspirations, alchemical medicine made a notable contribution to late medieval pharmacy. Alcohol-based preparations could be used to deaden pain, cleanse sores, and (like electuaries) broaden the range of potable commodities available to the practitioner. Utilising similar techniques, the production of therapeutic oils and perfumes also advanced by leaps and bounds. In the battle to contain and eliminate incipient *lepra* any weapon might prove useful, but none was sure of success.

It is, of course, important to remember that the medieval concept of 'a cure' was far less certain than our own. Patients as well as pilgrims could often expect

---

224 See, for example, BL, MS Sloane 3508B, fos 177v–178r; Bodleian Library, MS Ashmole 346, fo. 49r; M. Pereira, 'Alchemy and the Rise of Vernacular Languages in the Late Middle Ages', *Speculum*, lxxiv (1999), pp. 336–56.

225 BL, MS Sloane 428, fo. 18v.

226 Bodleian Library, MS Ashmole 1437, p. 62. I am grateful to Dr John Henderson for help with the Italian translation. The less affluent might content themselves with a simple water of fumitory: BL, MS Sloane 2948, fo. 73r. Murray Jones, *Medieval Medicine in Illuminated Manuscripts*, p. 67, reproduces a fifteenth-century drawing of distillation equipment, showing how calamint, fennel and other medicinal herbs would be processed. See also, Voigts, 'Master of the King's Stillatories', pp. 233–52.

227 I am grateful to Dr Peter Murray Jones for this information, presented in an unpublished paper on 'John Argentine and the Quintessence of Human Blood' at the University of East Anglia in March 2002. For Argentine's career, see *MPIME*, pp. 112–15; and D.R. Leader, 'John Argentein and Learning in Medieval Cambridge', *Humanistica Lovaniensia*, xxxiii (1984), pp. 71–85.

228 Hughes, *Arthurian Myths*, reassesses the role of alchemists and physicians at the Lancastrian and Yorkist courts.

little more than *relative* improvement, a temporary remission of symptoms or the restoration of partial mobility. Only too well aware of their limitations, physicians and surgeons routinely specified exactly what modest outcome a course of treatment might reasonably achieve, although such prudent measures did not always protect them from litigation.[229] The criteria for determining a successful cure from incipient *lepra* were rather different, in so far that the patient had a clear and certain goal. Having submitted to what was, at best, an uncomfortable and costly regimen of diets, medication, purges, baths, massage, bleeding, cupping and cauterisation, he or she hoped, like Nicholas de Ely, to walk again in public without shame. The distressing facial symptoms, which John of Gaddesden and most other leading medical authorities regarded with such concern, would have been eliminated or at least contained. Ulcers, nodules and discoloured patches would have disappeared or been rendered comparatively unobtrusive; there would be no hint of the foetid stench of leprosy, no untoward deformity or distortion of the features. That was the devout hope of every suspect. Some recovered, while others continued, like Bernard Gordon's perplexing patient, to defy diagnosis. But many were disappointed and had eventually to face the reality of segregation from society. What might they expect?

---

[229] Rawcliffe, 'Pilgrimage and the Sick', pp. 131–2.

# 6

## A Disease Apart?
## The Impact of Segregation

*It is natural but rather sad that people should be resigned to the fact of 250,000 of our fellow subjects dying of leprosy, but tremendously agitated when they find that there is an idea that the mutton chop they have bought in the meat-market may have been handled by a leper.*

*Edward Clifford*, Father Damien, *1889* [1]

Even at a distance of 500 years, Alice Dymock emerges from the Yarmouth leet rolls as an unusually feisty character. The litany of presentments made against her begins unremarkably enough, in the mid 1480s with charges of petty larceny, quarrelling with her neighbours and selling ale against the assize, all of which were common misdemeanours.[2] Her light-fingered husband, however, was already keeping a disorderly house; and in 1491 she herself was amerced as a procuress. She incurred a similar fine two years later, when her lover, one John Robbins, also ran into trouble for almost murdering her husband. We know that she and Robbins were conducting a liaison, because in the following year they were presented by the leet for adultery. Since she was fined 6*s.* 8*d.*, that is twice as much as he, for the offence, along with a further 6*s.* for harbouring suspicious persons, we can understand why she expressed some free and frank opinions about the ruling elite. For this she subsequently faced accusations of being a common scold. Patience in Yarmouth was clearly wearing thin: in 1496 she incurred exemplary fines of 16*s.* 8*d.* for promoting immorality, scolding and receiving her lover.

But Alice remained an unrepentant Magdalen. Still 'keeping and promoting debauchery and a brothel in her house' *and* selling ale without licence, she was back in court in 1498, and again in the following year, this time as a common whore and provoker of quarrels. By 1499 the now familiar catalogue of charges embraced keeping a suspicious house, bawdry and cursing her exasperated

---

1    Clifford, *Father Damien*, p. 149. He is referring to the national panic following reports that 'a leper with his hands distinctly infected by the disease' was working in a London market: *The Times*, 19 June 1889, p. 13.
2    NRO, Y/C4/189, rot. 13v; 191, rot. 16r.

neighbours.[3] A new century brought a new offensive on the part of the authorities. In 1500 Alice was presented as a leper, who committed a grave nuisance by mixing among adults and children. She was ordered to leave the borough within three months upon pain of £10, which was by far the highest fine ever imposed by any of the four leet courts up to that date. After a few defiant weeks of brothel keeping and sowing discord she packed her bags, but not before assaulting various individuals in her ill-governed house and – as a nice touch of bathos – milking her neighbours' cows.[4]

Alice's long history of antisocial behaviour, which branded her a spiritual if not a physical leper, provides a fascinating case study of the measures taken by the rulers of late medieval English towns to protect the urban environment from corruption. The connection between sexual misconduct and disease, and, indeed, the assumption that allegations of *leprosy* would hasten her removal, graphically illustrate the extent to which popular fears of infection had taken root. Had they known of it, Victorian authors such as H.P. Wright and Robert Liveing would have cited the case as an example of that 'high moral duty' which led to the compulsory segregation of lepers 'as among the dead'.[5] Predictably, however, medieval approaches to exclusion varied considerably, not only with the passage of time, but also according to the occupation, status and, of course, the personal repute of the individual concerned. As we shall see, official attempts to separate presumed lepers from society tended to occur during periods of crisis, when concerns about epidemic disease, disorder and vagrancy were running high. They are well documented in early fourteenth-century England, at which time a dramatic rise in population, followed by food shortages, cattle plagues and epidemics caused widespread social and economic dislocation.[6] Yet not all lepers were shunned, feared or required to depart for solitary places.

It was in 1327, just six years after the brutal pogrom against Jews and lepers in southern France, that Richard Wallingford became abbot of St Albans. A brilliant young mathematician and mechanical engineer, he promptly embarked upon a rigorous campaign of internal reform, coupled with a drive to enforce monastic rights over tenants and townsmen. Perhaps in response to stress, the first signs of leprosy soon appeared on his person. Initial attempts by a faction of disaffected monks to have him removed resulted in their excommunication, after which the rest of the community swung solidly behind him. By 1333, though, the disease had advanced so dramatically that an ambitious monk from Abingdon abbey, who had his eye on the next vacancy, petitioned the Pope to intervene. The ensuing commission of inquiry reported that Richard's condition caused such offence that he could no longer enter the chapter house or choir,

---

3  R.M. Karras, *Common Women: Prostitution and Sexuality in Medieval England* (Oxford, 1996), pp. 68–9, discusses Alice's case in the context of prostitution.
4  NRO, Y/C4/202, rot. 4v; 203, rots 7r, 9r. For the wider background, see M.K. McIntosh, 'Finding Language for Misconduct: Jurors in Fifteenth-Century Local Courts', in B.A. Hanawalt and D. Wallace, eds, *Bodies and Disciplines: Intersections of Literature and History in Fifteenth-Century England* (Minneapolis and London, 1996), pp. 87–122; and M.K. McIntosh, *Controlling Misbehaviour in England 1370–1600* (Cambridge, 1998), passim.
5  Liveing, *Elephantiasis Graecorum*, pp. 13, 23.
6  B. Harvey, 'Introduction: The "Crisis" of the Early Fourteenth Century', in B.M.S. Campbell, ed., *Before the Black Death* (Manchester, 1991), pp. 1–24.

and was manifestly unfit for the monastic life.[7] This was not, however, the view of his brethren, the larger and most intimidating of whom announced that they would personally chop the whistleblower into small pieces. 'He [Richard] meets with us daily', they protested, 'and as his works make manifest, he has borne himself with honour from the time he undertook his office, and he continues to do so, in matters both spiritual and temporal'.[8] The abbot died three years later, having been assisted in the final stages of his illness by a coadjutor, or deputy, who assumed many of his more arduous duties. With uncharacteristic warmth, the monastic chronicler, Thomas Walsingham, pronounced him patient and magnanimous in adversity, noting that his last years had been spent in constant pain.[9] That the monks were familiar with recent medical literature on the 'contagiousness' of *lepra*, through corrupt air and close proximity, seems almost certain, although they clearly deemed the risk of infection sufficiently slight to pose no real threat. Wallingford, who evidently could not bring himself to utter the word '*lepra*', gave thanks for their humanity in his prayers:

> And, moreover, though I be a man in an extreme state, and by thy providence smitten with a foul morphew (*mala morphea*), so that I am unworthy to have dealings with men, but by the law should be put out without the camp, yet Thou, O Lord ... so inclinest the hearts of the great towards me that they do not abhor my service, my speech, and the deformity of face and hands, but be pleased to partake of my company and to show their respect.[10]

Having, in his youth, succumbed to the pleasures of the flesh, Abbot Wallingford clearly felt that he deserved far worse. And such would, indeed, have been his fate had he been a creature of fiction rather than fact.

That the physical burden of leprosy would be accompanied by the even greater torment of ostracism, and in some cases forcible detention, had long been a common literary *topos*. We have already encountered Robert de Boron's tale of the future emperor, Vespasian, whose disease was reputedly 'so terrible and so foul' that he had to be 'shut away in a tower with neither window nor view, save a tiny casement, against which a ladder was set to give him food whenever need arose'.[11] This dark prison serves as an explicit metaphor for the young man's spiritual ignorance, which is dispelled by the healing light of Christianity, just as the leprosies of sin vanish upon exposure to the Veronica. The fourteenth-century English poem, *Titus and Vespasian*, describes the 'noble' hero as a voluntary exile, whose 'meselry' is divinely ordained as part of God's plan for vengeance against the Jews. But until the coming of Pope Clement and the Veronica he, too, remains an object of revulsion:

> The evell was on hym soo ranke
> That on his folke so foule stanke,

7   J.D. North, ed., *Richard of Wallingford* (3 vols, Oxford, 1976), ii, pp. 1–16.
8   North, *Richard of Wallingford*, i, p. 547.
9   Walsingham, *Gesta*, ii, pp. 201, 293.
10  North, *Richard of Wallingford*, i, p. 551. North translates '*morphea*' as plague, but Wallingford's precise choice of words is significant: see above, pp. 162, 163, 187 n. 145.
11  Boron, *Joseph d'Arimathie*, p. 120; and above, pp. 244–5.

From amonges his men he flegh [fled],
And helde is chambre biside negh,
That unnethe [none of] his men for his stynke
Mighte hym brynge mete or drynke,
At a vice [with a vice at the end of a stick] thei turnede in his mete
Whan he shulde anything ete.
And thus in bed he lay,
That he ne might out, nyght ny day.[12]

The didactic purpose of most medieval verse makes it unreliable as a source of evidence regarding the fate of real rather than literary lepers, not least because the grand themes of punishment, redemption and enlightenment, with which such writing deals, demanded stark treatment.

Had she retired to the secluded private quarters that customarily awaited a high-status leper, the proud and promiscuous Cresseid would have escaped retribution and forfeited self-knowledge. Only the indignity of public shame and destitution in a squalid suburban *leprosarium* will suffice. It is, however, worth noting that her life 'at the tounis end' is far from cloistered, taking her 'fra place to place' in search of alms, and permitting one final encounter with her former lover, Troilus.[13] Even in the pages of literature, seclusion was usually far from absolute (the repugnant Vespasian actually kisses one loyal retainer 'ofte, mouthe to mouthe'), while in reality the more draconian regulations were applied sporadically and often ignored. On the other hand, as Alice Dymock discovered, leprosy could serve as a useful catch-all for the elimination of misfits.

After examining the measures taken by the Church and the English common law to provide a secure legal framework for the support as well as the containment of lepers, we will assess the growing influence of medical ideas about miasma and contagion. Successive outbreaks of plague from 1349 onwards made urban communities increasingly vigilant on this score. As we shall see, however, attendant anxieties about prostitution and vagrancy contributed in equal measure to the hostility encountered by 'leprous' men and women who failed to conform to accepted social norms. Yet, as the last part of this chapter reveals, such concerns were not matched by an expansion in hospital places. On the contrary, far from being herded into the nearest *leprosarium*, even the most deserving often found it difficult to secure a bed. We conclude by exploring the gradual decline of institutional support, as many leper houses were obliged to sell accommodation to the healthy on the open market, and patrons jealously protected their spiritual investments by vetting admissions.

## Canon law

Convinced of the authenticity of the 'Leper Mass', many authors have excoriated the medieval Church for its repressive attitude towards the leper, or, more accurately, a range of social undesirables whom it branded as leprous. Its more

---

[12] J.A. Herbert, ed., *Titus and Vespasian: Or the Destruction of Jerusalem* (London, for the Roxburghe Club, 1905), p. 57.
[13] Henryson, *Testament of Cresseid*, pp. 23–49, 75–80.

trenchant critics have described this brutal approach as the ultimate expression of a repressive process of centralisation and even as a cynical attempt at the exploitation of lay benefactors for crude financial profit.[14] Like all other inhabitants of the Christian West, the sick were affected by a process of reform that greatly augmented the power of the Papacy and stamped the authority of Rome upon the faithful from their cradles to their graves. Since, however, a major plank of this programme hinged upon the improvement of pastoral care for vulnerable social groups, the picture was considerably less bleak than might at first appear. Scottish clergy were, for example, urged in the mid thirteenth century not to exacerbate the woes of lepers through the over-zealous enforcement of parochial rights, but to commiserate with their afflictions.[15]

As we have already seen, whether they were enshrined in the rulings of canon law or expressed in less formal ways, ecclesiastical responses to leprosy were profoundly influenced by the book of Leviticus. A belief that confirmed lepers should live 'outside the camp' did not, however, condemn them to banishment or neglect. Nor did it imply that they were to be incarcerated as prisoners. On the contrary, the conviction that God chastises those whom he loves the most, and that Christ himself had not only consorted with lepers but had actually come to resemble one in his final agony, bestowed a special status upon the inmates of *leprosaria*, which Christians ignored at their peril.[16] Indeed, although their numbers may already have begun to decline by the late thirteenth century, homiletic literature stressing the spiritual merits to be gained by caring for such men and women continued to circulate in ever increasing quantities. Food, drink, clothing, utensils, land and money were all welcome, but it was especially meritorious to provide the consolations of religion for pious souls whose full and active membership of the Church never came in question.

In a letter of 726 to the Anglo-Saxon missionary, St Boniface, Pope Gregory advised that 'lepers who belong to the Christian faith should be allowed to partake of the body of and blood of the Lord, but they may not attend sacred functions with people of good health'.[17] Such a ruling presupposed, at the very least, that separate services would be held for the sick, although from the standpoint of Mosaic law it seemed preferable to construct chapels where they would be free to worship together undisturbed. A belief that lepers could not reasonably be expected to withdraw from society *unless* they had regular access to the sacraments is, for example, clearly expressed in instructions sent by Louis VI of France (d. 1137) to the clergy of Compiègne,[18] and likewise prompted the benefactors of early English *leprosaria* to build or endow their foundations with substantial chapels. A fine example may still be seen at Sprowston on the outskirts of Norwich, where Herbert de Losinga built the city's first leper hospital [plate 28]. Standing two storeys high (to accommodate both men and women), the chapel measured approximately 8.5 m x 32 m, and thus allowed

14  Pegg, 'Le corps et l'autorité', pp. 265–87, and Watts, *Epidemics and History*, pp. 49–56.
15  Wilkins, *Concilia*, i, p. 617, canon lxxii.
16  See, for example, Merlet and Jusselin, *Cartulaire de la léproserie du Grand-Beaulieu*, nos 6, 19, 64.
17  C.H. Talbot, ed., *The Anglo Saxon Missionaries in Germany* (London, 1954), p. 82.
18  A. Luchaire, ed., *Louis VI le Gros: Annales de sa vie et de sa règne* (2 vols, Paris, 1890), ii, no. 631.

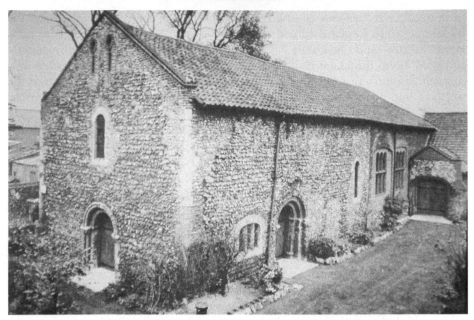

28. The *leprosarium* of St Mary Magdalen at Sprowston, on the outskirts of Norwich. Founded by Bishop Herbert de Losinga (d. 1119) in remission of his sins, the hospital has been greatly altered, although enough of the Norman fabric survives to reveal a substantial two-storey construction, which would have permitted a significant level of liturgical provision.

ample space for the daily performance of the *opus Dei* as well as the celebration of Mass.[19]

Yet the great majority of *leprosaria* had far less certain beginnings. Originating as small, informal gatherings of men and women who had left their homes once the disease became established, they boasted few facilities and little in the way of spiritual care. Often misinterpreted as a mandate for the exclusion of lepers from society, the twenty-third ruling of the third Lateran Council of 1179 was unambiguously designed to provide support for such communities, whose members were *already* obliged by Mosaic Law to live apart from the healthy (*qui cum sanis habitare non possunt*). It begins by stressing the Church's apostolic mission to the sick and deploring the fact that many had been deprived of succour, most notably for lack of chapels, clergy and proper burial facilities.[20] This lamentable neglect on the part of ecclesiastical authorities was to be addressed as a matter of urgency, always allowing for the parochial rights of established institutions. In addition, to provide much-needed financial assistance, Alexander III granted all *leprosaria* an exemption from the payment of tithes on agricultural produce. Archbishop Hubert Walter reiterated the decree

[19] Rawcliffe, *Hospitals of Medieval Norwich*, pp. 41–7; Gilchrist, *Contemplation and Action*, fig. 22, p. 47.
[20] J.D. Mansi, ed., *Sacrorum conciliorum nove et amplissima collectio* (53 vols, Venice, Florence and Paris, 1759–98), xxii, col. 230; Avril, 'Le IIIe Concile du Latran', pp. 21–76.

in its entirety at the Council of Westminster, in 1200; and fifty-six years later the papal nuncio to England agreed that Rome would demand no taxes from poor lazar houses and hospitals. Successive English parliaments subsequently remitted their fiduciary claims upon leper hospitals where the warden was himself 'meseal', this being a sure guarantee that such places still received the sick and had not (as papal tax collectors often alleged) been converted to other uses.[21]

Many communities benefited from these injunctions. Abbot Alvered of Saint-Pierre-sur-Dives was among the first to act, permitting the lepers of Bretford in Warwickshire to have their own chaplain, and allowing them to keep tithes of milk and of herbs from their garden.[22] Bishop le Puiset's foundation charter for his new hospital at Sherburn in County Durham (1184 x 89) refers to both a church *and* an infirmary chapel, which between them were to be served by three priests and four clerks.[23] Determined at this time to make decent provision for the lepers who congregated near the hot springs in Bath, Bishop Reginald Fitzjocelin entrusted their community to the care of the almoner of Bath priory. He also assigned woodland and grazing just outside the town for their sheep and appointed a chaplain to serve them under his personal direction.[24] Lay donors proved no less generous, providing property and rents to support chaplains, along with lights, vestments and plate to furnish the Mass.[25] Thus, for example, William de Aumari gave to the hospital chapel at Burton Lazars a grant of land to illuminate a lamp, which was to burn in the chapel during all services for the health of his immortal soul.[26]

Contrary to popular assumptions, the majority of these buildings were neither remote nor self-sufficient, while some even shared facilities with local congregations. The chapel of St Leonard's hospital, Leicester, was quite literally annexed to the eponymous parish church, which came under the patronage of the Benedictine abbot. This clash of jurisdiction gave rise, in the later Middle Ages at least, to repeated disputes about access and the celebration of Mass, in

---

21  D. Whitelock, M. Brett and C.N.L. Brooke, eds, *Councils and Synods I, Part II, 1066–1204* (Oxford, 1981), p. 1068; W.E. Lunt, *Papal Revenues in the Middle Ages* (2 vols, New York, 1934), i, p. 278; ii, pp. 162, 175, 182, 424; Strachey, *Rotuli Parliamentorum*, i, pp. 239–40, 442–3, 446, 451–2, 458–9; ii, pp. 426, 447. Practice did not, of course, always accord with precept, as the leprous sisters of Maiden Bradley found in their dispute with the canons of Notley: Cheney and Jones, *EEA, II, Canterbury 1162–1190*, no. 165; C.R. Cheney and E. John, eds, *EEA, III, Canterbury 1193–1205* (Oxford, 1986), no. 560.

22  M.J. Franklin, ed., *EEA, 16, Coventry and Lichfield 1160–1182* (Oxford, 1998), no. 91.

23  M.G. Snape, ed., *EEA, 24, Durham 1153–1195* (Oxford, 2001), no. 145. Richard Kellaw, bishop of Durham (1311–16), added another priest to serve a second chapel, which he built in order that male and female lepers could worship separately: Richardson, *Medieval Leper*, p. 125.

24  F.M.R. Ramsey, ed., *EEA, X, Bath and Wells 1061–1205* (Oxford, 1995), nos 77–81, 190–93; Manco, *Spirit of Care*, pp. 16–20. Episcopal concern about the provision of chapels in *leprosaria* continued. Thus, in the early fourteenth century, Bishops Dalderby and Burghersh of Lincoln issued a series of indulgences to assist the repair of chapels at St Giles's, Stamford, and St Leonard's, Bedford: LAO, Episcopal Registers iii, fos 67v, 287v, 416r; v, fos 281r, 302r.

25  For example, an inquisition of 1373 reported that the founder of the hospital at Corbridge, Northumberland, had set aside twenty-four acres of land to provide a chaplain 'to celebrate mass for the lepers every Sunday and feast day': *CIM, 1377–1388*, no. 76, pp. 50–51.

26  BL, MS Cotton Nero CXII, fo. 14r; and below, pp. 341–2.

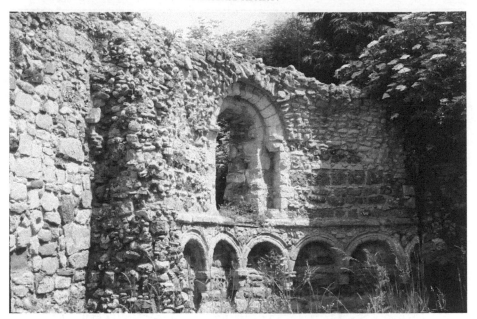

29. The imposing apse of the large Norman chapel of St James's leper hospital, Dunwich, suggests that the residents worshipped in some style. Those close to death would have been nursed in the nave, and would thus have enjoyed an uninterrupted view of the altar and of the Mass celebrated there.

which money rather than segregation proved the bone of contention.[27] The imposing Norman chapel assigned to the *leprosarium* at Dunwich, in Suffolk, stood in the graveyard of St James's parish church, immediately outside the town ditch [**plate 29**]. Its dominant position, at the intersection of two roads, within a short distance of the harbour and main gate, made it a prominent local landmark, which anyone entering the borough from the north-west had to pass [**map 3**].[28]

When endowing their chapels, patrons such as Herbert de Losinga made careful provision for the creation of an adjacent cemetery, where the hospital's dead could receive a proper burial in consecrated ground.[29] Although we lack sufficient evidence to be entirely certain, it looks as if the practice of burying lepers separately was a fairly recent development, associated with the creation of the first post-Conquest *leprosaria*.[30] The excavation of a parish cemetery at Timberhill in Norwich, which was abandoned just after the arrival of the Normans, revealed thirty-five identifiable victims of Hansen's disease, just over half of whom appear to have contracted lepromatous leprosy. Their symptoms had advanced sufficiently to affect the skeleton, and thus to render them imme-

[27] Nichols, *History and Antiquities of Leicester*, i, part 2, pp. 321–2.
[28] Comfort, *Lost City of Dunwich*, pp. 42, 104, 121.
[29] Rawcliffe, *Hospitals of Medieval Norwich*, p. 46.
[30] For pre-Conquest leper burials among the healthy, see Roberts and Cox, *Health and Disease*, pp. 120, 218–19.

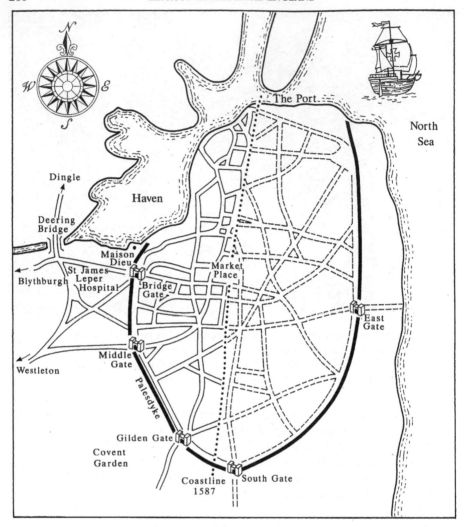

Map 3. Medieval Dunwich and its leper hospital (Phillip Judge)

diately recognisable as *leprosi*: indeed, a minimum of nineteen had sustained serious damage to the nasal area and jawbone. These individuals, who constituted a fifth of all excavated burials, may have lived in an informal community, on what would then have been the margins of the city. Yet they were interred alongside apparently 'healthy' people, sometimes in family groups.[31]

Over the following decades, many newly founded English hospitals for the sick poor acquired their own graveyards for the burial of patrons, staff and patients, although their existence often provoked quarrels with local parish churches and religious houses, which resented the loss of rights and income. In

---

[31] S. Anderson, 'Leprosy in a Medieval Churchyard in Norwich', in eadem, ed., *Current and Recent Research in Osteoarchaeology* (Oxford, 1998), pp. 31–7.

theory, at least, fewer such obstacles lay in the way of the creation of cemeteries in *leprosaria*, especially after 1179 when the third Lateran Council demanded it. The spread of Classical medical ideas about the dangers of mephistic air may have accelerated this trend, which also harked back to the Book of Leviticus. But we should not underestimate the more positive aspects of a measure designed to provide the spiritual solace of Christian rites for men and women whose condition merited sympathy as well as horror. Some authorities had, indeed, already stepped in to implement the seventh and last of the Comfortable Works.[32] Two decades earlier, for example, an *actum* of Bishop Alfred of Worcester ordered the consecration of a separate burial ground for those lepers who could not be interred in the monastic cemetery along with other local people.[33]

It would, nevertheless, be unwise to conclude that, in reality, lepers were any more isolated from the world in death than they had been in life. Reforms instituted in 1346 at the hospital of St Mary the Virgin, Ilford, insisting upon 'free burial by themselves' for the residents suggest that cupidity as well as laxity had long since undermined the papal ruling of 1179.[34] It is, moreover, apparent that, however anxious monastic houses such as Whitby and Bury St Edmunds may have been to remove leprous brethren from the cloister to hospitals specially endowed for the purpose, they expected to recover their bodies for burial in the heart of the community. The truncated funerary rites they devised may have been speedier and less elaborate than those performed for other religious, but the ties of shared profession clearly endured beyond the grave.[35] As we saw in chapter four, the presence of skeletons afflicted by Hansen's disease in late medieval urban cemeteries may, in part at least, be explained by the fact that some of these individuals were 'suspect' rather than 'confirmed' *leprosi*. Others may, however, have belonged to influential local families, who experienced few if any problems in conveying the remains of diseased relatives to the family tomb or plot. Excavations at the Dominican friary, Ipswich (1263 x 1538), for example, reveal a genetic relationship between leprous and 'healthy' skeletons buried in one of the town's most prestigious cemeteries.[36]

The burial of healthy individuals in the graveyards and chapels of *leprosaria* proved more contentious, not necessarily because of any reluctance on the part of the former to be interred alongside men and women whose earthly bodies had already begun to exhibit dramatic signs of decay. That the priests, nurses and

---

[32] C. Rawcliffe, 'The Seventh Comfortable Work: Charity and Mortality in the Medieval Hospital', *Medicina & Storia*, iii (2003), pp. 11–35.

[33] W.H. Hart, ed., *Historia et cartularium monasterii Sancti Petri Gloucestriae* (3 vols, RS, 1863–67), ii, p. 7. Easy access to established graveyards was equally important. In 1235, the lepers at Tweedmouth were allowed to retain 40s. a year in rents to repair the road to their cemetery: M.G. Snape, ed., *EEA*, 25, *Durham 1196–1237* (Oxford, 2001), no. 339.

[34] Dugdale, *Monasticon*, vi, p. 630. Excavation reveals that the cemeteries of *leprosaria* were deliberately situated in close proximity to roads, perhaps to underscore the inmates' transitory position between life and death, while also stimulating the gift of alms by travellers: Gilchrist and Sloane, *Requiem*, pp. 33–4.

[35] Page, *VCH Yorkshire III*, p. 334; A. Gransden, ed., *The Cartulary of the Benedictine Abbey of Bury St Edmunds in Suffolk* (London, 1973), appendix VIII; Atkinson, *Cartularium Abbathiae de Whitby*, ii, p. 515. The arrangement at Whitby was made before 1139.

[36] S.A. Mays, *Medieval Burials from the Blackfriars Friary, School Street, Ipswich, Suffolk* (Ancient Monuments Laboratory Report 16/1991, part 1), p. 61.

servants who ministered to the sick would expect to lie beside them in death is hardly surprising, especially as the humble and penitent leper seemed such a potent advocate. It is unfortunate that so little testamentary evidence survives from the twelfth and thirteenth centuries, when most *leprosaria* were founded, since there is good reason to suppose that pious men and women then appreciated the spiritual benefits of marching towards the Last Judgement alongside the poor of Christ. Continental examples are instructive. As early as 1153, clergy at Tournai were sufficiently concerned about the loss of burial fees to secure a ruling that only *conversi*, who acted as nurses and servants in the local leper house, might be permitted to share its cemetery.[37] Men such as Fulk de Grosslieu, who offered land to the hospital of the Grand Beaulieu, Chartres, in 1158, in return for burial just outside the church door, and Guillaume Aiguillon, who was interred there beside his wife a decade later, may have been far from unusual.[38] Nearer home, and at a later date, successive generations of the Twyer family were laid to rest in the chapel of St Sepulchre's hospital, Hedon, although the lepers were presumably buried in the graveyard, and thus at a respectful distance from their patrons.[39] Skeletal as well as documentary evidence suggests that the healthy were interred with the sick in the *leprosarium* of St James and St Mary Magdalen at Chichester.[40] Excavation of the hospital cemetery revealed a charnel pit and the existence of two stone-lined tombs, as well as the widespread use of coffins rather than the cheap shrouds deployed in most medieval hospitals. The funerary rites of the deceased were apparently accorded high priority.[41]

In practice, then, boundaries were predictably blurred. Local people might, for example, use the chapel and cemetery of a *leprosarium* in lieu of a parish church, as they were doing at St Leonard's, Northampton, well before 1282.[42] Conversely, lepers living in small communities without the benefit of spiritual services were able to request burial in the nearest parochial graveyard. This was certainly the case at another St Leonard's, just outside Norwich, where a persuasive combination of testamentary and skeletal evidence confirms that Lateran III was as much honoured in the breach as the observance by the later Middle Ages. St Margaret's, the nearest parish church, which lay just inside the walls in a poor part of the city, near the gallows, accepted leper burials, as did the neighbouring All Saints. Seven skeletons displaying advanced symptoms of lepromatous and tuberculoid leprosy, of the kind that any medieval surgeon would have instantly identified, and six others with treponemal infections (possibly syphilis), have

---

[37]  Avril, 'Le IIIe Concile du Latran', pp. 26, 29, 30, 37, 41.

[38]  Merlet and Jusselin, *Cartulaire de la léproserie du Grand-Beaulieu*, nos 46, 35.

[39]  Page, *VCH Yorkshire III*, pp. 309–10. See also below, p. 341.

[40]  J. Magilton, 'The Leper Hospital of St James and St Mary Magdalen, Chichester, and other Leper Houses', in Tabuteau, *Lépreux et sociabilité*, pp. 81–91. Such a conclusion rests, however, upon the assumption that Hansen's disease and medieval *lepra* were synonymous. Nor does Hansen's disease always affect the skeleton. For documentary evidence of 'healthy' burials in this cemetery, see W.D. Peckham, ed., *The Chartulary of the High Church of Chichester* (Sussex Record Society, xlvi, 1942–43), p. 7.

[41]  Magilton, 'Leper Hospital of St James and St Mary Magdalen, Chichester', in Roberts, *Burial Archaeology*, pp. 249–56.

[42]  R.M.T. Hill, ed., *The Rolls and Register of Bishop Oliver Sutton 1280–1299, II* (Lincoln Record Society, xliii, 1950), pp. 22–3.

been excavated from the cemetery of St Margaret's, which was closed in the 1460s.[43] Such arrangements were clearly not uncommon. The *leprosi*, Henry (d. 1448) and Richard Wellys (d. 1466), who may have been father and son, each made wills requesting burial in the graveyard of All Saints. Both were patients at St Leonard's hospital when they died. Henry actually left money for the construction of a new chapel there, which suggests that the inmates lacked facilities of their own and relied upon parochial clergy for support.[44]

The protection of the Church went beyond the simple provision of chapels, priests and cemeteries. As we have seen, the residents of monastic *leprosaria* either made a full – and entirely voluntary – profession or more commonly ranked as *conversi*, who, if not tonsured, were none the less bound by oaths of poverty, chastity and obedience. For this reason they could, in theory at least, expect to command the same respect as other religious. Waleran (d. 1166), count of Melun and founder of the *leprosarium* of St Gilles de Pont-Audemer, may have gone further than most patrons in actually ordering his tenants to treat the patients with the deference due to monks.[45] It was, however, common for the benefactors of early English leper houses to refer in fulsome language to the 'servants of God' who received their charity, and for the residents to describe themselves in similar terms.[46] At the hospital of St Mary Magdalen, Reading, which was founded in the early 1130s by abbot Ancher under a strict rule, the lepers were addressed as 'our brothers' by the monks, and even appeared in their bede roll, alongside members of other Benedictine communities, such as Ramsey and Durham.[47] That the Church sought to uphold the status of hospital inmates is reflected in one mid thirteenth-century English penitential, which threatened anyone who assaulted 'a religious person, such as a cleric, or a lay brother, or a monk, or a leper *de collegio*,' with excommunication.[48]

Elaborate admission ceremonies were staged in most of the larger *leprosaria* and hospitals of medieval Europe to mark each newcomer's entry into the reli-

---

[43] J. Bown and A. Stirland, *Criminals and Paupers: Excavations at the Site and Churchyard of St Margaret, Fyebridgegate, Magdalen Street, Norwich* (East Anglian Archaeology, forthcoming), chapter two.

[44] NRO, NCC, reg. Aleyn, fo. 9r; reg. Jekkys, fo. 43r. The antiquary, Francis Bloomefield, reports a local tradition that a north-facing tomb in the graveyard of St Clement's, Norwich, encased – and set apart – the body of a leper, who had been refused burial elsewhere. But he observes it 'is all an errour': *An Essay towards a Topographical History of Norfolk* (11 vols, 1805–10), iv, pp. 459–60.

[45] Mesmin, 'St Gilles de Pont-Audemer', ii, pp. 93–4; Avril, 'Le IIIe Concile du Latran', p. 26. Communal responses could be less charitable. In 1290, for example, it proved necessary to rescind a grant of the parish church of Reculver, Kent, made fourteen years earlier by Archbishop Kilwardby to the *leprosarium* at Harbledown, because the local people 'taking it ill to be subject to lepers', withheld their dues: *Calendar of Papal Registers: Papal Letters, 1198–1304*, p. 511.

[46] Numerous examples include: St Giles, Holborn (BL, MS Harley 4015, fos 187r–187v, 188v–189r), St James, Doncaster (BL MS Cotton Tiberius CV, fos 262r–264r, 265v, 267v, 268v), St Mary and St Matthew, Maiden Bradley (BL, Add. Charters 19137, 20423; MS Add. 37503, fos 6v, 9r–10r, 15v, 17v, 19v, 22v, 24r–25v, 27r, 28v, 30v), St Leonard, Lowcross (W. Brown, ed., *Cartularium Prioratus de Gyseburne, I* (Surtees Society, lxxxvi, 1889), pp. 173–94), St Mary Magdalen, Gaywood (*HMC, Eleventh Report, Appendix, Part III* (London, 1887), pp. 235–8).

[47] BL, MS Cotton Vespasian E V, fos 37r–38v. It was, presumably, here that Robert Leir of Burghfield took his vows, since a release of dower rights made to the monastic almonry by his wife, in about 1241, was effected 'post conversum dicti Roberti viri mei ad religionem leprosorum': Kemp, *Reading Abbey Cartularies*, ii, p. 63.

[48] J. Goering, 'The *Summa de Penitentia* of Magister Serlo', *Medieval Studies*, xxxviii (1976), pp. 1–53, at p. 9; and above, pp. 28–9.

gious life.[49] The festive aspect of these occasions complemented the solemnity of a ritual involving the acceptance of either monastic or quasi-monastic discipline. Some houses were more regimented than others. Until at least the 1320s, for example, all the sisters at Maiden Bradley had to take the habit as fully professed nuns,[50] whereas those at St James's, Canterbury did not. Indeed, the latter were assured in 1349 that, although they lived as a religious community, following all the customary observances, they were entirely 'free to leave, whenever they wished, just like other seculars (*sicut alie seculares*)'.[51] How many were actually leprous at this time cannot be determined, although it is important to stress that, far from attempting to detain unwilling or difficult residents, most *leprosaria* had always moved quickly to evict potential troublemakers.

The removal of an offender was, not surprisingly, a very public affair, designed to bring home the gravity of the lapse, while also setting a harsh example. At Ilford, for instance, a visitation by various 'great spyrytuall personnes' allegedly revealed that one leper had smuggled a prostitute into his room disguised as his sister. Barefoot and bareheaded, he was obliged to kneel on the altar steps during Mass, as a prelude to being symbolically stripped of his religious status and driven, like an unfrocked priest, from the church into a jeering crowd.[52] Smaller and more democratic institutions reserved the right to expel difficult residents. Inmates of the *leprosarium* at Lanlivery, Cornwall, who affronted their fellows 'in word or deed', were, for instance, to be deprived of their goods and removed until they made suitable amends.[53] Disputes with the patron could also result in ejection: '*les povere freres malades*' at the hospital of St Mary Magdalen, Colchester, complained to parliament in 1302 that the abbot had not only confiscated their records, but had forcibly ousted two of their number who had resisted him.[54]

New rules devised in 1344 by Abbot Mentmore of St Albans for the nearby leper hospital of St Julian imposed firm monastic discipline upon everyone but the very sick. All new entrants had to undergo an obligatory period of probation, 'during which time their morals and conversation [would] be manifestly revealed through their bearing and conduct'. Those whom the patron deemed suitable then took a formal oath of profession, sworn on the gospels in the hospital church before the entire community. They were, significantly, obliged to accept that incorrigible offences would be punished by expulsion 'like an

---

49  Below, pp. 302–3.
50  In 1321 the bishop of Salisbury ordered three new sisters at Maiden Bradley to take the veil, because they had been admitted before an episcopal inhibition on further professions: PRO, E135/22/50. As Bishop Montacute of Worcester observed in an *actum* of 1335, the poor and leprous nuns were especially deserving of charity: BL, MS Add. 37503, fo. 39r–39v; B. Kemp, 'Maiden Bradley Priory, Wiltshire, and Kidderminster Church, Worcestershire', in M. Barber, P. McNulty and P. Noble, eds, *East Anglian and other Studies Presented to Barbara Dodwell* (Reading Medieval Studies, xi, 1985), p. 102.
51  Duncombe and Battely, *Three Archiepiscopal Hospitals*, p. 431.
52  T.J. Pettigrew, 'On Leper Hospitals or Houses', *Journal of the British Archaeological Association*, xi (1855), pp. 9–34, 95–117, at p. 103. The account comes from a lost 'ledger' of Barking abbey, described and probably embellished by the antiquary, Arthur Agarde.
53  N. Orme, 'The Medieval Leper-House at "Lamford" Cornwall', *Historical Research*, lxix (1996), pp. 102–7, at p. 107.
54  Strachey, *Rotuli Parliamentorum*, i, p. 157.

apostate without any hope of return, other than by the special favour of the lord abbot'. As we shall see, regular chapter meetings in the hospital church undoubtedly strengthened communal life at St Julian's, especially as 'all seculars and unprofessed brothers' were automatically barred from these gatherings.[55]

Like many other hospital statutes, the regulations at St Julian's required the inmates to wear a sober habit of black and russet, which, with its long sleeves, ankle-length overcoat and voluminous hooded cape, would have made them immediately recognisable long before their deformed features or foetid breath became apparent [**plate 5**].[56] There was, however, no special 'uniform' or distinctive item of clothing designed to set lepers in general apart from healthy members of the English public, from the people who cared for them, or, indeed, from the brothers and sisters of other charitable institutions, who adopted a similar style of dress. They were certainly never expected to display a badge or garment of the sort that served from the thirteenth century onwards to identify Jews, heretics and prostitutes. Although the Council of Paris had ruled in 1212 that, where resources permitted, the inmates of hospitals and *leprosaria* should assume a habit and follow a rule, neither canon law nor local custom demanded that lepers ought to wear a *tabula*, striped hood or robe of a particular style or colour.[57]

It was for the founders or patrons of hospitals to stipulate how their beneficiaries should (or more usually should not) dress, their chief preoccupation being to emulate as far as possible the sombre and penitential garb of the monastic cloister. Indeed, the lepers of St Michael's hospital, Whitby, which came under the aegis of the nearby Benedictine house, actually wore the old or discarded robes of the Cistercians at Rievaulx. These were, appropriately, delivered each year on the feast of St Martin, who had shared his cloak with one leprous beggar and kissed another.[58] Residents of the hospital of St Mary Magdalen at Dudston were likewise expected to wear only the plainest robes of black, white or russet, avoiding the motley, or mixed, colours so often associated with persons of easy virtue.[59] They were, in short, subject to the same strictures as the clergy, whose fondness for gaudy secular apparel caused increasing alarm in an age preoccupied with the imposition of social and ecclesiastical order. It might be argued that lepers needed no distinguishing garment to warn the

---

55  Richards, *Medieval Leper*, pp. 131, 135–6. At Montpellier, the probationary period was just nine days, whereas at Noyon profession followed a year's trial: Le Grand, *Statuts*, pp. 182, 195.

56  Richards, *Medieval Leper*, pp. 131–2. These requirements may have been influenced by Archbishop Winchelsey's rules of 1299 for the Harbledown leper house. Both insisted upon the wearing of properly laced leather boots, perhaps as protection for ulcerated feet: Duncombe and Battely, *Three Archiepiscopal Hospitals*, p. 212.

57  Mansi, *Sacrorum conciliorum*, xii, cols 835–6; N. Vincent, 'Two Papal Letters on the Wearing of the Jewish Badge, 1221 and 1229', *Jewish Historical Studies*, xxxiv (1994–96), pp. 209–24.

58  Atkinson, *Cartularium Abbathiae de Whitby*, i, p. 330.

59  Kealey, *Medieval Medicus*, pp. 108–9. Leprous sisters and healthy brothers at St James's, Westminster, had to be clothed in either russet or black at all times: BL, MS Cotton Faustina A III, fo. 320r–320v. A similar colour scheme obtained at St Bartholomew's, Dover, and at St Nicholas's, York, where discipline began to slip in the mid thirteenth century: Bodleian Library, MS Rawl. B.335, fo. 4r; W. Brown, ed., *Yorkshire Inquisitions, II* (Yorkshire Archaeological Society, xxxiii, 1897), pp. 124–5. At St Nicholas's, Carlisle, russet was worn: *CPR, 1340–1343*, p. 121; and at Sherburn either white or russet: Richards, *Medieval Leper*, p. 126.

public of their presence, but that, once decently and protectively clad in the livery of a hospital, they became deserving objects of Christian compassion, whose search for alms was legitimised by membership of a religious community.[60]

Such garb clearly set them apart from the vagrant and ill-disciplined beggars whose presence troubled ecclesiastical and urban authorities alike.[61] Quite possibly, as uniforms tend to do, it intensified a more general sense of difference and separation, which some lepers may actually have welcomed. As we have already seen, a tranquil and regulated life, devoid of stress or anxiety, was recommended as part of the palliative regimen for suspect and confirmed cases of *lepra*. That victims of the disease would find the unsolicited attention of others unsettling was recognised by members of the medical profession, who observed the anguish it might cause. Although, as the author of one thirteenth-century text observed, lepers seemed willing to mix in public, 'if a healthy person who is also unacquainted with their ailment, as for example children, looks on them in the face, they are afraid, their faces are troubled and they despair'.[62]

Other forms of retreat were available for men and women of means, whose circumstances allowed them to live quietly out of the public eye. Members of the secular clergy encountered fewer problems in securing admission to *leprosaria* than most laymen, but some understandably chose to retain the security of their livings. The Church acknowledged a dual responsibility in such cases, which demanded the appointment of a coadjutor to serve the parish and the proper provision of support and accommodation for both the sick priest and his new assistant. In response to an inquiry from the bishop of Lincoln, Pope Lucius III ruled in 1183–84 that such arrangements should be adopted whenever the leprous priest could no longer minister to his flock 'without offence'.[63] His primary concern was to preserve the sanctity of the Mass. Although similar provision was made for deaf, blind and disabled clergy, as well as those deemed mentally incapable,[64] leprosy posed a particular problem, in so far that the ulcerated hands of an infected priest threatened to defile the Host with human blood.[65] This very dilemma was one of the factors leading, in 1215, to the canonical prohibition upon the practice of surgery by members of the higher clergy, and explains why use of the lancet or cautery was henceforth forbidden to them. Hands stained with the bodily fluids of the sick could not presume to touch the flesh of God.[66] That physical revulsion might drive worshippers away from

---

60  Abbot Mentmore's rules for St Julian's stress the importance of wearing a decorous and appropriate habit which would facilitate the collection of alms: Richards, *Medieval Leper*, p. 132.

61  Farmer, 'Beggar's Body', pp. 159–64.

62  C. Singer, 'A Thirteenth Century Clinical Description of Leprosy', *JHM*, iv (1949), pp. 237–9, at p. 238. Statutes of this date for the *leprosarium* at Coutances recognised that 'mixing too long with the healthy is burdensome for lepers': Avril, 'Le IIIe Concile de Latran', p. 71.

63  W. Holtzman and E.W. Kemp, eds, *Papal Decretals Relating to the Diocese of Lincoln in the Twelfth Century* (Lincoln Record Society, xlvii, 1954), pp. 52–3.

64  For the deaf, see LAO, Episcopal Register iii, fos 366v–367r; the decrepit, R.L. Storey, ed., *The Register of Gilbert Welton, Bishop of Carlisle, 1353–1362* (Woodbridge, 1999), no. 431; and the mentally ill, J.F. Kirby, ed., *Wykeham's Register, II* (Hampshire Record Society, xiii, 1899), pp. 467–8.

65  Some *leprosaria* would only permit communion if those parts of the body that touched the wafer remained healthy, and by implication less soiled with sin: Borradori, *Mourir au monde*, p. 80.

66  Amundsen, 'Medieval Canon Law', pp. 40–42. The appalling prospect that a leprous priest who had

church, and perhaps also cause them to question the authority of the priesthood, was another cause for vigilance.

Ecclesiastical authorities were therefore anxious to determine whether or not a suspect had deteriorated to such a point that 'because of the deformity of the disease and the horror of his parishioners' he could no longer administer the sacraments. It was for this reason that the rector of Castle Carrock had to appear before the bishop of Carlisle in 1357 and explain why he should not employ a coadjutor.[67] Some priests, such as Thomas Scot, a canon of Holywood who confessed himself to be too blind and leprous to continue with his ministry, were given a free hand to appoint – and dismiss – their assistants.[68] In other cases the authorities would act. An arrangement of 1314 made by Bishop Walter Stapledon on behalf of the vicar of St Neots in Cornwall reveals how much care was taken, by the standards of the age, to temper caution with compassion. The incumbent was to receive 2s. each week for food, drink and footwear (perhaps for ulcerated feet), and a further 20s. a year for clothing. He retained the best chamber and an adjacent dwelling, although the hall of the vicarage was henceforward to be out of bounds. On the ground that a leper could not live among the healthy 'without peril' (sine periculo), a new privy was to be constructed for his use, along with a separate doorway through which he might come and go as he wished.[69] The precise nature of the 'peril' is not specified, although a man with Stapledon's academic background would have been well aware of current medical theories about miasma.

If the attractions of the monastic leprosarium had begun to wane for members of the later medieval clergy, they proved even less compelling for the laity. Despite the fact that many such institutions allowed their inmates to maintain contact with friends and family, the celibate life they demanded was not for all. Men and women who had hitherto enjoyed the pleasures of a companionable marriage must have felt scant vocation for the cloister. Whether their healthy wives and husbands shared this enduring commitment to the vows of matrimony was, however, another matter, and one over which the Church stamped its supreme authority. The imposition of monastic rules and dress upon hospitals and leprosaria was but one aspect of a far wider programme of ecclesiastical reform. Being part of the same drive towards lay conformity and obedience, attempts to regulate the institution of marriage likewise had significant repercussions for lepers. Hospitals following a rule often demanded a vow of chastity from the healthy spouse as well as the sick one, since it was assumed that, in all other cases, conjugal ties would continue unbroken. Some clashes with established custom were inevitable. That leprosy, 'stinking breath' and impotence

---

lost sensation in his hands might drop the chalice after consecration must also have prompted concern: Vincent, *Holy Blood*, pp. 49–50.

[67] Storey, *Register of Gilbert Welton*, no. 203.

[68] *Calendar of Papal Registers: Papal Letters, 1458–1471*, pp. 310–11.

[69] F.C. Hingeston-Randolph, ed., *The Register of Walter de Stapledon, Bishop of Exeter* (London, 1892), p. 342. Leprous chantry priests, such as John Creed of Frome, who had no permanent residence, might, if they wished, be maintained as hermits. He was assigned a hermitage in Selwood forest, in 1448, 'in order to avoid the peril of infecting other persons': H.C. Maxwell-Lyte and M.C.B. Dawes, eds, *The Register of Thomas Bekynton I* (Somerset Record Society, xlix, 1934), p. 101.

traditionally constituted grounds for separation is apparent from early Welsh laws, whose principal concern was not the segregation of the leper but the protection of the fugitive wife's property rights.[70] But by the time that these rulings were codified, in the early thirteenth century, they seemed distinctly out of step with the Church's uncompromising approach to the question.

An initial willingness on the part of the papacy to allow divorce in cases of leprosy had by then given way to a conviction that marriage was indissoluble, whatever the circumstances. Once begun, sexual relations between the two parties created bonds of obligation that no earthly power could shatter.[71] As Pope Alexander III observed in a letter of *c.* 1175 to the archbishop of Canterbury:

> It has come to our attention that, whereas by general custom those who are afflicted by the disease of leprosy are separated from the society of men and transferred out of cities and towns to solitary places, wives are not following their sick husbands, nor are husbands following their wives, but are presuming to remain behind without them. Since man and wife are one flesh and ought not to live without each other, our command is that you should not delay in earnestly inducing the wives of husbands who are afflicted with leprosy, and the husbands of wives, to follow them, and minister to them with conjugal affection. If they cannot be induced to do this, you should strictly order both of them to remain continent for the rest of their lives. And if they refuse to obey your command you must excommunicate them.[72]

While accepting that an unconsummated marriage might be dissolved if one of the parties contracted leprosy or some other serious disease, the papacy insisted that illness, however repugnant, constituted no obstacle to the payment of the conjugal debt.[73]

Ordinary men and women faced by such a dilemma could not always summon the necessary reserves of self-sacrifice and dedication required by the canonists. A growing awareness of medical literature on the sexual transmission of *lepra* tended further to undermine the Church's position. During the early ninth century, the Muslim jurist Al-Shāf'i had argued in favour of divorce in such cases, largely because 'men of medical learning' considered the likelihood

---

70 Cule, 'Diagnosis, Care and Treatment', pp. 38–9. These laws contain no mention whatsoever of the risks of infection: Touati, 'Contagion', pp. 183–4.

71 J.A. Brundage, *Law, Sex and Christian Society in Medieval Europe* (Chicago, 1987), pp. 262, 269, 334–5; C. Duggan, *Decretals and the Creation of 'New Law' in the Twelfth Century* (Aldershot, 1998), chapter nine, pp. 59–87, notably p. 86.

72 A. Friedberg, ed., *Corpus iuris canonici* (2 vols, Leipzig, 1879–81), ii, pp. 680–91, *De coniugio leprosorum*, X.4.8.1. The archbishop apparently sought advice from Alexander before the Council of Westminster. One of thirty-seven proposals on the agenda was that 'lepers shall not in future live among the healthy', a matter which was taken no further: M. Cheney, 'The Council of Westminster of 1175: New Light on an Old Source', in D. Baker, ed., *The Materials, Sources and Methods of Ecclesiastical History* (Studies in Church History, xi, 1975), pp. 61–8.

73 Friedberg, *Corpus iuris canonici*, pp. 680–91, *De coniugio leprosorum*, X.4.8.2–3. The three papal decretals were brought together in the *Liber extra* in about 1234 and implemented by the ecclesiastical courts. In 1437, for example, Robert Place obtained a dispensation to marry his betrothed wife's sister on the ground that he had never consummated the first marriage, 'because she was a leper': *Calendar of Papal Registers: Papal Letters, 1427–1447*, p. 626. A similar situation obtained in cases of insanity: Pickett, *Mental Affliction*, pp. 41–5.

of infection so great. Both the healthy partner and any children he or she might produce faced what he believed to be an unacceptable risk.[74] These ideas did not surface in Western literature for another two or three hundred years, when, as we saw in chapter two, concern focused primarily on the generation of leprous offspring. Although the Church continued to uphold the sanctity of marriage and of the marriage debt, individual clerics, who kept abreast of developments in medicine, then began voicing cautious reservations. Raymond de Penafort, writing shortly after 1234, advised that, when one of the spouses was leprous, abstinence should be practised because of the threat to any future progeny. Other theologians, such as Henri de Suse (1253), were more circumspect, suggesting that the disease *might* be communicated from parent to child, but for the laity a hint was quite enough.[75] As fears of transmission through touch and miasma took hold in the fourteenth and fifteenth centuries it became even harder to persuade reluctant spouses to honour their obligations.

A striking example of the potential tensions between ecclesiastical and medical approaches to these problems arose in the Hanseatic port of Kampen in the late 1460s, when the merchant, Geert ten Starte, was diagnosed as a suspect leper. Since his wife, Fenne Bouster, wanted him despatched to a *leprosarium* and out of her life at the first opportunity, he commissioned a canon lawyer of his acquaintance to produce a tract 'On the Marriage of Lepers'. This spelt out her moral and conjugal obligations in terms that brooked no evasion. The ties of compassion and the bonds of Christian marriage alike demanded that the spouse of a leper should live with him or her until such time as hospitalisation seemed unavoidable. Even then, though, rights of access remained, and the union could only be dissolved by death.[76] Unlike Fenne, some wives put precept into practice, and actually followed their husbands into *leprosaria*. Those suburban houses which either did not adopt, or had effectively abandoned, a religious rule must have welcomed them as unpaid servants and nurses. Evidence from France certainly suggests that, as hospital accommodation grew less communal and more private, it became easier for married couples to adapt to institutional life.[77] Less formal arrangements were undoubtedly made by and for English couples who wished to remain together. The late fifteenth-century 'spytell howses' established by Robert Pygot near his home in Walsingham, Norfolk, were, for example, initially intended to accommodate one John Ederych '*leprosus de Norwico*' and his wife, for their joint lives, and then no more than one or two lepers of 'good conversation and honest disposition'.[78]

Women such as Fenne, who was quite prepared to challenge the competence of her husband's physicians, constituted a small, if vociferous, minority. Lack of opportunity and resources, as well, perhaps, as lower levels of anxiety about the contagiousness of *lepra*, meant that individuals at the bottom of the social hierarchy frequently appear to have stayed with diseased spouses. The case of John

74  Conrad, 'Discussion of Contagion', pp. 175–6.
75  Bergman, 'Hoping against Hope', n. 47, p. 48; Touati, 'Contagion and Leprosy', p. 192.
76  Bergman, 'Hoping against Hope', p. 38.
77  Jeanne, 'Saint-Lazare de Falaise', pp. 49, 54. See also, S. Bormans, ed., *Cartulaire de la Commune de Namur, 1429–1555* (Namur, 1876), no. 188.
78  NRO, Norwich Archdeaconry Court, reg. Fuller, fo. 204r.

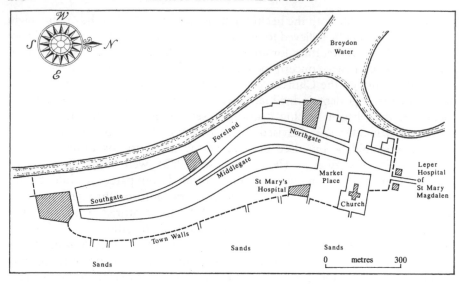

Map 4. Medieval Yarmouth and its leper hospital (Phillip Judge)

Eston, whose wife Beatrice was presented as a public nuisance for ten consecutive years by the jurors of Yarmouth before he reluctantly removed her in 1392, is, indeed, exceptional. Even so, at least twenty-one of the thirty-six female 'lepers' named in the borough leet rolls between 1369 and 1500 were currently living with their husbands, sometimes in defiance of previous orders from the court. [79] It is harder to determine how many of the thirty-seven men accused over the same period were married. In 1430, some five years after a local jury first pronounced her husband, Alexander, *leprosus*, Katherine Colkirke was forbidden under threat of a substantial fine from entering the market and touching the food on display there, evidently because of fears of contagion. She was clearly still caring for him, perhaps in lodgings on the sands just outside the walls, where most of the town's lepers elected to live [**map 4**].[80] Since the *leprosarium* at the north gate was small, selective and strictly segregated into male and female quarters, it clearly had little appeal for the likes of Katherine and Alexander, who wished to remain together.[81]

---

79   NRO, Y/C4/83–202. The other twenty were the wives of Robert Bastwyk (1369/72), Robert atte Gappe (1369/71), John de Wytton (1369/70), John Wayte (1381/82), John Melton (1386/88), John Dekene (1389/90), John Waryn (1392/93), Hugh Taillour (1399/1400), Roger Reynalde (1411/14), William Bryd (1418/19), John Faker (1418/19), William Boon (1420/21), Reginald Tynker (1420/26), Reginald Frenssh (1422/24), John Spitlyng (1429/31), Adam Tyler (1433/35), Reginald Knyght (1433/34), [ – ] le Glover (1480/81), John Mynne (1492/93) and Robert Knobbyng (1499/1500).

80   NRO, Y/C4/135, rots 10r–11r; 139, rot. 12v.

81   The women's quarters lay on one side of the road leading through the gate, and the men's on the other, which explains references to the 'two houses' of lepers there. The hospital boasted a priest and a chapel, and was supported by many local testators: H. Manship, *The History of Great Yarmouth*, ed. J. Palmer (London, 1854), pp. 432–4; above, p. 109.

## The common law

As we saw in chapter four, the suspect lepers of late medieval Yarmouth, and of all other English towns and villages, were subject to the rigours of the English common law and of local custom, which in some respects had a greater impact upon their lives than the surveillance of the Church. From a comparatively early date secular authorities in various parts of Europe had promulgated regulations defining the legal status of persons whose physical disability, gender, religious vocation or reduced mental capacity rendered them incapable of playing a full part in society. Early Welsh law, for example, banned lepers from taking possession of any inheritance that might come to them once they had been admitted to a *leprosarium*, and similarly barred any sons born *after* this date from succeeding to the leprous parent's property. The same prohibition applied to monks and priests, since, like lepers, they had entered religion, and were consequently divorced from the world by virtue of their vows. For this reason neither lepers nor religious could plead as individuals in a court of law. On the other hand, both enjoyed exemption from any legal obligations (such as the payment of compensation) that might be incurred after their profession, but not before.[82] Copies of these laws survive from the early thirteenth century onwards, by which time the compilation of similar reference works was well under way across the border.

The first attempt to produce a coherent guide to the laws and customs of England, *De legibus et consuetudinibus Angliae*, was credited to the royal justiciar, Ralph Glanville (d. 1190), founder of the *leprosarium* at West Somerton. A more detailed survey, bearing the same title, appeared in the 1220s or 1230s, its authorship being mistakenly attributed to the judge Henry de Bracton (d. 1268), who may have revised the original text.[83] This systematic exposition of the common law provides us with an authoritative account of the current legal position of English lepers, which was similar to that of their Welsh counterparts. Anyone who seemed so deformed and terrible of aspect that he or she had to be 'put out of the community of mankind' thereby forfeited his or her rights to plead, to inherit and to make contracts of any kind. As in Wales, a direct parallel may be drawn with 'the civil dead' who had entered religion.[84]

The law did, however, offer its full protection so far as the ownership of *existing* possessions was concerned, since these had been acquired or inherited before the disease became fully apparent. In such cases the leper continued to enjoy exactly the same rights as other subjects of the crown.[85] His or her property would either pass directly to the next of kin, be managed by designated

---

82  Cule, 'Diagnosis, Care and Treatment', pp. 38–41.
83  J.H. Baker, *An Introduction to English Legal History* (third edn, London, 1990), pp. 16, 201–2.
84  Thorne, *Bracton*, ii, pp. 51–2; iv, pp. 309–10. Pollock and Maitland, *History of English Law*, ii, p. 480, stress Bracton's comparison between the leper and the excommunicate (who has leprosy of the soul), although the latter's disease was infinitely worse. At some point before 1200, the corpse of a woman from Cheam, who had been excommunicated for adultery, was buried in the nearest leper cemetery because she could not be interred in her own parish: A. Heales, ed., *The Records of Merton Priory* (London, 1898), p. 57.
85  Thorne, *Bracton*, iv, p. 309.

trustees, or, in the case of tenants in chief, be let out to farm if the heir was under age.[86] As we shall see in the final section of this chapter, whatever the precise arrangements, care was taken to ensure the provision of appropriate support. We should also remember that, although the individual left secular society on entering a *leprosarium*, the legal status of all but the smallest hospitals was recognised by the courts. It was therefore possible for the residents to plead collectively, even against their patrons.

Legal 'death' was thus a relative concept, and, moreover, one liable to change over time. As late as 1170, for example, the sale and purchase of property by confirmed lepers did not apparently pose any difficulties, for it was then that one Martin *leprosus* disposed of his tenement in Goodramgate, York, to the archbishop.[87] By the early thirteenth century, though, leprosy, or at least an allegation to that effect, could certainly be advanced as a bar to pleading in the royal courts, as Cecilia de Tackely discovered when she tried to bring her brother's murderer to justice.[88] Assertions of this kind, which must often have been made by unscrupulous litigants, had, of course, to be proved. The recently widowed Agnes de Westwick was, for example, able to confound an attempt to deprive her of her dower by convincing the bench that her disease had neither prevented her from living with her late husband nor yet reached a stage at which it might be confidently diagnosed as leprous.[89] Not surprisingly, the actual date of confirmation, or more specifically of entry into hospital, could prove extremely contentious, as it marked the point at which an otherwise unimpeachable legal title might become invalid. Thus, a dispute over land in Suffolk, which reached the royal court at Westminster in the early 1220s, hinged upon whether or not a certain John de Whepstead had conveyed the property in question before or after being pronounced *extra communiam gentium*.[90]

The *Mirror of Justices*, a late thirteenth-century handbook for members of the judiciary, reiterated the ban on pleading. It also produced a list of people who were ineligible to serve on the bench, including women, serfs, idiots, attorneys, deaf mutes, lunatics, criminals, excommunicates and 'open lepers'.[91] By then, however, some of Bracton's pronouncements were already beginning to appear outdated. The common law was subject to constant development, not least with regard to the position of individuals who had little taste for the austerities of the monastic *leprosarium*. Men such as Adam de Gaugy, a tenant in chief 'smitten with leprosy', had presumably opted to remain in comparative seclusion at home rather than entering a hospital, for in 1279 he was allowed to inherit his

---

86  *Pipe Roll 1 John, Michaelmas 1199* (Pipe Roll Society, new series, x, 1933), pp. 16–17. The law also safeguarded the rights of spouses whose partners had entered *leprosaria*: R. Furley, *A History of the Weald of Kent* (2 vols, Ashford, 1871–74), ii, p. 64; and punished violent crimes against lepers. In 1240, for example, one William Franklin was imprisoned on suspicion of murdering the two children of 'a certain leper': *CCR, 1237–1242*, p. 216.

87  Lovatt, *EEA, 20, York 1154–1181*, no. 135.

88  *CRR, 1213–1215*, p. 199. See also, *CRR, 1201–1203*, p. 302.

89  *CRR, 1227–1230*, no. 247, cited in Thorne, *Bracton*, iv, p. 309.

90  *CRR, 1223–1224*, p. 204. See also, *CRR, 1233–1237*, no. 602.

91  Whittaker, *Mirror of Justices*, pp. 44–5, 47. See also F.M. Nichols, ed., *Britton* (2 vols, Oxford, 1865), i, pp. 223–4, 227, 322.

late brother's estates and pay homage in private to the king's steward.[92] Sir Edward Cooke's dictum that 'ideots, leapers, madmen, outlawes . . . or the like' might freely inherit, 'albeit it was otherwise holden in ancient time', had a longer history than he supposed.[93]

By 1302 the royal justices had no problem in dealing with a leprous plaintiff in a case involving an inheritance, their only requirement being that he should wait outside the court and appoint an attorney to plead on his behalf.[94] The right to bequeath and convey property seems also to have been recognised at about this time, even in hospitals committed to a strict rule. The revised statutes of St Julian's hospital (1344), assumed that each brother would not only enter the house with moveable possessions 'to ease his infirmity', but would be free to bequeath a third upon any person of his choice. To avoid any legal wrangles, the regulations even stipulated how and when his testament (along with triplicate sets of an accompanying inventory) was to be made, sealed and probated.[95] As noted above, by the fifteenth century the residents of modest suburban leper houses were drawing up wills. William Mannyng, a 'lazer' who died in the *leprosarium* by Monkbridge, York, in 1428, provided for his funeral and left the residue of a meagre estate to his wife. Notwithstanding his apparent poverty, he deemed it important to settle his affairs in the same way as other men.[96]

The full force of the common law was rarely employed to secure the removal of suspect lepers from society, although, as we saw in chapter one, a royal writ (known from sixteenth-century formularies by the title *de leproso amovendo*) might be issued in cases of individual intransigence. Since evidence of their use tends to survive only in contentious cases, such as that of Joanna Nightingale, it could be that many more directives were actually dispatched.[97] But, as it stands, the record is sparse, comprising about half a dozen. In 1420, for example, the court of King's Bench issued a reprimand to the sheriff of Lincolnshire because of his repeated failure to arrange for the examination of John Louth, a mercer from Boston. The text of the writ describes Louth as a leper, who

> commonly mingles with the men of the aforesaid town and communicates with them in public as well as private places and refuses to remove himself to a place of solitude, as is customary and as it behoves him to do, to the serious danger of the aforesaid men and their manifest peril on account of the contagious nature of the aforesaid disease (*propter contagionem morbi predicti*).[98]

---

92   *CFR 1272–1307*, p. 109.
93   Coke, *Institutes*, lib. I, sect. 1, 8A.
94   A.J. Horwood, ed., *Year Books of the Reign of King Edward the First, 30 and 31 Edward I* (RS, 1863), pp. 114–15. In 1204 it was ruled that one litigant who had sued out a writ of *mort d'ancestor* '*non debet summoneri quia leprosus est*': *Pipe Roll 6 John, Michaelmas 1204* (Pipe Roll Society, new series, xviii, 1940), p. 14. Coke considered it 'good law' for lepers to employ an attorney, because they had been separated from the community: *Institutes*, lib. II, sect. 11, 135b.
95   Richards, *Medieval Leper*, p. 132. The leprous sisters of St James's, Westminster, were censured in 1277 for bequeathing goods without the prior's authority: W. Page, *VCH London I* (London, 1909), p. 543.
96   J. Raine, ed., *Testamenta Eboracensia, I* (Surtees Society, iv, 1836), p. 414.
97   See above, pp. 186–7.
98   G. O. Sayles, ed., *Select Cases in the Court of King's Bench under Richard II, Henry IV and Henry V* (Selden Society, lxxxviii, 1971), pp. 247–8. Two similarly worded writs survive in a precedent book

The sheriff, who had allegedly passed the writ on to the bailiff of the honour of Richmond some time before, was ordered to execute it within the next two months, his dilatory approach contrasting sharply with the apparent anxiety of the authorities. A prompter reply came from the mayor and sheriffs of Lincoln, who returned a similar writ of May 1446 with admirable dispatch. In response to claims that John Hedon and his wife Alice were living publicly as lepers, they were able to report that the former had been pronounced free of disease, while the latter could not be found.[99] Were they in fact prepared to tolerate her continued presence? The case raises some interesting possibilities.

The writs themselves certainly demonstrate a growing fear of the risks of contagion (that is air-borne infection), which can likewise be detected in the changing vocabulary deployed by the rulers of English towns and cities. In response to a royal directive of 1331 concerning the number of lepers at large in Beverley, the bailiff listed five individuals who had been 'struck with leprosy by the grace of God and not otherwise', a turn of phrase which betrays no aware-ness of the possibility of infection, and little sense of urgency.[100] By the end of the century, however, the contaminated breath of lepers had become a matter of growing anxiety in England's major cities, and even the jurors of Yarmouth were complaining about the miasmas of disease. The scriptural proscriptions of Levit-icus were rapidly giving way to a more pressing and scientifically informed agenda of exclusion.

### The fear of miasma and contagion

Uneasiness about corrupt air and its potential for causing disease emerges from a wide variety of non-medical sources for at least two hundred years before the outbreak of the Black Death in 1349. Henry of Huntington's celebrated descrip-tion of Henry I's suppurating corpse, which reputedly caused the death of at least one of the men responsible for embalming it, proved a fitting obituary for this brutal monarch. But in observing how one of the surgeons wrapped wet linen around his head to protect himself from the stench, it also underscores contemporary beliefs about the dangers of inhaling foul smells.[101] Dead bodies were not the only perceived source of contamination, which also arose from sewage, stagnant water and, of course, the sick. It has been argued that the distancing of the infirmary from other monastic buildings in Cistercian houses, such as Fountains, reflects a desire to remove diseased and infectious monks from the rest of the community. The provision in 1262 of chalices for sole use by sick members of the order certainly suggests a degree of concern about physical as well as spiritual hygiene.[102] The Benedictine Abbess Euphemia (d. 1257)

---

kept by the clerk of the crown in Chancery. They relate to London and Hertfordshire but do not provide dates or names, beyond initials: PRO, C193/1, fos. 24v–25r.

99    PRO, KB145/6/24. I am grateful to Dr Hannes Kleineke for this reference.

100    *CIM, 1307–1349*, no. 1268.

101    D. Greenway, ed., *Henry, Archdeacon of Huntingdon: 'Historia Anglorum'* (Oxford, 1996), pp. 702–5. See also William of Newburgh's account of the plagues spread in 1196 by the foul air from unburied corpses: *Historia rerum Anglicarum*, ii, p. 481.

102    D.N. Bell, 'The Siting and Size of Cistercian Infirmaries in England and Wales', *Studies in Cistercian*

pursued a similar policy of sanitary reform at Wherwell in Hampshire. Among the many improvements effected during her thirty years in office were the disposal of 'noxious' matter from the precinct and the planting of gardens to sweeten the environment. She also constructed a new infirmary well away from the house, whence a subterranean watercourse removed 'all refuse that might corrupt the air'.[103]

In light of these general concerns about miasma, the 'stynking breath' and other malodorous symptoms of suspect and confirmed lepers inevitably provoked popular unease. Precisely when, and to what extent, this developed into a more concrete dread of infection (in the modern sense) is harder to establish. As we have already seen, medical assessments of *lepra* tended, on balance, to underplay the risks of short-term physical contact, whereas the ruling elite of later medieval England grew increasingly nervous on this score. Their motives were not, however, unmixed. Edward III's edict of 1346, ordering the removal of lepers from within the walls of London, constituted what was by English standards an unprecedented – and unique – warning of the hazards they presented. By infecting their victims 'as well in the way of mutual communications and by the contagion of their polluted breath, as by carnal intercourse with women in the stews and other secret places', the king asserted, some deliberately sought to contaminate the healthy. All victims of the disease were to leave for the country within fifteen days, while anyone who sheltered them was threatened with forfeiture. Since Edward was then attempting to clear 'certain malefactors and disturbers of the peace' from the streets of an unruly city before sailing on his next military expedition to France, it is tempting to regard this decree as pretext for the eviction of undesirables.[104] His recourse to such emotive language about the enemy within none the less marks a growing level of intolerance, which the Black Death and the national and regional epidemics that followed it at regular intervals for the next three hundred years further intensified.

The custom of burning the clothes of plague victims, and thus of destroying the miasmas of disease which allegedly clung to the fabric, was widely adopted during the fourteenth and fifteenth centuries.[105] It may already have been employed as a protective measure against *lepra*. Apparently dating from the reign of Alexander III (d. 1286), but probably somewhat later, regulations for the borough of Berwick-on-Tweed decreed that any leper who 'wilfully' forced his way through the gates was to be stripped of his upper garments, which were to be burnt, and sent away 'naked'. Although its primary purpose was to prevent vagrancy by obliging diseased paupers to gather in 'the proper place outside the town' where alms were regularly distributed by the authorities, this ruling

*Art and Architecture*, v (1998), pp. 211–38; M. Cassidy-Welch, *Monastic Spaces and their Meanings: Thirteenth-Century English Cistercian Monasticism* (Turnhout, 2001), pp. 142–3. The leprous Alice of Schaerbeck (d. 1250) was forbidden to take communion with others, '*propter periculum*': *Acta Sanctorum*, xx, June II (11 June), p. 474.
103  BL, MS Egerton 2104A, fos 43v–44r; J.C. Cox, ed., *VCH Hampshire II* (London, 1903), p. 133. For fears of miasma at the royal court, see *CLR, 1251–1260*, pp. 59, 507.
104  *CCR, 1346–1349*, pp. 54, 61–2; Riley, *Memorials*, pp. 365–6.
105  J. Henderson, 'The Black Death in Florence: Medical and Communal Responses', in Bassett, *Death in Towns*, pp. 136–50.

demonstrates an awareness of miasma theory and its specific application to leprosy. It appears, significantly, next to an order concerning the pollution of the river Tweed with dung and dirt.[106] Communities across the border grew increasingly vigilant after the onset of plague. In the late 1470s, for example, one Andrew Sauer was censored by the authorities at Prestwick for visiting the local *leprosarium*, 'daily and nigtly' with his wife and children. His practice of wearing 'the seik folkis clathis and bonnettis' seemed particularly reprehensible, since it threatened 'till infect the hale toune'.[107]

The steady proliferation of vernacular advice literature about the preservation of health made explicit the fact that 'from infected bodies comme . . . infectious and venomous fumes and vapours, the whiche do infecte and corrupte the aire'. The need to 'avoyde and eschewe all suche' assumed particular urgency during epidemics, but was generally regarded as a prudent measure.[108] As Thomas Forestier observed in his tract on the sweating sickness of 1485, it was always best 'not to be conversant myche with syke folkes or infecte'.[109] This had, paradoxically, long been the view of some medieval philanthropists, at least with regard to foundations for the indigent, which were traditionally selective about the type of patients they received. Pregnant women, lunatics, epileptics, the senile, victims of violence or serious injury, the terminally ill, and children were often singled out as undesirable. Moral and economic considerations carried particular weight, as did the likelihood of disruption to the daily round of services and prayers that patrons demanded. Lepers and sufferers from other 'intolerable' conditions (such as *fistulae*) might also be denied admittance, partly because they required intensive nursing, but also, one suspects, because they seemed so physically repugnant.[110] Staff or existing patients who contracted *lepra* would eventually be transferred to the nearest lazar house and assured of a stipend to provide whatever necessities they might require. Far greater trepidation on this score is, however, discernible after the pestilence of 1349, for, although some patrons continued to regard leprosy as just one of many potentially unacceptable conditions, others began to voice specific fears of infection.

Whereas the hospital of St Mary in the Newarke, Leicester, had, from its foundation in 1330, admitted patients with 'incurable diseases', apparently including lepers, new rules drafted in 1356 ordered their expulsion. Henry, duke

---

106  T. Smith, L.T. Smith and L. Brentano, eds, *English Gilds* (EETS, xl, 1870), p. 341; Thomson and Innes, *Acts of the Parliament of Scotland*, i, p. 92, cap. XVIII. There was a ritual element to this provision, since Mosaic Law decreed that 'leprous' cloth should be burnt [Leviticus 13, v. 52].

107  Simpson, 'Leprosy and Leper Hospitals', part 3, p. 419. At Chartres, the clothes of lepers were, from 1208 onwards, to be washed separately: Merlet and Jusselin, *Cartulaire de la léproserie du Grand-Beaulieu*, pp. 72–3, 154. At St Omer, in northern France, the inmates were told in 1463 not to remove any clothing, linen or sheets from the hospital, especially with the intention of pawning or selling them: Bourgeois, *Lépreux et maladreries*, p. 319. For Swedish examples, see Richards, *Medieval Leper*, pp. 56, 138.

108  M. Healy, 'Discourses of the Plague in Early Modern London', in J.A.I. Champion, ed., *Epidemic Diseases in London* (Centre for Metropolitan History, Working Paper Series 1, 1993), p. 21.

109  BL, MS Add. 27582, fo. 76v.

110  See, for example, Le Grand, *Statuts*, pp. 25 (Angers), 115, 119 (Troyes), 155 (Vernon); Rubin, *Charity and Community*, pp. 158, 300–01; H.E. Salter, ed., *A Cartulary of the Hospital of St John the Baptist* (3 vols, Oxford Historical Society, lxviii–lxix, 1914–16), iii, p. 3; Maxwell-Lyte and Dawes, *Register of Thomas Bekyngton*, i, p. 289.

of Lancaster, the founder's son, announced his intention to build a *leprosarium* 'at the end of the town', where they might be supported at his expense. The duke's well-documented interest in current medical theory may be further detected in his regulations concerning the ritual to be observed at the deathbed of hospital priests. Each of the canons was to exchange a kiss of peace with the dying man, unless there was a risk that sickness might spread from one to another in this way.[111] Because of anxiety about the 'helth and welfare' of Henry VI in plague time, the Commons in the parliament of 1439 likewise urged that the customary kiss of homage exchanged between him and his tenants in chief should be suspended. In order to avoid the transmission of 'an infirmite most infectif', they argued, 'the presence of suche so infect most be eschewed, as by noble fisisseanes and wise philosofors bifore this tyme pleynly it hath bene determined, and as experience dayly sheweth'.[112] Their arguments seemed no less applicable to leprosy, rendering even more heroic the behaviour of pious Christians such as Queen Matilda, and, no doubt, prompting a sharp decline in the practice of embracing victims of the disease.

A significant number of fifteenth-century almshouses, whose founders came from the ranks of the nobility, gentry and mercantile elite, instituted measures for the prompt removal of lepers and anyone else who posed a risk to health. Ordinances compiled in about 1424 for Richard Whittington's almshouse in London insisted that any such cases should be sent elsewhere at the hospital's expense 'lest they infect their fellows or provoke horror'.[113] Being, no doubt, familiar with these regulations, the duke and duchess of Suffolk incorporated them, almost verbatim, into their own lengthy statutes for God's House at Ewelme, Oxfordshire.[114] Indeed, such precautions, which combined long-established concerns about the leper's appearance with newer fears of miasma, now became a matter of routine. The almsmen who found refuge at Lady Margaret Hungerford's hospital in Heytesbury were, for instance, to live together 'on lesse than they be touched or infecte with a leeper or other infirmytees intollerabill, such as shulde infect or ennoy their felawship'.[115] Archbishop Henry Chichele went even further by insisting that all the almsmen at Higham Ferrers should be 'clenc . . . of theire bodies, without botches, biles [boils] or blanes [sores]', lest they prove 'noisome' to their companions.[116]

Were these measures always observed? The constant repetition of injunctions about contagious disease reflects the derivative nature of hospital statutes, which

---

[111] A.H. Thompson, *The History of the Hospital and New College of the Annunciation of St Mary in the Newarke, Leicester* (Leicester Archaeological Society, 1937), pp. 4, 17, 60.

[112] Strachey, *Rotuli Parliamentorum*, v, p. 31. The kiss was replete with moral as well as physical danger; an appropriate penance for 'erotic osculation' was kissing the hand of a leper: Brundage, *Law, Sex and Christian Society*, pp. 302–3.

[113] J. Imray, *The Charity of Richard Whittington* (London, 1968), p. 118. See also the 1447 rules for Ellis Davy's almshouse, Croydon, which was also supervised by the Mercers' Company: C. Harper-Bill, ed., *The Register of John Morton Archbishop of Canterbury 1486–1500*, I (Canterbury and York Society, 1987), no. 180.

[114] Goodall, *God's House at Ewelme*, pp. 249–50. Reiterated in the 1495 statutes of the almshouse of St John the Baptist, Lichfield: Bodleian Library, MS Ashmole 855, fo. 158v.

[115] Canon Jackson, 'Ancient Statutes of Heytesbury Almshouse', *Wiltshire Archaeological and Natural History Magazine*, xi (1869), pp. 289–308, at p. 301.

[116] BL, MS Lansdowne 846, fo. 78r.

often drew heavily upon existing models. Left to their own devices, some institutions may have been less particular about admissions than their benefactors wished. For the first sixty years of its history, St Giles's hospital, Norwich, excluded patients on grounds of gender alone. It was not until 1309 that one of its major patrons insisted that anyone suffering from 'an intolerable disease' should henceforth be refused admission, apparently because of the mounting pressure upon limited resources. Yet *ad hoc* care for such people clearly continued, despite this shift in policy. In 1440, for example, the master was presented in court for harbouring a leper named Geoffrey Skinner and ordered to remove him within the next few weeks under pain of a 20s. fine. Indeed, as late as 1596–97 the hospital provided nursing care for 'one supposed to be a leper' at a cost of 6d., although the patient had probably been assigned separate quarters.[117] Less than half a mile away to the north of Norwich, in 1374–75, one Richard Jobbe, leper, was said to be living in the precinct of St Paul's hospital, where he occupied a house. Perhaps the almswomen, some of whom also worked as nurses, had taken him under their wing in defiance of local opinion.[118]

The pressures of communal life are no less apparent in the monasteries of later medieval England, where a more stringent approach to segregation may also be linked to fear of pestilence. The miracles of Thomas Becket describe quite a few cases where monks, servants and young boarders had either been removed from or were about to be transferred out of religious houses because they seemed leprous. As was then the case in lay society, a decision ostensibly made in accordance with the precepts of Leviticus appears in practice to have been chiefly influenced by the readiness of individuals and communities to tolerate the presence of men and women whose symptoms became progressively more unpleasant. Initially obliged to live apart from the healthy young scholars at Abingdon abbey, one of Queen Eleanor's foundlings, who appeared '*elephantico morbo corrpetus*', was eventually expelled from the monastic complex altogether by Bishop Godfrey of St Asaph. This was because

> the tuberous face, weeping eyes, balding eyebrows, the spreading ulcers on the arms and thighs, which penetrated to the very bones, provoked nausea. His hoarse voice was barely audible to those standing near to him; his bandages had to be changed every day, or at least on alternate days, because of the flow of matter. All these things deterred others from living or conversing with him.[119]

Anxiety about infection seems to have played little, if any, part in the Bishop's decision, which (as was so often the case) hinged upon the distressing physical state of the young man. The presumed effects of nausea upon the beholder should not be underestimated, for such an assault upon the body's sensory mechanisms and vital spirits could inflict lasting damage. Yet the possibility of

---

117   Rawcliffe, *Medicine for the Soul*, p. 163; NRO, DCN 79/3 (Holme Street Leet, 18 Henry VI). Another leper was presented in 1443, but no specific place of residence was given: DCN 79/4 (Holme Street Leet, 21 Henry VI). Significantly, in 1440 (one year after a serious plague epidemic) there was also an offensive against prostitution.

118   Hudson, *Leet Jurisdiction*, p. 68.

119   Robertson, *Materials*, i, pp. 213–14.

transmission by breath, gaze or touch seems to have raised few concerns at this time. One of the first hints that English monastic communities harboured specific reservations on this score occurs a couple of decades later, when the novice mistress who had tended a leprous sister at Sempringham was shunned as a potential source of infection. 'Because she used to massage her with ointment', the scribe explained, 'she herself was avoided by the other nuns, who feared that they would contract the *maculae* [of leprosy] from her.' It is, however, note-worthy that, rather than living apart in a *leprosarium*, the patient had remained for years in the monastic infirmary, where she lay alongside other sick nuns.[120]

Had he been pronounced leprous, no such option would have been available in the 1450s to brother Richard Walsham of Norwich cathedral priory. As a senior monastic official, he might at best have hoped to remain, like Abbot Wallingford, in private quarters within the precinct. But attitudes had hardened in the aftermath of repeated epidemics, whose effects were all too apparent in shrinking communities with falling incomes.[121] Norwich was certainly not the only monastic house to monitor the health of its brethren, especially after the Black Death. A breviary from the Benedictine abbey of Muchelney in Somerset contains, alongside the conventional liturgical material, a copy of John of Bordeaux's popular tract on the pestilence, a dietary and a *regimen sanitatis*, geared to the demands of the religious life. This warns that the consumption of milk and wine together will increase the risk of leprosy, an admonition under-scored by the further addition of notes made in about 1500 on the diagnostic tests to be deployed on the blood and urine of suspects. Significantly, the author observes that medical authorities look first for signs in the face, the voice and the feet.[122] Fear that infection would cut a swathe through her cloister meanwhile led the abbess of Syon, in Middlesex, to petition Rome in 1487 for permission to remove a leprous monk without delay. Intensified, no doubt, by the recent outbreak of sweating sickness in southern England, her conviction that, once generated, the noxious effluvia of leprosy would create a potentially dangerous environment was by then commonplace. She was, indeed, empowered to segre-gate any other member of the house who might in future be afflicted 'either with leprosy or any other contagious disease'.[123]

Use of the word 'contagion' was, as we have seen, remarkably fluid during the medieval period, although a growing apprehensiveness about the dangers of physical contact clearly emerges from the documentary record. From a compar-atively early date, some of the larger, quasi-monastic *leprosaria* limited the freedom of lepers to enter rooms and offices where communal food was being stored or prepared.[124] Some also restricted their movements in church, desig-nating specific spaces for worship or even, as at Brives in 1259, providing service

120 Foreville and Keir, *Book of St Gilbert*, pp. 282–5.
121 Walsham's case is discussed above, pp. 185–6. For the impact of plague on the priory, see Rawcliffe, 'Threshold of Eternity', pp. 51–3.
122 B. Schofield, ed., *Muchelney Memoranda* (Somerset Record Society, xlii, 1927), pp. xxiii, 14–21, 53.
123 M.J. Haren, ed., *Calendar of Papal Registers: Papal Letters, XV* (Dublin, 1978), no. 76.
124 As, for example, at St Mary Magdalen, Gaywood: Owen, *Making of King's Lynn*, pp. 106–7; and the Grand-Beaulieu, Chartres: Merlet and Jusselin, *Cartulaire de la léproserie du Grand-Beaulieu*, nos 180, 359.

books for the sole use of leprous clergy, who were not supposed to handle any others.[125] Such rulings initially reflect a combination of fastidiousness and unease about ritual pollution rather than fear of contagion (in the modern sense). It was as a penance for the revulsion he felt towards his 'Christian brothers' that St Francis forced himself to share the same dish as a leper whose weeping sores bled into the food.[126] Evidently unaware of, or indifferent to, recent medical theories about the transmission of disease, his companions responded with squeamishness rather than alarm at such apparently reckless behaviour. Late as they are, Abbot Mentmore's rules of 1344 for St Julian's hospital express similar sentiments. He not only forbade the lepers from entering the mill or brewery without authority, but also prohibited physical contact with the bread or beer 'since it is not fitting (*cum non deceat*) for men with this disease to handle what is destined for the common use'.[127]

Questions of morality as well as defilement may have prompted further regulations of this kind, since the two were inextricably joined in the minds of those who believed that leprosy increased the libido. At the hospital of St Mary Magdalen, Reading, for example, orders banning the leprous brethren from the laundry (which appear in conjunction with regulations about sexual continence) were clearly intended to deliver them from temptation, manifest in the buxom form of the washerwoman.[128] The laundress herself came under scrutiny at St Julian's, where she had to be a woman of 'mature age and good conversation, about whom there may be no untoward suspicion'. Here, too, freedom of association was primarily linked to the snares of sexual promiscuity.[129] Yet other fourteenth-century clergy, such Bishop Stapledon, were more concerned about the health hazards arising from human contact, however legitimate. We may note that, by 1371, it was proving so difficult to get a suitable priest for St Nicholas's hospital at Harbledown, that the archbishop of Canterbury had to provide lodgings opposite the gates, where the incumbent could live at a safe distance from his congregation.[130]

A rising tide of public disquiet about the presence of suspect or confirmed lepers in urban markets confirms that here, too, moral and aesthetic concerns were giving way to other anxieties.[131] In 1366, for example, John Knight and his wife, both of whom were reputedly leprous, faced expulsion from Colchester. This, the borough court declared, was because of the danger they presented by

125  Le Grand, *Statuts*, p. 212.
126  Brooke, *Scripta Leonis, Rufini et Angeli*, pp. 125–7.
127  Walsingham, *Gesta*, ii, p. 506.
128  BL, MS Cotton Vespasian E V, fo. 39r; and above, pp. 122–3. Laundresses and others who washed away society's filth generally got a bad press: J. Le Goff, *Un autre moyen âge* (Paris, 1999), p. 91. See also Merlet and Jusselin, *Cartulaire de la léproserie du Grand-Beaulieu*, no. 359.
129  Walsingham, *Gesta*, ii, p. 507. Rules of 1372 from St Bartholomew's hospital, Dover, urged the leprous inmates to avoid unnecessary contact with the healthy, although, since the warden was himself a leper with an active administrative role, these strictures cannot have been systematically applied: Bodleian Library, MS Rawl. B.335, fos 2r, 4r.
130  Duncombe and Battely, *Three Archiepiscopal Hospitals*, pp. 209–10.
131  At Castres (Tarn) in 1346 lepers from the local hospital were forbidden from entering the town without a distinguishing white cloth and rattle, and were ordered not to handle food in the market. But they systematically ignored this rule: U. Robert, *Les signes d'infamie au moyen âge* (Paris, 1891), pp. 149–52.

roaming about the market, 'selling and buying victuals, and especially geese and capons'. Stray poultry was often killed in plague time because the miasmas of disease clung tenaciously to its feathers, although in this instance the principal risk seemed to lie elsewhere. John and Alice's habit of embracing and kissing children was the real bone of contention, since 'many people' feared that, like plague, the disease would spread more quickly among the young.[132] But victuallers inevitably came under scrutiny. John Mayn, the Londoner 'smitten with the blemish of leprosy', who incurred the displeasure of the corporation in 1372 was, significantly, a baker. The command that he should cease 'communicating with other sound persons by reason of the infection of that disease' must have assumed particular urgency because of his trade.[133] This was certainly true of the wife of an Exeter merchant named Richard Trymell, who was bound over in heavy securities of £100 in 1428 to ensure that she left the city within five weeks. He was, meanwhile, to keep her 'secrete et honeste' at home, and prevent her from either brewing or selling ale.[134] As the case of Katherine Colkirke reveals, the mere sight of lepers or their carers touching food on open display was too much for some authorities. The Norwich assembly ruled in 1473 that anyone buying provisions for the city leper houses might only point at wares in the market with a stick, and that stallholders who permitted otherwise would be fined.[135]

In April 1472, Edward IV had written sharply to the rulers of London about their apparent indifference to a recurrent threat of leprosy. Although 'many devout and weldisposid persones' had founded hospitals for men and women 'enfecte with the contagious and perilous siknes of lepour', the latter were apparently

> vagrant and walkyng contrarye to the will and entent of the edifiers and bilders of the same, aswel abought in this citee and suburbies of the same comenyng and medlyng daily with other people which ben of clene compleccon and not enfecte with the said sykynes, which, if it shuld be suffered shuld cause grete hurt, jerobardy and perell . . . For it is certaynly undirstond that the said siknes daily growith and encresith by suche medlyng and comynycacion, more than it hath doon in daies passed.[136]

Galvanised into action by the threat of a £500 fine, the citizens deemed it expedient to remind the gatekeepers of an old 'usage', whereby any 'persone enfecte' entering the gates of London was – like the lepers of Berwick – to be deprived of

---

132  I.H. Jeayes, ed., *Court Rolls of the Borough of Colchester* (3 vols, Colchester, 1938–41), ii, p. 185. For birds and miasma, see M. Jenner, 'The Great Dog Massacre', in W.G. Naphy and P. Roberts, eds, *Fear in Early Modern Society* (Manchester, 1997), pp. 44–61; and for the risk to children, Cohn, *Black Death Transformed*, p. 215.

133  See above, pp. 22–3.

134  Devon RO, Exeter Mayor's Court Roll, 6–7 Henry VI, rot. 34v. I am grateful to Dr Hannes Kleineke for this reference.

135  NRO, NCR, 16D, Assembly Proceedings 1434–1491, fo. 95v. This rule contrasts sharply with late thirteenth-century practice at Peterborough, where the servant in the monastic *leprosarium* was permitted to eat in the refectory on certain feast days: BL, MS Cotton Vespasian E XXII, fo. 4r.

136  CLRO, Journal 8, fo. 21r. The Latin text is on fo. 19v.

his upper garment and, if he were mounted, his horse.[137] Edward's anxiety may have been prompted by a suspect case of leprosy then under investigation at the royal court, although the previous autumn had been marked by a serious outbreak of pestilence, which clearly intensified fears about miasma.[138] When the citizens copied his mandate into their Journal, they placed it next to a statute, first passed by the parliament of 1388, for the removal of butchers' waste and dung lest it give rise to 'many sykenes and othere intolurable diseasez'. The juxta-position of these items is as striking as the sporadic nature of their enforcement, which tended to follow major epidemics and other crises in the body politic.[139]

We can observe this cyclical phenomenon at work in Yarmouth, where an almost unbroken run of leet records from 1366 onwards provides a remarkable insight into the measures for public health adopted by this once flourishing port. Between 1369 and 1501, at least 113 presentments were made against seventy suspect lepers, who defied the custom of the borough by living within the walls. The roll for 1440–41 eschews a firm diagnosis, referring simply to infirmities so grave that three other individuals could not remain among their neighbours. Such a sustained level of vigilance is understandable in light of previous experi-ence. Claims that over 7,000 residents died in the first outbreak of plague alone were clearly exaggerated, although losses in both 1349–50 and 1361 had a devas-tating impact upon an already depressed local economy.[140] It is easy to see why the earliest recorded attempts to remove lepers from the town coincided with what *The Anonimalle Chronicle* called England's 'third pestilence', in 1369–70.[141] A plague in Cambridge, in 1389, may have triggered off anxiety throughout Norfolk, for the burgesses of King's Lynn as well as Yarmouth were then back on the lookout.[142] Few years of the fifteenth century passed without some health scare, but it seems that the number of presentments generally rose during or immediately after epidemics: in 1400 at the time of another national outbreak;[143] in 1405–07, when the pestilence raged in London;[144] and again during a severe regional epidemic of 1420–21.[145] Renewed surveillance is likewise evident in

---

137  Sharpe, *Calendar of Letter-Book L*, pp. 102–3. Exactly a century earlier, following the case of John Mayn, the corporation had introduced measures for keeping the streets and river clear of dung and removing lepers from the city: R.R. Sharpe, ed., *Calendar of the Letter-Books of the City of London, Letter-Book G* (London, 1905), p. 301.

138  See above, p. 187. For the devastation caused by the 1471 plague, see N. Davis, ed., *Paston Letters and Papers of the Fifteenth Century* (2 vols, Oxford, 1971–76), i, pp. 440–41.

139  CLRO, Journal 8, fos 21v–22r; E.L. Sabine, 'City Cleaning in Medieval London', *Speculum*, xii (1937), pp. 19–43. In the 1531 *Registrum omnium breuium*, fo. 267r–267v, the writ *de leproso amovendo* appears next to that *de vicis et venellis mundandis*.

140  P. Rutledge, 'A Fifteenth-Century Yarmouth Petition', *Great Yarmouth District Archaeological Society Bulletin*, xlvi (1976), unpaginated. The poll tax returns of 1377 list 1,941 adults, which suggests a total population of just above 3,000: J.C. Russell, *British Medieval Population* (Albuquerque, 1948), p. 142.

141  NRO, Y/C4/83, rots 15v–16r (three presentments); V.H. Galbraith, ed. *The Anonimalle Chronicle, 1333 to 1381* (Manchester, 1927), p. 58.

142  J.M.W. Bean, 'Plague, Population and Economic Decline in England in the Later Middle Ages', *Economic History Review*, series two, xv (1963), pp. 423–37, at p. 428; Owen, *Making of King's Lynn*, p. 213; NRO, Y/C4/101, rot. 11r (two presentments for leprosy, one for receiving lepers).

143  NRO, Y/C4/110 (two presentments); Bean, 'Plague, Population and Economic Decline', pp. 428–9.

144  NRO, Y/C4/116, rot. 16r–16v; 117, rot. 9r (three presentments); *CCR, 1405–1409*, p. 297.

145  NRO, Y/C4/130, rot. 5r–5v (three presentments); Bean, 'Plague, Population and Economic Decline', pp. 428–9.

1425–26 and 1433–34, when disease threatened to spread from London;[146] in 1440, following the 'most infectif' outbreak of plague described above;[147] in 1446–47, when 'a great pestilence' struck Lincoln;[148] and in 1448–49 during visitations at Oxford and Westminster.[149]

By this date the borough authorities were well aware that *lepra* might also be engendered by 'corrupt mete, and of mete that is sone corrupt, as of mesel swynes fleische that hath pesen [eggs or lumps] therinne and is infecte with suche pesen and greynes'.[150] Like the rulers of other English towns, they moved fast to confiscate flyblown meat from 'pokky pigges'. Offenders who sold contaminated wares 'infected with leprosy . . . to the grave peril of the people' were threatened with exemplary fines of up to 20*s.*, which ranked on a par with the securities then demanded from suspect lepers.[151] As a port, Yarmouth was especially vulnerable to sea-borne infection, and its rulers may have reacted more forcefully to these threats than many inland towns. Yet it would be misleading to suggest that their preoccupation with public health was inspired simply by a dread of disease. The fact that roughly equal numbers of men and women were presented for *lepra* gives pause for thought in view of the widespread conviction that women's cooler humoral makeup offered them significant protection. Recent research in communities where the incidence of Hansen's disease is comparatively low and generally confined to adults suggests that over 80 per cent of sufferers are male.[152] We cannot, of course, now tell how many of the Yarmouth suspects had actually contracted Hansen's disease, and would be ill-advised to speculate too closely on this point, although the disparities are worth noting. The preponderance of female suspects before 1416, when no fewer than sixteen out of twenty-two presentments (almost 80 per cent) concerned women, seems especially striking. Does it reflect well-attested changes in the composition of the labour market after the Black Death?[153] As women became more visible in the workforce and began undercutting male rates of pay, resentment against them may have increased.

Irrespective of gender, the status of our seventy-three suspects also invites comment. With the exception of one member of the atte Gappe family, presented in 1369–70, *all* belonged to the lower strata of society.[154] A few practised recognised trades as websters, daubers, shipwrights, coopers, tailors,

---

146 NRO, Y/C4/135, rots 10r–11r (three presentments); 142, rots 14v, 15v (three presentments); Bean, 'Plague, Population and Economic Decline', pp. 428–9.

147 NRO, Y/C4/148, rot. 19r (three presentments); Strachey, *Rotuli Parliamentorum*, v, p. 31.

148 NRO, Y/C4/153, rot. 16r (two presentments); *HMC, Fourteenth Report, Appendix VIII* (London, 1895), pp. 10–11.

149 NRO, Y/C4/155, rots 14r–15r (four presentments); Bean, 'Plague, Population and Economic Decline', pp. 428–9.

150 Seymour, *On the Properties of Things*, i, p. 426; above, pp. 79–80.

151 NRO, Y/C4/186, rot. 15r.

152 Jacquart and Thomasset, *Sexuality and Medicine*, pp. 188–93; Ell, 'Diet and Leprosy', p. 117.

153 P.J.P. Goldberg, *Women, Work, and Life Cycle: Women in York and Yorkshire c. 1300–1520* (Oxford, 1992), pp. 336–7.

154 This was Joanna, wife of Robert atte Gappe. In 1379, about seven years after her departure from Yarmouth, another member of this mercantile family left 6*s.* 8*d.* to the nearby leper house at Gorleston, to which she may have retired: NRO, Y/C4/83, rots 15v, 16r; 84, rot. 2r–2v; A. Suckling, *The History and Antiquities of the County of Suffolk* (2 vols, London, 1846–48), i, p. 37.

butchers and, significantly, cooks. The great majority, however, followed no designated occupation. At least three were living as the tenants of another suspect, while two, and perhaps more, were Dutch, and thus quite literally alien members of the community. Some harboured criminal tendencies, although none could rival Alice Dymock's spectacular catalogue of misdemeanours.[155] Many English boroughs complained vociferously about poverty at this time, but claims of 1399 and 1407 that this once prosperous 'forte ville de guerre' was declining fast carry a ring of truth.[156] Were local juries more likely to pass judgement upon unsettled men and women who threatened to consume the town's slender resources?

## The wild and the tame

That lepers fell into two categories, the 'wild' and the 'tame', was a common perception among ecclesiastical and urban authorities, who were thus able to reconcile otherwise contradictory ideas about the disease. References to these leprosi extranei, lepreux forains, lepreux sauvages, veldzieken, akkerzieken and the like across Europe suggest that they presented a common problem, their numbers impossible to judge, but easy to exaggerate.[157] Some were truly peripatetic, wandering from one place to the next for as long as they were able, while others fetched up in ramshackle settlements on the outskirts of towns and cities. The Church's response to the more intractable among them, who stubbornly refused to modify their behaviour or accept the rule of religion, reflects a sense of moral panic any nineteenth-century eugenicist would have recognised and no doubt endorsed. The assumption that, left unchecked, the worst of these extranei were sexually voracious, and would contaminate the rest of society, served to focus an inchoate dread of the unruly and ungovernable poor. Concurrent with a desire to improve their material circumstances and provide at least rudimentary spiritual comforts, reformers expressed the need to impose order upon these marginal and potentially subversive characters. At the turn of the twelfth century, one senior Parisian cleric was urged to visit their communities as often as possible, not only to preach the word of God, but also to deal with 'vagrant, drunken and debauched lepers, who go about from place to place, from market to market, and gather together at night in [their] shanties, or even in other leprosaria, corrupting others by their bad example'.[158] The greatest immediate threat, however, lay in their association with common prostitutes, through whom, it was argued, contagion would rapidly spread throughout society. True to form, Langland's Lady Meed, who is 'as commune as the carte-wey to knaues and to alle', distributes her favours liberally among 'meseles in heggys'.[159]

---

155 The wife of Reginald Frenssh was first presented as a leper in 1422–23, and one year later for violent assault. In 1425–26 she was involved in another brawl and was also accused of theft: NRO, Y/C4/132, rot. 10r; 133, rot. 9r; 135, rot. 10r.

156 Strachey, Rotuli Parliamentorum, iii, pp. 254, 438, 620.

157 Uyttebrouk, 'Sequestration', p. 629; Borradori, Mourir au monde, pp. 79–80.

158 Avril, 'Le IIIe Concile du Latran', p. 70; Brundage, Law, Sex and Christian Society, p. 493. A general fear of vagabondage was expressed at this time: Le Goff, Autre moyen âge, p. 95.

159 W.W. Skeat, ed., Langland's Vision of Piers the Plowman Text C (EETS, liv, 1873), p. 51.

Men such as the two lepers 'of evil reputation' who were accused of rape in the royal court at Westminster in 1220 seemed to justify these dark suspicions. So too did the case of Adam Matte, *leprosus*, whose visit to what was obviously a brothel outside Temple Bar, London, ended tragically in the 1380s. Having declined his remarkably generous offer of 10s. for sex, the owner allegedly connived at the violent rape of 'a very beautiful maidservant', who became hysterical, lost her reason and later died.[160] Townsmen and women who offered hospitality to vagrant lepers were often tarred with the same brush as the landlords of disorderly taverns and houses of ill repute. In 1287, for example, the fair court at St Ives, Huntingdonshire, accused two such offenders of placing their neighbours and visiting traders at serious risk (*ad maximum periculum*). Since they were presented along with three brothel keepers, it looks as if this threat was deemed to be spiritual as well as physical.[161] The connection was made explicit in instructions for the holding of ward moots promulgated in London during the reign of Edward II, which ordered officers to inquire (among other nuisances) if 'any woman of lewd life . . . or common bawd, or courtesan . . . or any leper' was roaming the streets.[162] The customs of Bristol, confirmed by royal charter in 1331, bracketed such people together as persons who should not dwell within the walls, and the burgesses of Yarmouth clearly made a similar equation.[163]

In 1462–63, for example, William Powtwyn, William Cook and Robert Stacy, *leprosi*, and a pair of 'ill-governed' women were each told to depart the port under pain of a 20s. fine, the lepers within three weeks, the others within seven.[164] Alice Dymock was but one of many notorious females who trailed a moral as well as a physical miasma in their wake. The aptly named Magna Haughe stood charged in 1384 as a common receiver of lepers within the town. Her further offence of failing to wear a striped hood, which urban authorities throughout Britain used as a means of identifying prostitutes, must have seemed particularly heinous because of the threat she posed to unsuspecting males.[165] Indignation that a servant employed by the extra mural *leprosarium* had attempted, in 1399–1400, to blackmail married women into granting him their sexual favours was likewise compounded by the fear that he might himself be contagious. Similar concerns prompted the indictment in 1486–87 of John Cook the younger on a charge of illicitly keeping and frequenting the wife of a leper,

---

160  *CRR, 1220*, p. 199; Sayles, *Select Cases in the Court of King's Bench under Richard II*, pp. 45–6.
161  C. Gross, ed., *Select Cases Concerning the Law Merchant, I* (Selden Society, xxiii, 1908), p. 14. Two procuresses interrogated in King's Lynn in 1312 were said to be plying their trade 'ad damnum et periculum totius communitatis': Isaacson and Ingleby, *Red Register*, i, p. 64.
162  H.T. Riley, ed., *The Liber Albus: The White Book of the City of London* (London, 1861), pp. 290–92. The compiler of the *Liber* (1419) ended his work with an index whose layout is suggestive. 'Of Jews and lepers and of driving swine out of the city; and ordinances as to sturdy beggars' is followed by a section devoted to 'courtesans and other persons taken in adultery': pp. 508–10.
163  F.B. Bickley, ed., *The Little Red Book of Bristol* (2 vols, Bristol and London, 1900), i, pp. 33–4, no. 11. In 1213 the papal legate, Robert de Courson, had ruled that prostitutes, like lepers, should live 'outside the camp': Mansi, *Sacrorum conciliorum*, xxii, cols 835–6, 854.
164  NRO, Y/C4/167, rot. 21r–21v. Two of the leets threatened Powtwyn with a 100s. fine, which suggests that he was either very sick or very unpopular.
165  NRO, Y/C4/96, rot. 10r. For the wearing of hoods by Yarmouth prostitutes, see Y/C4/105, rot. 6v; and generally, Karras, *Common Women*, pp. 15, 18–22.

'by which infection may happen'.[166] Erasmus's warning that the good Christian should 'eschewe as a certayne pestylence the communycacion of corrupte and wanton persons' was all too familiar to generations of Englishmen and women who had smarted under the divine lash of plague.[167] The creeping contagion of sins committed by Alice and her kind seemed just as lethal as their contaminated bodies.[168]

Yet, powerful as it may have been, fear of physical and moral contagion was not the only – or indeed necessarily the overriding – motive behind attempts to impose social controls upon the vagrant leper. In 1860, on a visit to Madras, one British physician reported that

> The leper in this part of India, so long as he can work, or has money, is no outcast from the society of his fellow creatures, who live in the same house, partake of the same food, or even intermarry with him; but when the time arrives that he is unable to work, he becomes uncared for by all.[169]

Despite its apparently segregationist credentials, a bill of 1889 'to make provision for the isolation of lepers' in British India was, in fact, aimed solely at the indigent, whose aggressive begging posed more of a challenge to the authorities than the disease itself. The problem was hardly new. In medieval Europe the search for a hospital place often followed the same depressing sequence of events.[170] Once an individual grew too sick to work and became an extra mouth to feed, the chances of eviction increased exponentially, but until then families and neighbours were often far more tolerant than the authorities might have wished. This was certainly the case at Lakenheath in Suffolk, where, in the lean years between 1310 and 1336, at least nine individuals were presented as lepers and ordered to depart from the manor as custom decreed. Six were living with their parents and one with her husband. Did they seem an economic liability rather than a threat to health? Tellingly, a further six villagers stood charged with harbouring suspects to whom they were not related, and who may have perpetrated the double offence of being both outsiders and mendicants.[171] A similar pattern emerges at Ramsey, in Huntingdonshire, the home of William Bassesson, who doggedly remained in the bosom of his family for over a decade

166  NRO, Y/C4/110, rot. 5r; 191, rot. 15v.
167  Erasmus of Rotterdam, *Enchiridion militis Christiani*, ed. A.M. O'Donnell (EETS, cclxxxii, 1981), p. 191; Horrox, *Black Death*, chapter three. In some parts of Europe prostitutes as well as lepers were forbidden to touch food on sale in public places: Jacquart and Thomasset, *Sexuality and Medicine*, p. 231, n. 64; Jansen, *Making of the Magdalen*, p. 176 n. 34.
168  While he was still protector, in May 1483, Richard III issued an ordinance 'to eschew the stynkynge and horrible sin of lechery' by expelling prostitutes from London: J. Hughes, *The Religious Life of Richard III* (Stroud, 1997), p. 97. See also, P.J.P. Goldberg, 'Pigs and Prostitutes: Streetwalking in Comparative Perspective', in K.J. Lewis et al., eds, *Young Medieval Women* (Stroud, 1999), pp. 172–93.
169  Buckingham, *Leprosy in Colonial South India*, p. 35. For more recent parallels, see L. Navon, 'Beggars, Metaphors and Stigma', *SHM*, xi (1998), pp. 89–105.
170  Jeanne, 'Saint-Lazare de Falaise', p. 45.
171  Cambridge University Library, EDC 7–15–II–1–2; II–1–6, mm. 1, 12, 18, 33, 45; II–1–8, m. 19; II–1–9, mm. 26, 29, 30, 37, 42; PRO, SC2/203/95, m. 4. I am grateful to Professor Christopher Dyer for allowing me to consult his computerised indices to these records in Birmingham University Library.

in open defiance of the court.[172] But not all suspect lepers could rely upon such loyal support. For the disreputable, feckless or friendless, vagrancy was the sole alternative.

What might these itinerants expect? As we have already seen, during the twelfth and thirteenth centuries the sick mingled freely at shrines and travelled widely on pilgrimages. The more reputable among them were even received by pious householders, bent on performing the Seven Comfortable Works.[173] Some hospitals initially held a type of 'open day', usually on an appropriate festival, when wandering lepers could claim doles of food and clothing. Through the generosity of Queen Matilda, bread, ale, cod, salmon, cheese and butter were distributed among such visitors to St Nicholas's, York, each year on 29 June (the feast of Saints Peter and Paul), while the *leprosarium* of St Mary Magdalen at Gaywood offered food and overnight accommodation to them every Maundy Thursday.[174] Official sanction was, indeed, often bestowed upon their presence in busy thoroughfares and public buildings, especially in the years before unease about infection took hold of the popular imagination. Lepers then mixed among the thousands of paupers who flocked to the royal court for alms, sometimes even penetrating as far as the queen's private chambers.[175] They played a formal part in funerals, appearing as earthly representatives of Christ among the poor mourners, with whom they shared food, clothing and money. Having served as almoner to the pious Henry III, Walter Suffield, bishop of Norwich (d. 1257), left £5 to be distributed among the lepers in his diocese, whether they lived alone or in communities, and a further 2*d*. to each one present at his funeral.[176] The sound of their bells, rung loudly to solicit alms, certainly resounded through the public thoroughfares of East Anglia, for at about this time a synodial statute specifically forbade the practice. So much noise diverted respectful attention from priests carrying the Eucharist to the dying. As F.O. Touati has observed, bells and rattles were primarily designed to attract donations rather than frighten people away, especially if the leper had lost his or her voice and could not shout like other beggars.[177]

Secular authorities faced more immediate problems than bell ringing as population pressure reached crisis point and the crowd of mendicants flooding into towns increased. In an attempt to stem the tide, regulations set down by the rulers of London at the turn of the thirteenth century decreed that 'no leper shall

172 Bassesson, whose name suggests illegitimacy, was the most persistent offender, but six others were presented between 1308 and 1339: BL, Add. Rolls 34363Ar, 34364r, 34365r, 34770v, 39602r, 39603r; PRO, SC2/179/14, m. 2r; 179/22, m. 4r. See also, E.B. de Windt, ed., *The Court Rolls of Ramsey, Hepmangrove and Bury 1268–1600* (Subsidia Mediaevalia, xvii, 1990), pp. 19–56.

173 Raine, *Vita et miraculis S. Godrici*, p. 431.

174 *CCR, 1272–1279*, p. 280; Owen, *Making of King's Lynn*, p. 108. The *leprosarium* at Ripon initially offered overnight accommodation to transient lepers, but ceased to do so long before 1345 because of poverty: Raine, *Memorials of the Church of SS Peter and Wilfrid*, i, pp. 211–12, 224–32, 236–8.

175 See above, pp. 41, 146–7.

176 NRO, NCR, 24B/1. Bishop Giffard of Worcester (d. 1302) followed his example: J.W. Bund, ed., *The Register of William de Geynesburgh, Bishop of Worcester* (Oxford, 1907), p. 49.

177 F.M. Powicke and C.R. Cheney, eds, *Councils and Synods, II, 1205–1313, Part I, 1204–1265* (Oxford, 1964), p. 361; Touati, *Maladie et société*, pp. 417–20. An inventory of the goods of the hospital of St Mary Magdalen, Sprowston, recorded the ownership of a 'kynkebelle', or clapper for begging: Rawcliffe, *Hospitals of Medieval Norwich*, p. 46.

be going about in the city, or shall make any sojourn in the city . . . but [they] shall have a common attorney for themselves, to go each Sunday into the parish churches to collect alms for their sustenance'.[178] The appointment of proctors or agents to raise money on their behalf was a tactic already deployed by hospitals such as 'the Maudlyn' at Exeter, which, from the time of Bishop Bartholomew (d. 1184), if not before, had profited from collections made twice a week among the citizens by such an official.[179] Preaching offered a particularly effective means of attracting donations, although the Church expressed concern when laymen mounted the pulpit 'under the pretext of explaining the needs of lepers'. There were, moreover, ample opportunities for fraud.[180] Even so, the financial benefits likely to accrue from a properly co-ordinated and systematic approach to fund-raising explain why so many hospitals and *leprosaria* employed agents, especially during the troubled early years of the fourteenth century when numerous licences were issued by the crown, the episcopate and municipal authorities for this purpose.[181]

Having first approved the appointment of a collector for the hospital of St Mary Magdalen at this time, the bailiffs of Eye, in Suffolk, continued the practice for another two centuries. In 1528, for example, William Bennet was empowered by them to solicit 'pious and charitable alms from Christian people all around', to advertise and sell indulgences and to display the house's relics 'for the good and utility of the hospital and the said lepers living there'.[182] How many of the inmates were then leprous rather than pox-ridden is a moot point, although the authorities still chose to describe St Mary's as a *leprosarium*. The same was true of St Leonard's, Norwich, whose new proctor was chosen in 1539 by the Dean and Chapter for 'the sustentacon, releeff and comfourte of the prysoners of almyghty god, vexed with suche sykenes and diseases that they of necessitee ar constreyned and compelled to eschewe and avoyde oute and from the company of all peopyll'. Since several of them appeared 'grevously towched, smytten and vexed wyth the horybyll and hatefull dysease and sykenes of leprye', the Dean authorised William Hampton to beg on their account.[183] Not all such 'foregoers' or 'questors' were imposed from outside. The residents of some *leprosaria* chose and supervised their own agents, whose remit might well extend across the whole of England. In 1346, the leprous brothers and sisters of St Bartholomew's, Dover, authorised John de Chellesfelde to travel round the country offering an indulgence of 240 days to anyone who gave alms on their behalf; and as late as

---

178  Riley, *Liber Albus*, p. 238; R.R. Sharpe, ed., *Calendar of Letter-Books of the City of London, Letter-Book A* (London, 1899), p. 219.

179  F. Barlow, ed., *EEA, XI, Exeter 1046–1184* (Oxford, 1996), no. 98.

180  Powicke and Cheney, *Councils and Synods, II, 1205–1313, Part I, 1204–1265*, p. 386; G.R. Owst, *Preaching in Medieval England* (Cambridge, 1926), pp. 103–4.

181  Rawcliffe, *Medicine for the Soul*, pp. 65–6.

182  V. Brown, ed., *Eye Priory Cartulary and Charters, II* (Suffolk Records Society, Charters Series, xiii, 1994), no. 422, p. 134. For the activities and abuses of proctors acting for hospitals, see Owst, *Preaching*, pp. 100–02.

183  NRO, DCN 39/1. See also MSC 1/5, for a similar licence of 1529 for the nearby hospital of St Mary Magdalen and St Clement.

1539 'the house of lepers' at Bury St Edmunds appointed one Edward Hurste as a special nuncio nationwide.[184]

The award of such permits did not, however, preclude wayside begging by the residents of *leprosaria*, whose personal contribution remained vital to the survival of smaller houses. Any potential nuisance could be avoided through careful regulation. Some hospital statutes attempted to confine begging to the immediate vicinity of the precinct, while others established a rota system, to keep numbers in check.[185] As we have already seen, the assumption of a special robe, or habit, conferred both protection and respectability. The real problem, though, lay elsewhere, beyond institutional control, and prompted a more authoritarian response. This attempt at policing should be set against the social and demographic upheavals of the later Middle Ages. Whereas the run of early fourteenth-century famines and epidemics had caused hunger and homelessness on a massive scale, successive outbreaks of plague created what, from the government's perspective, was an army of overpaid and underemployed scroungers. And it was fear of a rebellious underclass tainted by the sins of sloth and envy that spawned what Michel Mollat has termed 'a generation frightened by pauperism'.[186]

This siege mentality found its most trenchant expression in mounting hostility towards outsiders, however apparently deserving. In 1367, for example, the rulers of London imposed a blanket ban upon mendicants, vagrants, pilgrims and lepers, without much apparent distinction.[187] Four years later, in the aftermath of war and pestilence, Charles V of France expressed grave concern over the 'quantity and number of leprous men and women infected by the malady of St Lazarus' who were pouring into Paris. Since healthy citizens could not go about their business without being waylaid for alms, he ruled that all lepers who had not been born in the city or did not live there should be immediately expelled. His decree refers to the perceived risks of infection (notably through mephistic air), but was primarily intended to address the problem of mendicancy. A subsequent ruling by the provost of Paris attempted vainly to limit entry into the city to those lepers who had written authority, and to prevent any of them from begging within the walls.[188] In this context it is interesting to return to the wording of measures instituted by the Scottish parliament of 1427 for the diagnosis and control of 'lippir folk'. The nineteenth-century isolationists who regarded them as a model of their kind employed a selective reading, for clause VIII specifically states:

> That no leper folk, neither men nor women, shall from henceforth enter any borough of the realm other than three times in the week: that is to say each Monday, each Wednesday and each Friday, from ten o'clock until two in the

---

184 Bodleian Library, MS Rawl. B.335, fos 97v–98r; Turner and Coxe, *Calendar of Charters in the Bodleian Library*, p. 442.

185 Le Grand, *Statuts*, p. 192; Avril, 'Le IIIe Concile du Latran', pp. 43, 52.

186 M. Mollat, *The Poor in the Middle Ages* (Yale, 1986), pp. 231–2; Clark, 'Social Welfare', pp. 396–7.

187 Sharpe, *Calendar of Letter-Book G*, p. 217.

188 M. de Lauriere et al., eds, *Ordonnances des roys de France* (23 vols, Paris, 1723–1849), v, pp. 451–2; Jeanselme, 'Comment l'Europe se protéga', pp. 18–19, 112.

afternoon. And when fairs and markets fall on these days, they should postpone their visits and come on the [following] morning to get their living.[189]

Twelve hours a week were thus set aside for them to collect authorised alms and purchase food, while freelance begging was henceforward confined to the town gates.

The effectiveness of such injunctions is hard to judge. Margery Kempe grew accustomed to the sight of lepers in her native King's Lynn, for she records how they reminded her of 'owr Lord Ihesu . . . with hys wowndys bledyng'. Her behaviour on such occasions must have been as disconcerting to them as it was to her neighbours ('than had sche gret mornyng & sorwyng for sche myth not kyssyn the lazerys whan sche sey hem in the stretys'), but it confirms that reactions were neither predictable nor uniform.[190] At about this time, in 1433, Henry Overton of Ramsey was fined by the local court for keeping savage dogs which attacked the lepers coming down the road from what was, presumably, their settlement outside the vill. It is interesting to note that a measure specifically for their protection had been passed at the previous assembly, whose deliberations, unfortunately, have been lost.[191] A grey area between the 'wild' lepers, who figured so prominently as objects of popular apprehension, and the docile residents of established *leprosaria* was inhabited by a variety of ill-documented, often anonymous individuals living alone or in small groups on the outskirts of towns and villages, and thus generally beyond the historical record.

What little evidence we have suggests that these people rarely conformed to the nineteenth-century image of the lonely outcast, abandoned by family and friends. St Milburga's most spectacular miracle concerns a leprous child, whose stepfather carried her 'decomposing' body on his shoulders all the way to Wenlock priory in search of a cure. The girl had been nursed since birth by her mother, who appears also to have cared for her previous husband until he died of the disease. Among the many lepers who were healed by Thomas Becket we find Richard Sunieve, whose mother 'followed him lest he should perish' and, with equal devotion, supplied all his wants. Others, like Mabel of Dudley, depended upon the regular visits and practical support of neighbouring monks and clergy. Although the blind and bedridden leper, Gympe, received precious little help from his parish priest (who bore the brunt of Becket's wrath as a result), 'many benefits' came his way from a charitable local landowner and, indeed, from the daughter who ran his errands.[192] At a later date, testamentary evidence provides enough examples of *ad hoc* relief to suggest that, however alarmed they may have been by the spectre of noisome vagrants, many people made provision for those lepers whom they knew personally and had assisted during their lifetimes. Thus, in 1380, the rector of Little Snoring in Norfolk left 3s. to an otherwise undocumented group of 'lepers living in my parish at Quenegate'. We know nothing of 'Margaret lyppar', to whom the widow, Agnes

189  Thomson and Innes, *Acts of the Parliament of Scotland*, ii, p. 16.
190  Meech, *Book of Margery Kempe*, p. 176.
191  BL, Add. Roll 39647r.
192  Edwards, 'St Milburga', p. 147; Robertson, *Materials*, i, pp. 338–9; ii, pp. 229–34, 245–7.

Alblastyr of Wortsed, bequeathed 1s. in 1524, save that she was almost certainly representative of many.[193]

A sense of the iceberg below the water emerges from the accounts presented in 1310 by the executors of Thomas Bitton, bishop of Exeter. In accordance with the terms of his will, they distributed about £29 among thirty-nine communities of lepers in Devon and Cornwall, mostly along southerly routes that the bishop himself would have travelled. Although some of the places named, such as Barnstaple, Exeter, Launceston, Tavistock and Totnes, possessed established leper houses, twenty-three apparently did not. Here the recipients of alms were clearly living in small, informal settlements, or even, as seems to have been the case at Sancreed, by themselves.[194] One century earlier St Hugh of Lincoln had assiduously visited the lepers dwelling on his estates, and although Bitton may have been less actively involved in the discharge of his pastoral duties, he, too, would almost certainly have helped to maintain these scattered groups.[195] The award of over 300 royal letters of protection and numerous indulgences for the support of struggling communities during the crisis years of the thirteenth and fourteenth centuries further underscores the fact that most lepers were almost certainly to be found *outside* the major *leprosaria* about which most is known. Thus, for example, Bishop Dalderby's grant of indulgences to 'the sick outside Horncastle' in 1309 and an obscure house of lepers at 'Walmesford' between 1307 and 1312 provides our only evidence of refuges in these places. For, paradoxically, given the rising levels of anxiety about infection and vagrancy, it could very hard to obtain institutional assistance.[196]

## Finding a hospital place

The difficulties of gaining prompt admittance to a hospital of one's choice are well known to users of today's National Health Service and were no less familiar to the sick poor of medieval England. Far from being rounded up and confined within secure walls, lepers – and their carers – had often to pull strings and grease palms to secure a coveted bed. Hints of the obstacles to be overcome survive from an early date, as we have seen in the case of the leprous mason who sought admittance into a community at York.[197] The *vita* of Godric of Finchale likewise describes how one desperate woman approached her parish priest for help in finding a place for her sick daughter. Significantly, in this instance, remarriage made it impossible for her to continue caring for the child, whose condition had deteriorated to such a point that her new husband recoiled in horror from her presence.[198]

193 R. Taylor, *Index Monasticus: The Diocese of Norwich* (London, 1821), p. 59; NRO, NCC, reg. Grundisburgh, fos 57r–58r. Nutton, 'Did the Greeks Have a Word', p. 160–61, detects a similar phenomenon in the Classical world.

194 Orme and Webster, *English Hospital*, pp. 172–7; M.I. Somerscales, 'Lazar Houses in Cornwall', *Journal of the Royal Institution of Cornwall*, new series, v (1965), pp. 61–99.

195 See above, p. 123.

196 Satchell, 'Emergence of Leper Houses', pp. 84–91; LAO, Episcopal Register iii, fos 122r, 149v, 231r, 257r.

197 Robertson, *Materials*, i, pp. 334–6.

198 Raine, *Vita et miraculis S. Godrici*, p. 456.

A variety of factors, including wealth, gender, religious vocation, place of residence, kinship and personal repute, determined whether a specific individual would succeed in his or her quest. Most of the larger English monasteries either established and managed their own *leprosaria*, or administered them on behalf of lay or ecclesiastical founders. Such institutions inevitably gave priority to leprous monks, their relatives, employees, tenants and friends.[199] Royal and baronial patrons, who paid the piper, naturally called the tune. On entering the hospital of St Leonard, Peterborough, in 1147, its chief benefactor, Robert de Torpel, not only secured a monk's annual allowance for himself, but even more generous support for the four servants who accompanied him and henceforward became pensioners of the abbey.[200] At about the same time, Roger, earl of Clare settled a generous endowment upon the monastery of Stoke-by-Clare, along with his son, Adam the leper, whom he made a monk there (*cum Adam, filio suo leproso, quem monachum fecit*), evidently on the assumption that either a hospital bed or other appropriate accommodation would be found for him.[201] Entry *ad succurrendum* into the religious life was, as we have seen, a common and accepted feature of monastic profession at this time, which clearly exercised a particular appeal for lepers. It carried a price, none the less, and thus constituted a potential act of simony. Since Gehazi, the archetypal 'simoniacal seller' [II Kings 5, vv. 20–27], had been struck down by leprosy as a punishment for greed, this moral dilemma was not without irony. In practice, though, the full force of canon law was rarely brought to bear in such cases, especially when the house in question could plead poverty.[202]

It might, indeed, be argued that the de Torpels and Clares of twelfth-century England were helping to subsidise accommodation for other sick religious. According to 'a private leiger' of later date, St Laurence's hospital was established on the outskirts of Canterbury in the second quarter of the twelfth century by the abbot of St Augustine's so that:

> If any monk of this monastery suffers a contagious disease (*morbum contagiosum*),[203] and especially leprosy, because of which he cannot live within the precincts of the monastery without causing offence to the brethren, he will be furnished in the aforesaid place with a suitable room, and will have there victuals and clothing, not from the assets of the hospital, but from this monastery, just as any other brother.[204]

---

[199] The monks of St Albans, members of their families, townspeople and relatives of the abbot were accorded preference at St Julian's: Richardson, *Medieval Leper*, p. 130.

[200] King, *Peterborough Abbey*, pp. 27–8. See also the endowment made upon Tavistock abbey in about 1205 by Reginald de Putte, in return for a leper's corrody, tenable for life: H.P.R. Finberg, ed., 'Some Early Tavistock Charters', *EHR*, lxii (1947), pp. 352–77, at p. 375.

[201] Harper-Bill and Mortimer, *Stoke by Clare Cartulary*, i, nos 37, 136–7. Juliana de Cirencester gave property to the nuns of Maiden Bradley when her daughter, who was presumably leprous, took the veil there: BL, MS Add. 37503, fo. 6v; and in about 1194 Elias de Amundeville conveyed land worth 60s. a year to Burton Lazars on the entry of his sick son: T. Bourne and D. Marcombe, eds, *The Burton Lazars Cartulary: A Medieval Leicestershire Estate* (University of Nottingham Centre for Local History, Record Series, vi, 1987), p. 24.

[202] Lynch, *Simoniacal Entry*, pp. 27–32, 66.

[203] 'Contagious' in this context almost certainly means 'putrefying': Touati, 'Contagion', pp. 188–9.

[204] Duncombe and Battely, *Three Archiepiscopal Hospitals*, p. 440. St Laurence's also received the sick or impoverished relatives of monks.

Similarly, Bishop Robert de Chesney of Lincoln (d. 1166) gave St Leonard's hospital at Clattercote, near Banbury, to the Gilbertine order as a refuge for diseased nuns. Any of their number who might be 'suffering from appalling sickness or shameful illness such as leprosy or the like', and had thus to be 'separated from the company of the healthy', could retire there. At first, the leprous sisters enjoyed priority over other applicants, but before long the house was reserved for their use alone.[205]

Not all of the *leprosaria* run under monastic supervision were so selective, although they still screened applicants in a variety of ways. As might be expected, preference was often accorded to unbeneficed clergy, whose condition prevented them from celebrating the Mass, and whose neglect would have brought the entire priesthood into disrepute.[206] Thus, for example, Abbot Anselm (d. 1148) of Bury St Edmunds reputedly founded St Peter's hospital outside the Risby gate for sick and leprous priests, who had certainly begun to occupy these agreeable quarters by the late twelfth century.[207] The plight of individual clergy also inspired compassion, as in 1342, when Edward III ordered the master of St Nicholas's hospital, Scarborough, to admit a chaplain named John de Burgh. The latter had been 'suddenly struck by the disease of leprosy' and was 'unable through shame to beg among Christians'. Whether his humiliation sprang from the disease or his reduced circumstances is unclear, although he clearly presented a deserving case.[208]

Residential qualifications were widely adopted by lay and ecclesiastical authorities alike.[209] The thirteen leprous inmates of the hospital of St Mary Magdalen, Ilford, were supposed to come from estates belonging to the abbess of Barking, who exercised rights of patronage there. Applicants from the town itself were accorded equal priority from at least 1346 onwards, when it was agreed that the burgesses could nominate alternate candidates.[210] In return for doles of food assigned from the borough, the hospital of St Giles, Maldon, likewise undertook from the mid twelfth century to maintain any resident who became leprous, and who, in theory, was thus assured of a free place.[211] Yet in practice members of the urban elite clearly exercised a powerful right of veto. We can see this process in operation at Beverley, in 1394, when one Margaret Taylor appeared before the twelve keepers of the town to solicit a bed in the *leprosarium* outside Keldgate 'by

---

205 B. Golding, *Gilbert of Sempringham and the Gilbertine Order c.1130–c.1300* (Oxford, 1995), pp. 235. By the mid thirteenth century the house had become a priory of canons.

206 See Rawcliffe, *Medicine for the Soul*, pp. 27–8, for a fuller discussion of the institutional care offered to sick, blind and aged clergy.

207 Harper-Bill, *Medieval Hospitals of Bury St Edmunds*, pp. 7–9.

208 *CCR, 1341–1343*, p. 650.

209 This was often in response to the demands of individual patrons, such Henry and Elena de Tarbock, who granted land in Ridgate to Burscough priory, Lancashire, in 1277, on the condition that it would always support a leper from the earl of Lincoln's fee at Widnes. Elena's grandfather had originally given the property to an obscure group of lepers living there: L.C. Loyd and D.M. Stenton, eds, *Sir Christopher Hatton's Book of Seals* (Oxford, 1950), no. 406.

210 Dugdale, *Monasticon*, vi, pp. 629–30. Residential qualifications were often extremely specific: Jeanne, 'Saint-Lazare de Falaise', p. 42.

211 J. Sayers, 'The Earliest Original Letter of Pope Innocent III for an English Recipient', *BIHR*, xlix (1976), pp. 132–5; *CCR, 1402–1405*, pp. 17–18.

way of charity'.[212] She proved successful, although others were doomed to disappointment. In an age of falling rents and rising wages, the ability to make some monetary contribution towards precarious hospital budgets seemed increasingly desirable.

The search for financial help did not always sit easily with the imposition of strict religious discipline. The hospital of St Bartholomew, Dover, was reputedly founded in 1141 by a local landowner for two of his brothers and any other canons from the neighbouring Augustinian priory who contracted leprosy. By the early 1370s, however, it also accepted celibate laymen and women, whose ability to pay 106s. 8d. on entry (and a further 3d. to each resident for a special dinner) fostered a rather different type of exclusivity. On the other hand, if it was ever fully implemented, the heavy round of suffrages expected of all but the sickest inmates must have deterred those who preferred a less regimented existence.[213] A basic level of religious knowledge was, of course, essential, but could not necessarily be taken for granted. The lepers at Harbledown near Canterbury had to know the *Pater Noster, Salve Regina, Ave* and *Credo* by heart, and were tested on admission to ensure that they could play a full part in the house's intercessionary activities.[214] As we have seen, St Julian's hospital, which was run under the direct supervision of St Albans abbey from the mid twelfth century onwards, maintained an equally stringent vetting procedure. The revised statutes of 1344 insisted that the abbot should personally approve all new entrants, perhaps after a private interview.[215]

Lay benefactors of *leprosaria*, who retained control of their foundations rather than surrendering them to monastic houses or town councils, were equally careful to keep an eye on admissions. Like other aspects of 'good lordship', the provision of beds for friends, family or retainers could prove highly contentious, especially when places were in short supply. In 1204, for example, Roger de Rosel successfully defended his right to a *maladaria* in Newton, Yorkshire, from which a leper nominated by him had been ejected. The rival claimants had substituted a patient of their own, whose sojourn proved distressingly brief.[216] It is easy to see why, in 1258, Sir Thomas Tracy, patron of the leper house of St Mary Magdalen at Lanlivery in Cornwall, stipulated that none of the six places were henceforth to be filled without his consent, or that of his successors. Beyond the expectation that newcomers would provide 2s. for a dinner to mark their entry, as well as donating other unspecified 'gifts' to the house, we

212  A.F. Leach, ed., *Beverley Town Documents* (Selden Society, xiv, 1900), p. 41.
213  Bodleian Library, MS Rawl. B.355, fo. 1r.
214  Duncombe and Battely, *Three Archiepiscopal Hospitals*, p. 212. Rules of 1415 at St James's, Canterbury, giving priority to young, literate and docile women, probably marked the house's final transition from a leper hospital to a home for distressed gentlewomen, but some form of selection had probably obtained from the date of its foundation in the twelfth century: ibid., p. 433.
215  Richards, *Medieval Leper*, pp. 130–31. Such arrangements were common. At the hospital of St Mary Magdalen, Colchester, the master filled empty places with the assent of the abbot, who exercised rights of visitation. The five leprous inmates may also have been tested on their knowledge of the liturgy, as they had to perform a strenuous round of suffrages: J.L. Fisher, ed., 'The Leger Book of St John's Abbey, Colchester', *Transactions of the Essex Archaeological Society*, new series, xxiv (1951), pp. 77–127, at pp. 119–22. The abbot of Whitby likewise nominated patients at St Michael's hospital: Atkinson, *Cartularium Abbathiae de Whitby*, ii, p. 515.
216  *CRR, 1203–1205*, p. 90.

know nothing of Tracy's desiderata. Such intangibles as personal acquaintance and moral calibre must, however, have carried a good deal of weight.[217] Quite possibly he followed the example of other landowners in making specific provision for relatives or tenants. The leper hospital of St Sepulchre in Hedon, was, for instance, established in the late twelfth century by Alan Fitzhubert, with widespread support from his family, 'to receive any afflicted person allied to the founder or his heirs within the fourth degree of blood and sufficiently provide for him'.[218]

As was the case in hospitals for the sick poor, individuals of more modest means could purchase the title to a single bed, or beds, which thereby became their own private property. Ownership of the bed next to the door of the infirmary hall at St Bartholomew's, Dover, cost a benefactor named Herlewyn over £5, an investment which guaranteed that he and his heirs would always have a place, either for themselves or a worthy candidate of their choice. In this way, families were able to reserve accommodation and engage in pious works without the expense and trouble of endowing an entire hospital.[219] Sometimes the founder of a *leprosarium* would retain limited rights of presentation after entrusting all its other possessions to a local religious house. Thus, the Huttons of Guisborough kept a bed at St Leonard's, Lowcross, electing at least once to recommend an 'infirm' candidate who was not leprous. Although Hugh Hutton forbade his descendants from capitalising financially from this potentially lucrative asset, others were quite prepared to do so.[220] At some point in the early thirteenth century, for example, Hugh de Moreville paid handsomely for the hereditary right to present 'three poor persons, lepers or others' and a chaplain to St Nicholas's hospital, Carlisle.[221] Since another patron subsequently annexed two more beds, and the mayor of Carlisle also required the hospital to accept lepers from the city in return for weekly doles of food, there must have been brisk competition for places. Even so, 'the custom that when any would give goods for the sustenance of a brother or sister ... he or she would be received as such' appears to have worked reasonably well until a series of corrupt masters pocketed the funds and began turning away patients.[222]

Whatever the admissions policy adopted by specific institutions, leading benefactors, both lay and ecclesiastical, expected preferential treatment for their own nominees. Some had a more legitimate case than others. In 1287, for instance, Archbishop John le Romeyn asked the master of the Sherburn hospital, Durham (founded a century earlier by one of his predecessors), to receive a leprous nun who could not remain in her community because of fears of conta-

---

217  Orme, 'Leper-House at "Lamford" Cornwall', p. 107.
218  G. Poulson, *The History and Antiquities of the Seigniory of Holderness* (2 vols, Hull, 1841), ii, pp. 193–6.
219  Bodleian Library, MS Rawl. B.335, fos 36v–37r.
220  Brown, *Cartularium Prioratus de Gyseburne*, i, pp. 193–4. John Hutton relinquished his right to the prior of Guisborough, who ran the hospital.
221  R.L. Storey, ed., *The Register of John de Kirkby, Bishop of Carlisle, II* (Canterbury and York Society, 1995), pp. 27–8.
222  *CPR, 1340–1343*, p. 121; J. Wilson, ed., *VCH Cumberland II* (London, 1905), p. 199. Abuses began in about 1327, and were exacerbated by warfare along the border.

gion but still had to follow the religious life.[223] At its height, the hospital main-tained sixty-five lepers of both sexes in comfortable circumstances, but smaller houses struggled to accommodate placemen or women, however deserving. Such pressures were certainly apparent at the hospital of the Holy Innocents, Lincoln. According to a charter of Henry I, this modest institution was supposed to take ten lepers from the city (*de ejectibus civitatis Lincolniae*) on the recom-mendation of 'the mayor and other good men' of Lincoln, as well as anyone who contracted the disease while serving in the royal household and thus enjoyed the king's personal support.[224]

Attitudes to such people varied. On the positive side, they sometimes came bearing valuable gifts and annuities. In 1230, for example, Henry III despatched a leprous servant to Lincoln's other hospital (St Giles's), along with a donation of 20*s.* so that he could provide the residents with 'a pittance', or celebratory meal, of the kind often held to mark a new arrival.[225] Any *leprosarium* would have welcomed a patient such as Brito, a royal yeoman 'tainted with leprosy' who was assigned an annual pension of over £6 for the next four years in 1244, or Alice de Costentin, whose more modest stipend of 1*d.* a day came initially from the earl of Chester and then, after 1241, the king.[226] Yet not everyone was either sick or financially independent. Many were elderly or disabled, and quite literally ate into the slender resources of vulnerable institutions. It thus became necessary to attract alternative funding through a move to privatisation. By 1335 the number of designated lepers at the hospital of the Holy Innocents had dwin-dled as the proportion of healthy, fee-paying sisters (*quae non intraverunt per viam rectam sed per viam pecuniae*) rose. It even transpired that the single leper then in residence had been obliged to pay the warden 100*s.* for his place, in contravention of the original statutes.[227]

At St Giles's, Holborn, a royal foundation leased from 1299 by the Order of St Lazarus, the situation was unusually complex because of the triangular conflict of interests at stake. Notwithstanding its grant to the Order, the crown continued to abuse its residual rights of patronage by awarding 'liveries', or subsidised accommodation, there to aged but otherwise able-bodied servants from the royal court. A petition of 1315 from the master to parliament for redress was granted on the ground that such individuals could not fittingly be lodged alongside lepers (*sani inter leprosos conversari non debent*), but this did

---

223  W. Brown, ed., *The Register of John le Romeyn, Archbishop of York, 1286–1296, I* (Surtees Society, cxxiii, 1913), p. 163; Allan, *Sherburn Hospital,* unpaginated.

224  Dugdale, *Monasticon,* vi, pp. 627–8.

225  *CLR, 1226–1240,* p. 163. Another royal servant 'infected with the stain of leprosy' was given 20*s.* in 1256 on his entry into a *leprosarium* (probably St Julian's) at St Albans, 'where he proposes to end his days': *CLR, 1251–1260,* p. 303. Yet William de Wherewell, a leper who had previously served the king, arrived empty-handed at St Giles's in 1300 with nothing but the royal mandate: *CCR, 1296–1302,* p. 376.

226  *CLR, 1240–1245,* pp. 90, 211. Contributions towards support were apparently expected at St Giles's hospital, Chester, which admitted royal and baronial nominees, as well as local burgesses: B.E. Harris, ed., *VCH Chester III* (London, 1980), p. 178.

227  Dugdale, *Monasticon,* vi, pp. 627–9; Strachey, *Rotuli Parliamentorum,* v, p. 472; W. Page, ed., *VCH Lincolnshire II* (London, 1906), pp. 230–31. An inquiry of 1316 revealed numerous abuses, including the sale of corrodies for significant sums, with the result that 'the devotion of the surrounding people' had declined: *CIM, 1307–1349,* no. 293.

not end the problem.[228] Indeed, the Lazarites themselves were not above reproach, at least according to the rulers of London, who claimed – without any legal justification – that 'a certain person of the said city suffering from the disease' had founded the hospital, and (more truthfully) that many other charitable citizens had invested heavily in it. Having failed in their initial attempts to wrest the patronage from the crown, the mayor and Corporation in turn complained to parliament in 1348 and again, with added urgency, six years later about the Order's many derelictions. These included the sale of corrodies (board and lodging) on a commercial basis and the virtual abandonment of any responsibilities to the truly sick. As a result, they argued, 'the said poor diseased folk' were forced to roam the streets, where they posed a threat to healthy men and women. Driven, no doubt, by current fears of pestilence and vagrancy, an agreement whereby the warden of St Giles's would always maintain a complement of fourteen lepers from the city and suburbs at the nomination of the mayor and commonality was brokered at this time.[229] Successive royal inquiries revealed a continuing history of mismanagement, intensified by the fact that leading Londoners, such as the fishmonger, Nicholas Exton, did not scruple to lease well-appointed retirement homes in the precinct. Yet some lepers remained, and it was ostensibly for their benefit that the hospital briefly came under new management at the close of the fourteenth century.[230] During the 1460s St Giles's and the 'maladerie' of the Holy Innocents, Lincoln, were alike exempted from parliamentary acts of resumption because they still received 'certeyn lepers of oure meniall servauntes', which suggests some continuity of purpose and perhaps also of abuse.[231]

The proliferation of corrodies in hospitals and *leprosaria* had already incurred the censure of the Council of Paris, which protested in 1212 about the waste of resources and corruption of morals occasioned by the presence of so many idle dependants.[232] The problem was rife across Europe, and is well documented in England. Condemn it as they might, royal commissioners, borough authorities and ecclesiastical visitors were powerless to halt a long-standing trend that gained rapid momentum during the later Middle Ages.[233] As early as the 1160s 'sound and healthy women' were competing for the twenty-five places reserved for leprous sisters (*mulieres leprosae*) at the hospital of St James, near Canter-

228 Strachey, *Rotuli Parliamentorum*, i, p. 310; *CPR, 1313–1317*, p. 300.
229 E. Williams, ed., *Early Holborn and the Legal Quarter of London* (2 vols, London, 1927), ii, nos 1624–6; Sharpe, *Calendar of Letter-Book G*, pp. 27–9; Marcombe, *Leper Knights*, pp. 161–6.
230 *CPR, 1374–1377*, p. 99; *1396–1399*, p. 47; Williams, *Early Holborn*, nos 1615–23, 1627–54, covers the various royal inquiries in detail. For the parlous state of the lepers in 1401, see R.R. Sharpe, ed., *Calendar of the Letter-Books of the City of London, Letter-Book I* (London, 1909), pp. 13–14.
231 Strachey, *Rotuli Parliamentorum*, v, pp. 472, 520–21, 602. Optimism triumphed over experience in 1457, when the crown handed over Holy Innocents to the Lazarites, on the understanding that they would support three lepers from the royal household or nearby crown estates: Marcombe, *Leper Knights*, pp. 166–8.
232 Mansi, *Sacrorum conciliorum*, xii, cols 835–6. The ruling had little effect, as reforms of 1257 at Chartres and of 1349 at Paris highlighted this abuse: Merlet and Jusselin, *Cartulaire de la léproserie du Grand-Beaulieu*, no. 345; Le Grand, *Statuts*, p. 245. See also, Lynch, *Simoniacal Entry*, pp. 168, 213–14.
233 Risse, *Mending Bodies*, pp. 168–9, notes cases where men and women disguised themselves as lepers to gain admittance.

bury. Managed by the monks of Christ Church, who selected all the patients, this wealthy hospital must have attracted the widows and daughters of affluent burgesses. Pope Alexander III himself intervened to halt the practice, on the ground that it was diverting support from the lepers who badly needed it, but market forces prevailed.[234] Indeed, by the fourteenth century some corrodies appear to have become hereditary, although the master did, to his credit, resist attempts by Queen Philippa to secure a place for one of her servants.[235] Similar complaints about the indiscriminate award of board and lodging to unsuitable people surfaced at the nearby hospital of St Nicholas, Harbledown, in 1298–99. On this occasion, concern not only focused upon the threat to the leprous poor, but also to the religious life of the hospital where, it was feared, the round of intercessionary prayer would be disrupted. Significantly, no reference was made in either place to the risks of infection.[236]

Even after such fears became entrenched, the more affluent English *leprosaria* remained a tempting prospect for elderly men and women in search of sheltered accommodation. In 1334, for example, one 'healthy' married couple sued the master of William le Gros's hospital at Hedon for a corrody comprising a private chamber, a daily allocation of pottage and bread, twenty-eight gallons of ale every fortnight, a generous assignment of pittances, 300 turves a year, and a consignment of thatch, straw and pasturage for their sheep.[237] It is now hard to determine the extent to which arrangements of this kind actually deprived the sick of necessary support, since many houses were by then reporting a fall in the number of applicants. But central and local authorities, disturbed by the potential threat of miasmatic disease and vagrancy, continued to wring their collective hands over the problem. A royal commission of inquiry addressed in 1376 to the mayor of Bristol expressed concern about the excessive award of corrodies at St Lawrence's hospital, which could no longer support the lepers 'and other infirm persons' who were supposed to live and worship there.[238] Another of 1391 revealed that St Bartholomew's, Oxford, had been ruined through aggressive asset stripping.[239]

No less pernicious was the imposition of entry fines, or one-off payments charged for admittance into a *leprosarium* or hospital. The case of the leprous mason healed by Thomas Becket suggests that the practice was already well established by the 1170s, if not earlier.[240] Tacitly accepting that a degree of commercialisation was inevitable, the bishop of Exeter ruled at this time that he and his successors would vet all applicants for admission to the city's leading leper house whether they paid or not.[241] Ecclesiastical visitors, who inspected hospitals such as St Nicholas's, York, reiterated complaints about the subversion

---

234  *HMC Eighth Report* (London, 1881), p. 325; Brigstocke Sheppard, *Literae Cantuarienses*, iii, pp. 75–6.
235  W. Page, ed., *VCH Kent II* (London, 1926), p. 209. The crown was not always successful in placing its nominees. In 1374, the master of St Mary the Virgin, Ilford, successfully stood his ground: Page and Round, *VCH Essex II*, p. 186.
236  Duncombe and Battely, *Three Archiepiscopal Hospitals*, p. 212.
237  Page, *VCH Yorkshire III*, pp. 308–9.
238  *CPR 1374–1377*, p. 310; *CIM, 1387–1393*, no. 313.
239  *CIM, 1387–1393*, no. 313.
240  Robertson, *Materials*, i, pp. 334–6.
241  Barlow, *EEA, XI, Exeter 1046–1184*, no. 98.

of religious life and discipline. An inquiry of 1291 into the alleged mismanagement of this once affluent royal foundation revealed that, between 1264 and
1274, four lepers had been admitted free, *pro Deo*, but other brothers and sisters
had been obliged to pay a flat fee of about £13 each. By the 1280s, however, *all*
newcomers were being charged up to £15 for entry, irrespective of health. Since
the hospital was supposed to accommodate lepers, along with 'the old and feeble
of the city', out of charity, such abuses incurred particular censure and were
henceforward forbidden. It is easy to see how the abandonment of the monastic
habit, financial malpractices and 'disorderly conversation' followed insidiously
from the sale of hospital places. Men and women who paid for the comfortable
private lodgings that had been constructed at St Nicholas's by the early fourteenth century were disinclined to accept the harsh strictures of communal
life.[242] Potential benefactors, who expected a spiritual return from their investment, meanwhile turned elsewhere.

A type of ongoing means test may also have obtained, whereby relatives were
expected to employ the assets of sick family members to provide for their
support.[243] Evidence of such an *ad hoc* arrangement emerges, for example, in
1203, when the royal court decreed that the uncle and next heir of a young man
named Daniel, who had entered the *leprosarium* at Castle Rising, Norfolk,
should pay to keep him there as well as supplying whatever essentials he might
need.[244] Some thirty years later, a similar verdict was passed in favour of one
Jordan the leper, whose property was sold to provide him with 'the necessary
victuals for life'.[245] As a man of moderate means, he too was obliged to
contribute towards his own upkeep. Some religious fraternities, which functioned as a type of mutual provident society, were certainly prepared to assist
long-term members who became leprous. The guild of the Virgin Mary in Chesterfield decreed that any brother who could not support himself 'through age,
loss of limb or leprosy' would either be given food and shelter or maintained 'in
a house of religion where he may stay during his life'. Such organisations, which
were extremely judgemental about self-induced hardship, did not apparently
regard *lepra* as a stigma where reputable artisans were concerned.[246]

However it was raised, a sum equivalent to the annual salary of a well-heeled
parish priest lay far beyond the means of most suspect lepers, who became
increasingly dependent upon outside help and favour in the search for accommodation. The register of Bishop Dalderby of Lincoln records the issue of indulgences on behalf of at least thirteen such men and women in the years between
1304 and 1316. Thus, for example, anyone who assisted Adam Gyliot of East
Deeping to raise the funds for a hospital bed could count upon twenty days'

---

242  Brown, *Yorkshire Inquisitions*, ii, pp. 122–32; and below, p. 332.
243  In *The Testament of Cresseid*, Robert Henryson observes that Cresseid gained admittance to a
     *leprosarium* because 'scho was of nobill kin'. Her father's generosity must have proved a further
     recommendation: ibid., pp. 44, 75.
244  D.M. Stenton, ed., *The Earliest Northamptonshire Assize Rolls* (Northamptonshire Record Society, v,
     1930), no. 836.
245  *CRR, 1233–1237*, no. 936B.
246  The guild dated from 1218, and the statutes were recorded in 1389: Smith, Smith and Brentano,
     *English Gilds*, p. 166.

relief from enjoined penance, and a corresponding improvement in the health of his or her immortal soul.[247] In addition, six other individuals 'struck by the disease of leprosy' secured indulgences for unspecific relief, although they may have been just as desperate for institutional help during this testing period of famine and economic dislocation. Among them was the especially unfortunate Nicholas of Norfolk, 'whose good limbs had been afflicted by diabolic fury', and whose wife and apparent keeper had recently died.[248] Rural communities that had previously been able to support one or two 'deserving' lepers and other sick or incapacitated individuals could evidently no longer bear the expense.

The predicament faced by the leprous hero of *Amis and Amiloun* must have been far from unusual at this time. Having first relegated him to 'the table's ende', and then to 'a litel loge' half a mile from her gate, his wife – a Fenne Bouster in the making – finally threw him out. Amiloun and his faithful page took to the road, eventually settling outside a busy market town where they survived on the alms provided by local people.

> Thai duelled there yeres thre,
> That child & he al-so,
> & liued in care & pouerte,
> Bi the folke of that cuntre,
> As thai com to & fro,
> So that in the ferth [fourth] yere
> Corn bigan to wex dere,
> That hunger bigan to go,
> That ther was noither eld no ying [old or young]
> That wald yif [give] hem mete no drink,
> Wel careful were thai tho.[249]

Aid for the leprous poor seems to have been offered on just such a personal basis, and thus to have been subject to the vagaries of boom and slump experienced by Amiloun in his wayside hut. As one survivor of the 1315 famine observed, 'such was the dearth in England that those who were accustomed to supporting themselves and their dependents in a suitable manner [now] travelled along streets and through places as beggars'.[250]

So far as we can tell, no English town adopted the practice that had, reputedly, obtained in the four Scottish boroughs of Berwick, Roxburgh, Edinburgh and Stirling since the twelfth century. Here any burgess of means who succumbed to leprosy was expected pay his or her own way 'in the spytaile of the burgh', while the resident poor received 20s. each from public funds to provide food, board and clothing there. Any subsequent shortfall would be made up by

---

247  LAO, Episcopal Register iii, fos 74v, 138r, 203v, 207r, 230v (Gyliot), 235v, 239r, 257v, 258r, 273v, 274r (two different people), 335v, 336r (the last two references concern the same person). Indulgences were also granted to the blind, deaf and paralytic, probably because of the biblical resonance of their condition: Register iii, fos 87r, 219v, 318v, 327v, 366v–367v, 427v; v, fos 261v, 283r, 341v, 362v.

248  LAO, Episcopal Register iii, fos 74r, 87r, 122r, 164v (Norfolk), 181v, 281v.

249  Leach, *Amis and Amiloun*, p. 72.

250  I. Kershaw, 'The Great Famine and Agrarian Crisis in England 1315–1322', *Past and Present*, lix (1973), pp. 3–50, at p. 11.

begging at the hospital gates, rather than in the streets of the town. In this way it was hoped to eliminate an annoying nuisance, while guaranteeing that places would be available for anyone who lived within the walls.[251] This, too, was the intention in Dublin, where the practice of charging for admission to St Stephen's hospital had apparently left many diseased citizens homeless. Perturbed by the threat to public health and order, the assembly ruled in 1491 that 'every fre man and woman of this cite enfected with lepyr [should] be received and take into the house of Saint Stewnes within the fraunches of this cite frely, without anny fyne paying to anny person or persones'. Offenders faced a substantial penalty of 40s., which may well reflect growing alarm at the twin spectres of vagrancy and disease as much as concern for the leprous.[252] Yet, despite the competition for beds and lack of subsidized support, many individuals, healthy as well as sick, eventually found refuge in the lazar houses of medieval England. Once regarded as little short of a living death, hospital life was demonstrably neither as cloistered nor as oppressive as might be supposed. Indeed, for some patients, at least, the struggle proved worthwhile. Did others face a less agreeable experience?

---

[251] Thomson and Innes, *Acts of the Parliament of Scotland*, i, p. 344. Some boroughs, such as Lydd, did, however, make *ex gratia* payments of a few shillings to deserving cases: *HMC, Fifth Report, Appendix* (London, 1876), p. 522.

[252] J.T. Gilbert, ed., *Calendar of Ancient Records of Dublin, I* (Dublin, 1889), p. 372.

# 7

## Life in the Medieval Leper House

*But my uncle's intentions went further: he was not only proposing to tend the bodies of the lepers but their souls too. And he was forever among them, moralizing away, putting his nose into their affairs, being scandalized, and preaching. The lepers could not endure him. Pratofungo's happy licentious days were over. With this thin figure on his one leg, black-dressed, ceremonious and sententious, no one could have fun without arousing public recriminations, malice and back-biting. Even their music, by dint of being blamed as futile, lascivious and inspired by evil sentiments, grew burdensome, and those strange instruments of theirs became covered with dust. The leper women, deprived of their revels, suddenly found themselves face to face with their disease and spent their evenings sobbing in despair.*

Italo Calvino, The Cloven Viscount, *1951* [1]

As described in the hospital cartulary of 1372, the ritual for admission into St Bartholomew's, Dover, must have made a striking impression upon all the participants gathered in the church to welcome a new addition to their select community.[2] The sub-prior of St Martin's abbey, who acted as warden, would already have examined the candidate to ensure that he or she was suitable. Because they were to take vows of religion, all the brothers and sisters had to be either single, widowed or married to a spouse who was prepared to embrace a life of chastity.[3] As we have seen, they were also required to pay a substantial entrance fee, while agreeing to provide the other inmates with a special meal to mark their arrival. Once these desiderata had been met, and the warden was satisfied as to the applicant's moral worth, the reception ceremony could proceed. It fell into two parts, the first of which took place at the church door, where the warden, fully robed, made many solemn demands of the newcomer. He or she was to be 'useful and faithful' to the hospital, obedient to the

1   Italo Calvino, *Our Ancestors* (London, 1995), p. 63.
2   Bodleian Library, MS Rawl. B.335, fos 1r–2v. How many newcomers were leprous at this time is a moot point, although the master had to be.
3   See above, pp. 267–8. Abbot Mentmore's statutes of 1344 for St Julian's hospital, St Albans, demanded that all married brethren *and* their wives should swear a formal oath of chastity on admission, before the probationary period began: Richards, *Medieval Leper*, p. 130. See also BL, MS Cotton Faustina A III, fos 323r–323v (St James's, Westminster); and Dugdale, *Monasticon*, vi, p. 629 (Ilford).

authorities and respectful to the other patients. Men and women alike were to conduct themselves chastely and soberly at all times, undertaking to leave one half of all their effects to the house after death. The entrant then swore on a missal to uphold these conditions, promising also to pray devoutly for the Church and realm of England, the king and queen and the monks of St Martin's; the burgesses of Dover and all the hospital's other benefactors, living and dead, rounded off the list. A blessing with holy water followed, after which it was at last possible to enter the sacred space of the church. As the postulant knelt at the high altar, the warden invoked God's blessing, praying that he or she would be enfolded in divine love forever, without spot or stain (*sine macula*). A black or russet habit was then blessed, and presented as a source of support, inspiration and protection. Just as God had promised to clothe his servants in garments of health and everlasting joy, so this robe should prompt humility and contempt for the world. After a final prayer for the preservation of his or her chastity, the entrant received the tonsure and, on bended knee, presented a burning candle and an offering of two pence at the altar. The service was over and the community could now move to the refectory for a feast.

Ceremonies of this kind took place in lazar houses and hospitals all over Europe.[4] We know comparatively little about the way they were conducted in England, although it is clear that most *leprosaria* of any size mounted some kind of ritual to mark the arrival of a new brother or sister. Even if it did not involve the bestowal of habit and tonsure, there were rules to be read and explained, promises to be made and, above all, a momentous stage of transition to be observed. At the *leprosarium* of St Mary Magdalen, Hedon, the entrant was to kneel at the altar, where the priest, in surplice and stole, demanded the obligatory oath of obedience to the master and statutes. He then recited a number of Latin prayers, psalms and invocations over the newest member of his flock, commending him or her to God.[5] The custom at Harbledown was rather different, since, in keeping with the general prominence accorded to weekly chapter meetings, the oath (which, in this mixed community, placed particular emphasis on chastity) was taken before a special assembly of residents, both male and female.[6] Perhaps because of the hospital's long history of mismanagement, the undertaking required, from at least 1344 onwards, of each *frater leprosus* at Ilford reflected some distinctly temporal concerns. Here, the newcomer swore on the gospels that, besides following the existing rules, he would accept no more than the prescribed number of lepers into the community, would alienate none of its property and would never condone the sale of pensions or corrodies. This meant that all the goods he brought with him would henceforward be shared in common, rather than passing to friends or family on his death.[7]

Whatever form it may have taken, induction was, of course, only the begin-

---

4   See above, p. 20 n. 21.
5   York Minster Library, MS B2 (3) a 5.
6   Duncombe and Battely, *Three Archiepiscopal Hospitals*, pp. 212–13.
7   Dugdale, *Monasticon*, vi, p. 630. See Orme, 'Leper House at "Lamford" Cornwall', pp. 104, 106–7, for further emphasis upon shared property.

ning. What could the hopeful petitioner expect once he or she had pledged compliance with the statutes and finally secured a much-coveted bed? Did entry into a *leprosarium* really mark an abrupt break with the outside world, as the joys of normal life became little more than a distant memory? Had a protracted death knell begun to sound with every shake of the bell or rattle? Partly because it served a segregationist agenda, the nineteenth-century view of institutional provision was depressingly bleak. As one early advocate of compulsory isolation maintained:

> The expulsion of lepers from society was effected with great energy; and what proves this are the thousands of *leprosaria* which were built in the Middle Ages, and the unremitting persecution which was directed against these wretches in order to exterminate them . . . We once again encounter this malady in all the places where isolation did not occur, or has not been implemented in a satisfactory manner . . . If [leprosy] had not completely disappeared in the Middle Ages – because isolation achieved this with a rigour that was terrible enough, although often exaggerated – it would never have been contained in modern times.[8]

However strongly they may have argued the case for forcible detention, subsequent generations of leprologists, such as Edouard Jeanselme, were obliged to concede that, in fact, medieval *leprosaria* had rarely, if ever, incarcerated their inmates. The most cursory perusal of the surviving statutes revealed an entirely different picture of voluntary seclusion little different from that of other charitable foundations and monastic houses. Even so, while accepting that the hospitalised leper might be lucky to secure a bed, scholars continued to stress the unique marginality of these 'antechambers of eternity', in both a topographical and spiritual sense. Jeanselme's view that 'therapeutics were totally excluded' from such places still remains current, despite the fact that the larger ones, at least, were fully equipped to offer the best and most effective medicine for the souls of patients as well as patrons.[9]

Indeed, although many hospitals lacked the resources to provide more than rudimentary physical care, others also did their best to fulfil the bodily and emotional needs of the sick. At St Bartholomew's, Dover, for instance, the sixteen brothers and sisters were promised regular assignments of candles, wheat for bread and barley for ale, along with oats, beans, peas and bacon for pottage.[10] Running the medieval equivalent of a workers' co-operative under the direction of their leprous master, they divided the produce of their gardens, dairy, mill and poultry farm equally between them, selling the rest for common profit. Eggs, milk, chicken and fresh bread (all of which were recommended in the

---

8    L. Drognat-Landré, *De la contagion seule cause de la propagation de la lèpre* (Paris, 1869), pp. 69–70.
9    See, for example, Agrimi and Crisciani, 'Charity and Aid', p. 193; Grmek, *Diseases in the Ancient Greek World*, p. 172; and, for Jeanselme, above, pp. 24–5.
10   Pottage was a nutritious type of porridge, to which legumes and vegetables such as leeks and cabbage would be added. It constituted a dietary staple among the medieval labouring classes: C. Dyer, *Standards of Living in the Later Middle Ages* (Cambridge, revised edn, 1998), pp. 58, 64, 134, 153, 157–8. Its popularity in the more affluent *leprosaria* may have been due to the fact that patients with damaged mouths and teeth would have found it easy to eat. At St Leonard's, Lancaster, which was poorer, the basic individual allocation in 1328 comprised a two-pound loaf every day and pottage three times a week: *CIM, 1307–1349*, p. 167.

treatment of *lepra*) must have been plentiful, because many of the hospital's rents were paid in kind. Since it owned osier beds and a stretch of water, we may assume that fresh fish were also available. Either from its own sheep or the flocks of its tenants, the house obtained wool to make some of the patients' clothing. Major feast days were marked not only by cash doles but also by the allocation of an extra four gallons of ale, and a strict rule about the distribution of alms and legacies meant that (in theory) everyone received a fair share of any incoming donations. Spiritual succour came in many guises, from the daily celebration of the Eucharist and canonical hours (which were illuminated by a lamp hanging in the church), to facilities for regular confession and, after death, for the commemoration of all departed brothers and sisters. One of the leprous brethren was charged with the task of keeping and cleaning the house's substantial collection of plate and ecclesiastical vestments, which suggests that the liturgy was observed with some solemnity.[11]

Standards clearly varied from place to place and over time, not least at Dover, where, after this auspicious start, the financial situation appears to have grown increasingly parlous.[12] But there can be little doubt that on parchment, at least, patrons and founders made strenuous efforts to ameliorate the last painful years of men and women whose sufferings were so acute. The analogous process of atrophy and decline that affected the majority of late medieval English *leprosaria* tends to obscure the careful planning that may initially have been devoted to such questions as location, layout and provisioning, each of which played a crucial part in the *regimen sanitatis*. Archbishop Lanfranc's decision to build a leper house at Harbledown, some distance from Canterbury was, for example, influenced by more than his knowledge of Leviticus. The hospital occupied a 'peculiarly healthful' site, much frequented by herbalists, who gathered there to collect medicinal plants.[13] As we shall see, a major thoroughfare ran just past the precinct, offering the residents ample opportunity to beg for alms [plate 30]. Even in this rural retreat, there were constant opportunities for human contact.

We have seen in previous chapters the extent to which religious beliefs determined how lepers should behave and, by the same token, how society should respond to their predicament. It is now time to focus upon the ways in which the Christian imperative of care for the sick might be translated into actual practice. Turning first to the reality of life 'outside the camp', we assess the degree to which leper communities were integrated into the wider fabric of English society. We then explore the provision of practical physical support, in the way of food, clothing, fuel and accommodation, before investigating the spiritual resources upon which a patient might draw in one of the richer and better documented English *leprosaria*. But it will also become apparent that even quite small institutions were originally able to exceed the basic requirements of canon law in fulfilling the needs of their residents.

---

11  Bodleian Library, MS Rawl. B.335, fos 2r–4v. Unfortunately, the last part of this cartulary, listing the plate and vestments, has been removed.
12  Sweetinburgh, *Role of the Hospital*, pp. 136–40, 170–75, discusses the hospital's economic problems.
13  Duncombe and Battely, *Three Archiepiscopal Hospitals*, p. 173. Burton Lazars, another hilltop location that boasted a healing spring, was also hailed for its 'uncommonly salubrious air' and abundant herbs: Marcombe, *Leper Knights*, pp. 142–6.

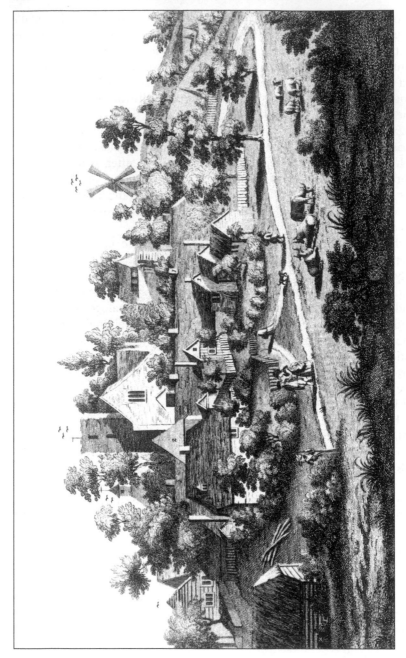

30. An eighteenth-century impression of the hospital at Harbledown, Kent, which was then an almshouse. Its salubrious position near the top of a hill in open countryside, the proximity of a main road and the availability of timber and farmland, made it an ideal site for Archbishop Lanfranc's pioneering foundation for lepers in the late eleventh century.

## Degrees of separation

Not all lazar houses enjoyed such a bracing environment as that offered by the slopes of Harbledown. Many were to be found in the suburbs of English towns, cheek by jowl with practitioners of unsavoury trades, such as dyeing, iron smelting and lime burning. Fires and thefts were common in rough areas frequented by criminals and prostitutes.[14] Yet such risks were hardly unique to civic *leprosaria*. Friaries, hostels and hospitals for the sick poor, which also needed land, water and ready access to transport, might likewise be found on the outskirts of major centres of population. At Toulouse, for example, most of the *leprosaria* occupied adjacent sites to general hospitals, being effectively paired with them at five of the city gates. Indeed, one lazar house was so hemmed in by urban development that it soon had to move further out of town.[15] A similar picture emerges at Bury St Edmunds, where the female *leprosarium* of St Petronilla was located near the Domus Dei and eventually merged with it. In this instance, though, it was the hospital not the leper house that had decamped from a central site to a more spacious and desirable extramural location.[16]

Suburban growth often caught up with communities that had once seemed secluded. At King's Lynn, for instance, the Cowgate leper house had originally commanded a fine site in open country near where the main east–west road met the ferry over the river Ouse. By 1432, however, it lay in the middle of a thriving commercial district, next to the Tuesday market and the common staithe.[17] The hospital of St John the Baptist at Thetford was similarly overtaken by development, although in this case a merger with the outlying house of St Mary Magdalen made it possible to move the lepers further out of town.[18] The relocation of St Laurence's hospital, Launceston, in the mid thirteenth century, may, perhaps, coincide with the promulgation of stricter rules, reputedly dating from 'time immemorial', for the exclusion of lepers from the borough. But the new eighteen-acre site boasted so many desirable features (including an abundant water supply, a chapel and cemetery) and occupied such a prime spot (next to a bridge and main road), that other, more positive considerations must also have prompted the prior of Launceston to facilitate the move.[19]

Many of the earliest *leprosaria* were deliberately situated in remote areas, far from the bustle of secular society. As common among female religious as it was among lepers, the desire for a return to the eremitical life of the desert fathers initially proved a powerful factor in determining the choice of location.[20] So too did more pragmatic considerations, such as the availability of land, the wealth of

14  In 1305, for example, the patrons of the *leprosarium* of St Mary Magdalen, Baldock, obtained permission to move it to a 'safer' site, because of fires and thieves: BL, Harley Charter 112 A 3; Rawcliffe, 'Passports to Paradise', pp. 10–13; Touati, *Archives*, p. 57.
15  J.H. Mundy, 'Charity and Social Work in Toulouse 1100–1250', *Traditio*, xxii (1966), pp. 203–87, at pp. 214 (map), 228–9.
16  Harper-Bill, *Hospitals of Bury St Edmunds*, pp. 3–9, 98–9.
17  Isaacson and Ingleby, *Red Register*, i, p. 156; ii, p. 90.
18  Page, *VCH Suffolk II*, p. 452.
19  Orme and Webster, *English Hospital*, pp. 200, 202; and above, p. 191.
20  The situation of nunneries and rural *leprosaria* was in many ways similar: R. Gilchrist, *Gender and Material Culture* (London, 1994), pp. 65–9. Indeed, one French bishop argued in the mid twelfth

the founder and the potential for expansion. We have already seen how many hospitals grew up next to the healing wells and springs that attracted people with skin diseases.[21] Some houses appear to have colonised hitherto uncultivated and marginal terrain, which, in the case of St Thomas's at Bolton in Northumberland, allowed ample scope for reclamation. In 1235, about a decade after its foundation, 120 acres of moor and 150 of alder wood had already been enclosed, although the land in question proved far from fertile.[22] Yet however strong their vocation may have been, the leprous brothers and sisters who joined these communities never quite abandoned the world. For all its apparent isolation in a wilderness of wood and scrubland, St Michael's, Whitby, stood conveniently near the 'spityllbrygd' over the river Esk which carried a regular flow of wayfarers and thus of alms past its gates.[23]

At first glance, the hospital of St Mary Magdalen on the Gaywood causeway, near King's Lynn, seems to have occupied an equally liminal position, on marshland interspersed with banks, dykes, fleets, saltpans and reed beds. Perhaps because drainage posed such a problem, the precinct was even surrounded by a moat. Yet it not only commanded one of the principal routes into Lynn but also stood close to the residence of its patrons, the bishops of Norwich, thereby proclaiming their pastoral zeal and Christian compassion.[24] Like all religious houses of any size, the more affluent English *leprosaria* were enclosed, usually with walls and ditches of the kind found at Burton Lazars (which was also partially moated).[25] The purpose of these structures was not to imprison the residents (although they clearly helped to maintain monastic discipline and keep livestock under control), but to exclude the malign influences of the outside world, which might so easily contaminate an environment of prayer and contemplation.[26]

As we saw in the previous chapter, most *leprosaria* relied heavily upon begging, which in some cases provided their staple income. Strategic proximity to heavily frequented roads and waterways, preferably at a point such as a gate, bridge or crossroads where travellers were likely to congregate was therefore essential.[27] The construction of a hospital chapel, at which prayers might be offered or thanks given for a safe journey, naturally helped to boost takings. Occupying a prime position about a mile south of Walmgate on the main road to Hull, St Nicholas's, York, clearly attracted substantial donations, not all of which reached their intended destination. Reforms of 1303 introduced a system of triple locks for the alms box in the chapel, which was henceforth 'to be opened before all' and the contents fairly distributed.[28] Seclusion, on the other hand,

---

century that lepers fled the world in order to avoid its temptations, and that their lonely places belonged as much to God as busy towns: Avril, 'Le IIIe Concile du Latran', pp. 27–8.

21  See above, pp. 228–9.
22  J.C. Hodgson, *A History of Northumberland VII* (London, 1904), pp. 202–4.
23  Atkinson, *Cartularium abbathiae de Whitby*, i, p. 329.
24  King's Lynn Borough Archives, C56/ 2, 4, 6, 12, 15, 16, 18; T. Pestell, *Landscapes of Monastic Foundation* (Woodbridge, 2004), pp. 187–8.
25  Marcombe, *Leper Knights*, p. 147; Gilchrist, *Contemplation and Action*, pp. 43–4.
26  Rawcliffe, *Medicine for the Soul*, p. 39.
27  Touati, *Archives*, p. 54.
28  Page, *VCH Yorkshire III*, p. 348.

spelt disaster. Patrons of St Laurence's hospital near the Swiss town of Lausanne soon realised their mistake in selecting 'a solitary place . . . devoid of all solace and passers by' for the lepers, and moved them to a more agreeable and populous location, where they could solicit alms.[29] Some apparently isolated sites none the less appear to have been especially well chosen for this purpose, as Erasmus and John Colet discovered when they travelled along the sunken road at Harbeldown and were unable to escape the importunate almsmen from the former leper house.[30] Yet access to a major thoroughfare could prove to be a mixed blessing. In the early 1330s, when many *leprosaria* were feeling the chill wind of economic recession, the infirm sisters of Maiden Bradley, 'wretchedly languishing through the affliction of leprosy', successfully petitioned Rome for assistance in a dispute over lapsed rights. Faced by a grim scenario of declining rents, falling yields and lapsed offerings, they were, none the less, still obliged to shoulder 'a heavy burden of hospitality' because of the hospital's position on the road through Selwood forest. The presence of leprous nuns evidently did little to deter travellers in search of food and a night's lodging.[31]

Although they often pre-dated the erection of boundary crosses, such as that raised in marble by the burgesses of King's Lynn 'on the causeway of Mawdelyn' in 1361–62, many *leprosaria* stood at or near important local landmarks and junctions.[32] If such an archetypically liminal situation underscored the leper's own tenuous position between life and death, it certainly did not signal his or her relegation, forgotten and despised, to the outer margins of society. On the contrary, the citizens of York registered their 'bounds and metes' by moving from one leper hospital and religious house to another: 'by a ditch and a marsh next to the spitalwell by way next the abbot of St Mary's . . . as far as the Maudeleyn spetell in the highway which leads from York to Clyfton . . . as far as the cross next the bridge beyond the mill of St Nicholas's hospital . . . next to the close of the hospital of St Nicholas aforesaid'.[33] It was virtually impossible to enter any major English town or city without encountering a similar ring of charitable institutions, which have now almost entirely vanished from sight. Their disappearance makes it easy to underestimate whatever impact they may have had, not least as a means of demonstrating the philanthropy and civic pride of their founders.

Before decline set in, some of the wealthier suburban *leprosaria* must once have seemed truly imposing. However fanciful it now appears, Matthew Paris's pen and ink drawing in his *Chronica majora* of St Giles's, Holborn, on the western approach to London, illustrates this point well [**plate 31**]. Its church

---

29  Borradori, *Mourir au monde*, p. 200.

30  Orme and Webster, *English Hospital*, p. 47. The hospital of St Mary Magdalen at Lyncombe, outside Bath, likewise commanded a 'hollow way', as well as being conveniently near a major fairground: Manco, *Spirit of Care*, pp. 22–6.

31  BL, MS Add. 37508, fos 38r–39v; Kemp, 'Maiden Bradley Priory', pp. 87–120.

32  H. Harrod, *Report on the Deeds and Records of King's Lynn* (King's Lynn, 1874), p. 79. Also in East Anglia, *leprosaria* at Langwade, Thetford (both St Mary Magdalen and St John the Baptist) and Sudbury stood by boundary crosses: W. Page, ed., *VCH Norfolk II* (London, 1906), pp. 440, 452; C. Dallas, *Excavations at Thetford by B.K. Davison* (East Anglian Archaeology, lxii, 1993), p. 217; Hodson, 'John Colney's Hospital', p. 268.

33  J.W. Percy, ed., *York Memorandum Book* (Surtees Society, clxxxvi, 1973), pp. 62–3. Similar practices obtained at Ipswich: Page, *VCH Suffolk II*, p. 139.

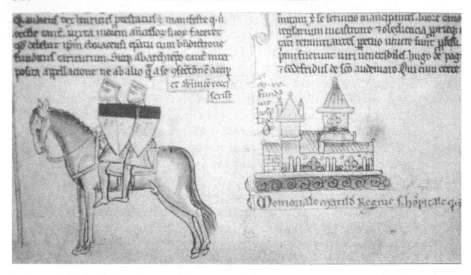

31. Matthew Paris's illustrations for his *Chronica majora* include a sketch of St Giles's hospital, Holborn, founded by Matilda, the first queen of Henry I. The hospital was eventually leased to the Knights of St Lazarus by the crown, but the figures on the left are Templars, so dedicated to poverty that they can afford only one horse. The hospital, which was later dogged by corruption and abuses, must initially have been a celebrated local landmark.

constituted a prominent landmark, well known to travellers who probably stopped there to make offerings. The ruins of St Giles's, Maldon, another twelfth-century foundation, reveal a cruciform structure of some size, while excavations on the site of St Nicholas's, York, have unearthed a stone-built and aisled hall of impressive proportions, as well as the above-mentioned chapel and cemetery. This mixed house of lepers and the aged poor was conceived on ambitious lines, as one would expect of a royal foundation initially intended for no fewer than forty patients.[34] With its two well-appointed chapels (one of which was over sixty feet long), the 'Maudlyn' at Exeter spoke equally well of the citizens whose testamentary bequests had been so conspicuously converted into stone and mortar, vestments and plate.[35] It is thus hardly surprising that certain houses became the focus of urban ceremonies and penitential rituals. The spectacular annual procession held at Norwich on the feast of Corpus Christi ended at the hospital of St Mary Magdalen, Sprowston, while a similar, if less ostenta-

---

[34] *Royal Commission on Historical Monuments, Essex II* (London, 1921), pp. 177–8; A. Clarke, 'Digging for Lepers', *Archaeology in York, Interim*, xix, no. 1 (1994), pp. 4–11; 'York Archaeological Trust Site Investigations, 148 St Lawrence Street, York, Summary and Assessment' (unpublished report, York Archaeological Trust, 1993/11). The leper house allegedly built by Hugh de Lacy at Kilbixy, in County Westmeath, during the twelfth century was 'a splendid piece of masonry' with walls as thick as those of the neighbouring castle: Lee, *Leper Hospitals*, p. 57.

[35] Orme and Webster, *English Hospital*, pp. 226–31. By 1363, the leper house at Romney was said to be 'truly destitute and devoid of men', but the buildings still suggested investment on a considerable scale: Brigstocke Sheppard, *Literae Cantuarienses*, ii, pp. 437–8.

tious, celebration at Grimsby was marked by a service for the mayor and all the burgesses at the *leprosarium* outside the walls.[36]

Since the travellers of medieval England were as reliant upon bridges as they were upon roads, the upkeep of both came to assume the same charitable status as care for the sick and needy. With its promise of a safe transition to paradise for both patient and patron, the *leprosarium* in turn represented a spiritual bridge, or roadway to heaven for those who had already endured their purgatory on earth. Like the anchoress, to whom he or she might so readily be compared, the medieval leper stood poised 'upon the bridge of heaven, above the sea of this world'.[37] The religious symbolism of this pleasing metaphor masks a more functional association between leper hospitals and bridges, which offered a host of practical benefits. The gatehouses and arches of suburban bridges provided shelter for those seeking alms in inclement weather, while the slow and congested traffic on approach roads promised rich pickings for the begging bowl. Wayfarers entering towns such as Banbury, Chester, Dunwich, Glasgow, Leicester, Newport Pagnell, Oxford, Wallingford and Wymondham would have encountered the more mobile residents of pontine *leprosaria* as they crossed over.[38] So crucial was the neighbouring bridge to the survival of St Leonard's hospital, Northampton, that the portcullis actually appears on its seal, below a figure the patron saint [**plate 32**], while the seal of the lazar house at Luanceston describes it as being '*inter aquas*', that is lying between the rivers Kemsey and Tamar.[39] Rural hospitals could be even more dependent upon the presence of a ford or bridge, which constituted their major connection with the outside world. Charters, statutes and other contemporary documents refer repeatedly to these important topographical features. Thus, for example, Bishop le Puiset's leper house at Sherburn stood '*iuxta pontem*'; and St Laurence's at Ickburgh, on the Norfolk-Suffolk border, was known as the '*domus leprosorum de novo ponte*', or 'newebrygge'.[40]

In practice, then, the requirement that lepers should dwell 'outside the camp' allowed a striking degree of physical proximity.[41] The residents of St Laurence's hospital, Bristol, lived near the east gate, within a few paces of the market, while those at Yarmouth colonised a similar site immediately to the north of the

---

36 W. Hudson and J.C. Tingey, eds, *The Records of the City of Norwich* (2 vols, Norwich, 1906–10), ii, p. 230; S. Rigby, 'Urban "Oligarchy" in Late Medieval England', in J.A.F. Thomson, ed., *Towns and Townspeople in the Fifteenth Century* (Gloucester, 1988), p. 67. French leper hospitals played an important part in the liturgical year of their communities: Jeanne, 'Group des lépreux', p. 56; E. Thevenin, 'La léproserie Saint-Lazare de Reims: Une espace de festivités', in Tabuteau, *Lépreux et sociabilité*; Kupfer, *Art of Healing*, pp. 144–5.

37 Salu, *Ancrene Riwle*, p. 107.

38 LAO, Episcopal Register iii, fo. 420v (Banbury); Baraclough, *Charters of the Anglo-Norman Earls of Chester*, no. 222 (Chester); Comfort, *Lost City of Dunwich*, p. 42 (Dunwich); Simpson, 'Lepers and Leper Hospitals', part 1, p. 306 (Glasgow); Nichols, *History and Antiquities of Leicester*, i (part 2), p. 323 (Leicester); *CPR, 1266–1272*, p. 114 (Oxford); P.H. Ditchfield, ed., *VCH Berkshire II* (London, 1907), p. 101 (Wallingford); and Blomefield, *Norfolk*, ii, p. 505 (Wymondham).

39 Markham and Cox, *Records of the Borough of Northampton*, ii, p. 333, and plate VI no. 5, facing p. 338; Orme and Webster, *English Hospital*, p. 200.

40 Snape, *EEA, 24, Durham 1153–1195*, no. 145; NRO, BRA/833/14/1. For Irish examples, see Lee, *Leper Hospitals*, pp. 35–6, 55; and for Wales, Cule, 'Diagnosis, Care and Treatment', p. 42.

41 Touati, *Archives*, pp. 60–64.

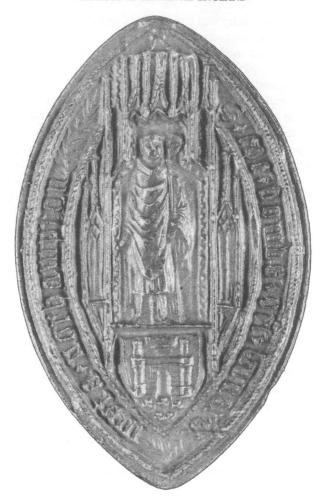

32. The connection between leper houses and bridges is underscored in the fifteenth-century seal of St Leonard's hospital, Northampton, which depicts the patron saint above, and the gate and portcullis of the neighbouring bridge below.

borough. Each of Norwich's five civic *leprosaria* commanded a gateway, with the result that anyone approaching from the north, west or south would have passed a hospital or some of its inmates [**map 5**].[42] That strong communal as well as familial ties flourished across walls and gates is apparent from the regulations passed in many English towns for the provisioning of adjacent *leprosaria*. Every Sunday, for example, the commonalty of Carlisle gave St Nicholas's hospital a 'pottle' of ale from each brewhouse in the city and a loaf of bread from each baker who had been trading there the previous day.[43] Comparable arrangements obtained at Guisborough in Yorkshire and at Shrewsbury, where, from the

[42] Rawcliffe, 'Topography of Suburban Hospitals', pp. 254, 256, 261.
[43] *CPR, 1340–1343*, p. 121.

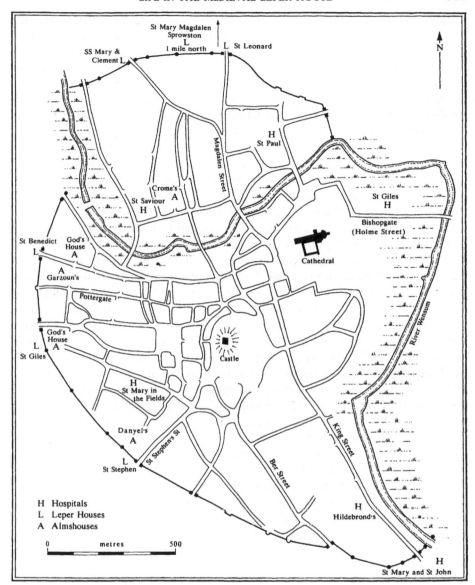

Map 5. Medieval Norwich and its hospitals for the sick, leprous and aged
(Phillip Judge)

twelfth century onwards, the lepers were allocated a double handful of corn and
a single one of flour from every sack opened for sale in the market.[44] Residents of
the hospital at Boughton, outside Chester, did even better, having been promised the right to exact a similar toll on all flour, grain, salt, cheeses, fish, fruit and

---

44  Page, *VCH Yorkshire III*, p. 314; A.T. Gaydon, ed., *VCH Shropshire II* (London, 1973), p. 106; Cullum,
   'Leperhouses and Borough Status', pp. 43–4.

other foodstuffs entering the city on horseback or by cart.[45] From the late twelfth century 'the Maudlyn' at Exeter, which benefited from a classic situation in fields at the city's southern gate, received three such tolls every week and additional ones on market days.[46] Urban guilds also offered support, both spiritual and temporal, to local leper houses, which might, of course, accommodate their own members. According to a local custom 'from a time beyond memory', the residents and staff of St Leonard's, Launceston, were permitted to join the town guild, whose dedication to St Mary Magdalen is, indeed, suggestive. Even their laundress belonged, although we cannot tell if the mandate that 'the prior of St Leonard's and his brother lepers cannot be rejected' actually permitted their physical presence at meetings. Regulations of the gild merchant at Southampton, confirmed in 1327, reserved two 'cestres' of ale to 'les meseaus de Maudeleyne' at every session, but this was for delivery to the hospital.[47]

Permission to stage an annual fair lasting up to a week on their property offered hospitals with parlous finances a useful way of earning money, both directly through the imposition of tolls and indirectly through the influx of people giving alms in cash or kind. To make the most of such a potentially lucrative opportunity the host institution needed plenty of open space, as well as freedom from the commercial restrictions that obtained within the walls of English towns and cities. A semi-rural situation, with easy access to major centres of population and production, was thus essential. Suburban leprosaria clearly fitted the bill in every respect. A hospital such as St Nicholas's 'in the fields beside Royston' could easily host the May fair approved by King John in 1213, since it had been assiduously enlarging its site through piecemeal acquisitions for some time. Royston's geographical position, right in the centre of the country, not far from St Albans, proved another advantage. St Bartholomew's, Dover, on the outskirts of an exceptionally busy port, drew great crowds to its annual fair, which survived into the nineteenth century. One of the most celebrated gatherings in England, the Stourbridge fair, held every spring near Cambridge, had its origins in a similar grant made by John to the local leper house [plate 33]. It was probably a recollection of his award of a fair to the leprosarium of St Mary Magdalen at Ipswich that prompted John Bale, a Carmelite friar turned evangelical Protestant, to eulogise the king as a model of Christian philanthropy. Bale was wrong to include Bury St Edmunds in his list of local lazar houses to benefit from John's largesse, as the grant of a fair to St Nicholas's hospital was actually made by his son. But he rightly appreciated the value of such privileges, which integrated many hospitals into the commercial life of the region.[48]

---

45  Baraclough, *Charters of the Anglo-Norman Earls of Chester*, no. 222. They were also entitled to a share of 'all packages of earthenware', of beasts sold at the horse fair and of bricks and timber carried by cart: Cule, 'Diagnosis, Care and Treatment', p. 45.

46  Barlow, *EEA, XI, Exeter1046–1184*, no. 98; Orme and Webster, *English Hospital*, pp. 226–7.

47  Somerscales, 'Lazar Houses in Cornwall', pp. 71–2; C. Gross, ed., *The Gild Merchant* (2 vols, Oxford, 1890), ii, p. 215. The chapel of St Nicholas's, Royston, which was unusually well appointed for a small house, may have been used as a guild chapel by the late fourteenth century, although the lepers had gone by then: Salzman, *VCH Cambridge II*, pp. 310–11.

48  These examples derive from Rawcliffe, 'Topography of Suburban Hospitals', pp. 267–8. Other *leprosaria* to benefit from the award of fairs include: St Mary Magdalen, Baldock, 1226 (S. Letters,

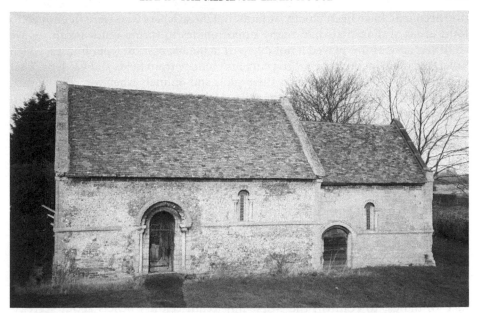

33. The chapel of the hospital of St Mary Magdalen, Stourbridge, which lay in the open fields outside Cambridge and was thus the ideal site for a major fair, celebrated throughout England.

Such concessions did not, however, always pass unopposed. Because of their location in exempt liberties under the jurisdiction of the Benedictine priory rather than the city, two Norwich *leprosaria* became embroiled in disputes with the authorities. The fair held annually at Sprowston from at least 1286 onwards generated particular friction, which twice erupted into armed conflict, while at yet another hospital, just outside one of the north gates, some of the lepers were selling substantial quantities of grain in contravention of the corporation's stringent rules about forestalling.[49] This kind of black market activity, which deprived the authorities of their tolls, must have been common and suggests that some local traders were prepared to do business with lepers if the price was right. Regulations for *leprosaria* at Dover (1372), Gaywood (before 1304), St Albans (1344) and York (1291) prohibited usury and other commercial activities undertaken for personal gain as 'monstrous in the eyes of God'.[50] The healthy

*Gazetteer of Markets and Fairs in England to 1516* (2 parts, List and Index Society, xxxii–xxxiii, 2003), i, p. 167); St Thomas, Bolton, Northumberland, 1226 (ibid., ii, p. 269); St Leonard, Chesterfield, 1196 (ibid., i, p. 91); St Mary Magdalen, Colchester, 1198 (ibid., i, p. 128); St James and St Denis, Devizes, 1208 (ibid., ii, p. 375); St Margaret, High Wycombe, 1229 (ibid., i, p. 63); St Mary the Virgin, Maiden Bradley, 1267 (ibid., ii, p. 372); St Mary Magdalen, Hedon, 1170 x 75 (ibid., ii, p. 399); St John the Baptist, Thetford, 1232 (ibid., i, p. 255); and St James, Westminster, 1290 (ibid., i, p. 237).

49   Rawcliffe, *Hospitals of Medieval Norwich*, pp. 46–7, 53. Such disputes were common. In 1302 the lepers of St Laurence's, Bodmin, were accused of levying illegal tolls at the fair: Orme and Webster, *English Hospital*, p. 188.

50   Bodleian Library, MS Rawl. B.335, fo. 4r (Dover); Owen, *Making of King's Lynn*, p. 107 (Gaywood); Richards, *Medieval Leper*, p. 131 (St Albans); Brown, *Yorkshire Inquisitions*, ii, pp. 127–31 (York).

brethren may have been chiefly at fault, but those lepers who were fit enough to tend crops and animals had many opportunities to turn a quick profit. As we shall see, agriculture played a notable part in the life of most leper houses, which bolstered their incomes by selling surplus produce from fields and gardens. That brethren should be free to visit their plots and animals whenever they wished was, for example, enshrined in the rules of the leper house at Lille, in northern France, and was implicit in the numerous grants of land, animals and grazing rights made to English hospitals.[51] However keen they may have been to remove suspects from within the walls, borough courts offered the same protection to lepers whose beasts or crops were stolen as they did to any other residents. In 1345, for example, the brethren of the hospital of St Mary Magdalen, Colchester, were involved in litigation over the ownership of six cows; and some thirty years later the Yarmouth authorities fined a local man 40*d.* for making off with sheep and cattle belonging to the *leprosarium* at the north gate.[52] As the Norwich records reveal, neighbours were always ready to join the hue and cry raised by a leper whose livestock had been misappropriated.[53]

Strict rules of enclosure, as at St Julian's, outside St Albans, where the gates were to be kept shut and entry and egress carefully monitored, appear, on the face of things, to confirm the worst nineteenth-century beliefs about segregation. Yet, if we examine the regulations of hospitals for the sick poor, such as St Thomas's, Southwark, we find identical (if not harsher) regulations for the brothers and sisters who made up the permanent staff, and whose lives were, in theory at least, subject to the same monastic discipline. Here, too, formal permission was necessary before anyone could leave the walled precincts, and then only with a designated companion on approved business.[54] Although they rarely encouraged it, the founders of England's larger, quasi-monastic *leprosaria* recognised that ambulant residents could not be prevented from getting out and about. Attempts to regulate their peregrinations were largely dictated by moral rather than hygienic considerations, since, as we have seen, pilgrimage remained a generally acceptable activity. Like the residents of other charitable institutions, lepers were generally forbidden to haunt taverns, eat in public places and, especially, to stay out after dark.[55] At Colchester they were not supposed to go

Allegations of usury were levelled against the residents of St Giles's hospital, Chester, in about 1300: Harris, *VCH Chester III*, p. 179.

51 Le Grand, *Statuts*, p. 201. At the *leprosarium* near Newton Bushell, Devon, the 'poor lazars' were to tend the gardens and grow vegetables, while fitter members of the community also helped the sick. The hospital was a very late foundation (1538), and its rules probably reflect general practice elsewhere: Orme and Webster, *English Hospital*, p. 251. Abbot Mentmore of St Albans specifically allowed the brother who supervised the agricultural labourers to leave the precinct whenever necessary: Richards, *Medieval Leper*, p. 135.

52 Jeayes, *Court Rolls of Colchester*, i, pp. 192, 196–7; NRO, Y/C4/85, rot. 1r.

53 Hudson, *Leet Jurisdiction*, p. 58. The case, which involved the illegal distraint, in 1312–13, of a female leper's beasts by a linen draper, suggests that the animals may have strayed onto one of the many drying grounds of suburban Norwich.

54 New College, Oxford, MS 3691, fo. 91v.

55 It is important to remember that the rules of *leprosaria* applied to the carers and priests as well as the sick. At St James's, Westminster, for example, the Augustinian canons were subject to equally strict regulations about eating and drinking outside: BL, MS Cotton Faustina A III, fo. 320r.

for a drink without the permission of the master, 'except as far as the cross standing at the end of a green which extends to New Hythe'.[56]

Aware that their charges might easily be diverted from the daily business of intercessionary prayer, ecclesiastical visitors did not make it easy for them to venture far afield without good reason. The inmates of St Bartholomew's, outside Dover, were constrained by a dual chain of command, whereby the master (who was himself leprous) could authorise leave of up to three days only. Anyone with more ambitious plans had to appeal directly to the sub-prior of Dover, whose verdict was final.[57] The hospital of St Mary Magdalen, Reading, was one of many others to require formal permission for extended periods of absence. Here also it was assumed that brethren would, from time to time, have good reason to travel, the only further *caveat* being that they might never do so alone. Indeed, *all* outings from the precinct, even to beg on the public highway, had to be made in twos or threes. This was, needless to say, a protective measure against spiritual contagion, lest any of the brethren succumb to the snares of the flesh, for which the penalty was immediate expulsion.[58] Lepers at Harbledown who went absent without leave more than twice, or persistently arrived home late, faced a similar punishment, although the statutes allowed modest amounts of outside recreation, as well as visits to the homes of relatives and friends.[59] Rules allegedly devised in 1154 for the hospital at Gaywood, near King's Lynn, permitted the residents two or three such outings annually. The threat of exclusion for a whole year should they stay away for too long must have deterred those who had hitherto abused the privilege. Certainly, the lepers were specifically warned to cease wandering about (*non sint vagabundi*), and to stop eating and drinking in the immediate environs of the house.[60]

Fear of abandonment into what was often a hostile and uncertain world must, in practice, have made hospital inmates tractable. Even so, undue intimidation or simple neglect provoked some spirited responses among the residents of English lazar houses. The catalogue of abuses to emerge in the 1290s during litigation in the court of King's Bench between the crown and the prior of Butley over the *leprosarium* at West Somerton was regarded by G.O. Sayles as proof of the wretched conditions customarily endured by 'the lonely, crippled and horrific leper'. These he compared to life in the Victorian workhouse.[61] The

---

56  Fisher, 'Leger Book of St John's Abbey', p. 122. At Dudston, Gloucester, the brothers had to return each day for vespers: Kealey, *Medieval Medicus*, p. 109.

57  Bodleian Library, MS Rawl. B.335, fos 3r, 4v.

58  BL, MS Cotton Vespasian E V, fo. 39r. Inmates of St Julian's hospital at St Albans had to obtain formal permission from the master for any outing, and from the archdeacon for an absence of more than twenty-four hours or a trip into 'the countryside'. Truants could not return without the abbot's pardon: Richards, *Medieval Leper*, p. 135. Similar rules obtained at St Mary Magdalen, Exeter: Barlow, *EEA, XI, Exeter 1046–1184*, no. 98.

59  Duncombe and Battely, *Three Archiepiscopal Hospitals*, pp. 211–13.

60  Owen, *Making of King's Lynn*, p. 107. The rule stipulates that 'if one of the sick absents himself for a month he will lose his support from the house for a year, and if [he is absent] for a year he will be expelled forever'. See Avril, 'Le IIIe Concile du Latran', pp. 50–51, 68–9, for concerns about excessive mobility, notably because of the opportunities it offered for sexual promiscuity; and Le Grand, *Statuts*, pp. 200–01, 227, 247–8, for similar instances in which miscreants faced a year's expulsion.

61  G.O. Sayles, ed., *Select Cases in the Court of King's Bench under Edward I, III* (Selden Society, lviii, 1939), p. c.

findings of a scandalised local jury and the subsequent rulings of the court suggest, however, that the prior's conduct was deemed reprehensible, and the forcible detention of lepers entirely unjustified:

> They [the jurors] said that all the lepers, before being admitted, swore an oath never to go out of the hospital, not to look over the walls, or climb trees to talk to their friends, or to complain in any way about their state, justly or unjustly . . . but to remain content with everything done to them without murmur or complaint. They said that no friend or stranger had access to the lepers, and that the prior had a large and strong dog tied up before the door of the hospital to prevent friends from enquiring into their condition or number, and assisting them in any necessity. Asked about the state of the house, the jurors said the chapel was roofless and very ruinous . . . After these disclosures, the prior was ordered to maintain, for nothing, the poorest and neediest lepers as the manor would support, to repair and maintain the buildings, *not to exact an oath in future, and to absolve those who had taken one.*[62]

The case did not end here. After what appears to have been a series of increasingly violent confrontations between the prior's men and the lepers, the latter staged a mutiny, aided and abetted by the parish priest and at least eleven of their neighbours. In October 1297 they looted the hospital, killed the guard dog and demolished the buildings which, they believed, had been erected by the prior for his own servants out of money that was rightfully their own. The ensuing legal battle resulted, like so many others, in stalemate, the lepers being pardoned any fine because of their poverty. Not surprisingly, the hospital itself never recovered, being left to collapse by the prior, whose guardianship had so demonstrably been found wanting.[63]

In less dramatic circumstances, the residents of smaller houses could up sticks altogether, and move on to a more appealing site. An inquisition of 1343 revealed that the lepers living in a tenement called 'le holdespitel' in Kingston, Surrey, founded by local people, had pulled down the buildings and transported them elsewhere.[64] The hospital of St Nicholas, Royston, seems to have been no more popular. Whereas Mass had once been celebrated regularly for the residents, it was found in 1359 that local lepers had 'for a great while past . . . refused to come and dwell there'.[65] Transience was, indeed, a feature of almost all England's smaller hospitals, which were rarely destined to survive unchanged from one century to the next.

A study of charitable provision in medieval Liège describes how the affluent, architecturally imposing and highly regulated civic *leprosaria*, to be found in the environs of Flemish towns, evolved from impoverished and uncertain begin-

---

62  BL, Harley Roll N 20; Mortimer, 'Prior of Butley', pp. 100–01. The prior had allegedly reduced the number of inmates from thirteen to eight so that he could pocket a greater share of the revenues. Although the house was supposed to take lepers 'in the greatest need', free of charge, one had paid over £8 for admission, while another had been nominated by the bishop of Norwich.

63  BL, Harley Roll N 20; Mortimer, 'Prior of Butley', pp. 101–3. By 1399, the annual value had fallen from £60 to about a tenth of that amount: *CPR, 1399–1401*, p. 114.

64  *CIM, 1307–1349*, no. 1859.

65  *CCR, 1354–1360*, p. 567.

nings.[66] Comparatively few suburban English leper houses developed in this way, the majority remaining at what might best be called an embryonic phase. Comprising a few cottages and outbuildings clustered around a chapel, they possessed neither the facilities nor the staff to impose even partial segregation upon what were essentially small, voluntary communities. Hospitals such as St Mary and St Lazarus, Sherburn, with its sixty-five beds and impressive complement of clergy, represented the summit of achievement; marshalled on the foothills beneath were lazar houses like Gilbert de Ley's late twelfth-century foundation not too far away at Witton, which could only support five patients.[67] The apostolic number of twelve, plus a warden (who was often either a priest or one of the lepers) generally constituted the optimum number.

Some houses bear comparison with the modest and short-lived *maisons Dieu* that sprang up across England during the fifteenth century as refuges for a few deserving individuals known personally to the donor.[68] John Kelle's petition of 1402 to the rulers of Beverley for permission to erect a *leprosarium* on a small plot of land adjoining a house at the north gate probably resulted from the need to provide for relatives, neighbours or servants. The 'lodge' in question cannot have long survived its first residents, for in 1494 another burgess proposed to rebuild it for a similar purpose.[69] Being both small and temporary, hostels of this kind are hard to trace and impossible to quantify. The late fifteenth-century 'spytell howses' established by Robert Pygot near his home in Walsingham, Norfolk, were, as we have seen, designed to accommodate a couple of lepers at most.[70] The *leprosarium* of St Leonard at Sudbury was not much bigger, but enjoyed a greater degree of security because its management had been entrusted to the mayor and corporation. The founder, John Colney, may himself have been leprous and was certainly the first warden. Significantly, although his statutes of 1372 threatened recalcitrant inmates with expulsion, the nineteenth-century antiquary who first transcribed them still felt obliged to note that victims of 'this loathsome disease' had to be strictly isolated.[71]

Did traffic move in the other direction? Recent research suggests that European leper hospitals were far from closed communities reserved for the sick and their carers. Together with the priests, servants, nurses and borders who lived in the precincts, there was a constant coming and going of outsiders, ranging from family members to administrators, ecclesiastical inspectors and business associates.[72] Indeed, whereas in many institutions the initial complement of lepers gradually dwindled as a combination of almsmen and fee-paying borders took

---

66  P. de Spiegler, *Les hôpitaux et l'assistance a Liège (Xe–XVe siecles): Aspects institutionels et sociaux* (Paris, 1987), pp. 59, 70, 74–5, 155, 158.

67  Snape, *EEA, 24, Durham 1153–1195*, no. 40.

68  P.H. Cullum, ' "For Pore People Harberles": What Was the Function of the Maisondieu?', in D.J. Clayton, R.G. Davies and P. McNiven, eds, *Trade, Devotion and Governance: Papers in Late Medieval History* (Stroud, 1994), pp. 36–54.

69  Leach, *Beverley Town Documents*, p. 42.

70  NRO, Norwich Archdeaconry Court, reg. Fuller, fo. 204r.

71  BL, MS Add. 19078, fo. 377r–377v; Hodson, 'John Colney's Hospital', pp. 268–74. The hospital accommodated just three lepers. On the death or removal of one, the other two chose his successor.

72  F.O. Touati, 'Les groupes de laïcs dans les hôpitaux et les léproseries au moyen âge', *Les mouvances laïcs des orders religieux* (Saint-Étienne, 1996), pp. 137–62; Tabuteau, *Lépreux et sociabilité*, passim.

priority, elsewhere there had always been a genuinely 'mixed' community where a few leprous individuals could be accommodated alongside elderly or disabled residents.[73] This was the plan of Archbishop Thurstan of York (d. 1140), who founded the hospital of St Mary Magdalen, Ripon, for the relief of blind priests and lepers from the liberty of 'Ripschire'. The former were to share one chamber, while the sick occupied a separate house conveniently near a bridge over the river Ure. As we have already seen, overnight accommodation was also available there for 'foreign' lepers, although by the 1340s both the detached house and the hospitality had long gone.[74] St Michael's, Whitby, and St Bartholomew's, Chatham, catered for a similar combination of the infirm and leprous, while at Gaywood, outside Lynn, the three sick residents were outnumbered by nine healthy brothers and sisters.[75] Even in the late fourteenth century, when fears of infection were rife, one Thomas atte Herst built a chapel and separate dwelling at Boughton-under-Blean for the shared benefit of 'lepers and other infirm persons'.[76]

Contact with the urban authorities responsible for managing the larger civic leper houses must have been frequent. The keepers or overseers of London's three principal *leprosaria* were exempted from other duties because of their obligation 'to go to the said places from day to day, to oversee the lazars and their houses there, and the rule and governance of the same and to chastise and punish offenders against their rule'. Allowance was also made during the late fourteenth century for the 'meritorious labour' and 'unpleasant and onerous occupation' involved, although attempts to keep the residents at home seem to have been at best sporadic.[77] It is harder to tell how far the officials of other English towns became personally involved in the routine administration of the leper houses at their gates. At Exeter, for example, one of the city council served as warden of St Mary's, being charged with the task of maintaining the fabric, drawing up accounts and paying the residents' weekly allowances.[78]

Less regular, but equally welcome, was the distribution of cash or goods which local people left to *leprosaria* and hospitals in their wills. A significant proportion of medieval testators made token gifts of a few pence or shillings to such institutions as a conventional act of piety, while others showed particular generosity to specific houses or individuals, whom they may have known. How were their alms allocated? Bishop Bitton's handsome bequest of 1307 to the lepers of his diocese was implemented by two officials, who visited forty different communities over a period of three years.[79] We may assume that they

---

[73] An inquiry at St Leonard's, Lancaster, in 1323, revealed three lepers and six paupers, although this is unlikely to have been the original complement: *CIM, 1307–1349*, no. 672.

[74] Raine, *Memorials of the Church of SS Peter and Wilfrid*, i, pp. 224–5, 228–9, 232, 236–8. St Thomas's, Bolton, another northern house, also received pilgrims and poor travellers: Hodgson, *Northumberland*, vii, pp. 202–3.

[75] Atkinson, *Cartularium Abbathiae de Whitby*, i, p. 329; Sweetinburgh, *Role of the Hospital*, pp. 70, 82 n. 62, 97; Owen, *Making of King's Lynn*, p. 106. St Nicholas's, York, was another 'mixed' house: above, pp. 298–9.

[76] *CPR, 1381–1385*, p. 448.

[77] Riley, *Memorials*, pp. 510–11; Sharpe, *Calendar of Letter-Book I*, p. 184; idem, *Calendar of Letter-Book K* (London, 1911), pp. 142–3.

[78] Orme and Webster, *English Hospital*, p. 227.

[79] See above, p. 291.

met and identified each recipient, soliciting prayers for the bishop's soul as they delivered his bounty. In Norwich, where, between 1370 and 1532, about a third of all testators left money to the five civic *leprosaria*, it is apparent that executors were often assigned this task. Aldermen William Loudon (d. 1493) and John Welles (d. 1495–96) both required that their executors should personally 'com thidre to vysett' the lepers and hand out alms, as did William Hayward, who died in 1507.[80] Such occasions no doubt served for the ritual commemoration of the deceased.

As we saw in chapter three, Christ's mandate that his followers should console the sick assumed particular relevance in the case of lepers, whose needs demanded succour from the living as well as the dead. Margery Kempe's desire to emulate the saints by kissing and exhorting the female patients in a lazar house near King's Lynn was, perhaps, unusual in an age so fearful of pestilential miasmas, although she followed in many eminent footsteps.[81] Notwithstanding the publicity accorded to the scores of medieval Magdalens who abased them-selves at the feet of lepers, most visits would have been less dramatic, but prob-ably more pleasurable for the residents. In contrast to the harsh regime at West Somerton, the *leprosarium* at Sherburn, County Durham, was extremely accom-modating about 'friends and well-wishers'. The latter were allowed 'to visit and comfort [the lepers] without hindrance, and stay overnight' if they had travelled far, although local people had to leave at curfew, when the gates were shut.[82]

Despite their general severity, Abbot Mentmore's rules for the hospital of St Julian likewise assumed that relatives and friends would wish to talk and eat together with the patients in privacy. Women of 'easy virtue and bad repute' were naturally banned, but arrangements could be made with the master for respectable female guests to be entertained in the residents' own quarters. Men of known probity needed no prior approval.[83] Smaller houses were less regu-lated. Pleadings in a case of assault at Sudbury, in 1265, revealed that two women and a youth were on their way to the local leper house (probably St Nicholas's) from the market at St Neots when a gang of malefactors (including a prostitute) tried to rob them. The incident certainly highlights the less salubrious aspects of suburban life, but it also suggests that local people may regularly have made this journey to call on friends and relatives.[84] Indeed, although regulations drawn up for the Scottish borough of Prestwick, in 1470, took the extreme and unusual step of prohibiting residents from visiting the nearby leper house, some people ignored them, and continued as before.[85]

The sale of indulgences kept many lazar houses afloat during periods of financial hardship. Although the great majority were probably bought from

---

[80] Rawcliffe, *Hospitals of Medieval Norwich*, p. 47; PRO, PCC Vox 5 (Loudon), 27 (Welles), Adeane 7 (Hayward).

[81] See above, p. 129.

[82] Richards, *Medieval Leper*, Appendix 2, at p. 127. Female relatives, but no other laywomen, were allowed to visit the *leprosarium* at Ilford, which explains why one resident allegedly disguised a prosti-tute as his sister: Dugdale, *Monasticon*, vi, p. 630; above, p. 264.

[83] Walsingham, *Gesta*, ii, p. 507; Richards, *Medieval Leper*, p. 134.

[84] C. Gross, ed., *Select Cases from the Coroners' Rolls, 1265–1413* (Selden Society, ix, 1896), pp. 1–2.

[85] Simpson, 'Lepers and Leper Houses', part 3, pp. 395, 418–19.

itinerant proctors, particular merit was to be gained from a personal visit to the hospital in question. Henry II may have been the most famous penitent to expiate his sins in an English *leprosarium*, but, as we saw in chapter three, he was certainly not alone. Like many other communities, the leprous nuns of Maiden Bradley offered forty days' remission of penance to contrite benefactors attending their church during the major feasts and their octaves [**plate 34**].[86] The lazar house at Preston, Lancashire, drew significant crowds with a more tempting promise of relief for five years and five *quadragene* (periods of forty days), which had been secured through the powerful patronage of Henry, duke of Lancaster. Unfortunately, not all the pilgrims who flocked to the chapel on high days and holidays displayed the humility and devotion expected on such occasions. In 1358, three years after the award of this valuable indulgence, a riot broke out, during which blows were exchanged and prisoners taken. The dispute appears to have arisen over claims by the rector of the nearby parish church to the takings, which in plague years exceeded £30 and were thus bound to attract predators.[87]

## Care of the body

The rule of St Benedict, which set the template for monastic life in the West, decreed that the sick should 'be served in the very deed as Christ himself', an especially poignant injunction in the case of lepers, whose sufferings seemed akin to crucifixion.[88] Since many of the *leprosaria* run under the aegis of religious houses gave priority to monks and their patrons, it is no surprise to discover that – in theory if not always in practice – the material wants of patients and carers were carefully addressed. Indeed, as we saw in chapter five, it was possible for the more affluent institutions to provide a palliative regimen of diet, bathing and environment that accorded well with current medical thought.[89] Although many communities experienced a precarious hand to mouth existence, others initially enjoyed a more than reasonable standard of living, well above the subsistence level at which a significant proportion of the medieval population was often obliged to survive. At Reading, for example, the abbot agreed to supply each leper with a basic daily allowance of half a two-pound loaf, a measure of grain and half a gallon of 'middling' ale (later increased to one loaf and a whole gallon). Five pence each month and regular oblations from the almoner on feast days enabled the patients to buy extra 'relishes', while the abbey also provided dairy cows, hay and equipment for the cart horse and support for

---

86  BL, Harley Charter 43 A 9.
87  W. Farrer and J. Brownbill, eds, *VCH Lancaster II* (London, 1908), p. 163; *Calendar of Papal Registers: Petitions, 1342–1419*, pp. 270–71. The hospital eventually won its case in 1364 after a hard fight and was allowed to keep 'the voluntary offerings wherein the revenues . . . chiefly consist': *Calendar of Papal Registers: Letters, 1362–1404*, p. 90. See also below, p. 349 n. 26, for a similar indulgence at St Giles's, Holborn.
88  J. McCann, ed., *The Rule of Saint Benedict* (London, 1921), pp. 258–9; Mesmin, 'Saint Gilles de Pont-Audemer', i, pp. 52–3, 193–7.
89  See Risse, *Mending Bodies*, pp. 184–90, for a general overview of the type of care provided by a prosperous European *leprosarium*, such as Melaten, near Cologne; and Horden, 'A Non-Natural Environment', for the application of the regimen in medieval hospitals.

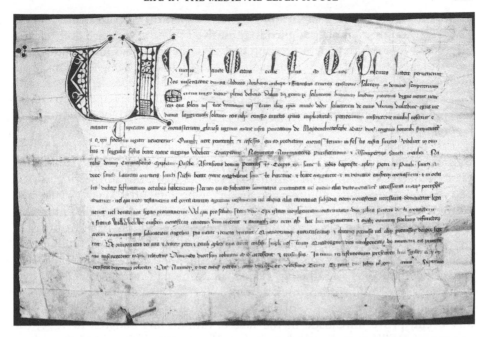

34. An indulgence of forty days' remission of enjoined penance, issued in March 1323–24 to the convent of St Mary, Maiden Bradley, a *leprosarium* for female religious, by the archbishop of Bar and the bishop of Ceneda. All confessed and penitent visitors to the house, as well as those giving alms or leaving legacies for its upkeep, might benefit.

the servants.[90] We know that meat was regularly eaten, because the disobedient forfeited their customary ration. Similar allocations were made at St Albans, where the award to each resident of a pig every year and an extra forty gallons of good ale at Christmas must have made Abbot Mentmore's strict rules easier to bear.[91]

Nor did monastic houses simply assist their own foundations. The hospital for lepers and the infirm established by Bishop Gundulf of Rochester (d. 1108) outside Chatham could rely on four quarters of corn and four of rye each year from Bexley abbey 'by way of charity'.[92] From at least 1275 onwards the almoner of Norwich cathedral priory recorded substantial handouts of bread and grain to the poor, sometimes specifically including the lepers at the city gates. It is now

---

[90] BL, MS Cotton Vespasian E V, fos 38r–39v. A two-pound loaf generated just over 2,000 calories and was often shared in medieval hospitals. Even if the ale was of the weaker variety consumed in London, a gallon a day was a generous allocation, on a par with that made to the Westminster abbey Benedictines: Rawcliffe, *Medicine for the Soul*, pp. 183–4; B. Harvey, *Living and Dying in England 1100–1540: The Monastic Experience* (Oxford, 1993), pp. 56–9.

[91] Each leper also received a quarter of oats and two bushels of salt every year: Richards, *Medieval Leper*, p. 133.

[92] Sweetinburgh, *Role of the Hospital*, p. 87 n. 82. Such arrangements were common. According to its foundation charter, the hospital of St Mary Magdalen, Exeter, was to receive fourteen loaves a week from the cathedral chapter, while the canons at Launceston gave seven to the nearby *leprosarium* in memory of an early benefactor: Orme and Webster, *English Hospital*, pp. 202, 226.

impossible to tell what proportion of the 139 quarters of corn distributed in 1279–80 was, for example, assigned to these five *leprosaria*, but such doles clearly offered a valuable safety net in testing times.[93] Other hospitals might sometimes help out, as was the case at St Leonard's, York, which set aside eight gallons of ale each day and eight 'messes' of meat on Sundays as an *opus leprosorum*. The master of St Nicholas's almshouse in Pontefract was likewise required to deliver either 15*s*. or a substantial consignment of oats every year to the community of lepers nearby.[94]

Lay patrons also expressed a lively concern about the long-term physical welfare of patients. Shortly before 1265, for instance, Sir William Legh settled over fifty acres of arable and pasture, supplies of marl, turf for heating, a reed bed and quarrying and milling rights upon the hospital of St Mary Magdalen at Allington, near Bridport, in return for daily prayers and masses for his immortal soul. In order to maintain acceptable standards of supervision, he then entrusted the house to the borough authorities, instructing them to conduct a full inspection twice a year in order to see that the chaplains were discharging their obligations and the lepers were being treated 'in a due and humane manner'.[95] As visitations and inquiries so often revealed, corrupt, incompetent or negligent administrators were prone to disregard the wishes of founders, which might, in any event, prove unrealistic in the face of diminishing budgets. In 1334, the master of William le Gros's hospital at Hedon stood charged with making wholesale cuts in what must once have been an extremely generous diet. Much to the inmates' annoyance, the daily ration of almost one gallon of ale and a 'mess' of beef, pork or mutton (herrings on fast days) had been reduced, while none of the twenty-four extra pittances due each year had materialised. Nor had the geese and piglets or the substantial quantities of pepper, cumin, salt, wax, oil, animal fat, cheese and butter to which they were entitled been distributed, even though many of these commodities could be put to medicinal use.[96] Dereliction of this kind had potentially serious consequences for the patron as well as the patient, since food and drink were often given in return for commendatory prayer. A grant to the *leprosarium* at Brook Street, Essex, of grazing rights and a tithe (tenth) of all the fodder, flax, cumin, geese, meat, cabbage, leeks, pears and onions deriving from specific properties of one William Doo, was intended to secure the remission of his own and his family's sins, and, significantly, those of his 'good lord' Geoffrey, earl of Essex, who had died excommunicate in 1144.[97]

Particular attention focused upon the provision of food for hospital patients

---

93 NRO, DCN 1/6/4. See also DCN 1/6/9 (1311–12), 26 (1395–96), 27 (1396–97). It seems likely that blanket references to 'the poor' in other accounts also included lepers.

94 Cullum, 'Hospitals and Charitable Provision', p. 30; A.F. Leach, ed., *Early Yorkshire Schools II* (Yorkshire Archaeological Society, Record Series, xxxiii, 1903), p. 6.

95 *HMC, Sixth Report* (London, 1877), Appendix, pp. 485–6. Concern about the physical welfare of patients was enshrined in the rules of some French leper houses, such as Meaux and Andelys: Le Grand, *Statuts*, pp. 186, 249.

96 York Minster Library, MS B 2 (3) a 5. Monastic patrons could be just as bad. In 1302, '*les povere freres malades*' of St Mary Magdalen, Colchester, complained to parliament that the abbot had destroyed the charter granting them 'bread, ale, cooked food and other types of victual': Strachey et al., *Rotuli Parliamentorum*, i, p. 157.

97 Fowler, *Registrum Simonis de Sudbiria*, i, pp. 210–12.

not only because this was a fundamental tenet of the *regimen sanitatis* but also, more immediately, because Christ had instructed his followers to feed the poor as a Comfortable Work. When founding a *leprosarium* at Newark for the soul of his late uncle, in the second quarter of the twelfth century, Alexander, bishop of Lincoln, provided the residents with a priest and a chapel for spiritual nourishment, and ninety-six baskets of grain, half of wheat and half of rye, each year from the episcopal estates to guarantee a regular supply of good quality maslin (mixed) loaves.[98] Whereas some hospitals derived the basic ingredients for bread, ale and pottage from market tolls, others were assigned tithes of particular crops, such as peas, wheat or barley from the granaries of benefactors like William Doo and his peers.[99] The more affluent houses, with significant landed holdings, either grew their own produce or were able to negotiate rents in kind, which might well include labour services as well as fuel and foodstuffs.[100] The late medieval shift from demesne cultivation to the leasing out of property for cash rents meant that, in some cases, a steady source of revenue was now assured, although the opportunities for peculation and mismanagement increased accordingly. So too did the vulnerability of struggling institutions to the economic upheavals of a market which demonstrably favoured the tenant rather than the landlord. As was the case in other hospitals, inspectors repeatedly criticised the failure to present and keep proper accounts and inventories, which in some *leprosaria* went hand in hand with deteriorating standards and falling revenues.[101] Inevitably, the few remaining patients suffered.

On paper, at least, once they could rely on a regular income from property or fee farms the better-endowed suburban leper houses tended increasingly to make a weekly allowance to residents, who were free to spend the money as they chose. At the Holy Innocents, Lincoln, for instance, the men were assigned one shilling a week and the women ten pence, which would have enabled them to live comfortably enough had the master not misappropriated a significant share of the profits.[102] The basic rate at St Bartholomew's, Oxford, stood at about 9*d.*, although here, too, a combination of asset stripping and laxity meant that, by 1391, certain customary doles were either overdue or had ceased altogether.[103]

98   Smith, *EEA, I, Lincoln 1067–1185*, no. 51.

99   As, for example, St Laurence's, Canterbury: Somer, *Antiquities of Canterbury*, Appendix part 1, no. x, p. 9; and both St Julian's and St Mary's at St Albans: BL, MS Cotton Nero D I, fo. 193r; Walsingham, *Gesta*, i, pp. 203–4.

100  St James's, Canterbury, faced serious problems when a dispute between the master and Archbishop Baldwin, in 1188, led to the confiscation of its oxen, sheep, ploughs and corn: Gervase of Canterbury, *Historical Works: The Chronicle of the Reigns of Stephen, Henry II and Richard I*, ed. W. Stubbs (2 vols, RS, 1879–80), i, p. 427. By 1343 the *leprosarium* owned the advowson of Bradgate church, worth £14 a year, over 170 acres of land and various properties in Canterbury, but faced poverty because of the injudicious award of corrodies: *CIM, 1307–1319*, no. 1830.

101  Hospital statutes often demanded the submission of annual or even quarterly accounts. See, for example, York Minster Library, MS B 2 (3) a 7 (Hedon); Orme, 'Leper-House at "Lamford" Cornwall', pp. 106–7; Richards, *Medieval Leper*, p. 128 (Sherburn); Rawcliffe, 'Passports to Paradise', pp. 13–15. French *leprosaria*, such as Pontoise, where the finances had been in a desperate state before reforms in 1315, made similar stipulations: Le Grand, *Statuts*, pp. 235–6, 243, 249.

102  *CIM, 1307–1349*, no. 293. Such rates compare favourably with the pensions paid by craft guilds to reputable members who could no longer work: Rawcliffe, *Hospitals of Medieval Norwich*, pp. 72, 87 n. 47.

103  *CIM, 1387–1393*, no. 313. Following an investigation into abuses at St Mary Magdalen, Hedon, in

As was the case at Norwich and Yarmouth, a servant or healthy brother would be dispatched to buy provisions in local markets and perhaps also help with cooking and cleaning.[104]

*Leprosaria* that followed a quasi-monastic rule were obliged, like all other religious houses, to observe certain dietary regulations initially established by St Benedict.[105] In such hospitals all food was supposed to be eaten in common at fixed times only, preferably in silence or to the accompaniment of sacred texts. Considerable variations none the less obtained from one place to another, a good deal of laxity being shown to the seriously ill, whose needs had, where possible, to be accommodated. At Dudston, outside Gloucester, all the patients were permitted to eat meat three times a week as well as on the major festivals, although they had to observe fast days (when fish or pottage would be served). Protests about the inadequacy of food and drink smacked of ingratitude ('on account of complaining the sons of Israel died in the desert') and could result, after three warnings, in the stoppage of the offender's substantial daily allowance of ale.[106] Enclosed communities were notoriously prone to grumble at mealtimes, and there may well have been a feeling that lepers, in particular, should be discouraged from giving rein to their grievances, lest they exacerbate an already serious imbalance of humours. Perhaps on account of their sex, the female residents of St James's, Westminster, incurred particular criticism in a visitation of 1267 because of their propensity to chatter loudly and appear at table without wearing the full monastic habit. The papal legate, Ottobon, who made the inspection, and found much else to deplore, recommended that readings from scripture should begin and end each meal in order to instil a proper sense of decorum.[107]

Freshly brewed ale from barley malt was not only a staple beverage but also a principal source of nutrition for all but the poorest households of medieval England. It formed a basic part of the daily diet in religious institutions for which evidence survives, *leprosaria* being no exception. Indeed, the physical deterioration of the leper's teeth and jaws must often have made it difficult for him or her to cope with solid food.[108] Ale might be purchased locally, supplied by a neighbouring monastic house or brewed on the premises. It came in varying strengths, the weakest (between 90 and 109 gallons per quarter) being drunk by

---

1475, the two remaining lepers were each promised 40s. a year for food and drink, while their servant was to have 33s. 4d. Six more lepers were to be accommodated, and £10 spent on much-needed repairs: York Minster Library, MS B2 (3) a 7.

[104] See above, p. 281. The servant of the leper house at Yarmouth was, in 1379–80, accused of stealing hens, and wandering about at night, perhaps on the hunt for other provender: NRO, Y/C4/91, rot. 10r.

[105] The first inmate of St Michael's, Whitby, who was a leprous monk, received a daily dish of meat or fish from the abbey, *secundum convenientiam dietae*, as well as ale and bread: Atkinson, *Cartularium Abbathiae de Whitby*, i, p. 329.

[106] Kealey, *Medieval Medicus*, pp. 108–9. Similar rules about complaints obtained at St Albans: Richards, *Medieval Leper*, p. 131. Meat was served three days a week and fish (or cheese and eggs) on four at Sherburn: ibid., p. 126. Benedictine regulations about diet, and the increasing disinclination to follow them, are discussed by Harvey, *Living and Dying*, pp. 38–41.

[107] BL, MS Cotton Faustina A III, fo. 320r.

[108] Dyer, *Standards of Living*, pp. 57–8. At Westminster abbey, ale provided 19 per cent of the energy value in the monastic diet: Harvey, *Living and Dying*, p. 58.

servants, artisans and the inmates of most hospitals and almshouses. In this, as in many other respects, the English leper had good reason to envy his or her French counterpart, who customarily drank wine, sometimes made on the premises from the hospital's vineyards. In the larger and more affluent establishments, such as the monastic house at Rouen, certain patients received up to a gallon each day, presumably for their servants as well. Largesse on this scale was unknown in England, but there were occasional bright spots in what must otherwise have been a somewhat monotonous regimen. During the 1240s, for example, the leprous nuns of Maiden Bradley received two tuns of good wine, shipped through the port of Southampton, as a gift from Henry III.[109]

Although, as we saw in chapter two, sub-standard meat and fish were consigned by urban custom to *leprosaria*, we should not assume that the residents were condemned to survive on a diet of contaminated foodstuffs. Rituals of this kind must often have served a largely symbolic purpose. Nor were founders and patrons indifferent to the quality as well as the quantity of the fare on offer. Clearly familiar with the *regimen sanitatis* and its emphasis upon the palliative benefits of proper nutrition, Bishop Kellaw insisted that fresh fish or good quality red herring (in season only) should be served at least once or twice a week at Sherburn. 'Particular care must be taken that nothing bad, mouldy or rotten is issued', he warned, urging that butter, eggs, cheese, beans and apples might be substituted if necessary.[110] Early founders such as William le Gros not only endowed their hospitals with land but also provided the livestock to guarantee a regular supply of fresh meat, dairy produce and poultry.[111] When entrusting the leper house outside Bath to the care of the priory in about 1095, Walter Hussey helped to ensure its self-sufficiency with a further gift of six oxen, four cows, sixty ewes and thirty rams.[112]

Thanks to their extramural situation, many of the major suburban houses were well placed to establish gardens, orchards, fishponds and home farms, with at least a few hens, pigs and geese, sometimes augmented by sheep and cattle. A list of possessions sequestered from the precinct of St Giles's, Holborn, in 1391, reveals that the hospital was still producing much of its own food, since the haul included eight horses, twelve oxen, two cows, four boars, twelve sows, 140 piglets, and an impressive number of geese, hens, capons and pullets. Most of these animals could have been kept in a relatively confined space, but the removal of four carts, two ploughs and quantities of agricultural equipment

---

109  Mesmin, 'Saint Gilles de Pont-Audemer', i, pp. 52–3; *CLR, 1240–1245*, p. 3; *1245–1251*, p. 126. At the *leprosarium* outside Noyon the punishment for certain offences, such as skipping Mass or leaving the precinct without permission, was loss of the daily wine allowance: Le Grand, *Statuts*, pp. 195–8.

110  Richards, *Medieval Leper*, p. 127.

111  See above, p. 105. In 1334 the master of William's hospital at Hedon was accused of removing stock and produce, including 360 sheep and a hundred quarters of barley, which suggests that it had, until then, farmed on a significant scale: York Minster Library, MS B 2 (3) a 7.

112  Manco, *Spirit of Care*, p. 24. Grants of land to *leprosaria* sometimes suggest intensive livestock farming. Thus, for example, Eudo Arsic and his widow together gave the Gaywood hospital, King's Lynn, thirty-seven acres of pasture and a fold course for 250 sheep: King's Lynn Borough Archives, KL/C56/2–3. Conversely, one thirteenth-century master of St Nicholas's, York, sold land in order to buy sheep, oxen, cows and other stock: Brown, *Yorkshire Inquisitions*, ii, p. 125.

suggests a more sustained investment in farming.[113] So too does the generous allocation of quantities of hay and straw harvested in the precinct and its adjoining meadows that was customarily made to corrodians, who were allowed to keep their own pigs alongside the hospital's herd. At least two of the leases recorded in the house's cartulary required tenants who were blacksmiths to maintain the ironwork on the ploughs and carts used in and around the precinct, while others contained clauses safeguarding rights of way for heavy agricultural implements.[114]

Gardens not only served a practical function for the production of herbs, fruit and vegetables, but also played a notable part in the *regimen sanitatis* as places for contemplation, gentle exercise and spiritual regeneration. It is now impossible to tell how often they were created for this use in English *leprosaria*, although one tantalising reference in Abbot Mentmore's rules for St Julian's suggests that their therapeutic value was clearly recognised. Here, the garden gate was to be kept locked in the interest of propriety, although any brother who had been phlebotomised or needed recreation because of his illness might have access. As we have seen, phlebotomy was generally discouraged in full-blown cases of *lepra*, but might be attempted topically, either to ease breathing problems or arrest facial damage. Since monastic infirmaries frequently possessed their own gardens for convalescent patients, it seems more than likely that leprous monks and their companions would have benefited from the same kind of tranquil and pleasing environment.[115]

Life in the more affluent English *leprosaria* did not, however, pass without more stimulating diversions. As in all monastic houses, special meals, libations and delicacies enlivened the liturgical round. The cellarer of Peterborough abbey was, for example, obliged to deliver four casks of ale to the lepers of St Leonard's to mark the major feast days, while extra dishes of fresh salmon and goose (a quarter each) then graced the table at Sherburn.[116] Anniversaries were notable occasions for dining as well as prayer. A generous master, such as Martin St Cross, would take practical steps to ensure that he was remembered with affection. On his death in 1259, he left 26s. 8d. for pittances to the lepers of Sherburn, along with 10s. a year for perpetual commemoration at a memorial dinner.[117] At Gaywood, the anniversary of the founder was marked by doles of 6d. *ad potandum*, similar sums being distributed on all the major feast days and on the death of a resident, so that the survivors could drink to his or her memory. Maundy Thursday, when Christ had washed the feet of His apostles, offered another opportunity for celebration. A steady flow of legacies from the burgesses

---

113 PRO, E315/38/171. What proportion of the fuel (1,000 faggots), oats, wheat, barley, malt, peas, beans and ale confiscated at this time would have been assigned to the lepers is uncertain, but the house seems to have been well stocked. It had evidently staged a recovery since 1355, when the outlook appeared bleak: below, p. 349.
114 BL, MS Harley 4015, fos 125r–125v, 131r; *CPR, 1374–1377*, p. 99; Williams, *Early Holborn*, ii, nos 1611, 1633, 1638, 1652.
115 Walsingham, *Gesta*, ii, p. 506; Rawcliffe, 'Threshold of Eternity', pp. 71–2; above, pp. 232–4.
116 BL, MS Cotton Vespasian E XXII, fo. 4r; Richards, *Medieval Leper*, p. 126.
117 J. Raine, ed., *Wills and Inventories I* (Surtees Society, ii, 1835), pp. 6–11. Not surprisingly, Archbishop Lanfranc's anniversary was observed in many Kent *leprosaria*, where doles of bread were distributed: Sweetinburgh, *Role of the Hospital*, p. 87 n. 82.

of Lynn, such as the butcher, Giles Grym, who in 1361 bequeathed one shilling to every inmate of the town's seven lazar houses, provided further comforts.[118] By then, however, the Gaywood hospital was experiencing financial difficulties, which made it increasingly dependent upon *ad hoc* outside support of this kind for subsistence rather than supplementary handouts.[119]

As might be expected, lepers living in the suburbs of London received some spectacular, if unpredictable, windfalls, largely because testators such as the former mayor, Robert Chichele (d. 1438), were rich enough to leave much larger bequests. Shared along with four other hospitals, his munificent legacy of £100 meant that the sick of St Giles's, Holborn, could rely on an extra two shillings each week for bread and ale for almost four years.[120] Conversely, the withdrawal of pittances proved an effective means of disciplining difficult patients, and ranked high on the list of grievances laid against corrupt masters. At the Grand-Beaulieu, Chartres, concerns were expressed in 1260 that the prior's failure to deliver them on time would undermine the house's religious ethos and alienate the inmates.[121]

As we saw in the previous chapter, the larger English *leprosaria* required all brothers and sisters to wear a habit or uniform, which, in theory at least, had to be replaced at regular intervals. High status lepers may well have been accorded a degree of laxity in such matters. As their health declined, the affluent female patients at Petit-Quevilly, near Rouen, were permitted by the bishop to own fur-lined cloaks and remain in bed during services.[122] Similar concessions almost certainly operated in English houses, although most inmates would have relied heavily upon whatever institutional provision could be made for them. Since clothing the poor ranked among the Seven Comfortable Works, it reflected badly upon the patron if they appeared ragged and dirty, like vagrants. On the other hand, ordinary medieval men and women did not accumulate large wardrobes or replace their clothing until strictly necessary. Even in royal and baronial households, where staff wore smartly coloured liveries, two sets of outer garments sufficed for the entire year. Such was the case at the hospital of St James and St Mary Magdalen, Chichester, where Bishop Seffrid assigned each of the eight lepers a linen tunic at Easter and a warmer woollen one for Christmas.[123] Residents of the monastic hospital at Reading fared rather better, each resident being entitled to a hood, a capacious tunic, a cloak and a blanket every year, and ten yards of linen for under garments whenever need arose. The

---

118  Owen, *Making of King's Lynn*, p. 108; King's Lynn Borough Archives, C12/5. For similar bequests see also C12/1/2, 3, 5, 8; C12/2, 7–9, 11; Isaacson and Ingleby, *Red Register*, i, pp. 2, 4, 76, 95, 116, 138, 149, 156, 158, 168, 171, 252.

119  *CPR, 1338–1340*, p. 412.

120  E.F. Jacob, ed., *The Register of Henry Chichele, Archbishop of Canterbury* (4 vols, Oxford, 1943–44), ii, p. 567. Bequests of 40s. or more to each London leper house were by no means uncommon.

121  Merlet and Jusselin, *Cartulaire de la léproserie du Grand-Beaulieu*, no. 354. At St James's, Westminster, in 1322, the master was ordered under pain of excommunication to assign all the customary pittances: BL, MS Cotton Faustina A III, fo. 322v.

122  Bériac, 'Fraternités des lépreux', p. 210. Complaints about negligence in the matter of dress voiced during a visitation of St James's, Westminster, in 1267 suggest that the sisters had grown extremely lax: BL, MS Cotton Faustina A III, fos 319v–320r.

123  BL, Ms Add. 24828, fo. 137r. This allowance contrasts favourably with the maintenance agreements negotiated by elderly peasants: Dyer, *Standards of Living*, pp. 175–6.

monks also presented a new girdle to each leper at Michaelmas and a pair of leather shoes at Easter. Interestingly, the annual entitlement also included a yard of serge to make stockings, which would have offered necessary protection for ulcerated legs. A laundress (who received board and two shillings in alms every year) was on hand to wash sheets, clothing and the long linen tablecloths also supplied by the monks.[124]

That filthy clothes and poor personal hygiene would exacerbate skin diseases was a lesson absorbed from the pages of medical literature.[125] We have already seen that hospital laundresses (and laundries) were viewed with ambivalence because of the temptations they offered, but such fears did not deter monastic *leprosaria* from engaging them. Since it was originally intended to accommodate sixty-five lepers of both sexes, Bishop le Puiset's hospital at Sherburn retained two washerwomen whose first duty every Saturday was to wash the patients' heads. Their clothing was to be laundered twice a week and their utensils cleaned every day. Such arrangements suggest that everyone possessed at least one change of garments, which the personal allowance of three ells of woollen cloth, six of linen and six of canvas (for towels) every year made possible. A tailor visited regularly to cut and sew the garments.[126]

Houses that enjoyed the relative security of a regular income were able to budget annually for whatever apparel might be needed. Thus, for instance, in 1267 the eight or so lepers of St Bartholomew's, Oxford, were together assigned almost £20 a year from the royal fee farm of the town, along with an additional sum of 65s. specifically for cloth.[127] Individual donations for the purchase of garments and furnishings are occasionally documented, one of the most generous being made by Henry III after the annexation of the earldom of Chester in 1237. Perhaps because the hospital of St Giles, Chester, had fallen upon hard times, or, more probably as an expression of his customary generosity to royal foundations, Henry settled an annual allowance of £5 upon it, while also authorising a number of supplementary grants over the years. These included two separate gifts of £20 and £10, made in 1243 and 1252, for clothing 'and other necessities', which by any standards represented a handsome subvention.[128]

---

124  BL, MS Cotton Vespasian E V, fo. 38r. At St James's, Westminster, the female lepers were ordered in 1267 to wear their linen or wool shirts in bed, rather than sleeping naked, which implies that undergarments were allocated: BL, MS Cotton Faustina A III, fo. 320v. Old linen towels were used as bandages in the royal household, a practice that probably obtained in many *leprosaria*: Myers, *Household of Edward IV*, pp. 124–5.

125  See above, pp. 226–7. When preaching to hospital staff, Jacques de Vitry stressed the importance of hygiene, lest squalid surroundings make their patients' health even worse: J. Bird, ed., 'Texts on Hospitals', in Biller and Ziegler, *Religion and Medicine*, pp. 102–3.

126  Richards, *Medieval Leper*, pp. 126–7. Water from a nearby spring, to which all the lepers had free access, was used for washing. At Ilford, the laundress was one of the few women allowed entry to the precinct: Dugdale, *Monasticon*, vi, p. 630. We know very little about the systems of water supply and waste removal in *leprosaria*, although some probably had drains: Gilchrist, *Contemplation and Action*, p. 43.

127  *CPR, 1266–1272*, p. 27. Bishop Alexander of Lincoln allocated £4 in annual rents to clothe the lepers of Newark: Smith, *EEA, I, Lincoln 1067–1185*, no. 51. At St Julian's, near St Albans, the individual allowance stood at 4s. a year: Richards, *Medieval Leper*, p. 133. The residents of St Leonard's, Peterborough, received forty ells of cloth annually from the abbot rather than cash: BL, MS Cotton Vespasian E XXII, fo. 4r.

128  *CLR, 1240–1245*, p. 205; *1251–1260*, p. 93. When confirming Queen Matilda's endowment of St

More typical is the endowment made at about this time by Scientia de la Gaye upon St Peter's, Bury St Edmunds, to which she promised 10s. a year in return for weekly Masses to be celebrated for her soul, the souls of her ancestors and of brethren dying in the hospital. Any spare cash was to be spent on new shoes for the residents.[129]

In practice, clothes must often have been recycled. Few medieval men and women expressed any scruples about wearing second- or third-hand garments, which were commonly passed from one person to another until they fell apart. Monastic cast-offs proved especially adaptable, irrespective of gender. Each of the thirteen sisters of St Mary's leper house, St Albans, not only received bread, ale and cooked food daily from the Benedictine cellarer, but was also promised a monk's pelisse and robe every year.[130] Whereas by the fourteenth century fears about infection meant that few healthy people would willingly have worn a leper's habit, no such concerns attached to the redistribution of items within a *leprosarium*. At Gaywood, for instance, every resident's best robe, cowl and chest passed, automatically, to another when he or she died.[131] Friends and benefactors must also have made *ad hoc* gifts of unwanted garments and money to buy new ones. At the hospital of the Holy Innocents, Lincoln, legacies, offerings from pilgrims and gifts were kept in a chest and shared among the residents as a clothing allowance until the master made off with the key.[132] As we have seen at St Nicholas's, York, abuses of this kind were fairly common, and demanded an effective system of shared accountability. To avoid fraud or theft, the lepers at Gaywood traditionally retained custody of the seal, relics, plate and books, while the healthy brethren managed the alms box, which had three separate locks for added security.[133]

In chilly north European climates, clothing the naked was rarely enough. Proper heating was for vital for all hospitals, which also needed a regular supply of fuel for cooking, brewing and washing. Some, such as Archbishop Lanfranc's foundation at Harbledown, actually owned substantial tracts of woodland (in this case over thirty acres), but others were dependent upon charity.[134] This useful and comparatively inexpensive type of alms proved extremely popular with founders and patrons, who, like Sir William Legh, often made specific

Giles's, Holborn, Henry II assigned an annual sum of 60s. to the lepers for better clothing: BL, MS Harley 4015, fo. 5r.

[129] *HMC, Fourteenth Report, Appendix VIII*, p. 156. Gilchrist, 'Christian Bodies', p. 14, suggests that lepers may have been obliged to go barefoot as a mark of penitence, although, with the notable exception of St Albans (see above, p. 129 n. 102), the documentary record provides no evidence of such practices. Skeletal evidence that some individuals interred in a leper cemetery at High Wycombe were 'ill-shod' and dirty almost certainly reflects either institutional poverty or previous neglect rather than deliberate abjection: M. Farley and K. Manchester, 'The Cemetery of the Leper Hospital of St Margaret, High Wycombe, Buckinghamshire', *Medieval Archaeology*, xxxiii (1989), pp. 82–9, at p. 87.

[130] Walsingham, *Gesta*, i, p. 203. The lepers at Whitby also wore second-hand monastic robes: see above, p. 265.

[131] Owen, *Making of King's Lynn*, pp. 107–8.

[132] *CIM, 1307–1349*, no. 293. Similarly, one Richard de Marsh left tithes to St Laurence's, Canterbury, to buy linen cloth: Somer, *Antiquities of Canterbury*, pp. 39–40, and part 1, Appendix XI b.

[133] Owen, *Making of King's Lynn*, p. 107.

[134] The lepers at Harbledown were also permitted by Henry II to remove cartloads of timber from royal woodland: Duncombe and Battely, *Three Archiepiscopal Hospitals*, pp. 205–6, 227–31.

allocations of turf, peat or kindling from their own estates. An early grant to the lepers of St James's, Doncaster, for example, included the right to mill grain free of charge and to take whatever wood they might need for building, fuel and the making of fences or hedges.[135] In 1259 the leprous sisters of Maiden Bradley laid claim to rights of 'oldewode underfotes' in Witham, which, along with common pasture in the woodland, had been settled upon them by a benefactor and was worth over £7 a year.[136] Hospitals such as St James's, Bridgnorth, which stood on the edge of royal forests, benefited from the ready availability of windfalls, as well as game abandoned by poachers. From 1224 onwards, Henry III allocated the residents a daily load of kindling, as well as occasional gifts of dead trees. A few years later he made a similar award from his woods at Condover to the lepers of St Giles's, Shrewsbury.[137] Generous as ever, Henry also recognised how valuable free timber could be for building projects. He granted the lepers at Wilton a single oak with which to repair their chancel, gave the *leprosarium* at High Wycombe ten, allocated fifteen to the community at Marlborough and no fewer than twenty to the nuns of Maiden Bradley, who enjoyed his particular support.[138]

Variations in size and wealth make it impossible to generalise about the standards of accommodation offered by English *leprosaria*, which might comprise little more than a few ramshackle roadside huts or cottages, but also included a number of substantial open-ward infirmaries lined with beds.[139] At one extreme stands St Nicholas's, York, where recent excavation has revealed an early twelfth-century aisled hall, at least twenty metres long and ten wide. Solidly built in limestone, it boasted two storeys at the western end, giving onto a communal area of open hearths at the eastern. The discovery of substantial deposits of chicken and fish bone suggests that the patients consumed sufficient quantities of protein (augmented occasionally by beef and bacon) from the outset. The arrival of fee-paying patients none the less demanded a more varied and high-status diet, which included teal, partridge, woodcock and a wide range of freshwater fish. This development seems to have coincided with the construction of a series of private chambers, a phenomenon deplored on both sides of the Channel, but one that ecclesiastical visitors were powerless to halt.[140]

Less impressive, but far more typical, were 'the seven cottages in which leprous people dwell' immediately outside the St Giles's gate of Norwich, which were acquired for their use by a local merchant in 1318. Another dwelling '*pur*

---

135  BL, MS Cotton Tiberius C V, fo. 255r–255v. Bishop Kellaw's revised rules of 1311 x 16 for Sherburn contain detailed instructions about allocations of peat, logs, straw and reeds for the lepers, additional provision being made for those near death: Richards, *Medieval Leper*, p. 126.

136  BL, Harley Roll N 23; *CPR, 1266–1272*, pp. 378–9.

137  *CCR, 1227–1231*, p. 509; *1231–1234*, p. 67; Gaydon, *VCH Shropshire II*, pp. 100, 106.

138  *CCR, 1231–1234*, pp. 6, 44; *1251–1253*, p. 358; *1268–72*, p. 220; *CLR, 1226–1240*, p. 23.

139  For the infirmary halls of St Margaret's, Taunton, and St Mary Magdalen, Glastonbury, see Gilchrist, *Contemplation and Action*, pp. 45–6. St Mary Magdalen, Hedon, had a hall lined with beds: York Minster Library, MS B2 (3) a 5.

140  Clarke, 'Digging for Lepers', pp. 4–11; 'York Archaeological Trust Site Investigations, 148 St Lawrence Street, York, Summary and Assessment'. By the 1260s each patient (only three of whom were lepers) 'had his own chamber by himself': Brown, *Yorkshire Inquisitions*, ii, p. 124. See Merlet and Jusselin, *Cartulaire de la léproserie du Grand-Beaulieu*, p. 176, for criticisms of the creation of private quarters, made in 1452.

*gentz feruz en la maladie de lepre'* stood nearby, on land in the city ditch, and was purchased by the authorities some twenty-five years later. It therefore looks as if a significant, but loosely organized, community congregated here. The other four extramural *leprosaria* would have looked roughly the same, since they each comprised a few cottages, maintained and supervised by a keeper who was, in turn, answerable to the mayor. One of these officials was reprimanded in the early sixteenth century for enclosing areas of land near the St Augustine's gate with hedges and ditches, which suggests that the residents had previously been obliged to make do with fairly modest plots and some common grazing for sheep.[141] On the other hand, as we have seen, they could rely on a steady stream of alms and legacies, as well as the occasional grant of timber for repair work.

Because of their concern about the availability of spiritual services, patrons were naturally anxious to fund the construction of chapels and decent lodgings for the priests who staffed them. A house as small as St Leonard's, Brackley, which accommodated just three male lepers in a separate dwelling, aimed to support two chaplains, one of whom served as master. The patron, Lady Zouche, did her best to ensure that all the buildings were well maintained, and had, by 1291, made an endowment sufficient to keep the fabric in a proper state of repair and the patients adequately fed.[142] Solicitude for the immortal souls of leprous men and women often marched hand in hand with practical improvements, although the former invariably assumed priority. In 1249, for instance, Henry III assigned the *leprosarium* outside Windsor ten marks to build a house for the chaplain, followed three years later by a gift of forty marks (just over £26) for substantial work 'in the court of the leprous women' who had settled there.[143] The provision of discrete quarters for men and women was, of course, essential in mixed houses, being one of the first things that Eadmer observed about Archbishop Lanfranc's two pioneering foundations outside Canterbury. The wooden houses constructed on the hillside at Harbledown were segregated so that the women remained some distance apart.[144] Although the ambulant brothers and sisters at Sherburn shared the same chapel, they too lived in separate 'houses', the female patients being under firm instructions to shut their door after services and keep to themselves. Similar rules obtained at Dudston, near Gloucester, and at St Bartholomew's, Dover, where the hall door that separated the male and female quarters was to be locked at night as a further precaution.[145]

In contrast with our relatively detailed knowledge of the possessions owned by the inmates of late medieval French leper houses, little can be ascertained about the type of goods and utensils that an English hospital patient was

---

141 Rawcliffe, *Hospitals of Medieval Norwich*, pp. 47–55; NRO, NCR, 16B, Norwich Assembly Book, 1491–1553, fo. 101v.

142 Or so it then seemed. In 1304, the bishop of Lincoln issued an indulgence to support 'the poor and sick' in the hospital: Hill, *Register of Bishop Oliver Sutton*, ii, pp. 93–5; LAO, Episcopal Register iii, fo. 64r.

143 *CLR, 1245–1251*, pp. 252, 334.

144 Eadmer, *Historia novorum in Anglia*, ed. M. Rule (RS, 1884), pp. 15–16.

145 Richards, *Medieval Leper*, p. 125; Kealey, *Medieval Medicus*, p. 108; Bodleian Library, MS Rawl. B.335, fo. 4r. At Amiens, female servants were not allowed to make the beds in the male dormitory until the patients had vacated the room. Anyone who needed constant nursing would be removed elsewhere so that a woman could attend him with propriety: Le Grand, *Statuts*, p. 227.

expected to provide, or might hope to be given, on admission.[146] The strict monastic rules concerning shared property and communal life that had initially obtained in the larger *leprosaria* must often have been ignored. Abbot Mentmore's recognition that the standard annual allowance at St Julian's did not suffice to provide all necessities, and that the residents might supplement this deficiency with their own goods, undoubtedly sanctioned a widespread practice. So long as they were honestly acquired and passed into common ownership on the death of the patient, he felt that a few creature comforts would help to mitigate the rigours of disease.[147] The patrons of England's larger hospitals certainly intended their foundations to be well stocked, although the temptation to sell or steal equipment was hard to resist, especially when inventories had not been properly kept. Bishop Kellaw expected that the kitchen at Sherburn would contain a hearth and 'appropriate utensils', comprising a lead cistern, earthenware pots, a table, a vessel for wine and bowls and basins for beer and for washing. Other tubs, cisterns pans and tripods would be used for brewing ale and laundering clothes. By the early fifteenth century, however, the house had been sadly depleted, for, as the number of lepers dwindled, administrative standards plummeted and abject poverty ensued. At St Mary Magdalen, Hedon, where just two lepers remained in 1475, one of the chaplains likewise reported attempts to sell off goods, such as brass pots, brewing vats and even bells, for personal profit.[148]

As the proliferation of royal and episcopal letters of protection reveals, most of England's smaller hospitals and *leprosaria* faced serious financial problems by the late thirteenth century, but we cannot automatically assume that all their residents were destitute. Richard Wellys, *leprosus*, whom we met in the previous chapter, was able to dispose of about £10 in cash and over £3 in uncollected debts, as well as unspecified moveables that were to be sold by his executors for pious uses. His kinsman, Henry, who had preceded him into the leper community at Fye bridge, Norwich, appointed two other *leprosi* to administer his estate in 1448, instructing them to discharge his debts, pay for his funeral and perform whatever charitable works they thought most beneficial for his soul. At just 11s., his cash bequests were far more modest, but not negligible.[149]

The level of personal autonomy evidently enjoyed by the residents of at least some late medieval extramural leper houses contrasts sharply with the regime still, theoretically, in force at places bound by the strictures of a religious rule. Here the imposition of monastic discipline was, from the outset, designed to create an atmosphere conducive to spiritual regeneration and collective intercession. Most houses about which evidence survives adopted a clear command

---

[146] French *leprosaria*, such as those at Meaux, Noyon, Pontoise and Andelys, often provided a list of necessary possessions, including a bed, linen and utensils, which either the hospital or the leper had to supply on entry: Le Grand, *Statuts*, pp. 188–9, 198–9, 236–7; Wellcome Library, Western MS 5133/1. One such sixteenth-century list survives from Launceston, but we cannot tell how old this practice was: Orme and Webster, *English Hospital*, p. 204.

[147] Walsingham, *Gesta*, ii, pp. 507–8.

[148] Richards, *Medieval Leper*, p. 127; Allan, *Sherburn Hospital*, unpaginated, sub 'Bishop Langley's Statutes'; York Minster Library, MS B 2 (3) a 7.

[149] NRO, NCC, reg. Jekkys, fo. 43r (Richard); Aleyn, fo. 9r (Henry).

structure headed by a master or warden, who might himself be leprous. As was the case at St Bartholomew's, Dover, he would, in that event, often work in tandem with a healthy colleague, who could discharge whatever tasks it was no longer possible or appropriate for him to perform.[150] Such a position was particularly suitable for a priest or member of a religious order who had himself contracted the disease. In 1392, for example, Thomas Wyke, a friar who had to leave his convent because of leprosy, was granted a dispensation either to be master of 'a poor hospital', become a hermit or occupy a benefice (presumably without the cure of souls).[151] In the larger mixed houses, such as Dover and Sherburn, a leprous 'prioress' would assume authority over the sisters, being answerable to the master for their good behaviour, while a 'prior' managed the men.[152]

Expulsion was, as we have seen, the ultimate penalty for serious misconduct, but there were many other ways of imposing order. A few houses, including St James's, Westminster, followed the monastic practice of chastising offenders with the rod, although the seriously ill were clearly exempt from such draconian treatment. Because it had to employ tonsured priests (there were eight Augustinian canons in 1267) to provide spiritual services for patrons as well as the sixteen sisters, and also needed a substantial staff of male and female servants, the risks of sexual incontinence seemed especially great in this type of establishment. Revised statutes of 1267 threatened miscreants, whether leprous or healthy, with a hard beating before the entire chapter, which was then left to impose a suitable act of penance.[153] Bishop Kellaw felt that the best way of enforcing the rules at Sherburn would be to give the lepers 'a stick which their prior should look after like a schoolmaster, with which he is to correct the disobedient and those who break the rules'. Recognising that some residents would refuse to be punished in this way, he did, however, institute an alternative penalty of fasting on bread and water.[154] A prescribed period on short commons seems to have been widely adopted, sometimes being invested with a ritual element of public shame and contrition. At Reading, for example, the meal that had been forfeited was placed on the middle of the common table and shared among the others, while the offender himself had to sit apart (probably on the floor) and consume his bread and water from the bench, without a tablecloth.[155] Defamation of, or disobedience to, the master, lying, wrath, pride, obduracy or noisy behaviour could each incur this humiliating penalty, while sexual activity, as we have seen, led to immediate ejection. Significantly, though, at St Albans the

---

150 Bodleian Library, MS Rawl. B.335, fo. 2r.

151 *Calendar of Papal Registers: Papal Letters, 1362–1404*, p. 454.

152 Bodleian Library, MS Rawl. B.335, fo. 2v; Richards, *Medieval Leper*, p. 125.

153 BL, MS Cotton Faustina A III, fo. 320v. Fasting on bread and water was the customary penalty for lesser crimes. The catalogue of abuses recorded at St James's during the fourteenth century suggests that such penalties either had little effect or were seldom enforced. Since the house cannot then have accommodated more than the token leper, the presence of so many healthy sisters must have encouraged misconduct: ibid., fo. 322r; Page, *VCH London I*, pp. 542–5.

154 Richards, *Medieval Leper*, p. 127. After the third such fast, the offender would be ejected. A similar choice between beating or fasting obtained at Dudston: Kealey, *Medieval Medicus*, p. 109.

155 BL, MS Cotton Vespasian E V, fo. 39r. This was a standard form of punishment in many French leper houses: Le Grand, *Statuts*, pp. 183, 185, 196, 200–02, 228–30, 248.

principal incentive to meek compliance constituted the prospect of loss of liberty, since breaches of the many regulations meant confinement within the precinct for a period commensurate with the offence.[156]

The successful management of any *leprosarium* depended, in the final resort, upon a degree of consensus, or at least malleability, on the part of the residents, which in larger houses was achieved in regular chapter meetings of all but the permanently bedridden. Lest anyone should claim ignorance of the rules, the statutes of many hospitals required that they should not only be explained carefully to each new entrant two or three times *before* admission, but also declaimed 'clearly in the common tongue' by the master at specific intervals before the whole community. Visitations of St James's, Westminster (1267), and of St Mary's, Ilford (1346), revealed so many problems that it seemed necessary to undertake this exercise at least four times a year, while at the Grand-Beaulieu, Chartres, monthly expostulations were required.[157] Chapters generally met once a week, as at Harbledown, where, according to regulations of 1298–99, their principal items of business were the public confession of sins and correction of lapses, notably with regard to breaches of the statutes and any failure to discharge the requisite burden of suffrages. Because of their gravity, cases of sexual incontinence were to be determined by a separate tribunal, comprising the prior, the prioress, two brothers and two sisters.[158] In most houses, however, the attribution of blame and choice of punishment were issues for collective rather than individual action, not least because one sin contaminated the entire community. The master of St Nicholas's, York, had clear instructions to correct any transgressions 'by counsel of the brothers and sisters', while at St Albans the leprous brethren maintained a strong sense of cohesion by holding 'common councils' where any matters of concern to their fellowship were discussed privately in the church.[159] Men or women who betrayed the secrets of the chapter invited retribution, which at Reading entailed a protracted fast on bread and water, with all the attendant ignominy involved.[160]

Chapters were not summoned simply for the imposition of discipline. Important business concerning their hospital and its possessions would often be transacted before all the assembled residents, while accounts and inventories had, in principle, to be rendered at prescribed intervals and managerial problems addressed.[161] Some communities, such as St Nicholas's, exercised a veto on

---

156   Richards, *Medieval Leper*, p. 135.
157   BL, MS Cotton Faustina A III, fo. 319v; Dugdale, *Monasticon*, vi, p. 630; Merlet and Jusselin, *Cartulaire de la léproserie du Grand-Beaulieu*, p. 155. The relevant parts of the rules at St Albans were also to be read in English four times a year: Richards, *Medieval Leper*, p. 136. Such a task was thirsty work, as the regulations of 1239 for the *leprosarium* at Lille recognised. They assigned two pints of wine as a reward: Le Grand, *Statuts*, pp. 202–3.
158   Duncombe and Battely, *Three Archiepiscopal Hospitals*, pp. 211–13. After two similar offences, recidivists at St James's, Westminster, were to be corrected by the abbot, rather than the chapter: BL, MS Cotton Faustina A III, fo. 320r.
159   Brown, *Yorkshire Inquisitions*, ii, p. 124; Richards, *Medieval Leper*, pp. 135–6. At Colchester, the chapter decided upon appropriate punishments: Fisher, 'Leger Book of St John's Abbey', p. 122.
160   BL, MS Cotton Vespasian E V, fo. 39r.
161   At the hospital of St Mary Magdalen, Hedon, for instance, the master was required to present an annual account 'to the brethren of the place' for audit before their chapter: York Minster Library, MS B 2 (3) a 7. Similar rules obtained at Brives from 1259 onwards, where a supplementary statement of

admissions and protested when masters or patrons acted without proper consul-tation.[162] Being understandably inclined to prefer affluent candidates who could contribute to general funds, the lepers themselves were, as we have seen, warned to eschew the financial blandishments of ineligible persons.[163] But not all meet-ings dealt with such routine issues. A major triumph by the nuns of Maiden Bradley over the rector of Kidderminster, who had attempted to withhold twenty marks a year from their ecclesiastical revenues, was, for example, cele-brated in 1341 at a special assembly of their commonalty. In the presence of all the sisters, both leprous and healthy, and their priests, this *homo ingratus* made a solemn oath upon the Evangelists that he would henceforward pay the money without demur.[164]

Although many English leper houses fell distressingly short of the standards expected by their founders and early benefactors, at least some appear to have made continuous efforts to address the physical requirements of the sick. Yet this was not their primary objective. As every good Christian knew, the rules and mechanisms that ensured the smooth running of hospitals and all other terres-trial institutions were a necessary consequence of the Fall, when disorder and wilful disobedience had first reared their ugly heads, along with disease. In contrast to mankind's faltering attempts to achieve a semblance of good govern-ment, the City of God required neither regulations nor remedies. With their sights set firmly upon this heavenly Jerusalem, patrons – and no doubt many of the patients – were inevitably more exercised about the fate of the immortal soul than its perishable shell. Such, indeed, was the message regularly preached to the residents of French (and almost certainly English) *leprosaria*, who were coun-selled to model themselves upon the saints, and embrace suffering rather than seeking an earthly cure.[165]

## Care of the soul

When commending the work of the new orders of hospitallers in his *Historia Occidentalis*, Jacques de Vitry singled out their selfless devotion to the spiritual health of the sick. 'Their chaplains minister to the indigent and invalids', he observed approvingly,

> . . . instruct the ignorant with the word of divine preaching, console the faint hearted and feeble, and exhort them to long suffering and actions of thanks with every humility and devotion. By night and day, they continually celebrate the divine offices in a common chapel so that all the infirm can hear them from their beds. They also assiduously and solicitously hear the ailing's confessions, supply

receipts and expenses was to be submitted on three further occasions during the year: Le Grand, *Statuts*, p. 210.

162 Brown, *Yorkshire Inquisitions*, ii, p. 126.

163 See above, p. 303; and Risse, *Mending Bodies*, pp. 168–9.

164 BL, MS Add. 37503, fos 55r–56r; Kemp, 'Maiden Bradley Priory', pp. 105–6. Such meetings occurred in French houses, too: Merlet and Jusselin, *Cartulaire de la léproserie du Grand-Beaulieu*, no. 114; Mesmin, 'Saint Gilles de Pont-Audemer', ii, pp. 121–5, 206–7.

165 Bériou and Touati, *Voluntate Dei leprosus*, pp. 42, 58, 67.

them with extreme unction and other sacraments, and give a fitting burial to the dead.[166]

In these few words, de Vitry provides a succinct account of an ideal towards which all but the most humble and destitute of hospitals aspired. For, however moribund the patients might be, their souls (and, of course, the souls of their benefactors) were always capable of redemption.

Ecclesiastical authorities stressed the importance of preaching the word of God in *leprosaria*, both as a source of comfort and as an exhortation to patience and penitence. The subject matter of sermons delivered by Humbert de Romans (d. 1277) and others, with its growing emphasis on repentance and abjection, strikes modern sensibilities as harsh. From a contemporary standpoint, though, the exercise might be compared to the way a firm but skilful physician introduced his patient to the rigours of a life-saving new regimen. Indeed, however robust their message, preachers were as sensitive as medical practitioners to the physical and psychological state of their congregations, and aware of the damage that an ill-judged word or phrase might cause. Thus, for example, Humbert advised clergy who were unused to addressing lepers:

> Let us take care, when we speak to them, never to describe their malady by the name of leprosy, because this distresses them greatly. We should only speak of it in general terms. And let us avoid, in the same way, anything which may exasperate them. It is important to speak to them with gentleness and compassion.[167]

As we saw in chapter three, the first step upon the road to spiritual health was through confession, a sacrament administered at some hospitals upon arrival, so that the patient would be ready to start at once upon the process of recovery. An early thirteenth-century *Summa pastoralis*, written for the guidance of an unnamed archdeacon of Paris, urged him to preach regularly in person for the education and *salus* of lepers, and to pay attention to the appointment of suitable confessors. The latter were to be 'good, humble and patient', notable for their loathing of *spiritual* rather than physical leprosy, 'which our Saviour never regarded with abomination, He who touched with his hand and cured the leper'.[168]

The cure of souls posed something of a challenge in outlying areas.[169] Ambulant inmates of St Thomas's, Bolton, were required, along with all the other villagers, to travel three times a year to Edlingham parish church to make a confession, although Mass was celebrated for the entire local community in the hospital chapel three times a week.[170] Where possible, however, measures were

---

166  Bird, 'Texts on Hospitals', p. 110.
167  N. Bériou, 'L'image de l'autre: le lépreux sous le regard des predicateurs, au moyen âge', *L'Histoire Aujourd'hui* (Liège, 1988), p. 5. Sensitivity on this score is invariably regarded as a modern reaction against medieval 'barbarism' and stigmatisation: Gould, *Don't Fence Me In*, p. 35. Yet it was far from uncommon in the Middle Ages.
168  Avril, 'Le IIIe Concile du Latran', pp. 72–3.
169  At Corbridge, in Northumberland, for example, a chaplain was required 'to celebrate mass for the lepers' every Sunday and major feast day, but by the fourteenth century it was hard to find one: *CIM, 1377–1388*, no. 76.
170  Hodgson, *Northumberland*, vii, pp. 205–6. Patients at the *leprosaria* outside Lille and Brives had also

taken to keep the leprous safely near home, especially once fears of contagion became established. As the new statutes for St Mary's, Ilford, explained in 1346: it was perilous for the healthy to consort with *leprosi*, and a scandalous dereliction on the part of the authorities that they should, in any event, be forced to leave the precinct in search of necessary consolation. To this end, an earlier arrangement for the appointment of two priests and a clerk to serve in the hospital was confirmed, their duties being to hear confessions, impose penance, grant absolution, celebrate the Eucharist, deliver the *viaticum* to those near death and bury them afterwards.[171] Anxious to implement the ruling of the Fourth Lateran Council with regard to annual confession, and acutely aware of the need to remove all traces of moral pollution from their wards, the larger English *leprosaria* watched over the spiritual hygiene of their patients.[172] The legate Ottobon's insistence that, at St James's, Westminster, each of the sisters should make a public confession once a week and take communion four times every year far exceeded the Council's requirements, and was subsequently modified.[173] But many houses shared his vigilance on this score. Bishop Kellaw's revised statutes for Sherburn specifically required one of the four priests to minister to the sick, provide the solace of the confessional and read the gospel on feast days and festivals in the *domibus leprosorum* to those who were too ill to go to church. He also built a chapel especially for the patients, where a solemn Mass of the Blessed Virgin was offered daily 'for the benefit of the brothers too weak or ill to arise early' and attend the main services.[174]

The bishop's concerns underline the centrality of the Mass in medieval hospital life. Described by St Ambrose as 'the sure protection and health of soul and body, and the remedy for all spiritual and physical ills', it was in every sense a *medicina sacramentalis*, suffused with occult power.[175] We saw in chapter two what a potent effect the sight of the Host at the moment of elevation might have upon the body's vital spirits, and, although the leper could not hope for much in

---

to confess and take communion three times a year, while those at Amiens were expected to confess frequently to an approved priest: Le Grand, *Statuts*, pp. 202, 209, 226; Bériou and Touati, *Voluntate Dei leprosus*, pp. 42, 58, 67.

171 Dugdale, *Monasticon*, vi, pp. 630.

172 Financial interests were also at stake in the wealthier hospitals, since each patient would customarily make an offering on important occasions in the ecclesiastical year. At Launceston, for example, the parochial chaplain, rather than the hospital priest, celebrated Mass on principal feast days and heard confessions during Lent, thereby pocketing all the proceeds: Orme and Webster, *English Hospital*, p. 202.

173 BL, MS Cotton Faustina A III, fo. 319v. A later visitation report of 1322 stressed that the sick should always confess to the same priest, who would be aware of their spiritual failings: ibid., fo. 321r. See also Bodleian Library, MS Rawl. B.335, fo. 4v, for similar concerns at Dover; and Avril, 'Le IIIe Concile du Latran', pp. 54–65.

174 Richards, *Medieval Leper*, pp. 125, 127. At Harbledown, in 1371, the priest was instructed to hear the patients' confessions and minister the sacraments by day and night in the church: Duncombe and Battely, *Three Archiepiscopal Hospitals*, no. 34.

175 P. Camporesi, *The Fear of Hell: Images of Damnation and Salvation in Early Modern Europe* (Oxford, 1991), p. 146. St Jerome described Christ as the *solus medicus*, who was both 'the physician and the medication': A.S. Pease, 'Medical Allusions in the Works of St Jerome', *Harvard Studies in Classical Philology*, xxv (1914), pp. 73–86. When accompanied by appropriate marks of penance, such as fasting, certain Masses, such as that of St Anthony, were believed to offer protection against *lepra* and other diseases: W.G. Henderson, ed., *Missale ad usum insignis ecclesiae Eboracensis, II* (Surtees Society, lx, 1872), pp. 233–4.

the way of physical improvement, his or her soul might still derive inestimable benefits from regular exposure to the body and blood of Christ [plate 5]. Few English *leprosaria* possessed the financial resources to support more than a single priest (which effectively reduced the number of Masses to one a day), and many had to rely upon visits from parochial clergy, who were expected to address the spiritual needs of less structured communities. Yet, where possible, efforts were made both by ecclesiastical and lay benefactors to fulfil the most pressing and meritorious of all their obligations to the poor of Christ. Not surprisingly, some patrons used their influence to secure papal exemptions from interdicts, which permitted the celebration of Mass in an unobtrusive manner, without bells or music, even though other places were forbidden to administer any of the sacraments.[176]

The rich and powerful were not alone in their desire to ensure that the round of religious observance ran smoothly and effectively. Several comparatively small hospitals accumulated collections of liturgical furniture that far exceeded the basic requirements deemed necessary to honour the Eucharist. A royal commission of inquiry held at Lincoln in 1316 revealed that, despite its sad history of decline, the *leprosarium* of the Holy Innocents still retained a silver chalice, a 'good' breviary, two 'good' psalters, two antiphoners, various vestments, lights and a thurible. Unfortunately, two missals had vanished and the chapel roof needed repairs.[177] The outlook seemed brighter at St Mary Magdalen, Sprowston, where, in the mid fourteenth century, the *leprosi* confirmed that nothing had been removed from their well-appointed chapel. An inventory of church goods then made by the archdeacon of Norwich records an impressive array of equipment (including processionals, antiphoners, graduals, books of sequences, silver gilt chalices and other plate, candlesticks, lamps, altar cloths, linen and vestments), as well as a cloth decorated with an image of the patron saint, which was used to decorate the lectern.

Significantly, whereas the masters of the Holy Innocents had abused their position, at St Mary's they presented a number of gifts to enhance the divine office.[178] Not all senior officials were bent on lining their own pockets. Martin St Cross, whose generosity in the matter of pittances has already been noted,

---

176	The hospital of St Mary Magdalen, Hedon, secured such a concession from Innocent III in 1200: York Minster Library, MS B 2 (3) a 5. See also Mesmin, 'Saint Gilles de Pont-Audemer', i, p. 44.

177	*CIM, 1307–1349*, no. 293. Such items were often bequeathed in wills, but are otherwise hard to trace. The gift by Henry III of two sacring bells and a set of vestments to the lepers at Ospringe in 1253 is probably representative of many more that went unrecorded: *CLR, 1251–1260*, p. 133. One of the grievances aired by the few remaining inmates of St Bartholomew's, Oxford, in 1391, was the fact that the fellows of Oriel College had not only cut down their timber, but had also removed a number of valuable relics. These allegedly included a piece of skin from the patron saint, a comb belonging to St Edmund, one of St Peter's ribs and some of St Stephen's bones. English *leprosaria* did not generally house such impressive collections, but the residents may be forgiven for exaggerating their losses: *CIM, 1387–1393*, no. 313.

178	A. Watkin, ed., *Inventory of Church Goods Temp. Edward III* (Norfolk Record Society, xix, 2 parts, 1947–48), part 1, pp. 33–4. An impressive list of goods, including two chalices, many books and vestments, various relics and a statue of the Magdalen, survives from the hospital of St Mary Magdalen, Winchester, but its late date of *c.* 1400 suggests that all the leprous inmates must by then have gone: BL, MS Harley 328, fos 28v–29r. More than adequate provision also appears to have been made at St Giles's, Holborn, at about this time: PRO, E315/38/171.

proved even more liberal where church goods were concerned. His bequests to the house at Sherburn, where he was buried, comprised: a set of cloth of gold vestments; a silver chalice; a book mounted in silver; two new graduals; two new antiphoners complete with psalters and hymnals and a third with a hymnal; a legendary and calendar; a customary; a silk altar frontal; and a black cloth to display the paten. He also owned a book on medicine, which was certainly in keeping with the hospital's commitment to proper physical as well as spiritual care.[179] The ownership of such valuable items explains why hospitals were so often dogged by crime. In 1455–56, for example, the *leprosarium* at Gaywood, outside King's Lynn, was robbed of a silver chalice and paten, allegedly worth 30s., a manual valued at 26s. 8d., eight service books and other vestments.[180]

Size was certainly no guide to the quality of furnishing and equipment. Henry Tangmere's modest foundation in Cambridge, which reputedly still accommodated male and female lepers in the early sixteenth century, was then fully stocked with plate, vestments and ornaments. They undoubtedly reflect the generosity of the local burgesses for whom prayers were to be said. One John Grene had, for example, donated a painted altar frontal depicting the patron saints, a wooden 'ymage' of the Virgin, 'new paynted', and another with three smaller 'ymages' enclosed inside it.[181] Most hospital chapels would have been decorated in some way, either with rolls of 'stayned' cloth, which could be hung on the walls in the manner of stage scenery, and changed in accordance with the principal feasts of the liturgical year, or with permanent wall paintings. Traces of paint have survived at Harbledown and at the *leprosarium* near Wimborne, in Dorset, reflecting what must once have been a common feature of the built environment.[182] Themes such as Christ's cure of the ten lepers, Dives and Lazarus, the trials of Job and *Christus quasi leprosus* would clearly reinforce the message preached in sermons and expounded in the confessional.

Having built, decorated and equipped a chapel or altar, benefactors were anxious to illuminate the divine office, and if possible any adjacent ward as well, so that the patients could see the monstrance and find comfort in the dark. Meticulous as ever, Bishop Kellaw insisted that, at Sherburn, a flame should always burn 'in the presence of the Lord's body and blood' and that at least two candles should also be lit during the Mass.[183] Even a small rural *leprosarium*, such as that at Ickburgh, was able to keep a lamp burning in its wayside chapel, while a major civic house, like St Mary Magdalen, Exeter, maintained a number of lights from at least the 1230s onwards.[184] In this way men and women of

---

[179] Raine, *Wills and Inventories*, i, pp. 6–7.

[180] Owen, *Making of King's Lynn*, p. 430.

[181] Palmer, *Cambridge Borough Documents*, i, p. 56.

[182] P.H. Newman, 'Notes on the Preservation of Some Ancient Wall Paintings', *Proceedings of the Society of Antiquaries*, xx (1903–5), pp. 41, 46.

[183] Richards, *Medieval Leper*, p. 126. Similar arrangements obtained at St Bartholomew's, Dover, from at least 1372, when it was established that a lamp would burn in the church before the cross during Mass, as well as in the hall: Bodleian Library, MS Rawl. B.335, fo. 4r. D. Postles, 'Lamps, Lights and Layfolk', *Journal of Medieval History*, xxv (1999), pp. 97–114, discusses the liturgical context, but does not consider the therapeutic value of *seeing* the Eucharist.

[184] NRO, BRA/833/14/1; Blomefield, *Norfolk*, ii, pp. 239–40; Orme and Webster, *English Hospital*, p. 228. Henry II's personal endowment upon St Giles's, Holborn, included 30s. 5d. a year to maintain lights: BL, MS Harley 4015, fo. 5r.

comparatively limited means could make a signal contribution, which had the added attraction of greatly augmenting their store of celestial merit. In the reign of Henry II, for example, Salomon de Whepstead left rents worth a shilling a year to illuminate one of the altars at St Peter's, outside Bury St Edmunds.[185] Twice this sum was set aside by a Cirencester burgess in order that the leprous nuns of Maiden Bradley could 'sustain the light in the church', his reward being perpetual membership of the hospital's fraternity, and a share in its manifold spiritual benefits.[186]

Failure to celebrate Mass on a regular basis exercised residents as much as ecclesiastical visitors and benefactors. Keenly alive to the fact that complaints on this score would strengthen their cause more than any others, the lepers at West Somerton made much of their spiritual neglect when fighting their battle against the prior of Butley.[187] Similar protests were voiced at St Bartholomew's, Oxford, where Mass was reputedly being celebrated twice a week rather than once a day by 1391, and sometimes not at all.[188] Such concern was fully justified, since to expire soon after looking upon the Host, and especially after receiving the *viaticum*, constituted a particular blessing, and ranked high among the benefits in which the hospitalised leper placed his or her trust. Conversely, though, the prospect of dying unconfessed generated fear and despondency. Indeed, one of the principal attractions offered by the more affluent medieval hospitals to long-stay patients was the provision made for death, burial and commemoration, each of which played their part in easing the soul's passage through purgatory.[189] Although, in theory, the leper had less need for anxiety on this score than any other sinful mortal, many sought the additional reassurance that a *leprosarium* could provide. Robert de Torpel's desire to be clad in the habit of a monk on his deathbed reflects the value placed by him and his contemporaries upon membership of a religious order, or at least of a community of lepers bound by a similar rule.[190] As the doctrine of purgatory developed, the need to make a 'Good Death' in the arms of the Church assumed even greater importance, as, of course, did the redemptive power of post-mortem prayers and intercession.[191]

We have already examined the measures taken by senior ecclesiastics to ensure that *leprosaria* were provided with graveyards as well as chapels, and need only note here that a Christian burial was by no means the final service provided for the departed brother or sister. Arrangements varied from one institution to

---

185  *HMC Fourteenth Report, Appendix VIII*, pp. 155–6. See also, BL, MS Cotton Tiberius C V, fo. 268r (St James's, Doncaster).

186  BL, MS Add. 37503, fo. 16v; see also Add. Charter 20423, for a similar grant. Small plots of land served equally well. At some point before 1271, one donor gave three acres of land to maintain a lamp at the Stourbridge *leprosarium*, outside Cambridge: Salzman, *VCH Cambridge II*, pp. 307–8.

187  The assertion that the prior used their revenues to maintain his own house and chapel in the precinct, keeping lavish hospitality there 'with many pages, horses and greyhounds', was almost as scandalous as the claim that women were regularly permitted to stay overnight. Significantly, when the lepers attacked these buildings, they took away various vestments, a chalice, a breviary and a missal: BL, Harley Roll N 20.

188  *CIM, 1387–1393*, no. 313.

189  C. Rawcliffe, 'Seventh Comfortable Work', pp. 11–35.

190  King, *Peterborough Abbey*, pp. 27–8.

191  Binski, *Medieval Death*, pp. 33–47.

another, but all of the larger houses made some kind of intercessionary provision for deceased residents. At the Gaywood *leprosarium* they were promised a trental, or requiem Mass on the thirtieth day after their funerals, and an annual service of commemoration. When a resident of the hospital of St Mary Magdalen, Colchester, died, each of the survivors was required to intone one hundred *Pater Nosters* on his behalf every day for the next month, while the master had to visit the grave after every Mass and pronounce absolution throughout the same period.[192] Sometimes a collection would be made on behalf of the deceased. At Dudston, for instance, all the other residents offered six psalters for the departed, gave a half penny each as alms for his or her soul and provided half a pound of wax for memorial candles.[193] In this way, the common bonds that had been forged over what may have been years of hospital life persisted far beyond the grave.

Under ideal circumstances, the settled routine of the *leprosarium* should have proved quieter and less stressful for the newcomer than his or her previous experience of life in an increasingly suspicious and intolerant society. Freed at last from the costly and painful struggle to arrest, or at least camouflage, the relentless progress of physical decay, the leper could enjoy the security and protection of a religious community, whose membership offered spiritual as well as physical support.[194] Thanks to the benefits of a nourishing diet, warm clothing and a settled regimen of prayer and light gardening duties, he or she may even have found solace in the cloistered environment of the precinct and its estates. Yet there were still plenty of contacts with the outside, as visits were exchanged with friends and family, whose welcome gifts eased the somewhat Spartan rigours of a rule based upon monastic principles of discipline and renunciation. Above all, though, as death approached he or she had ample opportunity to shed any residual burden of sin, to receive the sacraments of confession and the last rites, and expire in the arms of the Church. The reality of daily life in England's *leprosaria* was, of course, often very different, especially during the fourteenth and fifteenth centuries. Although a few new houses were established during this period, their modest size and limited resources stand in sharp contrast to the endowments originally made on older foundations, such as those at Holborn, Ripon, Sherburn and York. By then, however, these once prosperous hospitals accommodated no more than one or two leprous individuals at most, and had effectively been transformed into chantry chapels or almshouses. Does this dramatic decline reflect the steady retreat of *lepra* as a threat to the health of the English people? And, if so, why did the disease still occasion so much interest and anxiety?

---

192  Owen, *Making of King's Lynn*, pp. 107–8; Fisher, 'Leger Book of St John's Abbey', p. 121. Bishop Kellaw felt that each deceased brother and sister at Sherburn merited three hundred *Pater Nosters* a day for the month following his or her demise: Richards, *Medieval Leper*, p. 128. Lepers dying at the hospital outside Lille could expect 101 *Pater Nosters* and the same number of *Aves*: Le Grand, *Statuts*, p. 202.

193  *HMC Twelfth Report, Appendix IX*, pp. 426–7. At St James's, Westminster, where discipline was notoriously lax, vigils for the dead appear to have become disorderly because of 'drinking and unseemly noise': Page, *VCH London I*, p. 543.

194  This was, for example, the belief of the leprous poet, Jean Bodel: Raynaud, 'Congés', p. 237.

# Conclusion

*Many parts of the world are still wrapped in that ignorance of leprosy which characterised Europe in the Middle Ages. And so long as sufferers from leprosy are regarded by their fellow-creatures as either cursed (because of sin) or so dangerous to other human beings that they must be shut away from normal people, leprosy will continue to exist.*

Anthony Weymouth, Through the Leper-Squint, *1938* [1]

With a few notable exceptions, nineteenth-century physicians and polemicists found it easy to explain the disappearance of lepers and *leprosaria* from the British Isles. Drawing no distinction between medieval *lepra* and the disease they encountered in the colonies, they believed that an epidemic of dangerous proportions had most probably begun on the return of infected crusaders from the Holy Land.[2] Only a strict policy of isolation, implemented through the compulsory detention of suspects in leper houses, had saved the population from contagion, eventually removing the threat altogether. Advocates of the 'hereditary' theory of transmission, no less than those who accepted the more recent ideas of microbiologists such as Koch and Hansen, were convinced that segregation had been both systematic and effective, if only because it prevented lepers from reproducing. Paradoxically, however, the archival research that both lobbies hoped would provide ammunition for a revived policy of sanitary policing did not unearth the evidence they required. As we have seen, it soon became apparent that the medieval English leper was far from being a reluctant prisoner, locked away behind high walls, or relegated to some distant settlement miles from human habitation.

Indeed, as they discovered more about the insidious nature of *Mycobacterium leprae* and the long incubation period of Hansen's disease, leprologists recognised that confinement, however strict, would have proved almost totally useless. Even had confirmed cases been banished from medieval society, diagnosis at such an advanced stage would have been akin to locking the stable door

---

1   Weymouth, *Through the Leper Squint*, p. 24.
2   For the most recent and convincing demolition of this theory, see P.D. Mitchell, 'The Myth of the Spread of Leprosy with the Crusades', *PPL*, pp. 171–6.

after a bolting horse.[3] Once it was understood that suspects must have been spreading the *Mycobacterium* for years before their condition attracted attention, the focus of inquiry concentrated instead upon the relative capacity of the community at large to resist infection. Factors such as improved nutrition, better housing and increased immunity seemed to offer far more plausible explanations for the retreat of Hansen's disease from medieval England than historically dubious arguments about exclusion ever could. The onset of colder and wetter weather at the beginning of the fourteenth century has also been suggested as a possible curb upon the spread of the *Mycobacterium* outside the human body, although the local impact of climate change is difficult to judge.[4]

As Keith Manchester has demonstrated, the capacity to withstand a disease such as leprosy may be either innate or acquired. In the first instance, strong, healthy and well-nourished individuals living in clean and spacious conditions will be far less vulnerable than hungry paupers whose surroundings are cramped and squalid.[5] Medieval physicians observed that certain families were more susceptible to *lepra* than others, and there is now a widespread consensus that a person's genetic make-up may also determine the extent to which he or she can overcome the *Mycobacterium*. In addition, protracted and early exposure across successive generations will confer extra protection, and explains why tuberculoid leprosy eventually develops in communities that initially experienced the more aggressive and incapacitating lepromatous strain. This is because members of the host population acquire a degree of 'cell mediated immunity' and can thus better defend themselves against the *Mycobacterium* through the production of an enzyme that kills the invader. Rising standards of living and improvements in immunological status can thus, together, bring about a steady reduction in cases, until the number falls below the minimum necessary for sustainability. According Manchester, this trend was greatly accelerated in medieval England by the spread of tuberculosis. Transmitted by pathogens from the same genus as *Mycobacterium leprae*, this highly infectious disease also flourishes in crowded and unsanitary conditions. Infants who survived an attack of pulmonary tuberculosis (which affects the young at an earlier age than leprosy) would, he believes, have thereby gained a significant level of additional protection through the acquisition of cross-immunity.[6]

The effectiveness of his persuasive argument none the less depends upon the establishment of a clear chronology for both diseases, which at present remains an elusive prospect. A condition known as *ptisis*, 'tisik' or 'consumpcioun', characterised by the spitting of blood and other familiar symptoms, figures prominently in medieval remedy books and medical treatises. Its fatal effects upon the

---

3    Manchester, 'Tuberculosis and Leprosy: Evidence for Interaction of Disease', p. 33. Individuals with sub-clinical leprosy, who display no visible symptoms, can also carry the *Mycobacterium*.

4    K. Duncan, 'Climate and the Decline of Leprosy in Britain', *Proceedings of the Royal College of Physicians of Edinburgh*, xxiv (1994), pp. 114–20; Manchester, 'Leprosy: The Origin and Development of the Disease', pp. 31–49.

5    Although Ell, 'Diet and Leprosy', pp. 116–17, suggests that a diet high in cholesterol and rich in saturated fats would increase susceptibility among high status individuals.

6    Manchester, 'Tuberculosis and Leprosy: Evidence for Interaction of Disease', pp. 23–35. See also Grmek, *Diseases in the Ancient Greek World*, chapter eight.

human body and the difficulty of containing it were, for example, spelt out by Bartholomaeus Anglicus in his celebrated encyclopaedia.[7] Such evidence does not, however, tell us very much about the actual prevalence of pulmonary tuberculosis in later medieval England. Like leprosy, *ptisis* posed a considerable challenge to practitioners, and may thus have attracted a disproportionate amount of attention, not least because so many Classical authorities had already written about it. Moreover, as in the case of *lepra*, we soon encounter the manifold problems posed by variations in nomenclature and uncertainty about definitions. John Mirfield began the section on *ptisis* in his *Breviarium Bartholomaei* by observing that the term could be used generally to denote any wasting disease or fever, or more specifically with regard to a potentially fatal disorder occasioned by ulceration of the lung. He also notes that misdiagnosis was common, even by experts.[8] Since, unlike lepers, suspect *ptisisci* were never expected to live apart from the community, or enter designated institutions, we cannot even tell how seriously the population at large regarded the disease. Nor, as yet, can the palaeopathologist provide much assistance in this respect. Because tuberculosis affects the human skeleton in only a small percentage of cases, its effects upon the inhabitants of medieval England at any given time remain a matter of speculation.[9]

In the final resort, although Manchester's research greatly extends our knowledge of Hansen's disease, his findings do not necessarily elucidate or even accord with historical perceptions of *lepra*. Whereas he regards the sharp decline in leper house foundations after 1400 as proof positive that Hansen's disease was on the retreat, medieval magistrates took a less sanguine view of the phenomenon.[10] From the perspective of the royal court in the 1470s, or the rulers of Yarmouth at the close of the fifteenth century, suspect *leprosi* posed an even greater threat to public health than they had in the years before the Black Death. We must therefore look beyond the study of *Mycobacterium leprae* if we are fully to understand the chequered history of English medieval *leprosaria* and their inmates. It is apparent from skeletal evidence that a significant number of the latter were indeed suffering from Hansen's disease, having quite possibly been diagnosed by the expert practitioners whose capacity to recognise advanced cases of lepromatous and tuberculoid leprosy can hardly be questioned. But their presence goes only part of the way to account for the surge of endowments before about 1300, as does their disappearance for the striking fall in numbers afterwards.

The common assumption that the dramatic spate of new leper houses between about 1100 and 1250 constituted a response to a major epidemic of Hansen's disease is in itself highly suspect. As we learned in chapter two, definitions of *lepra* gradually changed during this period from the comprehensive terminology of the Book of Leviticus, which embraced a wide range of dermatological conditions, to a far more stringent set of diagnostic criteria

---

7   Seymour, *On the Properties of Things*, i, pp. 374–7.
8   Horton-Smith Hartley and Aldridge, *Johannes de Mirfeld*, pp. 74–89.
9   Roberts and Cox, *Health and Disease*, pp. 230–32, survey the late medieval skeletal evidence.
10  Manchester, 'Tuberculosis and Leprosy in Antiquity', p. 172.

adopted by Muslim physicians and their translators. In other words, as medical knowledge spread throughout society, fewer men and women with ready access to a trained practitioner or empiric were likely to be deemed leprous than before. Since these were the very people who would previously have secured entry to one of the larger, quasi-monastic *leprosaria*, such as Sherburn or Maiden Bradley, it is easy to see why contraction set in. We should also remember that many leper houses, along with other institutions for the sick and indigent, were the outcome of a growing enthusiasm for monastic endowments that reached its peak in the twelfth century. They were subject to changing fashions in lay piety and philanthropy, which inevitably found new outlets with the passage of time. Although the cult of *Christus quasi leprosus* continued to flourish, along with concern for the hospitalised leper, much of the initial enthusiasm for conspicuous displays of devotion to the sick abated. This may be attributable to falling numbers, but growing fears of contagion, concerns about the rootless poor and the changing religious *milieu* of the later Middle Ages also played their part. So too did legal developments. The Statute of Mortmain of 1279, which forbade the alienation of land to the Church without royal licence, proved especially detrimental for *leprosaria*, since permits were expensive, while the risks of attempting to evade the law could result in even costlier attempts at damage limitation.[11]

The gradual loosening of feudal ties between lords and tenants, which had previously obliged many of the latter to follow the lead of their superiors, engendered a greater freedom in the matter of charitable effort.[12] The available options also increased. As Benedictine chroniclers such as Matthew Paris bitterly complained, the arrival in England of the mendicant orders diverted a substantial proportion of secular wealth into the hands of the newcomers. The construction of the great English friaries, which, like *leprosaria*, were ideally sited for the collection of alms on the outskirts of towns, posed a threat to existing institutions, especially as the new orders exercised so much influence through preaching and the medium of the confessional.[13] Since many small suburban leper houses also depended for survival upon begging, the competition placed them at a serious disadvantage.[14] On the other hand, the friars could present themselves as natural agents for the administration of poor relief, especially as so many hospitals and *leprosaria* seemed to have failed in their obligations, not least through recourse to fee-paying patients. It is unfortunate that the early work of English mendicants among the sick is so badly documented, since laymen and women may initially have been drawn to them *because* their pastoral brief included the care of lepers and other vulnerable individuals.[15]

Particularly evident in urban communities, the popularity of the friars was

---

11  S. Raban, *Mortmain Legislation and the English Church 1279–1500* (Cambridge, 1982), chapters one and two; Sweetinburgh, *Role of the Hospital*, pp. 82–3.
12  Thompson, 'From "Alms" to "Spiritual Services" ', p. 233.
13  C.H. Lawrence, *Medieval Monasticism* (London, 1989), chapter twelve.
14  Sweetinburgh, *Role of the Hospital*, pp. 73–4, 83.
15  Although, according to Geoffrey Chaucer and other critics, some of their number preferred more congenial company in taverns to that of 'a lazar or a beggestere': *The Canterbury Tales*, Benson, *Riverside Chaucer*, p. 27.

equalled, if not outdone, by a growing sense of attachment to the parish, which became a principal focus of lay piety and corresponding levels of financial investment. When they were not engaged in schemes for the refurbishment and decoration of their churches, late medieval benefactors generally directed their more conspicuous charitable efforts into public works. Prominent among them were roads and bridges, the creation of modest almshouses for the *deserving* elderly poor and the foundation of schools, often in buildings that had once housed the sick and leprous. Indeed, it was through the reception of pupils, often as choral scholars, that several urban hospitals took on a new lease of life in the years after the Black Death.[16] Like the older monasteries, long-established hospitals, whatever their remit, exercised fewer attractions unless they could offer patrons a high level of liturgical provision, which involved a considerable outlay on buildings, staff and equipment.[17] Prospective patients also seem to have turned elsewhere, often electing to live in private quarters at home if they could afford to do so. This may have been a natural consequence of the general decline in the appeal of the monastic vocation, which had once gathered so many *leprosi* into the fold. As Abbot Mentmore of St Albans observed, when drawing up the statutes of St Julian's hospital in 1343, 'there are hardly enough lepers to be found who are prepared to come to the hospital and lead a life bound by its regulations'.[18] Yet the abbot would have been as reluctant to admit some of the indigent and morally dubious characters whom we encountered in chapter six as they would have been to accept the discipline of the cloister. Many presumed lepers were too poor, too intransigent or too disreputable to gain entry to such places.

Deplore it as they might, the ecclesiastical and urban authorities of late medieval England faced a constant visual reminder that many refuges for pilgrims, sick paupers, the homeless and lepers were falling into disrepair, if not actually vanishing from the landscape. The *leprosarium* at Ripon had allegedly been demolished by 1341, doles and hospitality for passing lepers being by then little more than a distant memory.[19] A similar picture of devastation emerges shortly afterwards at Royston, where the hospital of St Nicholas and its chapel had been laid waste. The chapel of St John's, by the bridge at Stony Stratford, was also by then 'for the most part in ruins', as were the once impressive buildings at New Romney, which had been totally deserted. The chapel there was rebuilt as a chantry for two priests, who replaced the lepers in 1363, any surplus profits being diverted for the support of Magdalen College, Oxford.[20] There can be little doubt that the process of decline gained rapid momentum from about 1300

---

16  C. Rawcliffe, 'The Eighth Comfortable Work: Education and the Medieval English Hospital', in C.M. Barron and J. Stratford, eds, *The Church and Learning in Later Medieval Society* (Donington, 2002), pp. 371–98. By 1414, for instance, the former leper hospital of St James, near Canterbury, was taking well-behaved young people capable of learning: Duncombe and Battely, *Three Archiepiscopal Hospitals*, p. 433.
17  Rawcliffe, *Medicine for the Soul*, chapter four.
18  Richards, *Medieval Leper*, p. 130.
19  Raine, *Memorials of the Church of SS Peter and Wilfrid*, i, pp. 211–12, 224–5.
20  *CCR, 1354–1360*, p. 587; *CPR, 1350–1354*, p. 303; Brigstocke Sheppard, *Literae Cantuarienses*, ii, pp. 437–8.

onwards. Here too, though, a number of socio-economic as well as epidemiological factors were at work.

The proliferation of royal and episcopal letters of protection, often for the specific purpose of fund-raising, constitutes a useful barometer of institutional hardship. A steady stream of such awards was made to *leprosaria* by the crown between 1201 and 1350, most (but not all) being recorded on the patent rolls. They suggest that many houses had already begun to feel the chill wind of recession well before the end of the thirteenth century.[21] But worse was to come. As we saw in chapter six, the combined effects of population pressure, crop failures, bad weather, disease and economic dislocation during the early fourteenth century were to threaten the very survival of many hospitals as well as that of innumerable solitary paupers. In his study of the great famine of 1315–22, Ian Kershaw has calculated that over one hundred such letters were granted to hospitals, leper houses and small monasteries in the first year of dearth alone. Some never weathered the storm, while others, such as St James's, Westminster, emerged badly damaged by 'the mortality of animals and poverty of their resources'.[22] Since even comparatively wealthy houses for the sick poor, such as St Giles's, Norwich, then faced serious economic problems, we can readily appreciate what a devastating effect these difficult years would have had upon small and under-funded *leprosaria* that relied heavily upon alms from local communities.[23] Not surprisingly, the award of papal and episcopal indulgences in return for financial support increased exponentially, not merely in terms of numbers but also with regard to the profusion of spiritual benefits offered.

Hospitals on the Scottish and Welsh borders faced the additional threat of raiding parties and endemic warfare. An inquiry of 1320 revealed, for example, that the *leprosarium* at Hexham, which traditionally accommodated poor husbandmen and the sick, as well as lepers, had lost all its archives, most of its rents and a good deal of stock in the previous round of hostilities. Doles from the neighbouring monastery had also dwindled, leaving the few remaining patients with only a fraction of the bread and ale customarily allocated to them by the monks.[24] For *leprosaria* that were already in decline, plague might prove the *coup de grace*. In some cases the blow was, indeed, dramatic. All of the few remaining inmates of St James's, Westminster, died in the Black Death of 1349–50, leaving the once spacious buildings unoccupied and available for lease.[25] In most cases, however, a long period of morbidity ensued, as a combination of falling rents and rising prices took its toll on failing institutions. At St Giles's, Holborn, an inquiry of 1355 revealed that debt, fire and 'the horrible mortality' had left its home farm uncultivated and its rented properties empty.[26]

---

[21] Satchell, 'Emergence of Leper-Houses', pp. 84–6.

[22] Kershaw, 'Great Famine', p. 31.

[23] Rawcliffe, *Medicine for the Soul*, pp. 84–90.

[24] J. Raine, ed., *The Priory of Hexham II* (Surtees Society, xlvi, 1865), pp. 130–32.

[25] Page, *VCH London I*, p. 545. The hospital eventually became part of the endowment upon Eton College.

[26] The Pope then awarded a major indulgence of five years and five *quadragene* to anyone who visited and gave alms: *Calendar of Papal Registers: Petitions, 1342–1419*, p. 270.

Disputes with the crown and citizens of London over patronage, as well as a litany of financial irregularities, greatly exacerbated the problem.

It is now impossible to tell whether the allegations of embezzlement, incompetence and neglect that dogged so many late medieval hospitals and *leprosaria* were a contributory cause or an inevitable consequence of this process of decline. Deteriorating economic conditions clearly brought out the worst in some masters, who were prepared to exploit any available source of revenue for their own personal advantage. Just a few examples from a depressingly long list will here suffice. At St Leonard's, Northampton, for instance, reforms of 1505 revealed that the house had been 'mysse used and evyll governed and gevyn awey'.[27] Only one leper and a female pauper allegedly remained by the Dissolution, which was a marginally better situation than obtained at St Mary Magdalen, Reading, 'wherof th'abbott taketh the profyttes and hathe taken downe the seyd chapell and all the howsys ther to apperteynyng, and so ther be no poer people relevyd'.[28] Successive priors of Southampton had been so remiss in maintaining the port's leper house, that by 1401 most of the buildings were ruinous, although they continued to pocket rents of over £16 for another century.[29]

A readiness to adapt could, nevertheless, ensure survival. Some places, such as St Mary Magdalen, Colchester, were re-founded during the fifteenth century to accommodate a mixture of 'poor persons and lepers', should any actually seek admission.[30] After a long period of decay, the once affluent *leprosarium* at Sherburn was set on its feet in 1434 by Bishop Langley of Durham as a modest refuge for thirteen paupers and two lepers 'if so many could be found', run in conjunction with a lavishly appointed chantry chapel.[31] Like many former leper houses, St John's at Blyth, Nottinghamshire, also concentrated upon the development of spiritual services, its staff of three resident chaplains being in part funded by the fee-paying corrodians who were recruited specifically to support them.[32] Other hospitals were merged in order to pool resources and save on running costs. Such a pragmatic solution was adopted at Thetford and Ipswich, in East Anglia, and at Ludlow, where the local *leprosarium* was converted into an almshouse under the aegis of the town's largest hospital.[33]

Many leper houses responded to the transformation in English society that

---

27  J.C. Cox, ed., *Records of the Borough of Northampton, II* (Northampton, 1898), pp. 331–2.
28  BL, MS Add. 6214, fo. 22r (pencil foliation).
29  Cox, *VCH Hampshire II*, p. 167. The offenders were by no means all monastic. At St Mary Magdalen, Exeter, a civic *leprosarium* which became an almshouse for 'poure people', a catalogue of abuses by the master came to light in 1500: *HMC, Report on the Records of the City of Exeter* (London, 1916), pp. 398–9.
30  Fisher, 'Leger Book of St John's Abbey', p. 120.
31  Despite further abuses, the house was still worth £142 a year at the Dissolution, which suggests that it must once have been very prosperous indeed: W. Page, ed., *VCH Durham II* (London, 1907), pp. 115–16. Bishop Repingdon of Lincoln likewise refounded St Leonard's, Newark, as a chantry with one priest, two poor bedesmen and a master: idem, ed., *VCH Nottingham II* (London, 1910), p. 167.
32  Page, *VCH Nottingham II*, p. 165.
33  Page, *VCH Norfolk II*, p. 452; idem, *VCH Suffolk II*, p. 139; Gaydon, *VCH Shropshire II*, p. 101. The hospital of St John, Brackley, and the nearby *leprosarium* were merged, and St Nicholas's, York, was annexed to the priory of Holy Trinity: Serjeantson and Adkins, *VCH Northampton II*, p. 154; Page, *VCH Yorkshire III*, p. 348.

occurred during a century of famine and plague by offering care for the elderly. The rapid fall in population experienced between 1315 and 1380 witnessed an appreciable rise in living standards among the survivors. Improvements in housing and diet produced men and women who were fitter, better nourished and, relatively speaking, more affluent. Such individuals naturally tended to live longer and thus to need sheltered accommodation. They, rather than the unemployed and vagrant poor, who were now more likely to incur censure than pity, became a priority. For this reason, some of the larger *leprosaria*, including those at Harbledown, Peterborough and Winchester, gradually assumed a new role. Indeed, by 1546, it was assumed that Lanfranc's pioneering foundation outside Canterbury had always existed 'for the releiffe and maintenance of almsfolk', the lepers being long forgotten.[34]

Like the *maisons Dieu* then springing up across England for the benefit of an ageing population, none of the twenty or so *leprosaria* that were founded or at least first mentioned after about 1350 appear to have been particularly large [**map 6**]. Some, such as John Colney's at Sudbury, Robert Pygot's at Walsingham and William Pole's in Highgate, were specifically geared to the needs of no more than two or three named residents.[35] Together with the few surviving institutions that continued to receive the occasional leper, they apparently sufficed for the reception of suitable cases. We cannot necessarily assume that such individuals were among the very last to contract Hansen's disease in England, since (with the exception of William Pole) we do not know how accurately they may have been diagnosed. But it is worth noting that the rise in living standards and attendant increase in the amount of meat and dairy produce consumed by the working classes after 1350 would, in fact, have created precisely those conditions in which Manchester believes greater resistance to *Mycobacterium leprae* would develop.[36] Changes in diet may also have encouraged the transmission of tuberculosis. As we have seen, urban authorities were well aware of the health risks posed by contaminated milk and meat, which possibly spread bovine tuberculosis – and thus, perhaps, a heightened resistance to Hansen's disease – among those now prosperous enough to eat beef on a regular basis.

The dissemination of medical knowledge may have led to the adoption of stricter diagnostic criteria, but it also encouraged a mounting fear of contagion, greatly intensified after 1350 by anxieties about the onset of plague. It was for this reason, along with distrust of the idle and ungovernable poor, that the spectre of leprosy continued to haunt so many English towns and cities. We have

---

[34] C. Cotton, ed., *The Canterbury Chantries and Hospitals in 1546* (Kent Records, supplement, 1934), pp. 38–44. For Peterborough (which maintained eight 'poor men' in 1535) see W.T. Mellows and P.I. King, eds, *The Book of William Morton, Almoner of Peterborough Monastery 1448–1467* (Northamptonshire Record Society, xvi, 1954), p. xxviii; and for Winchester, Cox, *VCH Hampshire II*, pp. 197–200.

[35] Those not listed by Satchell, 'Emergence of English Leper-Houses', pp. 250–399, are: Boughton-under-Blean, Kent, 1384 (*CPR, 1381–1385*, p. 448); Cambridge, by 1361 (Rubin, *Charity and Community*, pp. 122–3); Highgate, Middlesex, 1473 (*CPR, 1467–1477*, p. 373); Ipswich, Suffolk, by 1510 (Suffolk RO, Ipswich, IC/AA2/5/220; PRO, PCC Kidd 90); Newton Bushell, Devon, 1538 (Orme and Webster, *English Hospital*, pp. 250–51); Sudbury, Suffolk, 1372 (Hodson, 'John Colney's Hospital', pp. 268–74).

[36] Dyer, *Standards of Living*, chapters six and seven.

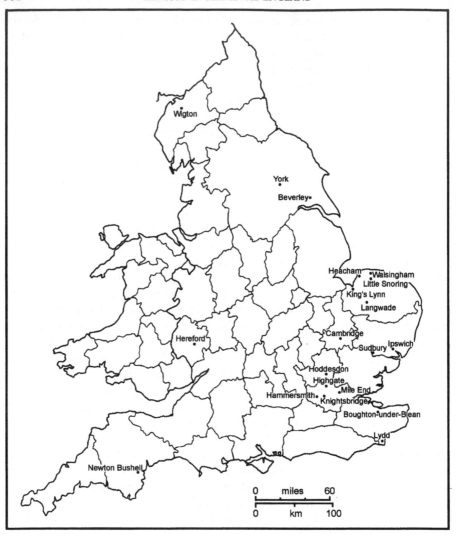

Map 6. English leper houses founded after *c.* 1350 (Phillip Judge)

no means of telling how far the presentments of *lepra* brought before four-teenth- and fifteenth-century borough courts were simply a means of removing undesirable individuals such as the notorious Alice Dymock from the commu-nity, and certainly cannot now determine how many suspects, if any, were actu-ally suffering from Hansen's disease. Medical practitioners believed that laymen were prone to make over-hasty judgements on the basis of a few contentious symptoms, although there was no shortage of readily available information about approved diagnostic procedures, which any competent local barber or empiric could undertake.[37] On balance, it seems that, in some cases at least,

---

[37] See chapter four, above.

juries were far less scrupulous where the morally disreputable, the unproductive and outsiders were concerned. Yet they were often slow to enforce regulations for the removal of lepers until an outbreak of plague or some other epidemic galvanized them into action.

The arrival of the *morbus Gallicus* at the close of the fifteenth century provided the rulers of English towns with a coherent and pressing agenda for the control of infected paupers, as the focus now shifted from a few suspect lepers to a growing army of pox-ridden mendicants. A far more aggressive programme of segregation began two or three decades later, specifically in order that 'the foulness [would] all be restricted to one place, and the rest of body not infected'.[38] The influential Ypres scheme for poor relief of 1525 was in many respects heir to the late medieval ideas about physical and moral contagion discussed in chapter six of this book. It aimed to put them into practice by removing from the streets all beggars 'arayed with skorfe and fylthynesse', who threatened others with their 'stynkynge sycknesses'.[39] The authors proudly reported that 'the dysfygured syghtes of these vysured [facially damaged] pore men . . . all roughe and scouruy and ronnynge with matter bothe vgely to loke on and euyll smellynge to the nose' had disappeared from the city because of improvements in public health. Instead, reputable citizens could now congratulate themselves that 'the contagyouse folkes are by theymselfe whose infection often times priuely crepynge as a canker hathe caused moche deth in the people'.[40]

It is interesting to observe how far suspicion still lighted upon men and women 'diseased in their faces', who were the first to attract attention. The Ypres scheme was translated into English during the 1530s, and had a profound effect upon the formulation of the Tudor poor law, as well as upon sanitary reforms in cities such as London, Norwich and York.[41] Designated by badges, and removed to buildings that had once served as suburban *leprosaria*, the sick poor were subject to greatly increased levels of surveillance and control, not least so that they might be cured and sent back to work. Occasional references to 'lepers' still surface in sixteenth-century sources, and medical texts books continued to discuss the problem of diagnosis and treatment for some time. But, as we saw in chapter two, fears about leprosy had now been subsumed into an expanding body of lore and literature concerning the pox. The Protestant physicians and magistrates of Tudor England were rarely disposed to regard disfiguring and repugnant illnesses as a source of spiritual authority or mark of divine election. Idleness, promiscuity and an addiction to strong drink seemed far more likely causes. Their anxieties eventually resurfaced three centuries later and seized the Victorian imagination in a contorted and sensationalised form which medieval men and women would have found perplexing and sometimes incomprehensible.

---

38 F.R. Salter, ed., *Some Early Tracts on Poor Relief* (London, 1926), p. 17. See also Arrizabalaga, Henderson and French, *The Pox*, pp. 155–70.

39 Salter, *Early Tracts*, pp. 42, 66.

40 Salter, *Early Tracts*, p. 69. The comparison with cancer also echoes medieval writing on *lepra*: see above, p. 170.

41 G.R. Elton, 'An Early Tudor Poor Law', *Economic History Review*, second series, vi (1953–54), pp. 55–67; P. Slack, *Poverty and Policy in Tudor and Stuart England* (London, 1988), pp. 118–19.

We have now returned to our starting point. This study of leprosy in medi-eval England began with an exploration of the process of distortion that gave birth to a miserable outcast, shunned and dreaded by healthy members of society. During the later nineteenth century a potent combination of factors, ranging from advances in the science of microbiology to the spread of imperi-alism, generated a fear of, and fascination with, leprosy among the intellectual elite of Europe and America. This rapidly inspired a genre of popular literature and evangelical propaganda that has continued, even today, to influence writers of medieval history, as well as scholars working in many other disciplines. Epito-mised by an enduring – but entirely unfounded – belief that the medieval leper was subject to a variety of cruel and bizarre rituals of exclusion, these myths and misunderstandings have largely obscured a far more complex and revealing picture of responses to human suffering.

The sheer diversity of medieval reactions to a disease called *lepra*, no less than the constant refinement and change to which they were subject from the mid twelfth century onwards, became apparent when we turned, in chapter two, to ideas about causation. A society convinced of the symbiotic connection between body and soul will inevitably be disposed to associate sickness with sin, although few medieval theologians – and even fewer medical practitioners – adopted such a crude, 'one size fits all', approach to aetiology. As in Victorian times, both clergymen and *medici* (who, in medieval England, were often indistinguishable) tended to regard sexual incontinence as a prime suspect. Yet the list of potential causes was sufficiently long and comprehensive to accommodate the holiest of saints as well as the most dissolute of reprobates. Indeed, a growing preoccupa-tion with the macerated body of Christ, along with the scorching fires of purga-tory, meant that, for many people, the leper seemed to have been blessed rather than cursed by God. However assiduously it may have been propagated by nine-teenth- and early twentieth-century advocates of segregation, the conviction that leprosy was deemed highly infectious *throughout* the Middle Ages seems equally untenable.[42] Theories about contagion by miasmatic air spread gradually from the 1250s onwards, but urban communities did not begin consistently to display an understanding of the medical literature and an attendant anxiety about sources of corruption until after the Black Death. Their efforts were, none the less, sporadic, and fears of communication by touch, breath or gaze never eclipsed a catalogue of other explanations that embraced heredity, diet, climate, stress and the impact of malign planetary forces.

Given the prominence accorded by medical authorities to humoral theory and the unique balance of every single individual, such apparent inconsistency is hardly surprising. The Church, too, demonstrated an ambivalent, if not some-times contradictory, response to *lepra*, influenced on the one hand by Old Testa-ment concepts of ritual pollution and exclusion, and on the other by the Christian imperatives of charity and compassion. The former obliged suspects to

---

[42] In one of his 1873 Goulstonian lectures, for example, Robert Liveing asserted: 'The belief that existed in the Middle Ages in the infectious character of leprosy . . . was at the root of all the laws and regula-tions affecting lepers, and . . . explains why, for many centuries, they were so carefully shunned by all except those who desired to perform some signal act of penance': *Elephantiasis Graecorum*, p. 16.

live 'outside the camp', while the latter prompted untold numbers of men and women to dedicate themselves, or at least some of their resources, to the care of the sick. Partly because of their attachment to such fictions as the 'Leper Mass', historians have tended to regard *leprosi* as the victims rather than the beneficiaries of ecclesiastical authority, especially after the sweeping reforms of Pope Innocent III. There can be little doubt that the ostentatious displays of largesse which funded almost 300 English *leprosaria* began to decline from then onwards, although, as we have just seen, there were many reasons for this phenomenon. Spared the association with heresy that led to vilification and persecution on the continent, English lepers did not invariably suffer from the advent of a confessional society, as has often been supposed. The widespread propensity to distinguish between the 'wild' and the 'tame', the penitent and the unregenerate, the rich and the poor, the well connected and the friendless, the vagrant and the settled, meant, in practice, that responses remained as heterogeneous as ideas about causation. In short, leprosy holds up a glass in which one can observe the most elevated spiritual aspirations as well as the deepest anxieties of medieval society.

The authority of the Church was greatly strengthened by the important diagnostic role accorded to the priesthood. Although they may often have had an agenda of their own (such as the promotion of a healing shrine or the enforcement of moral discipline), members of the clergy who assumed this responsibility were often equipped with specialist medical information and impressive levels of practical expertise. Changing diagnostic criteria, which grew more consistent and specific as newly translated texts percolated into Western Europe from the Muslim world, had a profound effect upon the way *lepra* was defined, detected and perceived. At first confined to an educated cadre of physicians, surgeons and priests, many of these works, and others based upon them, were eventually adapted for the benefit of a lay vernacular readership whose grasp of Classical theories about the preservation of health grew exponentially. The identification of suspects thus became a communal concern, as panels of medical experts and local juries assumed a role sanctioned by the courts. An increasing emphasis upon facial symptoms, without which confirmation was unlikely, meant that, in principle, only the most advanced cases would now be deemed leprous. Conversely, though, it became easier for magistrates to take action against social undesirables, whose marginal position prevented them from questioning an unfavourable verdict.

If fewer individuals of high or middling status were now likely to end their lives in a *leprosarium* or private retreat, far more became preoccupied by the need to camouflage or eradicate any alarming symptoms. As we saw in chapter five, a general consensus that immediate recourse to medical care and a good regimen might halt the spread of such a debilitating disease meant that the demand for both advice literature and a range of prophylactic treatment increased by leaps and bounds. The rapid expansion of international markets, accompanied by the arrival of Islamic texts on pharmacology, prompted a hitherto unparalleled growth in the range of available *materia medica*. A study of the stratagems adopted by putative lepers (many of whom were clearly suffering from a variety of curable dermatological and venereal diseases) provides an illuminating insight into medieval therapeutics. Prescribed for the rectification of humoral imbalances, remedies ranged from comparatively innocuous herbal beverages, baths and poultices to invasive mineral compounds, aggressive surgical procedures and esoteric alchemical preparations. It might, indeed, be argued that the struggle to combat *lepra* reveals the healing profession at its most inventive and pragmatic. A tendency on the part of previous generations of medical historians to deride these holistic measures, along with the diagnostic techniques adopted by practitioners, as 'superstitious' and 'primitive' now seems both misplaced and anachronistic.

Those who lost their battle against the disease faced the prospect of segregation from friends, family and neighbours, although, like the concept of *lepra* itself, the experience took many forms. The evidence presented in chapter six confirms that Victorian advocates of mandatory isolation generally (and perhaps sometimes wilfully) misunderstood both the context and purpose of medieval provisions for the removal and care of lepers. Neither canon nor common law, for example, was as draconian as they maintained, while the motives for excluding low status suspects from towns and cities often reflected economic, demographic or social pressures rather than fears of contagion. It is, however, striking to observe the close connection between outbreaks of plague and the introduction of measures for public health, which in turn reflects the spread of medical knowledge among the ruling elite of fourteenth- and fifteenth-century England. Paradoxically, though, institutional support was by then hard to come by and often reserved for a select group of acceptable individuals. Indeed, the larger medieval English *leprosaria*, which so many medical historians and journalists have portrayed as detention centres for the confinement of suspects, were always extremely particular about admissions.[43] Applicants who could not make a financial contribution or were reluctant to accept the constraints of a communal, quasi-monastic existence were unlikely to prove successful. Freedom of movement and association was, in any event, often determined by moral rather than hygienic considerations, and might well allow for periods of extended leave to visit relatives or go on pilgrimage.

In theory, at least, the assumption that most *leprosaria* were little more than staging posts for the next world, where patients languished far from the public eye without proper care or attention, seems equally hard to sustain. Situated in close proximity to towns, cities, roads, bridges, markets, fairs and ferries, the leper house was a ubiquitous feature of the twelfth- or thirteenth-century landscape. Founders and early patrons made careful provision for the physical welfare of inmates, ensuring that proper food and other resources would be readily available. Some were demonstrably aware of the recommendations about diet, cleanliness and exercise made by the physicians who produced tracts on the detection and treatment of *lepra*. Although the great majority of benefactors were understandably concerned for their own salvation, a general recognition

---

[43] Paolo Zappa, for instance, describes medieval leper houses as 'prisons where the sufferers, withdrawn from society and torn from the affection of their families, deprived of liberty and the enjoyment of their possessions, were relentlessly shut up and forbidden any contact with the outside world': *Unclean! Unclean!*, p. 72.

that patients, however sick, might also profit from the availability of spiritual services is apparent throughout our period. The ceaseless round of intercessionary prayer and Masses that marked life in the larger monastic hospitals may, in practice, have reduced the patient to little more than 'a liturgical appendage', but we should remember that the *regimen sanitatis* regarded it as a valuable means of regulating the accidents of the soul.

Despite the best efforts of hospital visitors and, occasionally, the complaints of the residents themselves, it proved impossible to maintain the standards set by the men and women who regarded the foundation of *leprosaria* as the best means of negotiating their speedy passage through the torments of purgatory. But this process of decline does not detract from the strength of the initial impulse, which reflects a combination of motives from compassion to fear and self-promotion to humility. Once we put aside our own preconceptions about the role of the hospital in today's highly medicalised society, and begin to regard these institutions through medieval eyes, the picture seems very different. As this book has argued, the same approach holds good of any study of historical responses to disease, which must venture far beyond the scrutiny of a particular virus or microbe and its impact upon bone and tissue. It must embrace, as far as the sources allow, the spiritual and intellectual *milieu* of the afflicted, and assess on their own terms the various stratagems with which they fought, individually and collectively, for survival. If the picture that emerges is sometimes contradictory, challenging and fragmented then it surely reflects the nature of human life itself.

# Bibliography

**Manuscript Sources**

*Bodleian Library, Oxford*
Ashmole 340, 346, 855, 1437, 1443, 1505
Bodley 484, 618, e Mus 19
Laud Misc. 156
Rawl. B.335

*Borthwick Institute of Historical Research, York*
Dean and Chapter Act Books

*British Library, London*
Add. 6214, 8195, 19078, 19112, 19674, 24828, 27582, 29895, 32098, 37503, 37508
Add. Charters 19137, 20423
Add. Rolls 34363A, 34364–5, 34770, 39602–3, 39647
Arundel 42
Cotton Claudius E IV, Faustina A III, Nero C XII, Nero D I, Tiberius C V, Vespasian
    E V, Vespasian E XXII
Egerton 1995, 2104A, 2572
Harley 3, 45, 328, 1736, 4012, 4015, 4431
Harley Charters 43 A 9, 58 I 39, 112 A 3
Harley Rolls N 20, N 23
Lansdowne 846
Royal 8 C I, 12 G IV, 17 D I
Sloane 4–6, 282, 428, 963, 1315, 1736, 2272, 2948, 3124, 3489, 3508B, 3983

*Cambridge University Library*
EDC 7–15–II–1–2, 6, 8, 9 [indexed on a database in Birmingham University Library]

*Cornwall Record Office*
Launceston Borough Records, B/Laus/285

*Corporation of London Record Office*
Journal 8
Plea and Memoranda Roll A40

*Devon Record Office*
Mayor of Exeter's Court Roll, 6–7 Henry VI

*King's Lynn Borough Archives*
KL/C7/2
KL/C12/1/2, 3, 5, 8; C12/2, 3, 5, 7–9, 11
KL/C56/2–6, 12, 15, 16, 18

*Lincoln Archive Office*
Lincoln episcopal registers iii and v

*New College, Oxford*
MS 3691

*Norfolk Record Office*
BRA/833/14/1
Bradfer Lawrence MS IX d
DCN 1/6/4, 9, 26, 27
DCN 35/7, 39/1, 79/3–4
DN, reg. 6, book 11
Le Strange MS DA6
MSC 1/5
NCC, registers Aleyn, Brosyard, Grundisburgh, Jekkys
NCR, 8A/1–2
NCR, 16B, Assembly Book, 1491–1553
NCR, 16D, Assembly Proceedings, 1434–1491
NCR, 24B/1
Norwich Archdeaconry Court, register Fuller
Y/C4/70, 83–203

*Public Record Office (National Archives)*
C1/46/158
C193/1
C115/K2/6683 I
E135/22/50, 38/171
KB145/6/24
PCC Adeane, Chayne, Kidd, Vox
SC2/179/14, 22, 203/95

*Suffolk Record Office, Ipswich*
IC/AA2/5/220

*Trinity College, Cambridge*
MSS O.I.9, O.I.13, O.I.77, O.9.28, R.14.32, R.15.21

*Wellcome Institute Library, London*
Western 408, 507, 510, 517, 548, 552, 784, 5133/1, 8004

*York Minster Library, York*
MS XVI.E.32
MS B2 (3), a 4–5, 7

## Printed Primary Sources

Abbott, E.A., ed., *St Thomas of Canterbury: His Death and Miracles* (2 vols, London, 1898)

*Acta Sanctorum* (69 vols, Rome, Paris and Brussels, 1863–1940)

Adelard of Bath, *Adelard of Bath: Conversations with His Nephew*, ed. C. Burnett (Cambridge, 1998)

Aegineta, Paulus, *The Seven Books of Paulus Aegineta*, ed. F. Adams (3 vols, Sydenham Society, London, 1844–47)

Aelred of Rievaulx, *Opera omnia*, PL, cxcv (Paris, 1855)

———, *Life of Edward the Confessor*, ed. J. Bertram (Guildford, 1990)

Albucassis, *Albucassis on Surgery and Instruments: A Definitive Edition of the Arabic Text with English Translation and Commentary*, eds M.S. Spink and G.L. Lewis (London, 1973)

Alcabitius, *Al-Qabisi (Alcabitius) The Introduction to Astrology*, eds C. Burnett, K. Yamamoto and M. Yano (Warburg Institute Studies and Texts, ii, 2004)

Alexander III, *Opera omnia: Epistolae et privilega*, PL, cc (Paris, 1855)

Alexander of Tralles, *Oeuvres médicales d'Alexandre de Tralles*, ed. F. Burnet (2 vols, Paris, 1933–36)

Allan, G., ed., *Collections Relating [to] Sherburn Hospital* (Durham, 1771)

Andersen, J.G., ed., *Studies in the Mediaeval Diagnosis of Leprosy in Denmark* (Copenhagen, 1969)

Anon, *A Litil Boke whiche Trayted and Reherced Many Gode Thinges Necessaries for the . . . Pestilence* (John Rylands Facsimiles, iii, 1910)

Aretaeus, *The Extant Works of Aretaeus, the Cappadocian*, ed. F. Adams (London, Sydenham Society, 1856)

Arnald of Villanova, *Le tresor des pauvres selon Maistre Arnoult de Ville Noue . . . et plusieurs aultre docteurs de medicine de Montpellier* (Lyon, 1512)

———, *Epistola Magistri Arnaldi Catalani de Villanova . . . de sanguine humano* (Basle, 1561)

———, *De dosi tyriacalium medicinarum*, in M.R. McVaugh, ed., *Opera medica omnia, III* (Barcelona, 1985)

Arnold, T., ed., *Memorials of St Edmunds Abbey* (3 vols, RS, 1890–96)

Atkinson, J.C., ed., *Cartularium Abbathiae de Whitby* (2 vols, Surtees Society, lxix, 1878, and lxii, 1881)

Audelay, John, *The Poems of John Audelay*, ed. E.K. Whiting (EETS, clxxxiv, 1931)

Aurelianus, Caelius, *Tardarum passionum libri V*, ed. G. Bendz (Berlin, 1993)

Avicenna, *Liber canonis* (Venice, 1507, reprinted Hildesheim, 1964)

Bacon, Roger, *De retardatione accidentium senectutis cum aliis opusculis de rebus medicinalibus*, eds A.G. Whittle and E. Withington (British Society of Franciscan Studies, xiv, 1928)

Banester, John, 'The Natvre & Propertie of Quick Siluer', in William Clowes, *Briefe and Necessarie Treatise Touching the Cure of the Disease called Morbus Gallicus* (London, 1585)

Banks, M.M., ed., *An Alphabet of Tales, I, A–H* (EETS, cxxvi, 1904)

———, *An Alphabet of Tales, II, I–Z* (EETS, cxxvii, 1905)

Baraclough, G., ed., *The Charters of the Anglo Norman Earls of Chester c. 1071–1237* (Lancashire and Cheshire Record Society, cxxvi, 1988)

Barlow, F., ed., *The Life of King Edward* (Oxford, 1992)

———, *EEA, XI, Exeter 1046–1184* (Oxford, 1996)

Bartholomaeus Anglicus, *On the Properties of Things: John Trevisa's Translation of*

*Bartholomaeus Anglicus' De proprietatibus rerum*, ed. M.C. Seymour (3 vols, Oxford, 1975–88)

Bataille, Henri, *Ton sang précédé de la lépreuse* (Paris, 1898)

Bede, *Ecclesiastical History of the English People*, eds B. Colgrave and R.A.B. Mynors (Oxford, 1969)

Bellaguet, M.L., ed., *Chronique du religieux de Saint-Denys* (6 vols, Paris, 1839–52)

Berg, W.S. van der, ed., *Antidotarium Nicolai* (Leiden, 1917)

Bériou, N., and Touati, F.O., eds, *Voluntate Dei leprosus: Les lépreux entre conversion et exclusion aux XIIème et XIIIème siècles* (Testi, Studi, Strumenti, iv, Spoleto, 1991)

Berjeau, J.Ph., ed., *Biblia pauperum* (London, 1859)

Béroul, *The Romance of Tristan*, ed., N.J. Lacy (New York, 1989)

Best, M.R., and Brightman, F.H., eds, *The Book of Secrets of Albertus Magnus* (Oxford, 1973)

Bickley, F.B., ed., *The Little Red Book of Bristol* (2 vols, Bristol and London, 1900)

Bird, J., ed., 'Texts on Hospitals', in P. Biller and J. Ziegler, eds, *Religion and Medicine in the Middle Ages* (Woodbridge, 2001)

Blamires, A., ed., *Woman Defamed and Woman Defended* (Oxford, 1992)

Bokenham, Osbern, *Legendys of Hooly Wummen*, ed. M.J. Serjeantson (EETS, ccvi, 1938, reprinted 1971)

Bonaventure, *Bonaventure: The Soul's Journey into God; The Tree of Life; The Life of St Francis*, ed. E. Cousins (Toronto, 1978)

Bond, E.A., ed., *Chronica Monasterii de Melsa* (3 vols, RS, 1866–67)

Boorde, Andrew, A *Compendyous Regyment or a Dyetary of Healthe* (London, 1547)

———, *The Breuiary of Healthe* (London, 1552)

Bormans, S., ed., *Cartulaire de la Commune de Namur, 1429–1555* (Namur, 1876)

Bouquet, Dom., ed., *Vie de Saint Louis par le confesseur de la Reine Marguerite: Rerum Gallicarum et Francicarum scriptores, XX* (Paris, 1840)

Bourne, T., and Marcombe, D., eds, *The Burton Lazars Cartulary: A Medieval Leicestershire Estate* (University of Nottingham Centre for Local History, Record Series, vi, 1987)

Bradshaw, Henry, *Life of Saint Werburge*, ed. C. Horstmann (EETS, lxxxviii, 1887)

Brandeis, A., ed., *Jacob's Well* (EETS, cxv, 1900)

Brie, F.W.D., ed., *The Brut* (EETS, cxxxi, 1906)

Brigstocke Sheppard, J., ed., *Literae Cantuarienses* (3 vols, RS, 1887–89)

Brodin, G., ed., *Agnus Castus: A Middle English Herbal* (Upsala, 1950)

Brooke, R.B., ed., *Scripta Leonis, Rufini et Angeli sociorum S. Francisci* (Oxford, 1990)

Brown, V., ed., *Eye Priory Cartulary and Charters, II* (Suffolk Records Society, Charter Series, xiii, 1994)

Brown, W., ed., *Cartularium Prioratus de Gyseburne, I* (Surtees Society, lxxxvi, 1889)

———, *Yorkshire Inquisitions, II* (Yorkshire Archaeological Society, xxxiii, 1897)

———, *The Register of John le Romeyn, Archbishop of York, 1286–1296, I* (Surtees Society, cxxiii, 1913)

Buch, J.A.C., ed., *Ouvrages historiques de Polybe, Hérodien and Zozine* (2 vols, Paris, 1836)

Buchanan, Robert Williams, *The Complete Poetical Works of Robert Williams Buchanan* (London, 1901)

Bund, J.W., ed., *The Register of William de Geynesburgh, Bishop of Worcester* (Oxford, 1907)

Burton, Robert, *The Anatomy of Melancholy*, eds T.C. Faulkener et al. (6 vols, Oxford, 1989–2000)

Caesarius of Heisterbach, *The Dialogue of Miracles*, eds H. von E. Scott and G.G. Swinton Bland (2 vols, London, 1929)

*Calendar of Close Rolls, 1277–1476* (58 vols, London, 1892–1953)

*Calendar of Fine Rolls, 1272–1509* (22 vols, London, 1911–63)

*Calendar of Inquisitions Miscellaneous . . . Preserved in the Public Record Office* (8 vols to date, London, 1916–)

*Calendar of Liberate Rolls, 1226–1267* (5 vols, London, 1917–61)

*Calendar of Papal Registers: Letters and Petitions, 1198–1492* (15 vols, London, 1894–1961)

*Calendar of Patent Rolls, 1216–1477* (41 vols, London, 1894–1916)

Caley, J., and Hunter, J., eds, *Valor Ecclesiasticus* (6 vols, London, 1810–34)

Calvino, Italo, *Our Ancestors* (London, 1995)

*Catalogue of Seals in the Department of Manuscripts of the British Museum I* (London, 1887)

Celano, Thomas, *Vita prima*, in *Analecta Franciscana, legendae S. Francisci Assisiensis, X* (Florence, 1941)

Celsus, Aulus Cornelius, *De medicina*, ed. W.G. Spencer (3 vols, London, 1935–38)

Chaucer, Geoffrey, *The Canterbury Tales*, in L.D. Benson, ed., *The Riverside Chaucer* (Boston, 1987)

Cheney, C.R., and Jones, B.E.A., eds, *EEA, II, Canterbury 1162–1190* (Oxford, 1986)

———, and John, E., eds, *EEA, III, Canterbury 1193–1205* (Oxford, 1986)

Cigman, G., ed., *Lollard Sermons* (EETS, ccxciv, 1989)

Clay, C.T., ed., *Early Yorkshire Charters, VII: The Honour of Skipton* (Yorkshire Archaeological Society, Record Series, extra series, v, 1947)

Cockayne, O., ed., *Leechdoms, Wortcunning and Starcraft in Early England* (3 vols, RS, 1864–1866)

Coke, Sir Edward, *The First Part of the Institutes of the Laws of England* (London, 1794)

Coleridge, Samuel Taylor, *The Rime of the Ancient Mariner*, ed. P.H. Fry (Boston, Mass., 1999)

Collins, A.J., ed., *Manuale ad usum percelebris ecclesie Sarisburiensis* (Henry Bradshaw Society, xci, 1958)

Constantine the African, trans., *Liber Pantegni* (Lyon, 1515)

———, *Tratado médico de Constantino el Africano: Constantini liber de elephancia*, ed. A.I. Martín Ferreira (Valladolid, 1996)

Copeland, Robert, trans., *Questyonary of Cyrurgyens* (London, 1542)

Cotton, C., ed., *The Canterbury Chantries and Hospitals in 1546* (Kent Records, supplement, 1934)

Cox, J.C., ed., *Records of the Borough of Northampton II* (Northampton, 1898)

*Curia Regis Rolls . . . Preserved in the Public Record Office* (18 vols to date, London, 1922–)


Danby, H., ed., *The Code of Maimonides, Book Nine: The Book of Offerings* (New Haven and London, 1950)

———, *The Code of Maimonides: Book Ten, The Book of Cleanness* (New Haven and London, 1954)

Dante Alighieri, *The Comedy of Dante Alighieri: Purgatory*, ed. and trans. D.L. Sayers (Harmondsworth, 1955)

———, *Hell*, trans. S. Ellis (London, 1994)

Davis, N., ed., *Paston Letters and Papers of the Fifteenth Century* (2 vols, Oxford, 1971–76)

Dawson, W.R., ed., *A Leechbook of the Fifteenth Century* (London, 1934)

Dembowski, P.F., ed., *Ami et Amile: Chanson de Geste* (Paris, 1969)

Diekstra, F.N.M., ed., *Book for a Simple and Devout Woman* (Groningen, 1998)

Douglas, D.C., and Greenaway, G.W., eds, *English Historical Documents, II, 1042–1189* (London, 1953)

Douie, D.L., and Farmer, H., eds, *Magna vita Sancti Hugonis: The Life of St Hugh of Lincoln* (2 vols, London, 1961–62)

Downer, L.J., ed., *Leges Henrici Primi* (Oxford, 1972)

Dugdale, W., *Monasticon Anglicanum*, eds J. Caley et al. (6 vols, London, 1817–30)

Duggan, A.J., ed., *The Correspondence of Thomas Becket, Archbishop of Canterbury, 1162–1170* (2 vols, Oxford, 2000)

Duvernoy, J., ed., *Le registre d'inquisition de Jacques Fournier, évêque de Pamiers* (3 vols, Toulouse, 1965)


Eadmer, *Historia novorum in Anglia*, ed. M. Rule (RS, 1884)

Easting, R., ed., *St Patrick's Purgatory* (EETS, ccxcviii, 1991)

Easting, R., ed., *The Revelation of the Monk of Eynsham* (EETS, cccxviii, 2002)

Eco, Umberto, *Baudolino* (London, 2002)

Edwards, A.J.M., ed., 'An Early Twelfth Century Account of the Translation of St Milburga of Much Wenlock', *Transactions of the Shropshire Archaeological Society*, lvii (1961–64), pp. 134–51

Erasmus of Rotterdam, *Enchiridion militis Christiani*, ed. A.M. O'Donnell (EETS, cclxxxii, 1981)


Farrer, W., ed., *Early Yorkshire Charters* (3 vols, Edinburgh, 1914–16)

Finberg, H.P.R., ed., 'Some Early Tavistock Charters', *EHR*, lxii (1947), pp. 352–77

Fisher, John, *The English Works of John Fisher*, ed. J.E.B. Mayor (EETS, extra series, xxvii, 1876)

Fisher, J.L. ed., 'The Leger Book of St John's Abbey, Colchester', *Transactions of the Essex Archaeological Society*, new series, xxiv (1951), pp. 77–127

Fitzherbert, Anthony, *The New Natura Brevium of the Most Reverend Judge Mr Anthony Fitzherbert* (London 1677)

Flaubert, Gustauve, *Salammbô* (Paris, 1970)

———, *La légend de Saint Julien l'Hospitalier illustrée de vingt-six compositions par L.O. Merson* (Paris, 1895)

———, *Oeuvres complètes de Gustave Flaubert: Correspondance: cinquième série, 1862–1868*, eds R. Dumesnil, J. Pommier and C. Digeon (Paris, 1929)

———, *Oeuvres complètes de Gustave Flaubert. Correspondance: supplément 1864–1871*, eds R. Dumesnil, J. Pommier and C. Digeon (Paris, 1954)

Fletcher, Joseph, *Christes Bloodie Sweat, or the Sonne of God in His Agonie by I.F.* (London, 1613)

Ford, A.E., ed., *La vengeance de Nostre-Seigneur* (Toronto, 1984)

Foreville, R., and Keir, G., eds, *The Book of St Gilbert* (Oxford, 1987)

Fowler, R.C., ed., *Registrum Simonis de Sudbiria* (2 vols, Oxford, 1927–28)

Francis, W. Nelson, ed., *The Book of Vices and Virtues* (EETS, ccxvii, 1942)

Franklin, M.J., ed., *EEA, 16, Coventry and Lichfield 1160–1182* (Oxford, 1998)

Friedberg, A., ed., *Corpus iuris canonici* (2 vols, Leipzig, 1879–81)

Furnivall, F.J., ed., *The Book of Quinte Essence* (EETS, xvi, 1866, reprinted 1965)

———, ed., *The Babees Book* (EETS, xxxii, 1868)

———, ed., *The Digby Plays* (EETS, extra series, lxx, 1896, reprinted 1967)

Galbraith, V.H., ed., *The Anonimalle Chronicle, 1333 to 1381* (Manchester, 1927)

Galen, Claudius, *Claudii Galeni opera omnia*, ed. C.G. Kühn (20 vols, Leipzig, 1821–33, reprinted Hildesheim, 1964–65)

———, *Galeni de optimo medico cognoscendo*, ed. A.Z. Iskander (Berlin, 1988)

Garton, C., ed., *The Metrical Life of St Hugh of Lincoln* (Lincoln, 1986)

Gascoigne, Thomas, *Loci e libro veritatum*, ed. J.H. Thorold Rogers (Oxford, 1881)

Gervase of Canterbury, *Historical Works: The Chronicle of the Reigns of Stephen, Henry II and Richard I*, ed. W. Stubbs (2 vols, RS, 1879–80)

Gilbert, J.T., ed., *Calendar of Ancient Records of Dublin, I* (Dublin, 1889)

Gilbertus Anglicus, *Compendium medicine* (Lyon, 1510)

———, *Healing and Society in Medieval England: A Middle English Translation of the Pharmaceutical Writings of Gilbertus Anglicus*, ed. F. Getz (Wisconsin, 1991)

Gordon, Bernard, *Opus lilium medicine* (Lyon, 1574)

Gower, John, *The English Works of John Gower*, ed. G.C. Macaulay (2 vols, EETS, extra series, lxxxi, 1900, and lxxxii, 1901)

Gransden, A., ed., *The Cartulary of the Benedictine Abbey of Bury St Edmunds in Suffolk* (London, 1973)

Grant, E., ed., *A Source Book in Medieval Science* (Cambridge, Mass., 1974)

Grant, M., ed., *Galen on Food and Diet* (London, 2000)

Green, M., ed., *The Trotula* (Philadelphia, 2001)

Greene, Graham, *A Burnt-Out Case* (London, 1974)

Grisdale, D.M., ed., *Three Middle English Sermons from the Worcester Chapter Manuscript F.10* (Leeds School of English Language Texts and Monographs, v, 1939)

Gross, C., ed., *The Gild Merchant* (2 vols, Oxford, 1890)

———, *Select Cases from the Coroners' Rolls, 1265–1413* (Selden Society, ix, 1896)

———, *Select Cases Concerning the Law Merchant, I* (Selden Society, xxiii, 1908)

Grosseteste, Robert, *Roberti Grosseteste episcopi quondam Lincolniensis epistolae*, ed. H.R. Luard (RS, 1861)

Gruner, O. Cameron, ed., *A Treatise on the Canon of Medicine of Avicenna* (London, 1930)

Guernes de Pont Sainte Maxence, *La vie de saint Thomas le Martyr, poème historique du XIIe siècle*, ed. E. Walberg (London, 1922)

Guy de Chauliac, *The Cyrurgie of Guy de Chauliac*, ed. M.S. Ogden (EETS, cclxv, 1971)


Haas, E. de, and Hall, G.D.G., eds, *Early English Registers of Writs* (Selden Society, lxxxvii, 1970)

Habig, M.A., ed., *St Francis of Assisi: Writings and Early Biographies* (London, 1973)

Hall, H., ed., *The Red Book of the Exchequer* (3 vols, RS, 1897)

Halliwell, J.O., ed., *The Miracles of Simon de Montfort* (CS, old series, xv, 1840)

Hanna, R., and Lawton, D., eds, *The Siege of Jerusalem* (EETS, cccxx, 2003)

Hardyng, John, *The Chronicle of Iohn Hardyng*, ed. H. Ellis (London, 1812)

Haren, M.J., ed., *Calendar of Papal Registers, Papal Letters, XV* (Dublin, 1978)

Harper-Bill, C., and Mortimer, R., eds, *Stoke-by-Clare Cartulary* (3 vols, Suffolk Records Society, Charter Series, iv–vi, 1982–84)

———, *The Register of John Morton Archbishop of Canterbury 1486–1500, I* (Canterbury and York Society, 1987)

———, *EEA, VI, Norwich 1070–1214* (Oxford, 1990)

———, *Charters of the Medieval Hospitals of Bury St Edmunds* (Suffolk Records Society, Charter Series, xiv, 1994)

Hart, W.H., *Historia et cartularium monasterii Sancti Petri Gloucestriae* (3 vols, RS, 1863–67)

Hatton, Sir Christopher, *Sir Christopher Hatton's Book of Seals*, eds L.C. Loyd and D.M. Stenton (Oxford, 1950)

Haydon, F.S., ed., *Eulogium historiarum sive temporis* (3 vols, RS, 1858–63)

Heales, A., ed., *The Records of Merton Priory* (London, 1898)

Helgaud de Fleury, *Vie de Robert le pieux*, eds R.H. Bautier and G. Labory (Paris, 1965)

Helmholz, R.H., ed., *Select Cases on Defamation to 1600* (Selden Society, ci, 1985)

Henderson, W.G., ed., *Missale ad usum insignis ecclesiae Eboracensis, II* (Surtees Society, lx, 1872)

Henri de Mondeville, *Chirurgie de Maitre Henri de Mondeville*, ed. E. Nicaise (Paris, 1893)

Henry of Huntingdon, *Henry, Archdeacon of Huntingdon: 'Historia Anglorum'*, ed. D. Greenway (Oxford, 1996)

Henry of Lancaster, *Le Livre de Seyntz Medicines*, ed. E.J. Arnould (Oxford, 1940)

Henry, A., ed., *The Pilgrimage of the Lyfe of the Manhode* (EETS, cclxxxviii, 1985)

———, ed., *The Mirour of Mans Saluacioun* (Aldershot, 1986)

Henryson, Robert, *Testament of Cresseid*, ed. D. Fox (London, 1968)

Herbert de Losinga, *The Life, Letters and Sermons of Bishop Herbert de Losinga*, eds E.M. Goulburn and H. Symonds (2 vols, Oxford, 1878)

Herbert, J.A., ed., *Titus and Vespasian: Or the Destruction of Jerusalem* (London, for the Roxburghe Club, 1905)

Herrtage, S.J.H., ed., *The Early English Version of the Gesta Romanorum* (EETS, extra series, xxxiii, 1879, reprinted 1962)

Higden, Ranulph, *Polychronicon Ranulphi Higden*, ed. J.R. Lumby (9 vols, RS, 1865–86)

Hildegard of Bingen, *Hildegard von Bingen's Physica*, ed. P. Throop (Rochester, Vermont, 1998)

———, *On Natural Philosophy and Medicine: Selections from the Cause et Cure*, ed. M. Berger (Woodbridge, 1999)

Hill, R.M.T., ed., *The Rolls and Register of Bishop Oliver Sutton 1280–1299, II* (Lincoln Record Society, xliii, 1950)

Hingeston-Randolph, F.C., ed., *The Register of Walter de Stapledon, Bishop of Exeter* (London, 1892)

*HMC, Fifth Report* (London, 1876)

*HMC, Sixth Report* (London, 1877)

*HMC, Eighth Report* (London, 1881)

*HMC, Eleventh Report, Appendix, Part III* (London, 1887)

*HMC, Twelfth Report, Appendix IX* (London, 1891)

*HMC, Fourteenth Report, Appendix VIII* (London, 1895)

*HMC, Report on the Records of the City of Exeter* (London, 1916)

*HMC, Report on the Hastings Manuscripts, I* (London, 1928)

Hoccleve, Thomas, *Hoccleve's Works: The Minor Poems*, ed. F.J. Furnivall (EETS, extra series, lxi, 1892)

Holmstedt, G., ed., *Speculum Christiani* (EETS, clxxxii, 1933)

Holtzman, W., and Kemp, E.W., eds, *Papal Decretals Relating to the Diocese of Lincoln in the Twelfth Century* (Lincoln Record Society, xlvii, 1954)

Horrox, R., ed., *The Black Death* (Manchester, 1994)

Horstmann, C., ed., *Yorkshire Writers: Richard Rolle and his Followers* (2 vols in 1, Woodbridge, 1999)

Horwood, A.J., ed., *Year Books of the Reign of King Edward the First, 30 and 31 Edward I* (RS, 1863)

Howlett, R., ed., *Chronicles of the Reigns of Stephen, Henry II and Richard I* (4 vols, RS, 1885–90)

Hudson, W., ed., *Leet Jurisdiction in the City of Norwich during the Thirteenth and Fourteenth Centuries* (Selden Society, v, 1892)

————, and Tingey, J.C., eds, *The Records of the City of Norwich* (2 vols, Norwich, 1906–10)

Hugh of St Victor, *Opera omnia*, PL, clxxv and clxxvii (Paris, 1879)

Hunt, T., ed., *Popular Medicine in Thirteenth-Century England* (Woodbridge, 1994)

————, *Anglo-Norman Medicine* (2 vols, Woodbridge, 1994–97)

Isaacson, R.F., and Ingleby, H., eds, *The Red Register of King's Lynn* (2 vols, King's Lynn, n.d.)

Jacob, E.F., ed., *The Register of Henry Chichele, Archbishop of Canterbury* (4 vols, Oxford, 1943–44)

Jacobus de Voragine, *The Golden Legend*, eds G. Ryan and H. Ripperger (London, 1941)

Jacques de Vitry, *The Life of Marie d'Oignies*, eds M.H. King and M. Marsolais (Toronto, 1993)

Jeayes, I.H., ed., *Court Rolls of the Borough of Colchester* (3 vols, Colchester, 1938–41)

Jocelin of Brakelond, *Chronicles of the Abbey of Bury St Edmunds*, eds D. Greenway and J. Sayers (Oxford, 1989)

John of Arderne, *Treatises of Fistula in Ano*, ed. D. Power (EETS, cxxxix, 1910)

John of Fordun, *John of Fordun's Chronicle of the Scottish Nation*, ed. W.F. Skene (Edinburgh, 1872)

John of Gaddesden, *Rosa Anglica practica medicine a capite ad pedes* (Pavia, 1492)

John of Salisbury, *Policraticus*, ed. C.J. Nederman (Cambridge, 1990)

John of Worcester, *The Chronicle of John of Worcester, III*, ed. P. McGurk (Oxford, 1998)

Johnson, C., and Cronne, H.A., eds, *Regesta Regum Anglo-Normannorum II* (Oxford, 1956)

Joinville, Jean, *The Life of St Louis*, ed. R. Hague (London, 1955)

Julian of Norwich, *A Book of Showings to the Anchoress Julian of Norwich*, eds E. Colledge and J. Walsh (2 vols, Toronto, 1978)

Kemp, B.R., ed., *Reading Abbey Cartularies* (2 vols, CS, fourth series, xxxi, 1986, and xxxxii, 1987)

Kemp, B.R., ed., *EEA, 19, Salisbury 1217–1228* (Oxford, 2000)

Kempe, Margery, *The Book of Margery Kempe*, ed. S.B. Meech (EETS, ccxii, 1940)

Kingdon, J.A., ed., *Facsimile of First Volume of Ms Archives of the Worshipful Company of Grocers of the City of London* (2 vols, London, 1886),

Kirby, J.F., ed., *Wykeham's Register, II* (Hampshire Record Society, xiii, 1899)

Knighton, Henry, *Chronicon Henrici Knighton monachi Leycestrensis*, ed. J.R. Lumby (2 vols, RS, 1889–95)

Lanfrank of Milan, *Lanfrank's 'Science of Cirgurie'*, ed. R. von Fleischhaker (EETS, cii, 1894)

Langland, William, *Piers Plowman Text B*, ed. W.W. Skeat (EETS, xxxviii, 1869, reprinted 1898)

————, *Langland's Vision of Piers the Plowman Text C*, ed. W.W. Skeat (EETS, liv, 1873)

Langtoft, Peter, *Peter Langtoft's Chronicle*, ed. T. Hearne (2 vols, Oxford, 1725, reprinted 1810)

Lauriere, M. de, et al., eds, *Ordonnances des roys de France* (23 vols, Paris, 1723–1849)

Lawn, B., ed., *The Prose Salernitan Questions* (Oxford, 1963)

Leach, A.F., ed., *Beverley Town Documents* (Selden Society, xiv, 1900)

————, ed., *Early Yorkshire Schools II* (Yorkshire Archaeological Society, Record Series, xxxiii, 1903)

Leach, M., ed., *Amis and Amiloun* (EETS, cciii, 1937)

Le Baker, Geoffrey, *Chronicon Galfridi le Baker de Swynebroke*, ed. E.M. Thompson (Oxford, 1889)

Le Grand, L., ed., *Statuts d'hôtels Dieu et léproseries* (Paris, 1910)

Lemay, H.R., ed., *Women's Secrets: A Translation of the Pseudo-Albertus Magnus's De secretis mulierum with Commentaries* (Albany, New York, 1992)

Lloyd, G.E.R., ed., *Hippocratic Writings* (Harmondsworth, 1983)

Lovatt, M., ed., *EEA, 20, York, 1154–1181* (Oxford, 2000)

Love, Nicholas, *The Mirror of the Blessed Life of Jesus Christ*, ed. M.G. Sargent (New York, 1992)

Lowell, James Russell, *The Poetical Works of James Russell Lowell*, ed. W.M. Rossetti (London, 1879)

Luchaire, A., ed., *Louis VI le Gros: Annales de sa vie et de sa règne* (2 vols, Paris, 1890)

Lull, Ramon, *The Book of the Ordre of Chyvalry*, trans. William Caxton, ed. A.T.P. Byles (EETS, clxviii, 1926)

Lydgate, John, and Burgh, Benedict, *Lydgate and Burgh's Secrees of Old Philisoffres* (EETS, extra series, lxvi, 1894)

————, *The Minor Poems of John Lydgate*, ed. H.N. MacCracken (EETS, cxcii, 1934)


McCann, J., ed., *The Rule of Saint Benedict* (London, 1921)

McCarthy, A.J., ed., *Book to a Mother* (Elizabethan and Renaissance Studies, xcii, Salzburg, 1981)

McNamara, J.A., and Halborg, J.E., eds, *Sainted Women of the Dark Ages* (Durham and London, 1992)

McNeill, J., and Gamer, H.M., eds, *Medieval Handbooks of Penance* (New York, 1938, reprinted 1990)

MacQueen, J., ed., *St Nynia* (Edinburgh, 1990)

Macray, W.D., ed., *Chronicon Abbatiae de Evesham* (RS, 1863)

————, *Chronicon Abbatiae Rameseiensis* (RS, 1886)

Maistre, Xavier de, *La jeune Sibérienne et le lépreux de la cité d'Aoste: A Literal Translation from the French* (Kelly's French Classics, London, 1886)

Mansi, J.D., ed., *Sacrorum conciliorum et amplissima collectio* (53 vols, Florence and Paris, 1759–98)

Manzalaoui, M.A., ed., *Secreta secretorum: Nine English Versions* (EETS, cclxxvi, 1977)

Map, Walter, *De nugis curialium*, ed. M.R. James, revised C.N.L. Brooke and R.A.B. Mynors (Oxford, 1983)

Markham, C.A., and Cox, J.C., eds, *The Records of the Borough of Northampton* (2 vols, Northampton, 1898)

Matarasso, P.M., ed., *The Quest of the Holy Grail* (Harmondsworth, 1969)

Maxwell, H., ed., *The Chronicle of Lanercost, 1272–1346* (Glasgow, 1913)

Maxwell-Lyte, H.C., and Dawes, M.C.B., eds, *The Register of Thomas Bekyngton, I* (Somerset Record Society, xlix, 1934)

Mayr-Harting, H., ed., *The Acta of the Bishops of Chichester 1075–1207* (Canterbury and York Society, 1964)

Mellows, W.T., and King, P.I., eds, *The Book of William Morton, Almoner of Peterborough Monastery 1448–1467* (Northamptonshire Record Society, xvi, 1954)

Menner, R.J., ed., *Purity, A Middle English Poem* (Yale Studies in English, lxi, 1970)

Merlet, R., and Jusselin, M., eds, *Cartulaire de la léproserie du Grand-Beaulieu, Chartres* (Chartres, 1909)

Mirk, alias Myrc, John, *Instructions for Parish Priests*, ed. E. Peacock (EETS, xxxi, 1868)

———, *Mirk's Festial: A Collection of Homilies*, ed. T. Erbe (EETS, xcvi, 1905)

Morris, R., ed., *An Old English Miscellany* (EETS, xlix, 1872)

———, *Old English Homilies of the Twelfth Century* (EETS, liii, 1873)

———, *Cursor Mundi, II* (EETS, lix, 1875, reprinted 1966)

Myers, A.R., ed., *The Household of Edward IV* (Manchester, 1959)


Nelson Francis, W., ed., *The Book of Vices and Virtues* (EETS, ccxvii, 1942)

Nichols, F.M., ed., *Britton* (2 vols, Oxford, 1865)

Nider, Johannes, *De morali lepra* (Nuremberg, c. 1470)

North, J.D., ed., *Richard of Wallingford* (3 vols, Oxford, 1976)


Oesterley, H., ed., *Gesta Romanorum* (Berlin, 1872)

Ogden, M.C., ed., *The Liber de diversis medicinis* (EETS, ccvii, 1969)

Old, H.O., ed., *The Reading and Preaching of the Scriptures, III, The Medieval Church* (Grand Rapids, Michigan, 1999)

Oliver, G., ed., *Monasticon dioecesis Exoniensis* (London, 1846)

Orderic Vitalis, *The Ecclesiastical History of Orderic Vitalis*, ed. M. Chibnall (6 vols, Oxford, 1969–80)

Orwell, George, *1984: A Novel* (London, 1949)

Owen, D.M., ed., *The Making of King's Lynn* (Records of Social and Economic History, new series, ix, 1984)


Palmer, W.M., ed., *Cambridge Borough Documents, I* (Cambridge, 1931)

Paris, Matthew, *Chronica Majora*, ed. H.R. Luard (7 vols, RS, 1872–84)

———, *The Life of St Edmund*, ed. C.H. Lawrence (Stroud, 1996)

Passy, L., ed., *Le livre des métiers de Gisors* (Pontoise, 1907)

Peckham, W.D., ed., *The Chartulary of the High Church of Chichester* (Sussex Record Society, xlvi, 1942–43)

Percy, J.W., ed., *York Memorandum Book* (Surtees Society, clxxxvi, 1973)

Peter Lombard, *Opera omnia, PL*, cxcii (Paris, 1880)

Phayer, Thomas, *Treatyse of the Pestylence* (London, 1546)

*Pipe Roll, 21 Henry II, 1174–1175* (Pipe Roll Society, xxii, 1897)

*Pipe Roll, 1 John, Michaelmas 1199* (Pipe Roll Society, new series, x, 1933)

*Pipe Roll, 6 John, Michaelmas 1204* (Pipe Roll Society, new series, xviii, 1940)

Pliny the Elder, *Natural History, VII*, ed. W.H.S. Jones (London, 1956)

Plummer, C., ed., *Bethada Náem Érenn: Lives of the Irish Saints* (2 vols, Oxford, 1922)

Potz McGerr, R., ed., *The Pilgrimage of the Soul: A Critical Edition of the Middle English Dream Vision* (New York, 1990)

Powell Harley, M., ed., *A Revelation of Purgatory by an Unknown Fifteenth-Century Woman Visionary* (Studies in Women and Religion, xviii, New York, c. 1985)

Powicke, F.M., and Cheney, C.R., eds, *Councils and Synods, II, 1205–1313, Part I, 1204–1265* (Oxford, 1964)

Prestwich, M., ed., *York Civic Ordinances, 1301* (Borthwick Papers, xlix, York, 1976)

Ptolemy, Claudius, *Tetrabiblos*, ed. F.E. Robbins (Cambridge, 1980)

Raine, J., ed., *Testamenta Eboracensia, I* (Surtees Society, iv, 1836)

———, *Wills and Inventories I* (Surtees Society, ii, 1835)

———, *Libellus de vita et miraculis S. Godrici, hermetiae de Finchale* (Surtees Society, xx, 1847)

———, *The Priory of Hexham, II* (Surtees Society, xlvi, 1865)

———, *Historians of the Church of York and its Archbishops* (3 vols, RS, 1879–94)

———, *Memorials of the Church of SS Peter and Winifrid, Ripon, I* (Surtees Society, lxxiv, 1881)

Ramsey, F.M.R., ed., *EEA, X, Bath and Wells 1061–1205* (Oxford, 1995)

Reginald of Durham, *Reginaldi monachi Dunelmensis libellus de admirandis beati Cuthberti*, ed. J. Raine (Surtees Society, i, 1835)

*Registrum Omnium Brevium* (London, 1531)

Reynes, Robert, *The Commonplace Book of Robert Reynes of Acle: An Edition of Tanner MS 407*, ed. C. Louis (New York, 1980)

Rhys Bram, J., ed., *Ancient Astrology: Theory and Practice* (Park Ridge, New Jersey, 1975)

Riley, H.T., ed., *The Liber Albus: The White Book of the City of London* (London, 1861)

———, *Memorials of London and London Life in the Thirteenth, Fourteenth and Fifteenth Centuries* (London, 1868)

Robert de Boron, *Joseph d'Arimathie*, ed. R. O'Gorman (Toronto, 1995)

Robert of Brunne, *Robert of Brunne's 'Handlyng Synne'*, ed. F.J. Furnivall, (EETS, cxix, 1901, and cxxiii, 1903, reprinted in one vol. 1973)

Robert of Flamborough, *Liber poenitentialis: A Critical Edition with Introduction and Notes*, ed., J.J.F. Firth (Toronto, Pontifical Institute of Medieval Studies, xviii, 1971)

Robert of Gloucester, *The Metrical Chronicle of Robert of Gloucester*, ed. W.A. Wright (2 vols, RS, 1887)

Robertson, J.C., ed., *Materials for the History of Thomas Becket* (7 vols, RS, 1875–85)

Roger of Howden, *Chronica Magistri Rogeri de Houedene*, ed. W. Stubbs (4 vols, RS, 1868–71)

Roger of Wendover, *Flores Historiarum*, ed. H.G. Hewlett (3 vols, RS, 1886–89)

Rolle, Richard, *English Writings of Richard Rolle*, ed. H.E. Allen (Oxford, 1963)

Ross, W.O., ed., *Middle English Sermons* (EETS, ccix, 1940, reprinted 1960)

Rothwell, W., et al., eds, *Anglo-Norman Dictionary* (London, 1992)

Rymer, T., ed., *Foedera, conventiones, literae et cuiuscunque generis acta publica, V* (The Hague, 1741)

Saint Anselm of Canterbury, *The Letters of Saint Anselm of Canterbury I*, ed. W. Frölich (Cistercian Studies, xcvi, 1990)

Saint Bernard of Clairvaux, *Opera omnia: Liber de modo bene vivendi*, PL, clxxxiv (Paris, 1854)

Saint Bridget of Sweden, *The Liber Celestis of St Bridget of Sweden: Volume I Text*, ed. R. Ellis (EETS, ccxci, 1987)

Saint Gregory the Great, *Opera omnia: Homiliarum in Evangelia*, PL, lxxvi (Paris, 1849)
————, *Morals in the Book of Job*, ed. J. Bliss (4 vols, Oxford, 1844–50)
Saint Isidore of Seville, *Opera omnia: Quaestiones in Vetus Testamentum*, PL, lxxxiii (Paris 1862)
————, *Isidori Hispalensis episcopi, etymologiarum sive originum libri XX*, ed. W.M. Lindsay (2 vols, Oxford, 1911)
Saint Ivo of Chartres, *Opera omnia*, PL, clxi (Paris, 1889)
Saint Jerome, *Opera omnia: Commentariorum in Isaiam prophetam*, PL, xxiv (Paris, 1845)
————, *Opera omnia: Commentariorum in Ezechielem*, PL, xxv (Paris, 1884)
Saint Thomas Aquinas, *Summa Theologica* (6 vols, Rome, 1894)
Salter, F.R., ed., *Some Early Tracts on Poor Relief* (London, 1926)
Salter, H.E., ed., *A Cartulary of the Hospital of St John the Baptist* (3 vols, Oxford Historical Society, lxviii–lxix, 1914–16)
Salu, M.B., ed. and trans., *The Ancrene Riwle* (Exeter Medieval English Texts and Studies, 1990)
Sayles, G.O., ed., *Select Cases in the Court of King's Bench under Edward I, III* (Selden Society, lviii, 1939)
————, *Select Cases in the Court of King's Bench under Richard II, Henry IV and Henry V* (Selden Society, lxxxviii, 1971)
Schofield, B., ed., *Muchelney Memoranda* (Somerset Record Society, xlii, 1927)
Schwob, Marcel, *Le roi au masque d'or, vies imaginaires, la croisade des enfants* (Paris, 1979)
Searle, E., ed., *The Chronicle of Battle Abbey* (Oxford, 1980)
Severus, Sulpicius, *Vie de Saint Martin*, ed. J. Fontaine (3 vols, Paris, 1967–69)
Sharpe, R.R., ed., *Calendar of Letter-Books of the City of London, Letter-Book A* (London, 1899)
————, *Calendar of Letter-Books of the City of London, Letter-Book D* (London, 1902)
————, *Calendar of Letter-Books of the City of London, Letter-Book G* (London, 1905)
————, *Calendar of Letter-Books of the City of London, Letter-Book I* (London, 1909)
————, *Calendar of Letter-Books of the City of London, Letter-Book K* (London, 1911)
————, *Calendar of Letter-Books of the City of London, Letter-Book L* (London, 1912)
Sharpe, R., et al., eds, *English Benedictine Libraries: The Shorter Catalogues* (Corpus of British Medieval Library Catalogues, iv, 1996)
Sheppard, J.B., ed., *Literae Cantuarienses* (3 vols, RS, 1887–89)
Shinners, J., and Dohar, W.J., eds, *Pastors and the Care of Souls in Medieval England* (Notre Dame, Indiana, 1998)
Small, J., ed., *English Metrical Homilies* (Edinburgh, 1862)
Smith, D.M., ed., *EEA, I, Lincoln 1067–1185* (Oxford, 1980)
Smith, T., Smith, L.T., and Brentano, L., eds, *English Gilds* (EETS, xl, 1870)
Snape, M.G., ed., *EEA, 24, Durham 1153–1195* (Oxford, 2001)
————, *EEA, 25, Durham 1196–1237* (Oxford, 2001)
Spector, S., ed., *The N-Town Play, I* (EETS, supplementary series, xi, 1991)
*Speculum humanae salvationis: The Miroure of Mans Saluacionne* (London, for the Roxburghe Club, 1888)
Spenser, Edmund, *Complete Poetical Works*, eds J.C. Smith and E. de Selincourt (Oxford, 1912)

*The Star*, iii, no. 10 (Carville, Louisiana, 15 October 1933); iv, nos 2 (July 1934), 3 (August 1934), 4 (September – October 1934)

Starkey, Thomas, *A Dialogue between Pole and Lupset*, ed. T.F. Mayer (CS, fourth series, xxxvii, 1989)

Stenton, D.M., ed., *The Earliest Northamptonshire Assize Rolls* (Northamptonshire Record Society, v, 1930)

Stevenson, J., ed., *Chronicon de Lanercost, 1272–1346* (Bannatyne Club, lxv, Edinburgh, 1839)

Stevenson, Robert Louis, *The Black Arrow: A Tale of the Two Roses* (London, 1901 reprint)

———, *The Works of Robert Louis Stevenson: Pentland Edition XV* (London, 1907)

Stevenson, W.H., ed., *Records of the Borough of Nottingham I* (Nottingham, 1882)

———, *Calendar of Records of the Corporation of Gloucester* (Gloucester, 1893)

Stone, B., ed. and trans., *The Owl and the Nightingale, Cleanness and St Erkenwald* (Harmondsworth, 1971)

Storey, R.L., ed., *The Register of John de Kirkby, Bishop of Carlisle, II* (Woodbridge, 1995)

———, *The Register of Gilbert Welton, Bishop of Carlisle, 1353–1362* (Woodbridge, 1999)

Stow, John, *A Survey of London by John Stow*, ed. C.L. Kingsford (2 vols, Oxford, 1908)

Strachey, J., et al., eds, *Rotuli Parliamentorum* (6 vols, London, 1783)

S[wadlin], T[homas], *Sermons, Meditations and Prayers upon the Plague 1636* (London, 1637)

Swinburne, Algernon Charles, *The Poems of Algernon Charles Swinburne, I, Poems and Ballads* (London, 1904)


Talbot, C.H., ed., *The Anglo Saxon Missionaries in Germany* (London, 1954)

Tanner, N., ed., *Decrees of the Ecumenical Councils* (2 vols, Georgetown, 1990)

Tennyson, Alfred, Lord, *The Poems of Tennyson*, ed. C. Ricks (3 vols, London, 1987)

Tertullian, *The Writings of Quintus Sept. Flor. Tertullianus*, eds A. Roberts and J. Donaldson (3 vols, Edinburgh, 1895)

Theoderic, *The Surgery of Theoderic*, eds E. Campbell and J.C. Colton (2 vols, New York, 1955–60)

Thomas de Chobham, *Thomae de Chobham summa confessorum*, ed. F. Broomfield (Louvain and Paris, 1968)

Thomas of Monmouth, *The Life and Miracles of St William of Norwich*, eds A. Jessopp and M. Rhodes James (Cambridge, 1896)

Thomas, A.H., ed., *Calendar of Select Plea and Memoranda Rolls Preserved among the Archives of the Corporation of the City of London, 1381–1412* (Cambridge, 1932)

———, *Calendar of Plea and Memoranda Rolls Preserved among the Archives of the Corporation of the City of London, 1413–1437* (Cambridge, 1943)

Thomson, T., and Innes, C., eds, *The Acts of the Parliament of Scotland* (12 vols, Edinburgh, 1844–75)

Thorne, S.E., ed., *Bracton on the Laws and Customs of England* (4 vols, Cambridge, Mass., 1968–77)

Thurston, H., ed., 'Visio monnachi de Eynsham', *Analecta Bollandia*, xxii (1903), pp. 225–319

Turner, G.J., ed., *Select Pleas of the Forest* (Selden Society, xiii, 1899)

Turner, W.H., and Coxe, H.O., eds, *Calendar of Charters and Rolls Preserved in the Bodleian Library* (Oxford, 1878)

Ulrich von Hutten, *De morbo Gallico*, trans. Thomas Paynell (London, 1533)

Vicary, Thomas, *The Anatomie of the Bodie of Man*, eds F.J. Furnivall and P. Furnivall (EETS, extra series, liii, 1888, reprinted 1973)

Voigts, L.E., and McVaugh, M.R., eds, 'A Latin Technical Phlebotomy and its Middle English Translation', *Transactions of the American Philosophical Society*, lxxiv, part 2 (1984), pp. 1–69

Voltaire, Francois Marie Arouet, *Oeuvres complètes de Voltaire*, 19, *Dictionnaire philosophique, III*, ed. L. Moland (Paris 1879, reprinted 1967)

Vriend, J. de, ed., *The Old English herbarium and medicina de quadrupedibus* (EETS, cclxxxvi, 1984)

Walker, D., ed., 'Charters of the Earldom of Hereford, 1095–1201', *Miscellany XXII* (CS, fourth series, i, 1964)

Walsingham, Thomas, *Gesta abbatum monasterii Sancti Albani*, ed. H.T. Riley (3 vols, RS, 1867–69)

———, *Ypodigma Neustriae*, ed. H.T. Riley (RS, 1876)

Wallace, Lewis, *Ben-Hur: A Tale of the Time of Our Lord* (New York, 1880)

A. Watkin, ed., *Inventory of Church Goods Temp. Edward III* (Norfolk Record Society, xix, 2 parts, 1947–48)

Watkiss, L., and Chibnall, M., eds, *The Waltham Chronicles* (Oxford, 1994)

Weatherby, E.H., ed., *Speculum sacerdotale* (EETS, cc, 1936)

Webber, T., and Watson, A.G., eds, *The Libraries of Augustinian Canons* (Corpus of British Medieval Library Catalogues, vi, 1998)

Wenzel, S., ed., *Summa virtutum de remediis anime* (Athens, Georgia, 1984)

———, *Fasciculus Morum: A Fourteenth-Century Preacher's Handbook* (Pennsylvania, 1989)

Whitelock, D., Brett, M., and Brooke, C.N.L., eds, *Councils and Synods I, Part II, 1066–1204* (Oxford, 1981)

Whittaker, W.J., ed., *The Mirror of Justices* (Selden Society, vii, 1895)

Wilde, Oscar, *The Picture of Dorian Gray*, ed. D.L. Lawler (London, 1988)

Wilkins, D., ed., *Concilia Magnae Britanniae et Hiberniae* (4 vols, London, 1737)

William of Malmesbury, *De gestis pontificum Anglorum*, ed. N.E.S.A. Hamilton (RS, 1870)

———, *The Vita Wulfstani of William of Malmesbury*, ed. R.R. Darlington (CS, third series, xl, 1928)

———, *The Chronicle of Glastonbury Abbey*, ed. J.P. Carley (Woodbridge, 1985)

———, *Gesta Regum Anglorum*, eds R.A.B. Mynors et al. (2 vols, Oxford, 1998–99)

William of Newburgh, *Historia rerum Anglicarum*, ed. R. Howlett (RS, 1885)

Williams, E., ed., *Early Holborn and the Legal Quarter of London* (2 vols, London, 1927)

Willis, Nathaniel Parker, *Complete Works* (3 vols, New York, 1846)

Wilson, R.McL., and Schneemelcher, W., eds, *New Testament Apocrypha, I* (SCM Press, 1973)

Windt, E.B. de, ed., *The Court Rolls of Ramsey, Hepmangrove and Bury 1268–1600* (Subsidia Mediaevalia, xvii, 1990)

Wood-Leigh, K.L., ed., *Kentish Visitations of Archbishop Warham and his Deputies 1511–1512* (Kent Archaeological Society, Kent Records, xxiv, 1984)

Wright, M., and Loncar, K., eds, 'Goscelin's *Legend of Edith*', in S. Hollis, ed., *Writing the Wilton Women: Goscelin's Legend of Edith and liber confortatorius* (Turnhout, 2004)

Wright, T., ed., *Political Poems and Songs Relating to English History* (2 vols, RS, 1859–61)

———, *The Book of the Knight of la Tour-Landry* (EETS, xxxiii, 1868, reprinted 1969)

Wycliffe, John, trans., *The Holy Bible . . . by John Wycliffe*, eds J. Forshall and F. Madden (4 vols, Oxford, 1850)

Zetterstein, A., ed., *The English Text of the Ancrene Riwle* (EETS, cclxxiv, 1976)

## Printed Secondary Sources

Adamson, M.W., *Medieval Dietetics: Food and Drink in the Regimen Sanitatis Literature from 800 to 1400* (Frankfurt and New York, 1995)

Agrimi, J., and Crisciani, C., 'Charity and Aid in Medieval Christian Civilisation', in M.D. Grmek, ed., *Western Medical Thought from Antiquity to the Middle Ages* (Cambridge, Mass., and London, 1998)

Albert, J.P., *Odeurs de sainteté: La mythologie Chrétienne des aromates* (Paris, 1990)

Alexander, J.W., 'Herbert of Norwich, 1091–1119: Studies in the History of Norman England', *Studies in Medieval and Renaissance History*, vi (1969), pp. 119–232

Alexandre-Bidon, D., 'Le coeur du Christ au pressoir mystique: le cas des céramiques du Beauvaisis au début du XVIe siècle', in D. Alexandre-Bidon, ed., *Le pressoir mystique* (Paris, 1990)

Alston, M.N., 'The Attitude of the Church towards Dissection before 1500', *BHM*, xvi (1944), pp. 221–38

Amundsen, D.W., 'Medieval Canon Law on Medical and Surgical Practice by the Clergy', *BHM*, lii (1978), pp. 22–43

———, *Medicine, Society and Faith in the Ancient and Medieval Worlds* (Baltimore, 1996)

Anderson, S., 'Leprosy in a Medieval Churchyard in Norwich', in S. Anderson, ed., *Current and Recent Research in Osteoarchaeology* (Oxford, 1998)

Anon, 'La lèpre et la castration', *Janus*, ii (1897–98), p. 289

Arbesmann, R., 'The Concept of "*Christus Medicus*" in Saint Augustine', *Traditio*, x (1954), pp. 1–28

Archibald, E., 'Did Knights Have Baths? The Absence of Bathing in Middle English Romance', in C. Saunders, ed., *Cultural Encounters in the Romance of Medieval England* (Studies in Medieval Romance, ii, 2005)

Ardsall, A. van, *Medieval Herbal Remedies* (London, 2002)

Arnold, D., 'Introduction: Disease, Medicine and Empire', in D. Arnold, ed., *Imperial Medicine in Indigenous Societies* (Manchester, 1988)

Arrizabalaga, J., 'Facing the Black Death: Perceptions and Reactions of University Medical Practitioners', in L. García-Ballester, R. French, J. Arrizabalaga and A. Cunningham, eds, *Practical Medicine from Salerno to the Black Death* (Cambridge, 1994)

———, Henderson, J., and French, R., *The Great Pox: The French Disease in Renaissance Europe* (New Haven and London, 1997)

———, 'Problematizing Retrospective Diagnosis in the History of Disease', *Asclepio*, liv, fasc. 1 (2002), pp. 51–70

Ashmead, A.S., 'Leprosy Overcome by Isolation in the Middle Ages', *Janus*, i (1896–97), p. 558

————, 'What a Leprosy Conference Should Be', *The Lancet*, cl, issue 3859 (14 August 1897), p. 414

————, *Suppression and Prevention of Leprosy* (Norristown, Pennsylvania, 1897)

Avi-Yonah, M., 'The Bath of the Lepers at Scythopolis', *Israel Exploration Journal*, xiii (1963), pp. 325–6

Avril, J., 'Le IIIe Concile du Latran et les communautés de lépreux', *Revue Mabillon*, lx (1981), pp. 21–76


Baker, D., 'A Nursery of Saints: St Margaret of Scotland Reconsidered', in D. Baker, ed., *Medieval Women* (Studies in Church History, Subsidia, i, 1978)

Baker, J.H., *An Introduction to English Legal History* (third edn, London, 1990)

Baker, P., *The Dedalus Book of Absinthe* (Sawtry, 2001)

Barber, M., 'Lepers, Jews and Moslems: The Plot to Overthrow Christendom in 1321', *History*, lxvi (1981), pp. 1–17

Barnes, D.S., *The Making of a Social Disease: Tuberculosis in Nineteenth-Century France* (Berkeley, California, 1995)

Barratt, A., 'Stabant matres dolorosae: Women as Readers and Writers of Passion Prayers, Meditations and Visions', in A.A. MacDonald et al., eds, *The Broken Body: Passion Devotion in Late Medieval Culture* (Groningen, 1998)

Bayer, H., 'Lepra Universalis: Neoplatonism (Catharism) and Judaism as Reflected in Twelfth and Thirteenth Century Literature', *History of European Ideas*, ix (1988), pp. 281–303

Bean, J.M.W., 'Plague, Population and Economic Decline in England in the Later Middle Ages', *Economic History Review*, series two, xv (1963), pp. 423–37

Beck, T., *The Cutting Edge: Early History of the Surgeons of London* (London, 1974)

Bell, D.N., 'The English Cistercians and the Practice of Medicine', *Citeaux*, xl (1989), pp. 139–74

————, 'The Siting and Size of Cistercian Infirmaries in England and Wales', *Studies in Cistercian Art and Architecture*, v (1998), pp. 211–38

Bergman, F., 'Hoping against Hope? A Marital Dispute about the Medical Treatment of Leprosy in the Fifteenth-Century Hanseatic Town of Kampen', in H. Marland and M. Pelling, eds, *The Task of Healing: Medicine, Religion and Gender in England and the Netherlands 1450–1800* (Rotterdam, 1996)

Bériac, F., 'Mourir au monde: Les ordines de séparation des lépreux en France au XVe et XVIe siècles', *Journal of Medieval History*, xi (1985), pp. 245–68

————, *Histoire des lépreux au moyen âge: une société d'exclus* (Paris, 1988)

————, *Des lépreux aux cagots: Recherches sur les sociétés marginales en Acquitaine médiévale* (Bordeaux, 1990)

————, 'Les fraternités des lépreux et lépreuses', in K. Elm and M. Parisse, eds, *Doppelklöster und andere Formen der Symbiose männlicher und weiblicher Religiosen in Mittelalter* (Berlin, 1992)

N. Bériou, 'L'image de l'autre: le lépreux sous le regard des predicateurs, au moyen âge', *L'Histoire Aujourd'hui* (Liège, 1988)

Bernabeu-Mestre, J., and Ballester-Artigues, T., 'Le Retour d'un péril: La lèpre dans l'Espagne, 1878–1932', *Annales de demographie historique: Epidémies et populations* (Paris, 1997), pp. 115–34

————, and ————, 'Disease as a Metaphorical Resource: The Fontilles Philanthropic Initiative in the Fight against Leprosy, 1901–1932', *SHM*, xvii (2004), pp. 409–21.

Berthelet, A., 'Sang et lèpre, sang et feu', in *Le sang au moyen âge: Actes du quatrième colloque international de Montpellier* (Cahiers du CRISIMA, iv, 1999)

Besserman, L.L., *The Legend of Job in the Middle Ages* (Harvard, 1979)

Biebel, E.M., 'Pilgrims to Table: Food Consumption in Chaucer's *Canterbury Tales*', in M. Carlin and J. Rosenthal, eds, *Food and Eating in Medieval Europe* (London, 1998)

Biernoff, S., *Sight and Embodiment in the Middle Ages* (London, 2002)

Biggs, D., 'The Politics of Health: Henry IV and the Long Parliament of 1406', in G. Dodd and D. Biggs, eds, *Henry IV: The Establishment of a Regime 1399–1406* (York, 2003)

Biller, P., 'Views of the Jews from Paris around 1300: Christian or "Scientific"?', in D. Wood, ed., *Christianity and Judaism* (Studies in Church History, xxix, 1992)

———, 'William of Newburgh and the Cathar Mission to England', in D. Wood, ed., *Life and Death in the Northern Church c. 1100–c.1700* (Studies in Church History, Subsidia, xii, 1999)

———, 'Introduction', in P. Biller and A.J. Minnis, eds, *Handling Sin: Confession in the Middle Ages* (York, 1998)

Binski, P., *Medieval Death: Ritual and Representation* (London, 1996)

Bird, J., 'Medicine for Body and Soul: Jacques de Vitry's Sermons to Hospitallers and their Charges', in P. Biller and J. Ziegler, eds, *Religion and Medicine in the Middle Ages* (York, 2001)

Blair, J., 'Saint Frideswide Reconsidered', *Oxoniensia*, lii (1987), pp. 71–127

Blomefield, F.B., *An Essay towards a Topographical History of Norfolk* (11 vols, London, 1805–10)

Bloomfield, M.W., *The Seven Deadly Sins* (Michigan, 1952)

Bonser, W., *The Medical Background of Anglo Saxon England* (London, 1963)

Borradori, P., *Mourir au monde: Les lépreux dans le pays de Vaud* (Cahiers Lausannois d'Histoire Médiévale, vii, 1992)

Bourgeois, A., *Lépreux et maladreries du Pas-de-Calais* (Arras, 1972)

Bown, J., and Stirland, A., *Criminals and Paupers: Excavations at the Site and Church-yard of St Margaret, Fyebridgegate, Magdalen Street, Norwich* (East Anglian Archaeology, forthcoming)

Brierre-Narbonne, J.J., *Le Messie souffrant dans la littérature rabbinique* (Paris, 1940)

Brody, S.N., *The Disease of the Soul: Leprosy in Medieval Literature* (Cornell, 1974)

Brown, E.A.R., 'Death and the Human Body in the Later Middle Ages: The Legislation of Boniface VIII on the Division of the Corpse', *Viator*, xii (1981), pp. 221–70

Brown, P., *The Body and Society: Men, Women and Sexual Renunciation in Early Christianity* (New York, 1988)

Brown, P., and Butcher, A., *The Age of Saturn: Literature and History in the Canterbury Tales* (Oxford, 1991)

Browne, S.G., *Leprosy in the Bible* (Christian Medical Fellowship, London, third edn, 1979)

Brundage, J.A., *Law, Sex and Christian Society in Medieval Europe* (Chicago, 1987)

Buckingham, J., *Leprosy in Colonial South India: Medicine and Confinement* (Basingstoke, 2002)

Butcher, A.F., 'The Hospital of St Stephen and St Thomas New Romney: The Documentary Evidence', *Archaeologia Cantiana*, xcvi (1981), pp. 17–26

Cadden, J., *Meanings of Sex Difference in the Middle Ages* (Cambridge, 1993)

Cameron, M.L., 'The Sources of Medical Knowledge in Anglo-Saxon England', *Anglo-Saxon England*, xi (1982), pp. 135–55

———, *Anglo-Saxon Medicine* (Cambridge, 1993)

Camille, M., *Image on the Edge: The Margins of Medieval Art* (London, 1992)

Camporesi, P., *The Incorruptible Flesh: Bodily Mutilation and Mortification in Religion and Folklore* (Cambridge, 1988)

———, *The Fear of Hell: Images of Damnation and Salvation in Early Modern Europe* (Oxford, 1991)

Carr, E.H., *What is History?* (London, 1961)

Carrasco, M., 'Sanctity and Experience in Pictorial Hagiography', in R. Blumenfeld-Kosinski and T. Szell, eds, *Images of Sainthood in Medieval Europe* (Ithaca and London, 1991),

Cartwright, F.F., *A Social History of Medicine* (London, 1977)

Cassidy-Welch, M., *Monastic Spaces and their Meanings: Thirteenth-Century English Cistercian Monasticism* (Turnhout, 2001)

Caviness, M.H., *The Windows of Christ Church Cathedral Canterbury* (London, 1981)

Cheney, M., 'The Council of Westminster of 1175: New Light on an Old Source', in D. Baker, ed., *The Materials, Sources and Methods of Ecclesiastical History* (Studies in Church History, xi, 1975)

Cholmeley, H.P., *John of Gaddesden and the Rosa Medicinae* (Oxford, 1912)

Cipolla, C.M., *Public Health and the Medical Profession in the Renaissance* (Cambridge, 1976)

Clanchy, M., *From Memory to Written Record: England 1066–1307* (Oxford, 1993)

Clark, E., 'Social Welfare and Mutual Aid in the Medieval Countryside', *Journal of British Studies*, xxxiii (1994), pp. 381–406

Clarke, A., 'Digging for Lepers', *Archaeology in York, Interim*, xix, no. 1 (1994), pp. 4–11

Classen, C., Howes, D., and Synnott, A., *The Cultural History of Smell* (London, 1994)

Clay, R.M., *The Mediaeval Hospitals of England* (London, 1909, reprinted 1966)

Clifford, E., *Father Damien: A Journey from Cashmere to His Home in Hawaii* (London, 1889)

Cochelin, I., 'Sainteté laïque: l'example de Juette de Huy (1158–1228)', *Le Moyen Age*, xcv (1989), pp. 397–417

Cohn, S., *The Black Death Transformed: Disease and Culture in Early Renaissance Europe* (London, 2001)

Colker, M.L., 'The Life of Guy of Merton by Rainald of Merton', *Medieval Studies*, xxxi (1969), pp. 250–61

Coletti, T., '*Paupertas est donum Dei*: Hagiography, Lay Religion and the Economics of Salvation in the Digby *Mary Magdalene*', *Speculum*, lxxvi (2001), pp. 337–78

Comfort, N., *The Lost City of Dunwich* (Lavenham, 1994)

Connor, S., *The Book of Skin* (Ithaca, New York, 2004)

Conrad, L.I., et al., *The Western Medical Tradition 800 BC to AD 1800* (Cambridge, 1995)

———, 'A Ninth-Century Muslim Scholar's Discussion of Contagion', in L.I. Conrad and D. Wujastyk, eds, *Contagion: Perspectives from Pre-Modern Societies* (Aldershot, 2000)

Constable, G., *Three Studies in Medieval, Religious and Social Thought* (Cambridge, 1995)

Coulton, G.G., *Medieval Panorama* (Cambridge, 1939)

Cownie, E., *Religious Patronage in Anglo-Norman England 1066–1135* (London, 1998)

Cox, J.C., ed., *VCH Hampshire II* (London, 1903)

Crane-Kramer, G.M.M., 'Was there a Medieval Diagnostic Confusion between Leprosy and Syphilis', *PPL*

Crawford, P., 'Attitudes to Menstruation in Seventeenth-Century England', *Past and Present*, xci (1981), pp. 47–73

Creighton, C., *A History of Epidemics in Britain, I, From AD 664 to the Great Plague* (London, 1894, reprinted 1965)

Crisciani, C., 'Teachers and Learners in Scholastic Medicine: Some Images and Metaphors', *History of Universities*, xv (1997–99), pp. 75–101

———, and Periera, M., 'Black Death and Golden Remedies: Some Remarks on Alchemy and the Plague', in *The Regulation of Evil: Social and Cultural Attitudes to Epidemics in the Late Middle Ages* (Micrologus' Library, ii, Turnhout, 1998)

Cule, J., 'The Diagnosis, Care and Treatment of Leprosy in Wales and the Border in the Middle Ages', *Transactions of the British Society for the History of Pharmacy*, i (1970), pp. 29–58

———, 'The Stigma of Leprosy: Its Historical Origins and Consequences with Particular Reference to the Laws of Wales', *PPL*

Cullum, P.H., 'Leperhouses and Borough Status in the Thirteenth Century', in P.R. Coss and S.D. Lloyd, eds, *Thirteenth Century England III* (Woodbridge, 1991)

———, ' "For Pore People Harberles": What Was the Function of the Maisondieu?', in D.J. Clayton, R.G. Davies and P. McNiven, eds, *Trade, Devotion and Governance: Papers in Late Medieval History* (Stroud, 1994)

Cunningham, A., 'Transforming Plague: The Laboratory and the Identity of Infectious Disease', in A. Cunningham and P. Williams, eds, *The Laboratory Revolution in Medicine* (Cambridge, 1992)

———, 'Science and Religion in the Thirteenth Century Revisited: The Making of St Francis the Proto-Ecologist', *Studies in the History and Philosophy of Science*, xxxi (2000), pp. 613–43; xxxii (2001), pp. 69–98

———, 'Identifying Disease in the Past: Cutting the Gordian Knot', *Asclepio*, liv, fasc. 1 (2002), pp. 13–34

Dalarun, J., *L'impossible sainteté: La vie retrouvée de Robert d'Arbrissel* (Paris, 1985)

Dallas, C., *Excavations at Thetford by B.K. Davison* (East Anglian Archaeology, lxii, 1993)

Damrosch, D., '*Non alia sed aliter*: The Hermeneutics of Gender in Bernard of Clairvaux', in R. Blumenfeld-Kosinski and T. Szell, eds, *Images of Sainthood in Medieval Europe* (Ithaca and London, 1991)

Daniell, C., *Death and Burial in Medieval England 1066–1550* (London, 1997)

Danielssen, D.C., *Traité de la spédalskhed ou éléphantiasis des Grecs* (Paris and London, 1848)

Davidson, C., 'The Fate of the Damned in English Art and Drama', in C. Davidson and T.H. Seiler, eds, *The Iconography of Hell* (Kalamazoo, 1992)

———, 'Heaven's Fragrance', in C. Davidson, ed., *The Iconography of Heaven* (Kalamazoo, 1994)

Debes, L.J., *A Description of the Islands and Inhabitants of Foeroe . . . Englished by J[ohn] S[tarpin] Doctor of Physick* (London, 1676)

Dekeyzer, B., *Layers of Illusion: The Mayer van den Bergh Breviary* (Ghent and Amsterdam, 2004)

Demaitre, L., *Doctor Bernard de Gordon: Professor and Practitioner* (Toronto, 1980)

———, 'The Description and Diagnosis of Leprosy by Fourteenth-Century Physicians', *BHM*, lix (1985), pp. 327–44

————, 'The Relevance of Futility: Jordanus de Turre (*fl.* 1313–1335) on the Treatment of Leprosy', *BHM*, lxx (1996), pp. 25–61

————, 'Medieval Notions of Cancer: Malignancy and Metaphor', *BHM*, lxxii (1998), pp. 609–37

————, 'The Art and Science of Prognostication in Early University Medicine', *BHM*, lxxvii (2003), pp. 765–88

Denery, D.G., ed., *Seeing and Being in the Later Medieval World* (Cambridge, 2005)

Ditchfield, P.H., ed., *VCH Berkshire II* (London, 1907)

Doka, K.J., *Fear and Society: Challenging the Dreaded Disease* (Washington DC, 1984)

Dols, M.W., 'Leprosy in Medieval Arab Medicine', *Journal of the History of Medicine and Allied Sciences*, xxxiv (1979), pp. 314–33

————, 'The Leper in Medieval Islamic Society', *Speculum*, lviii (1983), pp. 891–916

Doob, P.B.R., *Nebuchadnezzar's Children: Conventions of Madness in Middle English Literature* (Yale, 1974)

Douglas, M., *Purity and Danger: An Analysis of the Concepts of Pollution and Taboo* (London, 1966, reprinted 1994)

————, 'Witchcraft and Leprosy: Two Strategies of Exclusion', *Man*, new series, xxvi (1991), pp. 723–6

Drognat-Landré, L., *De la contagion seule cause de la propagation de la lèpre* (Paris, 1869)

Dugdale, W., *The Antiquities of Warwickshire* (2 vols, London, 1730)

Duggan, C., *Decretals and the Creation of 'New Law' in the Twelfth Century* (Aldershot, 1998)

Duncan, K., 'Climate and the Decline of Leprosy in Britain', *Proceedings of the Royal College of Physicians of Edinburgh*, xxiv (1994), pp. 114–20

Duncombe, J., and Battely, N., *The History and Antiquities of the Three Archiepiscopal Hospitals at and near Canterbury* (London, 1785)

Dutton, C.J., *The Samaritans of Moloka'i* (London, 1934)

Dyer, C., *Standards of Living in the Later Middle Ages* (Cambridge, revised edn, 1998)

Ehlers, E., *On the Conditions under which Leprosy Has Declined in Iceland* (London, 1895)

Ell, S.R., 'Blood and Sexuality in Medieval Leprosy', *Janus*, lxxi (1984), pp. 153–64

————, 'Diet and Leprosy in the Medieval West: The Noble Leper', *Janus*, lxxii (1985), pp. 113–29

Elton, G.R., 'An Early Tudor Poor Law', *Economic History Review*, second series, vi (1953–54), pp. 55–67

English, B., *The Lords of Holderness 1086–1260* (Hull, 1991)

Fabre-Vassas, C., *The Singular Beast: Jews, Christians and the Pig* (Columbia, New York, 1997)

Fabricius, J., *Syphilis in Shakespeare's England* (London, 1994)

Farley, M., and Manchester, K., 'The Cemetery of the Leper Hospital of St Margaret, High Wycombe, Buckinghamshire', *Medieval Archaeology*, xxxiii (1989), pp. 82–9

Farmer, S., 'The Beggar's Body', in S. Farmer and B.H. Rosenwein, eds, *Monks and Nuns, Saints and Outcasts: Religion in Medieval Society* (Ithaca and London, 2000)

————, 'The Leper in the Master Bedroom: Thinking through a Thirteenth-Century Exemplum', in R. Voader and D. Wolfthal, eds, *Framing the Family: Narrative and Representation in the Medieval and Early Modern Periods* (Arizona Center for Medieval and Reniassance Studies, 2005)

Farrer, W., and Brownbill, J., eds, *VCH Lancaster II* (London, 1908)

Farrow, J., *Damien the Leper* (New York, 1937)

Finucane, R.C., 'The Use and Abuse of Medieval Miracles', *History*, lx (1975), pp. 1–10

——, *Miracles and Pilgrims: Popular Beliefs in Medieval England* (New York, 1977)

Foreville, R., *Thomas Becket dans la tradition historique et hagiographique* (Variorum, London, 1981)

Foucault, M., *Madness and Civilisation: A History of Insanity in the Age of Reason* (London, 1971)

Foulon, C., *L'oeuvre de Jehan Bodel* (Paris, 1958)

Fowler, J., 'On a Window Representing the Life and Miracles of St William of York', *Yorkshire Archaeological and Topographical Journal*, iii (1873–74), pp. 198–348

French, R., 'Astrology in Medical Practice', in L. García-Ballester et al., eds, *Practical Medicine from Salerno to the Black Death* (Cambridge, 1994)

——, 'Foretelling the Future: Arabic Astrology and English Medicine in the Late Twelfth Century', *Isis*, lxxxvii (1996), pp. 453–80

Frost, R., 'The Urban Elite', in C. Rawcliffe and R.G. Wilson, eds, *The History of Norwich* (2 vols, London, 2004)

Furley, R., *A History of the Weald of Kent* (2 vols, Ashford, 1871–74)


Gaignebet, C., and Lajoux, J.D., *Art profane et religion populaire au moyen âge* (Paris, 1985)

García-Ballester, L., 'Changes in the *Regimina Sanitatis*: The Role of the Jewish Physicians', in S. Campbell, B. Hall and D. Klausner, eds, *Health, Disease and Healing in Medieval Culture* (Toronto, 1992)

Garnier, A., *Mutations temporelles et cheminement spirituel* (Paris, 1988)

Gaydon, A.T., ed., *VCH Shropshire II* (London, 1973)

Geremek, B., *The Margins of Society in Medieval Paris* (Cambridge, 1987)

Getz, F., 'Gilbertus Anglicus Anglicised', *Medical History*, xxvi (1982), pp. 436–42

——, 'Charity, Translation and the Language of Medical Learning in Medieval England', *BHM*, lxiv (1990), pp. 1–15

——, 'Medical Education in Later Medieval England', in V. Nutton and R. Porter, eds, *The History of Medical Education in Britain* (Amsterdam, 1995)

——, *Medicine in the English Middle Ages* (Princeton, 1998)

Gibbs, V., et al., *The Complete Peerage* (14 vols, London and Stroud, 1910–98)

Gilchrist, R., 'Christian Bodies and Souls: The Archaeology of Life and Death in Later Medieval Hospitals', in S. Bassett, ed., *Death in Towns: Urban Responses to the Dying and the Dead, 100–1600* (Leicester, 1992)

——, *Gender and Material Culture* (London, 1994)

——, 'Medieval Bodies in the Material World: Gender, Stigma and the Body', in S. Kay and M. Rubin, eds, *Framing Medieval Bodies* (Manchester, 1994)

——, *Contemplation and Action: The Other Monasticism* (Leicester, 1995)

——, and Sloane, B., *Requiem: The Medieval Monastic Cemetery in Britain* (London, 2005)

Gil-Sotres, P., 'Derivation and Revulsion: The Theory and Practice of Medieval Phlebotomy', in L. García-Ballester, R. French, J. Arrizabalaga and A. Cunningham, eds, *Practical Medicine from Salerno to the Black Death* (Cambridge, 1994)

——, 'The Regimens of Health', in M.D. Grmek, ed., *Western Medical Thought from Antiquity to the Middle Ages* (Cambridge, Mass., and London, 1998)

Ginzburg, C., *Ecstasies: Deciphering the Witches' Sabbath* (London, 1990)

Goering, J., 'The *Summa de Penitentia* of Magister Serlo', *Medieval Studies*, xxxviii (1976), pp. 1–53

Goldberg, P.J.P., *Women, Work, and Life Cycle: Women in York and Yorkshire c. 1300–1520* (Oxford, 1992)

———, 'Pigs and Prostitutes: Streetwalking in Comparative Perspective', in K. Lewis, N.J. Menuge and K.M. Phillips, eds, *Young Medieval Women* (Stroud, 1999)

Golding, B., *Gilbert of Sempringham and the Gilbertine Order c.1130–c.1300* (Oxford, 1995)

Goldwater, L.J., *Mercury: A History of Quicksilver* (Baltimore, 1972)

Gonthier, N., *Le châtiment du crime au moyen âge* (Rennes, 1998)

Goodall, J.A.A., *God's House at Ewelme* (Aldershot, 2001)

Goodich, M., *Other Middle Ages: Witnesses at the Margins of Society* (Philadelphia, 1998)

Goodman, L.E., *Avicenna* (London, 1992)

Gould, T., *Don't Fence Me In: From Curse to Cure, Leprosy in Modern Times* (London, 2005)

Graff, H.J., *The Legacies of Literacy: Communities and Contradictions in Western Culture and Society* (Bloomington and Indianapolis, 1987)

Greatrex, J., *Biographical Register of the English Cathedral Priories of the Province of Canterbury c. 1066–1540* (Oxford, 1997)

Green, A., *Flaubert and the Historical Novel: Salammbô Reassessed* (Cambridge, 1982)

Green, J.A., *The Aristocracy of Norman England* (Cambridge, 1997)

Greenslade, M.W., ed., *VCH Stafford III* (London, 1970)

Grigsby, B.L., *Pestilence in Medieval and Early Modern English Literature* (London and New York, 2004)

Groebner, V., 'Losing Face, Saving Face: Noses and Honour in the Late Medieval Town', *History Workshop Journal*, xl (1995), pp. 1–15

Grön, K., 'Leprosy in Literature and Art', *International Journal of Leprosy*, xli (1973), pp. 249–83

Grmek, G.D., *Diseases in the Ancient Greek World* (Baltimore, 1989)

Guenée, B., *La folie de Charles VI: Roi bien-aimé* (Paris, 2004)

Gussow, Z., and Tracy, G.S., 'Stigma and the Leprosy Phenomenon', *BHM*, xliv (1970), pp. 425–49

———, *Leprosy, Racism and Public Health: Social Policy and Chronic Disease Control* (Boulder, Colorado, 1989)

Gwynn, A., and Hadcock, R.N., *Medieval Religious Houses in Ireland* (London, 1970)


Habrich, C., Williams, J.C., and Wolf, J.H., eds, *Aussatz, Lepra, Hansen-Krankheit: Ein Menschheits Problem im Wandel* (Munich, 1982)

Hamilton, B., *The Leper King and his Heirs* (Cambridge, 2000)

Hammond, E.A., 'Physicians in Medieval English Religious Houses', *BHM*, xxxii (1958), pp. 105–20

Hansen, G.A., and Looft, C., *Leprosy in its Clinical and Pathological Aspects* (Bristol and London, 1895)

Harley, D., 'Rhetoric and the Social Construction of Sickness and Healing', *SHM*, xii (1999), pp. 407–35

Harper, S., *Insanity, Individuals and Society in Late-Medieval English Literature* (New York and Lampeter, 2003)

Harris, B.E., ed., *VCH Chester III* (London, 1980)

Harrod, H., *Report on the Deeds and Records of King's Lynn* (King's Lynn, 1874)

Harvey, B., 'Introduction: The "Crisis" of the Early Fourteenth Century', in B.M.S. Campbell, ed., *Before the Black Death* (Manchester, 1991)

——, *Living and Dying in England 1100–1540: The Monastic Experience* (Oxford, 1993)

Harvey, R.E., *The Inward Wits: Psychological Theory in the Middle Ages and the Renaissance* (Warburg Institute Surveys, vi, 1975)

Haskins, S., *Mary Magdalen: Myth and Metaphor* (London, 1994)

Hays, J.N., *The Burdens of Disease: Epidemics and Human Response in Western History* (New Brunswick, NJ, and London, 1998)

Hayum, A., *The Isenheim Altarpiece: God's Medicine and the Painter's Vision* (Princeton, 1989)

Healy, M., 'Discourses of the Plague in Early Modern London', in J.A.I. Champion, ed., *Epidemic Diseases in London* (Centre for Metropolitan History, Working Paper Series 1, 1993)

Henderson, J., 'The Black Death in Florence: Medical and Communal Responses', in S. Bassett, ed., *Death in Towns: Urban Responses to the Dying and the Dead, 100–1600* (Leicester, 1992)

Hepworth, M., and Turner, B.S., *Confession: Studies in Deviance and Religion* (London, 1992)

Hodgson, J.C., *A History of Northumberland VII* (London, 1904)

Hodson, W.W., 'John Colney's or S. Leonard's Hospital for Lepers at Sudbury', *Proceedings of the Suffolk Institute of Archaeology*, vii (1891), pp. 268–74

Hoeniger, F.D., *Medicine and Shakespeare in the English Renaissance* (Delaware, 1992)

Holcomb, R.C., 'The Antiquity of Congenital Syphilis', *BHM*, x (1941), pp. 148–77

Holister, C.W., *Henry I* (New Haven and London, 2001)

Hollis, S., 'Wilton as a Centre of Learning', in S. Hollis, ed., *Writing the Wilton Women: Goscelin's Legend of Edith and Liber confortatorius* (Turnhout, 2004)

Honeybourne, M.B., 'The Leper Hospitals of the London Area', *Transactions of the London and Middlesex Archaeological Society*, xxi (1967), pp. 1–55

Horden, P., 'Ritual and Public Health in the Early Medieval City', in S. Sheard and H. Power, eds, *Body and City: Histories of Urban Public Health* (Aldershot, 2000)

——, 'A Non-Natural Environment: Medicine without Doctors and the Medieval Hospital', in B. Bowers, ed., *The Medieval Hospital and Medical Practice* (Aldershot, forthcoming)

Horton-Smith Hartley, P., and Aldridge, H.R., *Johannes de Mirfeld: His Life and Works* (Cambridge, 1936)

Hughes, G., *Swearing: A Social History of Foul Language, Oaths and Profanity in English* (London, 1998)

Hughes, J., 'The Administration of Confession', in D.M. Smith, ed., *Studies in Clergy and Ministry in Medieval England* (Borthwick Studies in History, i, 1991)

——, *The Religious Life of Richard III* (Stroud, 1997)

——, *Arthurian Myths and Alchemy: The Kingship of Edward IV* (Stroud, 2002)

Hulse, E.V., 'The Nature of Biblical "Leprosy" and the Use of Alternative Medical Terms in Modern Translations of the Bible', *Palestine Exploration Quarterly*, cvii (1975), pp. 87–105

Huneycutt, L.L., 'The Idea of the Perfect Princess: The Life of Margaret in the Reign of Matilda II (1100–1118)', *Anglo-Norman Studies*, xii (1989), pp. 81–97

Hunnisett, R.F., *The Medieval Coroner* (Cambridge, 1961)

Hutchinson, J., *On Leprosy and Fish-Eating: A Statement of Facts and Explanations* (London, 1906)

Hyams, P., 'What Did Edwardian Villages Understand by "Law"?', in Z. Razi and R.M. Smith, eds, *Medieval Society and the Manor Court* (Oxford, 1966)

Imray, J., *The Charity of Richard Whittington* (London, 1968)

Irvine, W.C., 'Christian Teaching and Spiritual Work in Asylums', *Report of a Conference of Leper Asylum Superintendents and Others on the Leper Problem in India* (Calcutta, 1920)

Jackson, Canon, 'Ancient Statutes of Heytesbury Almshouse', *Wiltshire Archaeological and Natural History Magazine*, xi (1869), pp. 289–308

Jackson, J., *Lepers: Thirty-Six Years Among Them, Being the History of the Mission to India and the East 1874–1910* (London, 1910)

Jacquart, D., *Dictionnaire biographique des médecins en France au moyen âge* (Haute Etudes Médiévales et Modernes, series 5, xxxv, 1979)

———, *Le milieu médical en France du XIIe au XVe siècle* (Haute Etudes Médiévales et Modernes, series 5, xlvi, 1981)

———, and Micheau, F., *La médecine arabe et l'occident médiéval* (Paris, 1990)

———, and Thomasset, C., *Sexuality and Medicine in the Middle Ages* (Oxford, 1988)

———, *La médecine médiévale dans le cadre Parisien* (Paris, 1998)

———, 'A la recherche de la peau dans le discours médical de la fin du moyen âge', in *La pelle umana* (Micrologus' Library, xiii, Turnhout, 2005)

Jansen, K.L., *The Making of the Magdalen* (Princeton, 2000)

James, M.R., *The Ancient Libraries of Canterbury and Dover* (Cambridge, 1903)

Jeanne, D., 'Le group des lépreux à Saint-Lazare de Falaise aux XIVe et XVe siècles', in B. Tabuteau, ed., *Lépreux et sociabilité du moyen âge aux temps modernes* (Cahiers de GRHIS, xi, 2000)

Jeanselme, E., 'Comment l'Europe, au moyen age, se protéga contre la lèpre', *Bulletin de la Société Francaise d'Histoire de la Médecine*, xxv (1931), pp. 1–155

———, *La lèpre* (Paris, 1934)

Jenner, M.S.R., 'Underground, Overground: Pollution and Place in Urban History', *Journal of Urban History*, xxiv (1997), pp. 97–110

———, 'The Great Dog Massacre', in W.G. Naphy and P. Roberts, eds, *Fear in Early Modern Society* (Manchester, 1997)

Jessopp, A., *The Coming of the Friars and other Historic Essays* (London, 1890)

Johnstone, H., 'Poor Relief in the Royal Household of Thirteenth-Century England', *Speculum*, iv (1929), pp. 149–67

Jones, C., 'Discourse Entities and Medical Texts', in I. Taavitsainen and P. Pahata, *Medical and Scientific Writing in Late Medieval English* (Cambridge, 2004)

Jones, P. Murray, 'Medical Books before the Invention of Printing', in A. Besson, ed., *Thornton's Medical Books, Libraries and Collectors* (third edn, London, 1990)

———, 'Information and Science', in R. Horrox, ed., *Fifteenth-Century Attitudes* (Cambridge, 1994)

———, 'Harley MS 2558: A Fifteenth-Century Medical Commonplace Book', in M.R. Schleissner, ed., *Manuscript Sources of Medieval Medicine* (New York, 1995)

———, *Medieval Medicine in Illuminated Manuscripts* (London and Milan, revised edn, 1998)

———, 'Medicine and Science', in L. Hellinga and J.B. Trapp, eds, *The Cambridge History of the Book in Britain, III, 1400–1557* (Cambridge, 1999)

————, 'Music Therapy in the Later Middle Ages: The Case of Hugo van der Goes', in P. Horden, ed., *Music as Medicine: The History of Music Therapy since Antiquity* (Aldershot, 2000)

Jopling, W.H., *Handbook of Leprosy* (first edn, London, 1971)

Kalisch, P.A., 'An Overview of Research on the History of Leprosy', *International Journal of Leprosy*, xliii (1975), pp. 129–44

————, 'Tracadie and Penikese Leprosaria: A Comparative Analysis of Societal Response to Leprosy in New Brunswick, 1844–1880', *BHM*, xlvii (1973), pp. 480–512

Kantorowicz, E.H., *The King's Two Bodies: A Study in Medieval Political Theory* (Princeton, 1957)

Karras, R.M., *Common Women: Prostitution and Sexuality in Medieval England* (Oxford, 1996)

Kaufman, M.H., and MacLennan, W.J., 'Robert the Bruce and Leprosy', *Proceedings of the Royal College of Physicians*, xxx (2000), pp. 75–80

Kealey, E.J., *Medieval Medicus* (Baltimore, 1981)

Keene, D., *Survey of Medieval Winchester* (2 vols, Oxford, 1985)

Keiser, G., 'Scientific, Medical and Utilitarian Prose', in A.S.G. Edwards, ed., *A Companion to Middle English Prose* (Woodbridge, 2004)

Kemp, B., 'Maiden Bradley Priory, Wiltshire, and Kidderminster Church, Worcestershire', in M. Barber, P. McNulty and P. Noble, eds, *East Anglian and other Studies Presented to Barbara Dodwell* (Reading Medieval Studies, xi, 1985)

Kershaw, I., 'The Great Famine and Agrarian Crisis in England 1315–1322', *Past and Present*, lix (1973), pp. 3–50

Kieckhefer, R., *Unquiet Souls: Fourteenth-Century Saints and their Religious Milieu* (Chicago, 1984)

King, E., *Peterborough Abbey 1086–1310* (Cambridge, 1973)

King, H., *Hippocrates' Woman: Reading the Female Body in Ancient Greece* (London, 1998)

Kiple, K.F., ed., *Plague, Pox and Pestilence: Diseases in History* (London, 1997)

————, ed., *The Cambridge World History of Human Disease* (Cambridge, 1993)

Kipp, R.S., 'The Evangelical Uses of Leprosy', *Social Science and Medicine*, xxxix (1994), pp. 165–78

Kleinschmidt, H., *Perception and Action in Medieval Europe* (Woodbridge, 2005)

Klibansky, R., Panofsky, E., and Saxl, F., *Saturn and Melancholy* (London, 1964)

Knowles, M.D., Duggan, A.J., and Brooke, C.N.L., 'Henry II's Supplement to the Constitutions of Clarendon', *EHR*, lxxxvii (1972), pp. 757–71

Kristeva, J., *Powers of Horror: An Essay on Abjection* (Columbia, 1982)

Kuefler, M.S., 'Castration and Eunuchism in the Middle Ages', in V.L. Bullough and J.A. Brundage, eds, *Handbook of Medieval Sexuality* (New York, 1996)

Kupfer, M., *The Art of Healing* (Pennsylvania, 2003)

Kuryluk, E., *Veronica and Her Cloth: History, Symbolism and Structure of a 'True' Image* (Oxford, 1991)

Lacan, J., *Ecrits*, trans. A. Sheridan (London, 1977)

Lacroix, P., *Vie militaire et religieuse au moyen âge* (Paris, 1873)

Lambert, A., 'Leprosy Past and Present: I Present', *The Nineteenth Century*, xc (August 1884), pp. 210–27

————, 'Leprosy Past and Present: II Past', *The Nineteenth Century*, xc (September 1884), pp. 467–89

Lang, S.J., 'John Bradmore and his Book Philomena', *SHM*, v (1992), pp. 121–30

Laqueur, T., *Making Sex: Body and Gender from the Greeks to Freud* (Cambridge, Mass., 1992)

Lawler, T., 'On the Properties of John Trevisa's Major Translations', *Viator*, xiv (1983), pp. 267–88

Lawrence, C.H., *Medieval Monasticism* (London, 1989)

Leader, D.R., 'John Argentein and Learning in Medieval Cambridge', *Humanistica Lovaniensia*, xxxiii (1984)

Lechat, M.F., 'The Palaeoepidemiology of Leprosy: An Overview', *PPL*

Lee, A.G., *Leper Hospitals in Medieval Ireland* (Dublin, 1996)

Le Goff, J., *The Birth of Purgatory* (Chicago, 1984)

——, *Saint Louis* (Paris, 1996)

——, *Un autre moyen âge* (Paris, 1999)

Le Monnier, L., *History of St Francis of Assisi* (London, 1894)

Le Roy Ladurie, E., *Montaillou: Cathars and Catholics in a French Village 1294–1324* (Harmondsworth, 1980)

Letters, S., *Gazetteer of Markets and Fairs in England to 1516* (2 parts, List and Index Society, xxxii–xxxiii, 2003)

Levey, M., *Early Arabic Pharmacology* (Leiden, 1973)

Lewis, G., 'A Lesson from Leviticus: Leprosy', *Man*, new series, xxii (1987), pp. 593–612

Lewis, M.E., 'Infant and Childhood Leprosy: Present and Past', *PPL*

Lieban, R.W., 'The Field of Medical Anthropology', in D. Landy, ed., *Culture, Disease and Healing: Studies in Medical Anthropology* (New York, 1977)

Lieber, E., 'Old Testament "Leprosy", Contagion and Sin', in L.I. Conrad and D. Wujastyk, eds, *Contagion: Perspectives from Pre-Modern Societies* (Aldershot, 2000)

Liebman, C.J., 'La consécration légendaire de la basilique de Saint-Denis', *Le Moyen Age*, xlv (1935), pp. 252–64

Little, L.K., 'Pride Goes before Avarice: Social Change and the Vices in Latin Christendom', *American Historical Review*, lxxvi (1971), pp. 16–49

Liveing, R., *Elephantiasis Graecorum, or True Leprosy* (London, 1873)

Lobanov-Rostovsky, S., 'Taming the Basilisk', in D. Hillman and C. Mazzio, eds, *The Body in Parts: Fantasies of Corporeality in Early Modern Europe* (New York and London, 1997)

Lombard, C.M., *Xavier de Maistre* (Boston, Mass., 1977)

Lombard-Jourdan, A., *Saint-Denis: Lieu de mémoire* (Paris, 2000)

LoPrete, K.A., 'Adela of Blois and Ivo of Chartres: Piety, Politics and Peace in the Diocese of Chartres', *Anglo-Norman Studies*, xiv (1992), pp. 131–52

Luepnitz, D., 'Beyond the Phallus: Lacan and Feminism', in J.M. Rebate, ed., *The Cambridge Companion to Lacan* (Cambridge, 2003)

Lunt, W.E., *Papal Revenues in the Middle Ages* (2 vols, New York, 1934)

Lynch, J.H., *Simoniacal Entry into the Religious Life from 1000 to 1260* (Columbus, Ohio, 1976)

Lyttelton, George, Lord, *The History of the Life of King Henry the Second* (6 vols, London, 1769–73)

MacArthur, W., 'Mediaeval "Leprosy" in the British Isles', *Leprosy Review*, xxiv (1953), pp. 8–19

McCracken, P., *The Curse of Eve, the Wound of the Hero: Blood, Gender and Medieval Literature* (Pennsylvania Press, 2003)

McDannell, C., and Lang, B., *Heaven: A History* (New Haven and London, 1988)

MacDonald, M., 'Anthropological Perspectives on the History of Science and Medicine', in P. Corsi and P. Weindling, eds, *Information Sources in the History of Science and Medicine* (London, 1983)

MacDougall, S.C., 'The Surgeon and the Saints: Henri de Mondeville and Divine Healing', *Journal of Medieval History*, xxvi (2000), pp. 253–67

McIntosh, M.K., 'Finding Language for Misconduct: Jurors in Fifteenth-Century Local Courts', in B.A. Hanawalt and D. Wallace, eds, *Bodies and Disciplines: Intersections of Literature and History in Fifteenth-Century England* (Minneapolis and London, 1996)

———, *Controlling Misbehaviour in England 1370–1600* (Cambridge, 1998)

McMurray Gibson, G., *The Theater of Devotion* (Chicago, 1989)

Macnamara, C.N., *Leprosy: A Communicable Disease* (Calcutta, 1866)

McNeill, J.T., 'Medicine for Sin as Prescribed in the Penitentials', *Church History*, i (1932), pp. 14–26

McNiven, P., 'The Problem of Henry IV's Health, 1405–1413', *EHR*, c (1985), pp. 747–72

McVaugh, M.R., 'Quantified Medical Theory and Practice at Fourteenth-Century Montpellier', *BHM*, xliii (1969), pp. 397–413

———, 'Bedside Manners in the Middle Ages', *BHM*, lxxi (1997), pp. 201–23

———, 'Surgery', in M.D. Grmek, ed., *Western Medical Thought from Antiquity to the Middle Ages* (Cambridge, Mass., 1998)

———, 'Surface Meanings: The Identification of Apostemes in Medieval Surgery', in W. Bracke and H. Deumens, eds, *Medical Latin from the Late Middle Ages to the Eighteenth Century* (Brussels, 2000)

Magilton, J., 'The Leper Hospital of St James and St Mary Magdalen, Chichester', in C.A. Roberts, F. Lee and J. Bintoff, eds, *Burial Archaeology: Current Research, Methods and Developments* (BAR, British Series, ccxi, 1989)

———, 'The Leper Hospital of St James and St Mary Magdalen, Chichester, and other Leper Houses', in B. Tabuteau, ed., *Lépreux et sociabilité du moyen âge au temps modernes* (Cahiers de GRHS, xi, 2000)

Manchester, K., 'Tuberculosis and Leprosy in Antiquity: An Interpretation', *Medical History*, xxviii (1984), pp. 162–73

———, and Marcombe, D., 'The Melton Mowbray "Leper Head": An Historical and Medical Investigation', *Medical History*, xxxiv (1990), pp. 86–91

———, 'Tuberculosis and Leprosy: Evidence for Interaction of Disease', in D.J. Ortner and A.C. Aufderheide, eds, *Human Palaeopathology: Current Syntheses and Future Options* (Washington DC, 1991)

———, 'Leprosy: The Origin and Development of the Disease in Antiquity', in D. Gourevitch, ed., *Maladie et maladies: Histoire et conceptualisation* (Paris, 1992)

Manco, J., *The Spirit of Care* (Bath, 1998)

Manship, H., *The History of Great Yarmouth*, ed. J. Palmer (London, 1854)

Marcombe, D., *Leper Knights: The Order of St Lazarus of Jerusalem in England, c.1150–1544* (Woodbridge, 2003)

Marks, R., *Image and Devotion in Late Medieval England* (Stroud, 2004)

Marrow, J.H., *Passion Iconography in Northern European Art in the Late Middle Ages and Early Renaissance* (Kortrijk, 1979)

Martin, A., 'The Representation of Leprosy and of Lepers in Minor Art, Particularly in Germany', *The Urologic and Cutaneous Review*, xxv (1921), pp. 445–53

Mason, E., *St Wulfstan of Worcester c. 1008–1095* (Oxford, 1990)

Matsuda, T., *Death and Purgatory in Middle English Didactic Poetry* (Woodbridge, 1997)

Mayer, C.F., 'A Medieval English Leechbook and its Fourteenth-Century Poem on Bloodletting', *BHM*, vii (1939), pp. 381–91

Mehta, J., 'Social Reactions in the Past and Present of Leprosy', *PPL*

Mellinkoff, R., *The Mark of Cain* (Berkeley, California, 1981)

――――, *Outcasts: Signs of Otherness in Northern European Art of the Late Middle Ages* (2 vols, Los Angeles, 1993)

Mellor, R., *Tacitus* (London, 1994)

Merback, M.B., *The Thief, the Cross and the Wheel: Pain and the Spectacle of Punishment in Medieval and Renaissance Europe* (London, 1999)

Mercier, C.A., *Astrology in Medicine* (London, 1914)

――――, *Leper Houses and Medieval Hospitals* (London, 1915)

Michelet, J., *La sorcière* (2 vols, Paris, 1952)

*Middle English Dictionary* (Ann Arbor, 1956 onwards)

Miller, A.D., *An Inn Called Welcome: The Story of the Mission to Lepers 1874–1917* (London, 1964)

'Un Missionaire', *La lèpre est contagieuse* (Paris, 1879)

Mitchell, P., 'An Evaluation of the Leprosy of King Baldwin IV of Jerusalem', in B. Hamilton, *The Leper King and his Heirs* (Cambridge, 2000)

――――, 'The Myth of the Spread of Leprosy with the Crusades', *PPL*

Moblo, P., 'Blessed Damien of Moloka'i: The Critical Analysis of a Contemporary Myth', *Ethnohistory*, xliv (1997), pp. 691–726

Mollat, M., *The Poor in the Middle Ages* (New Haven and London, 1986)

Møller-Christensen, V., *Bone Changes in Leprosy* (Copenhagen, 1961)

Montero Cartelle, E., and Martín Ferreira, A.I., 'Le *De elephancia* de Constantin l'Africain et ses rapports avec le *Pantegni*', in C. Burnett and D. Jacquart, eds, *Constantine the African and 'Alī Ibn al 'Abbās al Maǧūsī* (Leiden, 1994)

Mooney, L.R., 'A Middle English Verse Compendium of Astrological Medicine', *Medical History*, xxviii (1984), pp. 406–9

Moorat, S.A.J., *Catalogue of Western Manuscripts on Medicine and Science in the Wellcome Historical Medical Library, I, Mss. Written before 1650 A.D.* (London, 1962)

Moore, R.I., 'Heresy as a Disease', in W. Lourdaux and V. Verhelst, eds, *The Concept of Heresy in the Middle Ages* (Mediaevalia Louaniensia, first series, iv, 1976)

――――, *The Formation of a Persecuting Society* (Oxford, 1987)

――――, 'Anti-Semitism and the Birth of Europe', in D. Wood, ed., *Christianity and Judaism* (Studies in Church History, xxix, 1992)

Mortimer, R., 'The Prior of Butley and the Lepers of West Somerton', *BIHR*, liii (1980), pp. 99–103

Mundy, J.H., 'Charity and Social Work in Toulouse 1100–1250', *Traditio*, xxii (1966), pp. 203–87

Munro, W., *Leprosy* (Manchester, 1879)

Murray, A., 'Religion among the Poor in Thirteenth-Century France: The Testimony of Humbert de Romans', *Traditio*, xxx (1974), pp. 285–324

――――, 'Counselling in Medieval Confession', in P. Biller and J. Minnis, eds, *Handling Sin: Confession in the Middle Ages* (Woodbridge, 1998)

Musacchio, J., *The Art and Ritual of Childbirth in Renaissance Italy* (New York, 1999)

Mustain, J.K., 'A Rural Medical Practitioner in Fifteenth-Century England', *BHM*, xlvi (1972), pp. 469–76

Musto, D.F., 'Quarantine and the Problem of AIDS', in E. Fee and D.M. Fox, eds, *AIDS: The Burdens of History* (Berkeley, Los Angeles and London, 1988)

Mynors, R.A.B., *Durham Cathedral Manuscripts to the End of the Twelfth Century* (Durham, 1939)


Nagy, P., *Le don des larmes au moyen âge* (Paris, 2000)

Navon, L., 'Beggars, Metaphors and Stigma', *SHM*, xi (1998), pp. 89–105

Newman, G., *On the History of the Decline and Final Extinction of Leprosy as an Endemic Disease in the British Isles* (London, 1895)

Newman, P.H., 'Notes on the Preservation of Some Ancient Wall Paintings', *Proceedings of the Society of Antiquaries*, xx (1903–5)

Nichols, J., *The History and Antiquities of the County of Leicester* (4 vols, London, 1795–1815)

Nicholson, R., *Scotland in the Middle Ages* (Edinburgh, 1974)

Nicoud, M., 'Les médecins Italiens et le bain thermal à la fin du moyen âge', *Médiévales*, xliii (2002), pp. 13–40

Niebyl, P.H., 'The Non-Naturals', *BHM*, xlv (1971), pp. 486–92

Nilson, B., *Cathedral Shrines of Medieval England* (Woodbridge, 1998)

Norri, J., 'Entrances and Exits in English Medical Vocabulary, 1400–1550', in I. Taavitsainen and P. Pahata, *Medical and Scientific Writing in Late Medieval English* (Cambridge, 2004)

Nutton, V., 'The Seeds of Disease: An Exploration of Contagion and Infection from the Greeks to the Renaissance', *Medical History*, xxvii (1983), pp. 1–34

———, 'Did the Greeks Have a Word for It? Contagion and Contagion Theory in Classical Antiquity', in L.I. Conrad and D. Wujastyk, eds, *Contagion: Perspectives from Pre-Modern Societies* (Aldershot, 2000)

———, *Ancient Medicine* (London, 2004)


Ober, W.B., 'Can the Leper Change his Spots? The Iconography of Leprosy', *The American Journal of Dermatopathology*, v (1983), pp. 43–58, 173–85

Oberhelman, S.M., 'Galen, On Diagnosis from Dreams', *Journal of the History of Medicine and Applied Sciences*, xxxviii (1983)

Obregón, D., 'Lepra, Exageración y Authoridad Médica', *Asclepio*, l (1998), pp. 125–48

Oliphant, Mrs [M.], *St Francis of Assisi* (London, 1868)

Orme, N., and Webster, M., *The English Hospital, 1070–1570* (New Haven and London, 1995)

———, 'The Medieval Leper-House at "Lamford" Cornwall', *HR*, lxix (1996), pp. 102–7

Osten, G. von der, 'Job and Christ', *Journal of the Warburg and Courtauld Institutes*, xvi (1953), pp. 153–8

Owst, G.R., *Preaching in Medieval England* (Cambridge, 1926)


Page, S., 'Richard Trewythian and the Uses of Astrology in Late Medieval England', *Journal of the Warburg and Courtauld Institutes*, lxiv (2001), pp. 193–228

Page, S., *Astrology in Medieval Manuscripts* (London, 2002)

Page, W., ed., *VCH Lincolnshire II* (London, 1906)

———, *VCH Norfolk II* (London, 1906)

———, and Round, J.H., eds, *VCH Essex II* (London, 1907)

———, *VCH Durham II* (London, 1907)

———, *VCH Suffolk II* (London, 1907)

————, *VCH Sussex II* (London, 1907)

————, *VCH London I* (London, 1909)

————, *VCH Nottingham II* (London, 1910)

————, *VCH Yorkshire III* (London, 1913)

————, *VCH Kent II* (London, 1926)

Palmer, R., 'The Church, Leprosy and Plague in Medieval and Early Modern Europe', in W.J. Sheils, ed., *The Church and Healing* (Studies in Church History, xix, 1982)

————, 'In Bad Odour: Smell and its Significance in Medicine from Antiquity to the Seventeenth Century', in W.F. Bynum and R. Porter, eds, *Medicine and the Five Senses* (Cambridge, 1993)

Pankhurst, R., 'The History of Leprosy in Ethiopia to 1935', *Medical History*, xxviii (1984), pp. 57–72

Parr, J., 'Cresseid's Leprosy Again', *Modern Language Notes*, lx (1945), pp. 487–91

Paravicini Bagliani, A., *Le corps du Pape* (Paris, 1995)

Paster, G.K., 'Nervous Tension: Networks of Blood and Spirit in the Early Modern Body', in D. Hillman and C. Mazzio, eds, *The Body in Parts: Fantasies of Corporeality in Early Modern Europe* (New York and London, 1997)

Payer, P.J., *The Bridling of Desire: Views of Sex in the Late Middle Ages* (Toronto, 1993)

Pease, A.S., 'Medical Allusions in the Works of St Jerome', *Harvard Studies in Classical Philology*, xxv (1914), pp. 73–86

Pegg, M.G., 'Le corps et l'autorité: La lèpre de Baudouin IV', *Annales*, xlv (1990), pp. 265–87

Pelling, M., 'Appearance and Reality: Barber-Surgeons, the Body and Disease', in A.L. Beier and R. Finlay, eds, *London, 1500–1700: The Making of the Metropolis* (New York and London, 1986)

Pereira, M., 'Alchemy and the Rise of Vernacular Languages in the Late Middle Ages', *Speculum*, lxxiv (1999), pp. 336–56

Pestell, T., *Landscapes of Monastic Foundation* (Woodbridge, 2004)

Pettigrew, T.J., 'On Leper Hospitals or Houses', *Journal of the British Archaeological Association*, xi (1855), pp. 9–34, 95–117

Peyroux, C., 'The Leper's Kiss', in S. Farmer and B.H. Rosenwein, eds, *Monks and Nuns, Saints and Outcasts: Religion in Medieval Society* (Ithaca and London, 2000)

Philip, L.B., 'The Prado *Epiphany* by Jerome Bosch', *Art Bulletin*, xxxv (1953), pp. 267–93

Pichon, G., 'Essai sur la lèpre du haut moyen âge', *Le Moyen Age*, fourth series, xxxix (1984), pp. 331–56

Pickett, R.C., *Mental Affliction and Church Law* (Ottawa, 1952)

Po-Chia Hsia, R., *The Myth of Ritual Murder: Jews and Magic in Reformation Germany* (New Haven and London, 1988)

Pollard, A.J., *Richard III and the Princes in the Tower* (Stroud, 1991)

Pollock, F., and Maitland, F.W., *The History of English Law* (2 vols, Cambridge, 1911)

Post, J.B., 'A Fifteenth-Century Customary for the Southwark Stews', *Journal of the Society of Archivists*, v (1977), pp. 418–28

Postles, D., 'Lamps, Lights and Layfolk', *Journal of Medieval History*, xxv (1999), pp. 97–114

Pouchelle, M.C., *The Body and Surgery in the Middle Ages* (Oxford, 1990)

Poulson, G., *The History and Antiquities of the Seignory of Holderness* (2 vols, Hull, 1841)

P[ryme], A.G. de La, 'Lundu, the Leper Isle', *Central Africa*, xxvii (1909), p. 214

Pugh, R.B., and Crittall, E., eds, *VCH Wiltshire III* (London, 1956)

Quétel, C., *History of Syphilis* (Oxford, 1990)

Quinlan, M., *Damien of Molokai* (London, 1909)

Raban, S., *Mortmain Legislation and the English Church 1279–1500* (Cambridge, 1982)

Rather, L.J., 'The Six Things Non-Natural', *Clio Medica*, iii (1968), pp. 337–47

Rattue, J., *The Living Stream: Holy Wells in Historical Context* (Woodbridge, 1995)

Rawcliffe, C., 'The Profits of Practice: The Wealth and Status of Medical Men in Later Medieval England', *SHM*, i (1988), pp. 61–78

———, *The Hospitals of Medieval Norwich* (Norwich, 1995)

———, *Medicine and Society in Later Medieval England* (Stroud, 1995)

———, 'Hospital Nurses and their Work', in R. Britnell, ed., *Daily Life in the Later Middle Ages* (Stroud, 1998)

———, *Medicine for the Soul: The Life, Death and Resurrection of an English Medieval Hospital* (Stroud, 1999)

———, 'Pilgrimage and the Sick in Medieval East Anglia', in C. Morris and P. Roberts, eds, *Pilgrimage: The English Experience from Becket to Bunyan* (Cambridge, 2002)

———, 'On the Threshold of Eternity: Care for the Sick in East Anglian Monasteries', in C. Harper-Bill, C. Rawcliffe and R.G. Wilson, eds, *East Anglia's History: Studies in Honour of Norman Scarfe* (Woodbridge, 2002)

———, 'Passports to Paradise: How English Medieval Hospitals and Almshouses Kept their Archives', *Archives*, xxvii (2002), pp. 2–22

———, 'The Eighth Comfortable Work: Education and the Medieval English Hospital', in C.M. Barron and J. Stratford, eds, *The Church and Learning in Later Medieval England* (Donington, 2002)

———, 'Master Surgeons at the Lancastrian Court', in J. Stratford, ed., *The Lancastrian Court* (Stamford, 2003)

———, 'The Seventh Comfortable Work: Charity and Mortality in the Medieval Hospital', *Medicina & Storia*, iii (2003), pp. 11–35

———, 'Sickness and Health', in C. Rawcliffe and R.G. Wilson, eds, *The History of Norwich* (2 vols, London, 2004)

———, 'The Earthly and Spiritual Topography of Suburban Hospitals', in K. Giles and C. Dyer, eds, *Town and Country in the Middle Ages: Contrasts and Interconnections* (Society for Medieval Archaeology, Monograph xxii, 2005)

———, 'A Case of Imputed Leprosy at Sparham, Norfolk', in R. Horrox and M. Aston, eds, *Much Heaving and Shoving: Late-Medieval Gentry and Their Concerns* (Lavenham, 2005)

———, 'Isolating the Medieval Leper: Ideas – and Misconceptions – about Segregation in the Middle Ages', in P. Horden, ed., *Freedom of Movement in the Middle Ages* (Donington, forthcoming)

Raynaud, G., 'Les congés de Jean Bodel', *Romania*, ix (1880), pp. 216–47

Resnick, I.M., 'Ps.-Albert the Great on the Physiognomy of Jesus and Mary', *Medieval Studies*, lxiv (2002), pp. 217–40

Rhodes, J.T., and Davidson, C., 'The Garden of Paradise', in C. Davidson, ed., *The Iconography of Heaven* (Kalamazoo, 1994)

Richards, J., *Sex, Dissidence and Damnation: Minority Groups in the Middle Ages* (London, 1991)

Richards, P., *The Medieval Leper and His Northern Heirs* (Cambridge, 1977, reprinted Woodbridge, 2000)

Riches, S., *Saint George: Hero, Martyr and Myth* (Stroud, 2000)

Riddle, J.M., 'Theory and Practice in Medieval Medicine', *Viator*, v (1974), pp. 158–84

Ridling, D.S., and Jopling, W.H., 'A Classification of Leprosy According to Immunity: A Five Group System', *International Journal of Leprosy*, xxxiv (1966), pp. 255–61

Rigby, S., 'Urban "Oligarchy" in Late Medieval England', in J.A.F. Thomson, ed., *Towns and Townspeople in the Fifteenth Century* (Gloucester, 1988)

Risse, G.B., *Mending Bodies, Saving Souls: A History of Hospitals* (Oxford, 1999)

Robbins, R.H., 'Medical Manuscripts in Middle English', *Speculum*, xlv (1970), pp. 393–415

Robert, U., *Les signes d'infamie au moyen âge* (Paris, 1891)

Roberts, C., 'Leprosy and *Leprosaria* in Medieval Britain', *MASCA Journal*, iv (1986), pp. 15–21

——, 'Treponematosis in Gloucester, England: A Theoretical and Practical Approach to the Pre-Colombian Theory', in O. Dutour et al., eds, *L'origine de la syphilis en Europe* (Paris and Toulon, undated, *c.* 1994)

——, and Manchester, K., *The Archaeology of Disease* (second edn, Stroud, 1995)

——, 'The Antiquity of Leprosy in Britain: The Skeletal Evidence', *PPL*

——, and Cox, M., *Health and Disease in Britain* (Stroud, 2003)

Roberts, G., *The Mirror of Alchemy: Alchemical Ideas and Images in Manuscripts and Books* (London, 1994)

Roose, R., *Leprosy and its Prevention* (London, 1890)

Rosser, G., 'Urban Culture and the Church 1300–1540', in D. Palliser, ed., *The Cambridge Urban History of Britain* (Cambridge, 2000)

Roueché, B, *Eleven Blue Men and other Narratives of Medical Detection* (New York, 1953)

——, *Annals of Medical Detection* (London, 1954)

*Royal Commission on Historical Monuments, Essex II* (London, 1921)

Rubin, M., *Charity and Community in Medieval Cambridge* (Cambridge, 1987)

Rubin, S., *English Medieval Medicine* (London and Vancouver, 1974)

Russell, J.C., *British Medieval Population* (Albuquerque, 1948)

Rutledge, P., 'A Fifteenth-Century Yarmouth Petition', *Great Yarmouth District Archaeological Society Bulletin*, xlvi (1976), unpaginated


Sabatier, P., *Life of St Francis of Assisi* (London, 1941)

Sabine, E.L., 'City Cleaning in Medieval London', *Speculum*, xii (1937), pp. 19–43

Sadie, S., ed., *The New Grove Dictionary of Music and Musicians* (29 vols, London, 2001)

Salzman, L.F., ed., *VCH Cambridge and the Isle of Ely II* (London, 1948)

Saunders, J., 'Quarantining the Weak-Minded: Psychiatric Definitions of Degeneracy and the Late-Victorian Asylum', in W.F. Bynum, R. Porter and M. Shepherd, eds, *The Anatomy of Madness, III, The Asylum and its Psychiatry* (London and New York, 1988)

Saunders, S., *'A Suitable Island Site': Leprosy in the Northern Territory and the Channel Island Leprosarium 1880–1955* (Darwin, 1989)

Sayers, J., 'The Earliest Original Letter of Pope Innocent III for an English Recipient', *BIHR*, xlix (1976), pp. 132–5

Schatzlein, J., and Sulmasy, D.P., 'The Diagnosis of St Francis: Evidence for Leprosy', *Franciscan Studies*, xlvii (1987), pp. 181–217

Schleiner, W., 'Infection and Cure through Women: Renaissance Constructions of Syphilis', *Journal of Medieval and Renaissance Studies*, xxiv (1994), pp. 499–517

Schmitt, J.C., *La raison des gestes dans l'occident médiéval* (Paris, 1990)

Serjeantson, R.M., and Adkins, W.R.D., eds, *VCH Northampton II* (London, 1906)

Shahar, S., 'Des lépreux pas comme les autres: L'ordre de Saint-Lazare dans le royaume latin de Jerusalem', *Revue Historique*, cclxvii (1982), pp. 19–41

————, *Growing Old in the Middle Ages* (London, 2004)

Shorter, E., *A History of Psychiatry* (New York, 1997)

Siena, K.P., *Venereal Disease, Hospitals and the Urban Poor* (Rochester, New York, 2004)

Sigal, P.A., *L'homme et le miracle dans la France médiévale* (Paris, 1985)

Silla, E., *People Are Not the Same: Leprosy and Identity in Twentieth-Century Mali* (Portsmouth and Oxford, 1998)

Simpson, J.Y., 'Antiquarian Notices of Leprosy and Leper Hospitals in Scotland and England', *The Edinburgh Medical and Surgical Journal*, clvi (1841), part 1, pp. 301–30; clvii (1842), part 2, pp. 121–56, part 3, pp. 394–429

Singer, C., 'A Thirteenth Century Clinical Description of Leprosy', *JHM*, iv (1949), pp. 237–9

Siraisi, N.G., *Taddeo Alderotti and his Pupils* (Princeton, 1981)

Slack, P., *Poverty and Policy in Tudor and Stuart England* (London, 1988)

————, *Medieval and Early Renaissance Medicine* (Chicago, 1990)

Smalley, B., *The Study of the Bible in the Middle Ages* (Oxford, 1952)

Smith, L., 'William of Auvergne and Confession', in P. Biller and A.J. Minnis, eds, *Handling Sin: Confession in the Middle Ages* (Woodbridge, 1998)

Smith, R.M., 'Modernistation and the Corporate Medieval Village Community in England: Some Sceptical Reflections', in A.R.H. Baker and D. Gregory, eds, *Explorations in Historical Geography: Interpretative Essays* (Cambridge, 1984)

Somer, W., *The Antiquities of Canterbury* (London, 1703)

Somerscales, M.I., 'Lazar Houses in Cornwall', *Journal of the Royal Institution of Cornwall*, new series, v (1965), pp. 61–99

Sontag, S., *Illness as a Metaphor* (London, 1990)

Spiegler, P. de, *Les hôpitaux et l'assistance a Liège (Xe–XVe siecles): Aspects institutionels et sociaux* (Paris, 1987)

Stannard, J., 'Dioscorides and Renaissance Materia Medica', *Analecto Medica-Historica 1: Materia Medica in the XVI Century* (Oxford, 1966)

————, 'The Herbal as a Medical Document', *BHM*, xliii (1969), pp. 212–20

Stein, M., 'La thériaque chez Galien: Sa preparation et son usage thérapeutique', in A. Debru, ed., *Galen on Pharmacology, Philosophy, History and Medicine* (Brill, 1997)

Stirland, A., 'Evidence for Pre-Columbian Treponematosis in Medieval Europe', in O. Dutour et al., eds, *L'origine de la syphilis en Europe* (Paris and Toulon, undated, c. 1994)

Strack, H.L., *Das Blut im Glauben und Aberglauben der Menschheit mit besonderer Berücksichtigung der "Volksmedizin" und des "jüdischen Blutritus"* (Munich, 1900)

Suckling, A., *The History and Antiquities of the County of Suffolk* (2 vols, London, 1846–48)

Swanson, R.N., 'Passion and Practice: The Social and Ecclesiastical Implications of Passion Devotion in the Late Middle Ages', in A.A. MacDonald et al., eds, *The Broken Body: Passion Devotion in Late Medieval Culture* (Groningen, 1998)

Sweet, A.H., 'The Library of St Radegund's Abbey', EHR, liii (1938), pp. 88–93

Sweetinburgh, S., *The Role of the Hospital in Medieval England* (Dublin, 2004)

Taavitsainen, I., 'Transferring Classical Discourse Conventions into the Vernacular', in I. Taavitsainen and P. Pahata, *Medical and Scientific Writing in Late Medieval English* (Cambridge, 2004)

Tachau, K.H., *Vision and Certitude in the Age of Ockham: Optics, Epistemology and the Foundations of Semantics 1250–1345* (Leiden, 1988)

Talbot, C.H., Hammond, E.A., *The Medical Practitioners in Medieval England* (London, 1965)

Tanner, N., *The Church in Late Medieval Norwich* (Toronto, 1984)

Taylor, R., *Index Monasticus: The Diocese of Norwich* (London, 1821)

Tentler, T.N., *Sin and Confession on the Eve of the Reformation* (Princeton, 1977)

Terrien, S., *The Iconography of Job through the Centuries: Artists as Biblical Interpreters* (Pennsylvania State University Press, Pennsylvania, 1996)

Tester, S.J., *A History of Western Astrology* (Woodbridge, 1987)

Thangaraj, R.H., and Yawalkar, S.J., *Leprosy for Medical Practitioners and Paramedical Workers* (Basle, 1986)

Thevenin, E., 'La léproserie Saint-Lazare de Reims: Une espace de festivités', in Tabuteau, B., ed., *Lépreux et sociabilité du moyen âge au temps modernes* (Cahiers de GRHS, xi, 2000)

Thin, G., *Leprosy* (London, 1891)

Thompson, A.H., *The History of the Hospital and New College of the Annunciation of St Mary in the Newarke, Leicester* (Leicester Archaeological Society, 1937)

Thompson, B., 'From "Alms" to "Spiritual Services": The Function and Status of Monastic Property in Medieval England', in J. Loades, ed., *Monastic Studies II* (Bangor, 1991)

Thorndike, L., *A History of Magic and Experimental Science* (8 vols, New York, 1923–58)

Touati, F.O., '*Facies leprosorum*: réflections sur le diagnostic facial de la lèpre au Moyen Age', *Histoire des Sciences Médicales*, xx (1986), pp. 57–66

———, 'Histoire des maladies, histoire totale?', *Sources: Travaux Historiques*, xiii (1988), pp. 3–14

———, 'Pharmacopée et thérapeutic contre la lèpre au moyen age: quelques réflexions méthodologiques', *Actes du 113e Congrés National des Sociétes Savantes, Strasbourg, 1988* (Paris, CTHS, 1991)

———, *Archives de la lèpre* (Paris, 1996)

———, 'Les groupes de laïcs dans les hôpitaux et les léproseries au moyen âge', *Les mouvances laïcs des orders religieux* (Saint-Étienne, 1996)

———, *Maladie et société an moyen âge* (Paris, 1998)

———, 'Contagion and Leprosy: Myth, Ideas and Evolution in Medieval Minds and Societies', in L.I. Conrad and D. Wujastyk, eds, *Contagion: Perspectives from Pre-Modern Societies* (Aldershot, 2000)

Townley, S., ed., *VCH Oxford XIV* (Woodbridge, 2004)

Trachtenberg, J., *The Devil and the Jews: The Medieval Conception of the Jew and its Relation to Modern Antisemitism* (New Haven and London, 1945)

Trease, G.E., and Hodson, J.H., 'The Inventory of John Hexham, a Fifteenth-Century Apothecary', *Medical History*, ix (1965), pp. 76–81

Turner, B.S., *The Body and Society: Explorations in Social Theory* (Oxford, 1984, London, 1996)

Turner, V., *The Ritual Process: Structure and Anti-Structure* (Chicago, 1969)

————, *Dramas, Fields and Metaphors: Symbolic Action in Human Society* (Ithaca, 1974)

————, *Image and Pilgrimage in Christian Culture: Anthropological Perspectives* (New York, 1978)

————, 'Betwixt and Between: The Liminal Period in Rites de Passage', in W.A. Lessa and E.Z. Vogt, eds, *Reader in Comparative Religion: An Anthropological Approach* (fourth edn, New York, 1979)

————, 'Social Dramas and Stories about Them', in W.J.T. Mitchell, ed., *On Narrative* (Chicago, 1981)

Uyttebrouck, A., 'Séquestration ou retraite volontaire? Quelques réflexions à propos de l'hérbergement des lépreux à la léproserie de Terbank-lez-Louvain', in *Mélanges offerts à G. Jacquemyns* (Brussels, 1968), pp. 615–32

Vaughan, M., *Curing their Ills: Colonial Power and African Illness* (Oxford, 1991)

Vigarello, G., *Concepts of Cleanliness: Changing Attitudes in France since the Middle Ages* (Cambridge, 1985)

Vincent, N., 'Two Papal Letters on the Wearing of the Jewish Badge, 1221 and 1229', *Jewish Historical Studies*, xxxiv (1994–96), pp. 209–24

————, 'The Foundation of Wormegay Priory', *Norfolk Archaeology*, xliii (1999), pp. 307–12

————, *The Holy Blood: Henry III and the Westminster Blood Relic* (Cambridge, 2001)

Voigts, L.E., 'A Doctor and His Books: The Manuscripts of Roger Marchall (d. 1477)', in R. Beadle and A.J. Piper, eds, *New Science Out of Old Books* (Scolar Press, 1995)

————, 'The Master of the King's Stillatories', in J. Stratford, ed., *The Lancastrian Court* (Stamford, 2003)

Walker Bynum, C., *Holy Feast and Holy Fast: The Religious Significance of Food to Medieval Women* (London, 1987)

————, *Fragmentation and Redemption: Essays on Gender and the Human Body in Medieval Religion* (New York, 1992)

Walker, S., 'Political Saints in Later Medieval England', in R.H. Britnell and A.J. Pollard, eds, *The MacFarlane Legacy: Studies in Late Medieval Politics and Society* (Stroud, 1995)

Ward, B., St Edmund, *Archbishop of Canterbury: His Life as Told by Old English Writers* (London, 1903)

Ward, B., *Miracles and the Medieval Mind* (Aldershot, 1987)

Watson, G., *Theriac and Mithridatum: A Study in Therapeutics* (London, 1966)

Watts, S., *Epidemics and History: Disease, Power and Imperialism* (Yale, 1997)

Waxler, N.E., 'Learning to be a Leper: A Case Study in the Social Construction of Illness', in E.G. Mishler, ed., *Social Contexts of Health, Illness and Patient Care* (Cambridge, 1981)

Wear, A., 'Fear, Anxiety and the Plague in Early Modern England', in J.R. Hinnells and R. Porter, eds, *Religion, Health and Suffering* (London, 1999)

Webb, D., *Pilgrimage in Medieval England* (London, 2000)

Wells, C., *Bones, Bodies and Disease* (London, 1964)

Weymouth, A., *Through the Leper Squint: A Study of Leprosy from Pre-Christian Times to the Present Day* (London, 1938)

White, G., *Natural History and Antiquities of Selborne* (London, 1906)

Wilkins, R., *The Fireside Book of Deadly Diseases* (London, 1994)

Wilkinson, J., *The Bible and Healing: A Medical and Theological Commentary* (Grand Rapids, Michigan, 1998)

Wilson, E., 'On the Nature and Treatment of Leprosy Ancient and Modern', *The Lancet*, lxvii, issue 1696 (1 March 1856), pp. 226–8

Wilson, J., ed., *VCH Cumberland II* (London, 1905)

Wood, C.T., 'The Doctor's Dilemma: Sin, Salvation and the Menstrual Cycle in Medieval Thought', *Speculum*, lvi (1981), pp. 710–27

Worboys, M., *Spreading Germs: Disease Theories and Medical Practice in Britain 1865–1900* (Cambridge, 2000)

Wormald, P., *The Making of English Law: King Alfred to the Twelfth Century I* (Oxford, 1999)

Wright, H.P., *Leprosy and Segregation* (London, 1885)

———, *Leprosy an Imperial Danger* (London, 1889)


Young, T.A., *Annals of the Barber-Surgeons of London* (London, 1890)


Zambaco, D.A., *Anthologie: La lèpre à travers les siècles et les contrées* (Paris, 1914)

Zappa, P., *Unclean! Unclean!* (London, 1933)

Ziegler, J., *Medicine and Religion c. 1300: The Case of Arnau de Vilanova* (Oxford, 1998)

———, 'Medicine and Immortality in Terrestrial Paradise', in P. Biller and J. Ziegler, eds, *Religion and Medicine in the Middle Ages* (York, 2001)

———, 'Skin and Character in Medieval and Early Renaissance Physiognomy', in *La pelle umana* (Micrologus' Library, xiii, Turnhout, 2005)

Zink, M., 'Le ladre, de l'exile au royaume', *Exclus et systemes d'exclusion dans la littérature et la civilisation médiévales* (Senefiance, v, Aix-en-Provence, 1978), pp. 69–88

## Unpublished Doctoral Theses and Archaeological Reports

Ayoub, L.J., 'John Crophill's Books: An Edition of British Library MS Harley 1735' (University of Toronto, PhD, 1994)

P. Cullum, 'Hospitals and Charitable Provision in Medieval Yorkshire 936–1547' (University of York, DPhil, 1990)

Liddiard, R., 'Landscapes of Lordship: The Landscape Context of Castles in Norfolk 1066–1506' (University of East Anglia, PhD, 2000)

Mays, S.A., 'Medieval Burials from the Blackfriars Friary, School Street, Ipswich, Suffolk' (Ancient Monuments Laboratory Report 16/1991, part 1)

Mesmin, S.C., 'The Leper Hospital of Saint Gilles de Pont-Audemer: An Edition of the Cartulary and an Examination of the Problem of Leprosy in the Twelfth and Thirteenth Century' (2 vols, University of Reading, PhD, 1978)

E.M. Phillips, 'Charitable Institutions in Norfolk and Suffolk c. 1350–1600' (University of East Anglia, PhD, 2001)

Satchell, A.E.M., 'The Emergence of Leper-Houses in Medieval England' (University of Oxford, DPhil, 1998)

'York Archaeological Trust Site Investigations, 148 St Lawrence Street, York, Summary and Assessment' (Unpublished report, York Archaeological Trust, 1993/11)

# General Index

This index covers personal names, places (other than individual leper houses, hospitals for the sick poor and almshouses which are listed separately by location in Index II) and the principal subjects mentioned in the text. To avoid the confusion that this book aims to dispel, separate headings have been created for leprosy as defined by today's clinicians (Hansen's disease) and for the disease as understood in biblical, Classical and medieval times. Saints may be found under their first names (e.g. Francis, Hugh), as may individuals whose names are toponyms (Robert de Torpel, William of Malmesbury). Members of the English peerage appear under their titles. Page numbers in **bold** type denote illustrations.

# Index of Leper Houses, Hospitals and Almshouses

Unless otherwise stated, all the institutions named are leper houses, a term which may denote transitory, informal communities as well as more established ones. Where possible, dedications have been provided, although many such places remain anonymous.